CARCINOGENS: IDENTIFICATION AND MECHANISMS OF ACTION

The University of Texas System Cancer Center
M. D. Anderson Hospital and Tumor Institute
31st Annual Symposium on Fundamental Cancer Research

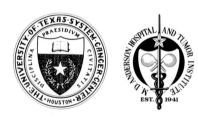

Published for
The University of Texas System Cancer Center
M. D. Anderson Hospital and Tumor Institute
Houston, Texas, by Raven Press, New York

The University of Texas System Cancer Center
M. D. Anderson Hospital and Tumor Institute
31st Annual Symposium on Fundamental Cancer Research

Carcinogens: Identification and Mechanisms of Action

Edited by

A. Clark Griffin, Ph.D.

Department of Biochemistry
The University of Texas System Cancer Center
M. D. Anderson Hospital and Tumor Institute
Houston, Texas

Charles R. Shaw, M.D.

Departments of Biology and Pediatrics
The University of Texas System Cancer Center
M. D. Anderson Hospital and Tumor Institute
Houston, Texas

Raven Press ■ New York

Raven Press, 1140 Avenue of the Americas, New York,
New York 10036

Library of Congress Cataloging in Publication Data

Symposium on Fundamental Cancer Research, 31st, Anderson
    Hospital and Tumor Institute, 1978.
    Carcinogens: identification and mechanisms of action.

    "Published for the University of Texas System Cancer
Center M. D. Anderson Hospital and Tumor Institute."
    Includes bibliographical references and indexes.
    1. Carcinogens—Congresses. 2. Carcinogenesis—
Congresses. I. Griffin, Amos Clark, 1918–
II. Shaw, Charles R. III. Anderson Hospital and Tumor
Institute, Houston, Tex. IV. Title.
RC268.6.S94 1978   616.9'94'071   78–23366
ISBN 0–89004–286–1

Editors' Foreword

Participation in the planning and organization of the Thirty-First Annual Symposium on Fundamental Cancer Research, the subject of this volume, has been a most rewarding experience. With the rapidly increasing evidence that environmental carcinogens may be responsible for much of human cancer, this meeting of outstanding scientists and contributors to this field is fortuitous and timely. The Symposium Committee, with the guidance of our respected advisors, felt that the major emphasis should be directed to the detection of these carcinogens and the mechanisms involved in their causing the normal cells, tissues, and organs of the body to become cancerous. This approach could provide the basis for cancer prevention by reduction of human exposure to these agents, by modification of their metabolism and mechanisms of action, and by the reversal of carcinogenesis at early stages.

The Symposium had excellent attendance; the presentations were of the highest caliber and were justly approved by those who had the opportunity to attend. We trust that the readers of this volume will be equally rewarded.

As cochairmen we acknowledge our appreciation to those many individuals who provided guidance and advice in all matters pertaining to this Symposium and this volume. The Symposium organizing committee members from The University of Texas System Cancer Center included: Ralph B. Arlinghaus, Biology; Frederick F. Becker, Pathology; James C. Chan, Virology; Roger R. Hewitt, Biology; Ronald M. Humphrey, Environmental Science Park; Thomas S. Matney, Biology; Rulon W. Rawson, Medicine; Earl F. Walborg, Jr., Biochemistry. The Planning Committee was given the best guidance and direction by our Advisory Committee: Vincent Allfrey, The Rockefeller University; Peter Emmelot, Antoni Van Leeuwenhoek-Huis, The Netherlands Cancer Institute; Joseph F. Fraumeni, Jr., National Cancer Institute; Alfred G. Knudson, Jr., Institute for Cancer Research, Philadelphia; Peter N. Magee, Fels Research Institute; James A. Miller, McArdle Laboratory for Cancer Research, University of Wisconsin Center for Health Sciences; G. Barry Pierce, University of Colorado Medical Center; Philippe Shubik, Eppley Institute for Research in Cancer, University of Nebraska Medical Center.

Special thanks and appreciation are given to Frances Goff and her staff for the many functions that they expertly and carefully planned and conducted. Also our thanks to the Coulter Electronics Scientific Company for providing funds for the hospitality rooms wherein the speakers and Symposium attendees could meet and discuss mutual interests. We are especially grateful to the National Cancer Institute and the Texas Division of the American Cancer Society for their continued support. We also wish to thank The University of Texas Health Science Center at Houston, Graduate School of Biomedical Sciences, for its assistance.

The Publications Office staff aided invaluably in all the matters pertaining to the information, announcements, and publications of the Symposium. Special acknowledgment is accorded Leslie Wildrick, who played a most important role in the completion of this volume.

Finally, we acknowledge with respect the sincere interest, concern, and guidance of Dr. R. Lee Clark in this the Thirty-First Annual Symposium, as he has shown for all of the preceding 30 years. It was through his vision and foresight that this series was initiated. Dr. Clark resigned as President of The University of Texas System Cancer Center M. D. Anderson Hospital and Tumor Institute in August 1978. This meeting and volume constitute the last of this outstanding series under his direct guidance. However, his dedication, concern, and interest will continue as long as these symposia that are concerned with the problems of cancer.

A. Clark Griffin, Ph.D.
Charles R. Shaw, M.D.
Co-Editors

Contents

Cellular and Molecular Markers of the Carcinogenic Process

Contributors

Nancy Acton
*National Institute of Arthritis,
  Metabolism, and Digestive Diseases
National Institutes of Health
Bethesda, Maryland 20014*

Vincent G. Allfrey
*Rockefeller University
New York, New York 10021*

James P. Allison
*The University of Texas System Cancer
  Center
Science Park - Research Division
Smithville, Texas 78957*

Manuel Altamirano
*Department of Microbiology
The University of Chicago
Chicago, Illinois 60637*

Marilyn S. Arnott
*Department of Biology
The University of Texas System Cancer
  Center
M. D. Anderson Hospital and Tumor
  Institute
Houston, Texas 77030*

Robert W. Baldwin
*Cancer Research Campaign Laboratories
University of Nottingham
Nottingham NG7 2RD England*

Frederick F. Becker
*Department of Pathology
The University of Texas System Cancer
  Center
M. D. Anderson Hospital and Tumor
  Institute
Houston, Texas 77030*

Isaac Berenblum
*The Weizmann Institute of Science
Rehovot, Israel*

Lidia C. Boffa
*Rockefeller University
New York, New York 10021*

Kallol Bose
*Department of Microbiology
The University of Chicago
Chicago, Illinois 60637*

Arnold Brossi
*National Institute of Arthritis,
  Metabolism, and Digestive Diseases
National Institutes of Health
Bethesda, Maryland 20014*

David Brusick
*Department of Molecular Toxicology
Litton Bionetics, Inc.
Kensington, Maryland 20795*

Ross G. Cameron
*Department of Pathology
University of Toronto
Toronto, Ontario, Canada*

R. Lee Clark
*The University of Texas System Cancer
  Center
M. D. Anderson Hospital and Tumor
  Institute
Houston, Texas 77030*

Edward M. Davis
*Biology Department
Yale University
New Haven, Connecticut 06520*

Michael J. Embleton
Cancer Research Campaign Laboratories
University of Nottingham
Nottingham NG7 2RD England

P. Emmelot
Division of Chemical Carcinogenesis
Antoni Van Leeuwenhoek-Huis
The Netherlands Cancer Institute
Amsterdam, The Netherlands

Emmanuel Farber
Department of Pathology
University of Toronto
Toronto, Ontario, Canada

Donald C. Fish
Frederick Cancer Research Center
Frederick, Maryland 21701

Paul B. Fisher
Division of Environmental Sciences, and
Institute of Cancer Research
Columbia University, College of
Physicians and Surgeons
New York, New York 10032

Joseph F. Fraumeni, Jr.
Environmental Epidemiology Branch
National Cancer Institute
Bethesda, Maryland 20014

Dezider Grunberger
Division of Environmental Sciences, and
Institute of Cancer Research
Columbia University, College of
Physicians and Surgeons
New York, New York 10032

Julie Harless
Section of Environmental Biology
Department of Biology
The University of Texas System Cancer
Center
M. D. Anderson Hospital and Tumor
Institute
Houston, Texas 77030

Curtis C. Harris
Experimental Pathology Branch
Carcinogenesis Research Program
Division of Cancer Cause and Prevention
National Cancer Institute
Bethesda, Maryland 20014

Charles Heidelberger
University of Southern California
Comprehensive Cancer Center
Los Angeles, California 90033

Roger R. Hewitt
Section of Environmental Biology
Department of Biology
The University of Texas System Cancer
Center
M. D. Anderson Hospital and Tumor
Institute
Houston, Texas 77030

John Higginson
International Agency for Research on
Cancer
Lyon, France

Douglas C. Hixson
The University of Texas System Cancer
Center
Science Park - Research Division
Smithville, Texas 78957

Robert J. Huebner
Laboratory of RNA Tumor Viruses
National Cancer Institute
Bethesda, Maryland 20014

Charles C. Irving
Veterans Administration Hospital and
University of Tennessee Center for the
Health Sciences
Department of Urology
Memphis, Tennessee 38104

Arthur E. Jacobson
National Institute of Arthritis,
Metabolism, and Digestive Diseases
National Institutes of Health
Bethesda, Maryland 20014

Alan Jeffrey
Division of Environmental Sciences,
and Institute of Cancer Research
Columbia University, College of
Physicians and Surgeons
New York, New York 10032

Dennis A. Johnston
Department of Biomathematics
The University of Texas System Cancer
Center
M. D. Anderson Hospital and Tumor
Institute
Houston, Texas 77030

Brian Laishes
Department of Pathology
University of Toronto
Toronto, Ontario, Canada

Lih-Syng Lee
Division of Environmental Sciences,
and Institute of Cancer Research
Columbia University, College of
Physicians and Surgeons
New York, New York 10032

Roy C. Levitt
Developmental Pharmacology Branch
National Institute of Child Health and
Human Development
National Institutes of Health
Bethesda, Maryland 20014

Jung-Chung Lin
Department of Pathology
University of Toronto
Toronto, Ontario, Canada

R. Stephen Lloyd
Section of Molecular Biology
Department of Biology
The University of Texas System Cancer
Center
M. D. Anderson Hospital and Tumor
Institute
Houston, Texas 77030

Jack Love
Section of Environmental Biology
Department of Biology
The University of Texas System Cancer
Center
M. D. Anderson Hospital and Tumor
Institute
Houston, Texas 77030

Alan Medline
Department of Pathology
University of Toronto
Toronto, Ontario, Canada

James A. Miller
McArdle Laboratory for Cancer Research
University of Wisconsin Center for Health
Sciences
Madison, Wisconsin 53706

Sukdeb Mondal
University of Southern California
Comprehensive Cancer Center
Los Angeles, California 90033

Daniel W. Nebert
Developmental Pharmacology Branch
National Institute of Child Health and
Human Development
National Institutes of Health
Bethesda, Maryland 20014

Dianne L. Newton
National Cancer Institute
National Institutes of Health
Bethesda, Maryland 20014

Katsuhiro Ogawa
Department of Pathology
University of Toronto
Toronto, Ontario, Canada

M. C. Paterson
Biology and Health Physics Division
Atomic Energy of Canada, Limited
Chalk River, Ontario K0J 1J0 Canada

Olavi Pelkonen
Developmental Pharmacology Branch
National Institute of Child Health and
Human Development
National Institutes of Health
Bethesda, Maryland 20014

Roman J. Pienta
Chemical Carcinogenesis Program
Frederick Cancer Research Center
Frederick, Maryland 21701

Malcolm V. Pimm
Cancer Research Campaign Laboratories
University of Nottingham
Nottingham NG7 2RD England

Donald L. Robberson
Section of Molecular Biology
Department of Biology
The University of Texas System Cancer
Center
M. D. Anderson Hospital and Tumor
Institute
Houston, Texas 77030

Umberto Saffiotti
Experimental Pathology Branch
Carcinogenesis Research Program
Division of Cancer Cause and Prevention
National Cancer Institute
Bethesda, Maryland 20014

E. Scherer
Division of Chemical Carcinogenesis
Antoni Van Leeuwenhoek-Huis
The Netherlands Cancer Institute
Amsterdam, The Netherlands

Philippe Shubik
Eppley Institute for Research in Cancer
University of Nebraska Medical Center
Omaha, Nebraska 68105

Robert Sklar
Department of Microbiology
The University of Chicago
Chicago, Illinois 60637

Joseph M. Smith
National Cancer Institute
National Institutes of Health
Bethesda, Maryland 20014

Dennis B. Solt
Department of Pathology
University of Toronto
Toronto, Ontario, Canada

Michael B. Sporn
National Cancer Institute
National Institutes of Health
Bethesda, Maryland 20014

James J. Starling
Department of Biochemistry
University of Florida
Gainesville, Florida 32611

Walter G. Sterling
Board of Regents
The University of Texas System
P. O. Box 2891
Houston, Texas 77001

Bernard Strauss
Department of Microbiology
The University of Chicago
Chicago, Illinois 60637

Kouichi Tatsumi
Department of Microbiology
The University of Chicago
Chicago, Illinois 60637

Giorgio Vidali
Rockefeller University
New York, New York 10021

Earl F. Walborg, Jr.
The University of Texas System Cancer
Center
Science Park - Research Division
Smithville, Texas 78957

Lee W. Wattenberg
Department of Laboratory Medicine and
Pathology
University of Minnesota
Minneapolis, Minnesota 55455

I. Bernard Weinstein
Division of Environmental Sciences, and
Institute of Cancer Research
Columbia University, College of
Physicians and Surgeons
New York, New York 10032

Michael Wigler
Division of Environmental Sciences, and
Institute of Cancer Research
Columbia University, College of
Physicians and Surgeons
New York, New York 10032

Hiroshi Yamasaki
Division of Environmental Sciences, and
Institute of Cancer Research
Columbia University, College of
Physicians and Surgeons
New York, New York 10032

Toshio Yamauchi
The University of Texas Medical School
at Houston
Houston, Texas 77030

SYMPOSIUM COMMITTEE

A. Clark Griffin, Cochairman
Charles R. Shaw, Cochairman
Ralph B. Arlinghaus
Frederick F. Becker
James C. Chan
Roger R. Hewitt
Ronald M. Humphrey
Thomas S. Matney
Rulon W. Rawson
Earl F. Walborg, Jr.
H. Rodney Withers

Ex Officio Members

George Blumenschein
Frances Goff
Felix L. Haas
Glenn R. Knotts
Joseph T. Painter
Grady F. Saunders
Stephen C. Stuyck

SESSION CHAIRMEN

Frederick J. de Serres
Environmental Mutagen Branch, National Institute of Environmental Health Sciences, Research Triangle Park, North Carolina

Peter Emmelot
Division of Chemical Carcinogenesis, Antoni Van Leeuwenhoek-Huis, The Netherlands Cancer Institute, Amsterdam, The Netherlands

Peter N. Magee
Fels Research Institute, Temple University School of Medicine, Philadelphia, Pennsylvania

Norton Nelson
New York University Medical Center, Institute of Environmental Medicine, New York, New York

G. Barry Pierce
Department of Pathology, University of Colorado Medical Center, Denver, Colorado

Charles R. Shaw
Departments of Biology and Pediatrics, The University of Texas System Cancer Center M. D. Anderson Hospital and Tumor Institute, Houston, Texas

ADVISORY COMMITTEE

Vincent Allfrey
  Rockefeller University, New York, New York

Peter Emmelot
  Antoni Van Leeuwenhoek-Huis, The Netherlands Cancer Institute, Amsterdam, The Netherlands

Joseph F. Fraumeni, Jr.
  National Cancer Institute, Bethesda, Maryland

Alfred G. Knudson, Jr.
  Institute for Cancer Research, Philadelphia, Pennsylvania

Peter N. Magee
  Fels Research Institute, Temple University School of Medicine, Philadelphia, Pennsylvania

James A. Miller
  McArdle Laboratory for Cancer Research, University of Wisconsin Center for Health Sciences, Madison, Wisconsin

G. Barry Pierce
  University of Colorado Medical Center, Denver, Colorado

Philippe Shubik
  Eppley Institute for Research in Cancer, University of Nebraska Medical Center, Omaha, Nebraska

Carcinogens: Identification and Mechanisms of Action, edited by A. Clark Griffin and Charles R. Shaw. Raven Press, New York © 1979.

Introduction

R. Lee Clark

The University of Texas System Cancer Center M. D. Anderson Hospital and Tumor Institute, Houston, Texas 77030

This 31st Annual Symposium on Fundamental Cancer Research is the third in the span of a dozen years that has addressed the answers of the scientific community to the challenge of carcinogenesis. During the 1971 symposium, Environment and Cancer, I made the statement, "In the history of this distinguished symposium series, there probably has not been a subject so finely attuned to the present." The topic of environmental carcinogenesis is becoming a progressively more urgent one, as we reveal the nature and multiplicity of the extrinsic impingement on the living cell.

During the last two decades, a sound scientific basis has been established for the identification and detection of carcinogens, chemical and physical, and equally well-designed studies have identified many of the metabolic pathways of activation and detoxification for the major types of chemical carcinogens, most of which require enzymes for activation. The corecipients of The University of Texas System Cancer Center's Bertner Award in 1971, Dr. Elizabeth C. Miller and Dr. James A. Miller, made a major contribution to these studies by proposing that most chemical carcinogens are either strong electrophilic reactants or are metabolically converted into such, thereby initiating the carcinogenic process in interaction with nucleophilic sites in macromolecules. Our current corecipients of the Bertner Award have contributed, among numerous other major works, the two-stage or multistage theory of carcinogenesis, upon which many subsequent studies have been based. Numerous other major contributions have advanced our knowledge through the fields of experimental pathology and through the study of histogenesis and its parallels between animal model and human organs and tissues and their functions, cellular and molecular biology, biochemistry, genetics, epidemiology, and, most recently, immunology.

The roles of DNA damage and repair mechanisms in the carcinogenic process are gradually being elucidated, as is the relationship of the wide range of individual genetic variations to the susceptibility to carcinogenesis. Equally important are the attempts at identification and exploitation of agents capable of inhibiting or reversing the biological mechanisms involved in initiation and promotion.

The increasing sociological impact of environmental carcinogens is most clearly revealed in national and international epidemiological studies. It appears that the majority of cancers are initiated by external agents, and, therefore, cancer may be primarily a preventable disease. Rapid technological advances, however, compound the problems of identification and control of the carcinogens. An informed populace must eventually decide on more carefully regulated technological development and more individual responsibility for health protection, or there will certainly be an increasing incidence of cancers and related diseases, including a wide range of birth defects. Unless current studies into chemoprevention and reversal of the carcinogenic process are successful, such decisions may be too late to benefit current generations who have already been and are exposed daily to both known and unsuspected carcinogens.

For the future, our research and developmental activities must concentrate on further elucidation of: (1) the exact biological mechanisms of carcinogenesis, (2) rapid, scientifically acceptable, and low-cost screening methods for identifying the potential for carcinogenesis of any suspect substance, be it naturally occurring or synthetically produced, (3) measures for the prevention and reversal of the carcinogenic process, (4) establishment of socially and medically acceptable low-risk levels of those carcinogens that cannot feasibly be eliminated from the environment, (5) identification of the population at risk for an environmentally induced cancer, (6) a national program that will strive to make more effective the National Clearinghouse on Environmental Carcinogens and implement a national network of laboratories (perhaps six to ten) wherein the above-mentioned goals can be accomplished and that will be associated with clinical and medical facilities for immediate human application.

Critical to all of the above is the unwavering availability of sufficient nationally derived funds to allow continued and enhanced productivity of the total cancer program.

The sequential elucidation of the current knowledge regarding carcinogenesis to be presented during this Symposium is the distillation of a generation of scientific excellence. The participants in this program represent a concentration of scientific pioneers rarely equalled. The members of the program committee, led by cochairmen A. Clark Griffin and Charles R. Shaw, feel deeply gratified and somewhat humbled by the enthusiastic response to their invitations.

The cosponsors of the 31st Symposium—the National Cancer Institute, the Texas Division of the American Cancer Society, The University of Texas System Cancer Center, the Board of Regents of The University of Texas, and the faculty of The University of Texas Health Science Center Graduate School of Biomedical Sciences—extend their appreciation to all of you, and particularly to Dr. Isaac Berenblum, who traveled the farthest, for sharing and exchanging knowledge on this occasion.

Carcinogens: Identification and Mechanisms of Action, edited by A. Clark Griffin and Charles R. Shaw. Raven Press, New York © 1979.

Welcome Address

Walter G. Sterling

Board of Regents, The University of Texas System, Houston, Texas 77030

Ladies and Gentlemen, on behalf of the Regents of The University of Texas System it is my pleasure to welcome you here to the 31st Annual Symposium on Cancer Research. The University of Texas System is proud of its M. D. Anderson Hospital and all of the work it has done in both research and patient care. We think it is a credit to the State and to the Nation.

To me there is only one sad note in this Symposium. This is the last one over which Dr. Lee Clark will preside, because he is retiring from his job as President of The University of Texas System Cancer Center M. D. Anderson Hospital and Tumor Institute. As you may know, he is the first and only President of Anderson. He has seen it grow from a few beds in a wooden shack on Brazos Street to the magnificent institution that it is now. We in Texas are very proud of him and his accomplishments, and we are heartily sorry that he is retiring.

Again on behalf of the Regents of The University of Texas System, I welcome you to this Symposium.

Carcinogens: Identification and Mechanisms of Action, edited by A. Clark Griffin and Charles R. Shaw. Raven Press, New York © 1979.

Keynote Address: Evolution, Chemical Carcinogenesis, and Mortality: The Cycle of Life

Frederick F. Becker

Department of Pathology, The University of Texas System Cancer Center M. D. Anderson Hospital and Tumor Institute, Houston, Texas 77030

The phenomenon of chemical carcinogenesis has intruded into the awareness of the scientific and lay public with rapidly increasing intensity, and with this intrusion there has arisen misinformation, fear, political intervention, and an adversarial relationship between scientists in the public arena. We have already witnessed what I call the saccharin backlash, and it is far from sweet. This state of disorder has resulted in part from the vast gaps in our understanding of the process of chemical carcinogenesis. The expertise of the scientists who will participate in this Symposium raises our hopes that these gaps will soon be filled. Therefore, my aim will not be so much to answer specific questions or to present extensively the abundant data available from our own studies and those of others but to offer a brief overview of chemical carcinogenesis, to identify themes that are currently influential, and, where possible, to identify those problems that make this area so complex. In many respects, the study of chemical carcinogenesis is akin to attempting to unravel the Gordian knot. As one traces a promising thread, it invariably leads to other mysteries and entanglements in daunting number, for, although we accept that the chronic exposure of a number of mammalian tissues to a variety of chemical agents often results in the evolution of the exposed cells to malignancy, there is no phase nor facet of this process, from its primary cellular interactions to its terminus in the death of the host, that is fully understood. We cannot state with certainty that the process results solely from the interaction of the suspected chemical agent with target cells, now that we understand the impact of the action of cocarcinogens or promoting agents, alterations of the host's immunological and hormonal modulating capacities, and the nagging possibility that the final common pathway might be the release of a genetic component—an oncogene—that lurks in the host's genome as a result of some ancient "miscegenation" with a wayward virus, a kind of biological original sin made manifest by a forbidden chemical agent.

You may recall that as the chosen Roman ascended the steps of the senate to be declared Caesar he was followed by another who continually reminded him of his fallibility by whispering, "Thou art mortal, thou art mortal." As part of this overview I have attempted to formulate a small number of rules. We could call them the *Thou Art Mortal* or TAM rules which are aimed at maintaining our sense of perspective, of emphasizing the dangers of sweeping assumptions and perhaps fostering an aura of humility in our search for the answer to unraveling this Gordian knot.

Having already disclaimed my obligation to restrict myself to comments supported by experimental results it is acceptable for me to ask, "Where did it all start?" Perhaps the best answer would be, "In the beginning," for there never has been a better milieu in which to achieve the alteration which we consider to be malignancy than in the formative days of earth. Bombarded by cosmic rays, steeped in the combustion products of volcanic activity, in anaerobic pools, at high temperatures, living macromolecules were formed. We might well ask if some of these progenitors of life are those primordial genes which, conserved for eons, need only exposure to the dimly remembered carcinogenic conditions of their genesis to reexpress themselves. Of the early stages of evolution Manfred Eigen (1971) wrote, "Under certain external conditions . . . there may result a macroscopic functional organization which includes self-reproduction, selection and evolution to where this system can escape the prerequisites of its origin and use the environment to its advantage." It strikes me that the evolution of those first macromolecules to a higher form and more complex organization, under the influence of the ultimate carcinogenic environment, bears a remarkable mirror image to the simplification of form and function undergone by mammalian cells under the influence of chemical agents in the process we term carcinogenesis. But, if true, then where did cancer lurk all those many years? Zimmerman (1977) has recently summarized the major studies of paleopathology with the conclusion that the absence of tumors in ancient times must be considered a reflection of a markedly lower incidence than that in modern populations. The fault, therefore, as Cassius to Brutus said, " . . . is not in our stars, but in ourselves. . . ." Perhaps common cancers began with the taking of snuff, or with the conversion from wood to coal for heat, accelerated with the burning of oil products, and finally climaxed with our ability to synthesize chemicals. In 1761, John Hill wrote in his paper entitled *Cautions Against the Immoderate Use of Snuff,* "Whether or not the tumors . . . which occur in snuff-takers are absolutely caused by that custom, or whether the principles of the disorder were there before, and snuff only irritated the parts, and hastened the mischief I shall not pretend to determine. Even supposing the latter only to be the case, the damage is certainly more than the indulgence is worth. No man should venture upon snuff who is not sure that he is not liable to cancer, and no man can be sure of that." Thus, Dr. Hill covered fairly well in 1761 the problems that we will approach in these several days.

Before we enter a discussion of chemical carcinogenesis let us skip briefly to end of the story, the malignant cell. The one major problem that continues to diminish the immediate importance of the results of every experiment in this field and casts a shadow of uncertainty on the relevance of every observation

TABLE 1. *Phenotypic comparison of transplantable hepatocellular carcinomas*

	GR_w	K	pp	AFP	Con A	Metast	MuLV p_{30}
311	2	39–41 (m)	4+	100 mg/ml	+	0	250
252	6	42–45	0	0	+	4+	<1.0
253	20	42	0	0	0	0	<1.0

is our inability to define the malignant cell and, further, to define that macromolecular characteristic which is the basis of malignancy. A vast amount of information exists that describes *what* this cell does and to a lesser extent *how* it does what it does . . . but the *why* evades us. Until now the malignant cell has been defined mainly in comparison with its normal version; the identification of an interesting metabolic control or macromolecular configuration in the normal cell compels us to seek it in the malignant. To overcome the impact of our ignorance of the basic nature of malignancy, many investigators have taken the approach of comparing cell characteristics that are identified at stages of the carcinogenic process with those of the malignant cell, suggesting that findings which are common to each are of particular significance. The dangers of this approach result in part from the incredible phenotypic diversity in malignant tumors and further from the logistics of tumor supply.

The tumors listed in Table 1 are three transplantable hepatocellular carcinomas (THC) induced by a single carcinogen in a single strain of inbred rats. I have included only 7 of the 13 methods that we have applied in an attempt to characterize these tumors. The three tumors range in growth rate (GR_w) from 2 to 20 weeks (Becker *et al.* 1973,1975). They were chosen to illustrate the phenotypic variation possible in tumors that have remained diploid, or near-diploid (K), with one containing a marker chromosome (m) (Becker *et al.* 1971,1973,1975, Wolman *et al.* 1972). Plasma protein synthesis (pp) by THC-311, as measured in vitro, exceeded that of normal livers; its production of alpha-fetoprotein (AFP) was equally vigorous, while the THC-252 and THC-253 produced neither (Becker *et al.* 1972,1973,1975). Agglutination of suspended cells by concanavalin A (Becker 1974, Becker and Shurgin 1975), their ability to metastasize (Becker 1978), and even the presence or absence of viral antigen were also varied and individual (Becker and Sherr 1978). The aggregate of these characteristics forms a fingerprint pattern for each tumor, but we did not identify any pattern that could be considered *the* malignant phenotype, nor did we find a single characteristic common in the more than 30 tumors studied.

Equally important was the finding that during transplantation there was a modeling of each tumor which resulted in accentuation or loss of primary tumor functions and significant alteration of other characteristics (Becker *et al.* 1973,1975). These findings should act as a warning, for the majority of studies that seek to identify *the* malignant characteristic are applied to cells which have undergone the selective processes of transplantation or tissue culture or to the "nth" degree of unnaturalness, ascites tumor formation. Our assumption that these cells display the original aberration which allowed the primary malignant cell to escape host control may be as aberrant as the function of the cell itself.

These findings have led to the first *Thou Art Mortal* rule. TAM #1: We cannot assume that the characteristics of cells which have undergone the selection of transplantation or explantation are valid parameters of malignancy, as that original cell arose in the host. Perhaps another definition of TAM #1 would be: "That ain't malignancy."

Invariably, exposure to carcinogenic agents is of a chronic nature, both in the experimental situation and in human experience. The administration of these carcinogens is limited by their toxicity, for they are indeed almost universally toxic, and by the life-span of the animals to which they are applied. We utilize small animals in order to increase the statistical likelihood of producing the sequences seen in humans; we maximize the dose to allow us to determine those sequences within the short life-span of these animals, and we are constantly limited by the desire to reduce the parallel, but perhaps unrelated, activities of these agents in inducing cell and host damage. The major obstacle to the identification of the crucial interactions and resultant alterations of chemical carcinogenesis results from the complexity of tissue alterations that invariably arise from chronic exposure and are most certainly composed of carcinogenic and noncarcinogenic components (see below). It is, therefore, of vital importance that we distinguish those alterations which are causally related to the induction of malignancy from the vast and complex array of biological and biochemical alterations that result from exposure to carcinogen. To increase our chances of achieving this goal we must identify those lesions or cells that are obligatory to the carcinogenic sequence. To study whole organs or even parts of organs is to risk dilution of vital alterations with the far more extensive changes that are *incidental*. To further achieve this goal of focusing our studies we must seek to identify crucial temporal alterations. Finally, where possible, we should examine primary malignancies before progression or artificial selection takes place.

Problems in analysis of carcinogenesis

---

1. Carcinogenic versus non-carcinogenic alterations
2. Population at risk for malignancy; premalignant
3. Time of irrevocable alteration; multiphasic sequence
4. Primary malignancy; as early as possible

Some years ago at New York University, Dr. George Teebor and I developed a model for the analysis of these alterations in liver (Teebor and Becker 1971). This model displays changes common to other combinations of chemical agents and tissues and will help us to review this process. To determine the effect of an intermittent regimen we fed the carcinogen acetylaminofluorene to rats for three-week cycles, interrupted by a week of normal diet. Small islands of cells first appeared that were proliferative and possibly clonal in origin. These foci, under the continued influence of carcinogen, grew and began to compress the surrounding cells. After three such feedings, grossly identifiable nodules may fill the liver, but if the carcinogen is then withdrawn, the majority of these nodules will disappear, even histologically, and the animals do not develop cancer. This, then, is reversibility in the morphological sense. The emphasis, however, is only on the morphological concept, since reversibility may not pertain to the biochemical or biological alterations. When these three-cycle animals were challenged with a subcarcinogenic dose of a second agent, dimethylnitrosamine, every rat produced multiple carcinomas in a relatively short period of time (Becker 1975). This is a good example of what has been described by Dr. Berenblum as a cocarcinogenic sequence of a synergistic type. The induction of malignancy by exposure to subcarcinogenic doses of multiple agents might also have considerable importance in human environmental conditions. However, the same effect can be achieved by the administration of one more cycle of acetylaminofluorene, at which time some process occurs that selects or alters a number of nodules in two ways. First, despite cessation of subsequent carcinogen administration, these nodules do not regress but persist until carcinomas appear. Therefore, not only are the nodules selected for a higher risk of malignancy and might be considered premalignant, but they are also selected for the persistence of a morphological alteration, an enlarged cell that in aggregate forms a nodule. This persistent nodule, with its high risk for malignancy, has many functional and morphological similarities to lesions that in other experimental systems and in humans are considered to be premalignant (see below).

Lesions at high risk for malignancy

Persistent mitotic activity
Loss of maturation—arrest of ploidy
                  —fetal proteins
Cytological atypia—negative/positive
Accumulation of cells—"tumor"
Abnormal architecture—cell to cell
                  —cell to vasculature
                  —cell to stroma

I have chosen to refer to these lesions as "at high risk for malignancy" rather than the more controversial and debatable term, premalignant. These lesions invariably demonstrate increased mitotic activity, and, equally important, cell division continues despite cessation of exposure to the carcinogen. The component cells demonstrate a lack of normal maturation. For example, we have demonstrated (with Dr. Wolman) (Becker *et al.* 1971) that the cells of the hepatic nodule remain diploid, while normal hepatocytes demonstrate increasing tetraploidy, or they may demonstrate the presence of fetal antigens or fetal enzymes.

Of interest, the majority of cells of these lesions may demonstrate cell enlargement and numerous alterations of cytoplasmic constituents, cytoplasmic more than nuclear atypia. The aggregate of these altered cells is a tumor—whether a nodule, papilloma, or polyp. Further, the architecture or polarity of these cells is atypical, whether in the relationship of cell to like cell or the distance to vessels or the distance to mesodermal constituents. These changes can be seen in the hepatic nodule of the rat, in the neurofibromas of von Recklinghausen's disease, in papillomas induced by chemical agents in the bladder, in the lesions induced in the mouse breast, in the papillomas of skin that arise from the classic initiation-promotion sequence, and in the polyps of familial colonic disease. Indeed, the similarity of these latter systems, illustrated by the papillomas of mouse skin with progression to cancer and also in colonic polyps and focal cancer of human familial disease, makes one wonder if the mouse is not the experimental equivalent of an everted colon or the latter, an inverted mouse. Despite the consistency of these alterations from system to system, none, as yet, has permitted us to identify that crucial factor which, during the lag period before the appearance of malignancy, predisposes these cells to progression. However, at least two possibly related proposals applicable to high-risk lesions must give rise to thoughts concerning the expression and progression to malignancy. Pierce and others have strongly emphasized the influence of the microenvironment on the expression of the malignant cell and its dormant period. In another vein, Riccardi has stressed the modification of the expression of the altered function of mutated cells by adjoining, nonmutated cells. It would appear to me, therefore, that progression to malignancy by cells of the high-risk lesions may be strongly influenced by the alterations in normal architectural relationships of these cells. An interesting mechanism for the effect of dimethylnitrosamine or the fourth feeding of acetylaminofluorene might be that of tumor promotion, recognizing the problem of applying this term as related to the action of a carcinogen. Similar effects have been achieved by the use of phenobarbital by Peraino *et al.* (1977) or the combination of other carcinogens by Farber *et al.* (1977). This would imply that at this juncture, the end of the third cycle, subsequent progression is not dependent on the accumulation of macromolecular events of the same kind as those which initiated the process. These findings lead to TAM #2: The disappearance of a given characteristic imparted by a carcinogen, especially a morphological characteristic, does not imply the reversion or repair of all others. Further, the carcinogenic process may represent an aggregate perturbation of the cell resulting from differing mechanisms and not simply an addition of identical macromolecular events; indeed, it may require more than one form of alteration to complete the carcinogenic-informational loop.

In summary, the discontinuous carcinogenic regimen has allowed us to identify lesions that illustrate the three major thematic concepts (the three S's), which I suggest characterize the process of chemical carcinogenesis: First, a *sequentiality* of alteration as exemplified by the replacement of one type of lesion or cell by another; second, the presence of *subpopulations,* for no matter how carefully we select a tissue for study we are dealing with a diverse population, in this case a variety of nodules, and these comprised of a diverse population of cells; and finally, the overriding influence of *stochastic* or chance selection.

For despite some evidence that tissues as focal as hepatic nodules may be derived from the clonal multiplication of a single cell, we now know that these nodules are internally heterogeneous, possibly as the result of differing pathways of differentiation by their component cells. These nodules demonstrate a variety of enzyme contents, fetoprotein production, variation in karyotype, differing susceptibility to antimitotic agents, and many other focal differences that indicate the presence of subpopulations. We are, therefore, chronically nagged by doubts concerning the significance of our analytic findings and further by the awareness that few of these cells have any likelihood whatsoever of eventuating as malignant. We know that the number of cells that demonstrate an initial alteration under the influence of any carcinogen is enormous compared to the number of morphologically identifiable lesions at each subsequent phase and that these continue to be lesser in number until one or two reach final presentation as a detectable carcinoma. Thus, the stochastic or chance concept must be added to our awareness of the difficulties in analyzing these tissues.

The almost overwhelming complexity imparted by the involvement of the three S's at every phase of this process, and at almost every level from the gross nodule to the location of chemical adducts, leads to TAM #3 and TAM #4. We must reduce to the least common denominator that which we examine in our attempts to identify the obligate alterations in a carcinogenic sequence, and we must also attempt to eliminate the coincidental but unrelated alterations resulting from the noncarcinogenic properties of an agent or the abscotropic or secondary effects resulting from alterations in nontarget organs.

Considerable progress along these lines of focusing our experiments has been achieved by the work of Warwick, Pound, and Craddock, using regenerating liver; Peraino, Farber, and Pitot and others using promoting agents, and a number of investigators in in vitro systems; all of which are, in effect, experiments which follow in the footsteps of the classic initiation-promotion studies of Berenblum and Shubik.

Many investigators have attempted to synthesize a pathogenetic sequence from the alterations that occur during chemical carcinogenesis. Most frequently, these have been described in terms of morphology, others in biochemical or biological terms. The most exciting result of this approach would be its complementation of one of the currently major themes of malignant causation-retrodifferentiation, escape from a deleterious environment, or the release of a cancer factor be it oncogene or other. The identification of other causative mechanisms by such a pathway would be equally welcome! My own approach has been to list the major characteristics of each phase, regardless of the method of observation, and from this aggregate derive functional compartments. The following outline of the phases of chemical carcinogenesis demonstrates this approach.

Phases of chemical carcinogenesis

Toxic
  Decreased RNA Polymerase Activity
  Decreased RNA Synthesis
  Decreased Plasma Protein Synthesis
  Decreased Cell Division (Spontaneous/Responsive)
  Increased AFP Synthesis
  Fetal Enzymes
Escape
  "Spontaneous" Cell Division (Focal)
  Responsive (Focal)
Growth
  Hepatic Nodules (Reversible)
  Functional Schizophrenia
Autonomy
  Growth/Maintenance
  Hepatic Nodules (Irreversible)
Malignant

One may thus envision an initial toxic phase, the extent of which is dependent on the agent-dose and other factors. This phase, most striking at the onset of exposure, is characterized mainly by an inhibition of functions, apparently resulting from the binding of the activated carcinogen-metabolites to crucial macromolecules. But simultaneously selected functions, such as the restitution of fetal characteristics, may occur, in all likelihood suggesting that the fetal functions and perhaps fetal macromolecules are more resistant to these toxic effects. The second phase, which I have termed escape, is that time during which selected cells can be identified by morphological and functional characteristics that differ from the normal cell. The single most important of these is persistent cell division. Subsequently, growth occurs as the most dominant feature of the process, resulting in the instance of hepatocarcinogenesis, in those nodules that I have termed simply—reversible—and further, with this growth there emerges a mixed phenotypic pattern, which I refer to as functional schizophrenia, wherein patterns of fetal and adult characteristics and those of injured and normal cells exist concurrently.

Although many authors including Potter, Markert, Anderson and others have emphasized the possible involvement of reexpression of fetal or embryonic character as a dominant factor in carcinogenesis, and while recently, Farber has expanded the work of Haddow and others to suggest that the evolution of the malignant cell may be dominated by its escape from the toxicity of carcinogens, no one has more graciously integrated the two factors than Uriel (1976), who wrote: " . . . the cells of metazoan organisms may escape from the effects of deleterious agents by retrodifferentiation and with this escape there is a progressive decrease in responsiveness to regulator signals which are normally operational. Retrodifferentiation thus results in a new stationary state adapted to a new, stressful environment." In accord with Uriel's proposal, the phase of autonomy is characterized by the ability of the component cells to escape some of the normal control mechanisms of the host, retaining their abnormal structure, phenotypic diversity, and their capacity to divide. For either these cells have now a supra-sensitivity to the normal stimuli to divide, or, more likely, they have achieved a threshold of momentum for cell division. I would suggest that the cells which are at high risk for malignancy are those that have reached a state of decreased vulnerability to the injurious environmental stress. I further propose that in achieving this new, and possibly less stable state, these cells are less capable of maintaining the oncogene, or cancer integrator, in a blocked condition. A similar instability might account for spontaneous transformation in culture. Unfortunately, although tantalizing, none of these hypotheses nor any available pathogenic sequence is sufficiently supported by experimental data to explain the why of malignancy. These thoughts lead to TAM #5: Give me a theory, and I'll give you a grant . . . and its converse, just because you have a grant doesn't mean you have a theory.

The mechanisms of action of chemical carcinogens and their resultant induction of alterations in target cells are, of course, the dominant theme of this program. I would like, however, to offer an outline of areas of interest related to this theme and present very briefly some data from our laboratory to illustrate points previously discussed. First, of course, the agent must arrive at and enter the target cell. This is not as simple as it sounds for there is evidence from Dr. Farber's laboratory that target cell permeability may be altered during exposure. The activation of these agents once within the target cell has been an important and exciting area of investigation (Miller and Miller 1977) with major studies emerging from the laboratories of the Millers, Weisburgers, Gelboin, Irving, and many others. It has also been reported by a number of investigators and solidified by the work of Farber that many of the factors responsible for normal drug metabolism and carcinogen activation are diminished by chronic exposure to carcinogens. But does the simple diminution of this capacity imply that the activation of carcinogen within the target cell no longer plays a role in the carcinogenic sequence, as has also been implied? One way of approaching this problem would be to examine the capability of this metabolic apparatus to activate the carcinogen and to produce some acceptable endpoint, such as bacterial revertants throughout the carcinogenic sequence. I use the term acceptable endpoint only in the broadest sense, for there is to date no final evidence

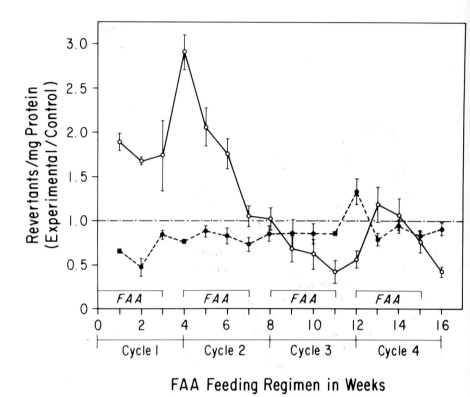

FIG. 1. The solid line represents the number of bacterial revertants produced when FAA was incubated with the microsome fraction and the dashed line N-OH-FAA with the cytosol. (Reproduced, with permission of Cancer Res., from Stout and Becker 1978.)

that the ability of microsomes to produce revertants in vitro is equatable with carcinogenicity, but similarly, there is no finite evidence that any other single measure, such as binding to a specific base, is significantly better. Our own approach to characterizing the changing metabolic capabilities of the liver was to isolate its microsomal compartment, the S9 fraction and cytosol, the S150, throughout exposure to 2-acetylaminofluorene (FAA) and to determine their capacity to activate respectively FAA or N-OH-FAA. This work performed with Dr. Daniel Stout (Figure 1) demonstrates an initial, pronounced activation of this capacity throughout the toxic phase and a portion of the escape phase. From that point onward, through the phases of growth and autonomy, the general trend was toward depression, and in this trend, the results correlate well with the published analyses of enzyme composition and P450. Interestingly, the activity of the soluble system in vitro was unaltered throughout the entire sequence. But let me use this brief presentation to make several points. First, due to our inability to isolate the focal lesions resulting from the first two cycles of feeding, the portion of this curve that demonstrates induced activity may reflect mainly the effect of the carcinogen on those cells that will not go on to other stages of malignant evolution. Comparison of isolated nodules and nonnodular parenchyma after the third or fourth cycle invariably demonstrated a more severe deficit in the nodules (once again illustrating the impact of TAM #3). Second, you will note that at the beginning of the most crucial phase of the entire process, the fourth cycle, an induction of enzyme activity occurred that would have been missed if only single points at the end of each cycle were determined. Further, I would emphasize that without knowing whether the vulnerability of the genome to mutagens is not also altered during exposure, we are still working in the shadow of the three S's. However, these findings lead to the formulation of TAM #6: Since the characteristics of the target cells are constantly altering under the influence of the carcinogen, no conclusions based upon data obtained at one stage of carcinogenesis, indeed from any single point, can be justifiably concluded to be implicated in any other.

For the moment let us accept the generally held belief that a major and crucial effect of carcinogen action is DNA damage. One of the most exciting and revealing areas of recent investigation has been the identification of various mechanisms for the repair of such damage (Roberts 1976). A failure of these mechanisms could take the form of a failure to excise the metabolites bound to DNA, replication of DNA inaccurately due to bound adducts, or an unfaithful replication of the DNA by altered polymerases. Our own studies, again with Dr. Teebor, have revealed that several of the crucial excision enzymes of repair are resistant to the effects of exposure to FAA (Teebor *et al.* 1977). More recently, Dr. John Chan and I have demonstrated that the beta form of DNA polymerase, the enzyme that some feel is involved in the replication of excised strips of DNA during repair, is similarly resistant. These findings are all the more striking when one considers the number of other enzymes, such as RNA polymerase, that are rapidly and significantly inhibited by the same regimen and suggest that this repair system has been selected evolutionarily for resistance—to defend DNA against a hostile environment.

In part, to emphasize the usefulness of the sequential carcinogenic system I will briefly present one other study by Dr. Chan and myself that relates to the fidelity of DNA synthesis by the alpha-polymerase under the influence of chemical carcinogens. When we examined the function of cytoplasmic DNA alpha-polymerase throughout chemical carcinogenesis, using the microincorporation assay of Loeb, a striking contrast with the results of the other DNA-related enzyme studies was evident. Thus, the fidelity of this enzyme decreases, reaching a significant degree of inaccuracy at the third cycle and remaining abnormal throughout the fourth cycle. However, to conclude from this experiment that this infidelity results in malignancy would necessitate ignoring the enormous complexity of the mammalian cell. It suggests only another possible loop in the complex matrix of carcinogen action and the importance of being aware of the constantly changing cellular environment that occurs under the influence of these agents.

From all of the above we can conclude that the field of chemical carcinogenesis is data and theory rich but answer poor, and we could ask, with justification, "Where do we go now?" The strategy seems clear. We must extend and refine methods for the identification of carcinogenic agents, and by analysis of their chemical and physical characteristics, we may be able one day to predict potential carcinogenicity prior to their introduction into the human environment. Next, we must continue to identify crucial interactions between these agents, metabolic pathways, and macromolecules of the target cells. Herein lies one of the most potentially fruitful goals in terms of human experience. If we can also identify those agents that would diminish these interactions by increasing the role of deactivating pathways or by interfering with the interaction of activated metabolites with crucial targets within the cell, we might, in a manner no more exotic than the elimination of goiter by added iodine, eliminate carcinogenicity.

We must also identify the alterations in cell structure and function induced by these reactions. For it is within an understanding of these phenotypic alterations that we may learn the *why* of malignancy, the *why* of its escape from normal control. It is in this very area that the exciting experiments suggesting reversal of this process by vitamin A analogs fall. We must seek objective means for identifying the functional basis of the morphological alterations of the carcinogenic sequence. We have wasted too much energy; we have created too much uncertainty by our willingness to fall victim to semantic traps baited with such terms as premalignant lesion, neoplastic nodules, in situ carcinoma, microinvasive, and even malignant, when objective evidence for many of these was lacking. This objective evidence will not be achieved by morphological examination alone but through the correlation of morphological appearance with measures of biological or biochemical activity. This leads to TAM #7: Lesions must only be designated by that biological function which can be conclusively associated with a given morphology.

Last, and perhaps of greatest importance, we must define malignancy, define those characteristics of cellular activity that permit the malignant cell to compete so effectively with normal cells and to destroy them.

The questions are often raised: "By which method are we most likely to solve this problem? . . . Are we too finite or not finite enough? . . . Should we lump, or should we split?" My answer is summarized in the last TAM #8: The goal of cancer prevention and cancer cure warrants the beat of different drummers, indeed the constant seeking of different tunes. For it is written that the solution to the Gordian knot came by means other than those conceived of by its originator, Gordius, King of Phrygia. It was Alexander who severed it with a single blow of his sword. Thus, as we pursue with dogged perseverance our goal of unraveling this fearful but fascinating problem, let us remain constantly alert to the possibility that a previously unexpected mechanism will become apparent as its basis. Let us remain constantly available to seize any clue with an open mind and hasten the conclusion of this important task.

REFERENCES

Becker, F. F. 1974. Differential lectin agglutination of fetal, dividing-postnatal and malignant hepato-cytes. Proc. Natl. Acad. Sci. USA 71:4307–4311.

Becker, F. F. 1975. Alteration of hepatocytes by subcarcinogenic exposure to N-2-fluorenylacetamide. Cancer Res. 35:1734–1736.

Becker, F. F. 1978. Patterns of metastasis of transplantable hepatocellular carcinomas. Cancer Res. 38:63–67.

Becker, F. F., R. A. Fox, K. M. Klein, and S. R. Wolman. 1971. Chromosome patterns in rat hepatocytes during N-2-fluorenylacetamide carcinogenesis. J. Natl. Cancer Inst. 46:1261–1269.

Becker, F. F., K. M. Klein, and R. Asofsky. 1972. Plasma protein synthesis by N-2-fluorenylaceta-mide-induced primary hepatocellular carcinomas and hepatic nodules. Cancer Res. 32:914–920.

Becker, F. F., K. M. Klein, S. R. Wolman, R. Asofsky, and S. Sell. 1973. Characterization of primary hepatocellular carcinomas and initial transplant generations. Cancer Res. 33:3330–3338.

Becker, F. F., and C. J. Sherr. 1978. Activation of endogenous type C viral p30 antigen in chemically induced rat hepatocellular carcinomas. Int. J. Cancer 21:756–761.

Becker, F. F., and A. Shurgin. 1975. Concanavalin A agglutination of cells from primary hepatocellu-lar carcinoma and hepatic nodules induced by N-2-fluorenylacetamide. Cancer Res. 35:2879–2883.

Becker, F. F., S. R. Wolman, R. Asofsky, and S. Sell. 1975. Sequential analysis of transplantable hepatocellular carcinomas. Cancer Res. 35:3021–3026.

Eigen, M. 1971. Molecular self-organization and the early stages of evolution. Q. Rev. Biophys. 4:149–212.

Farber, E., D. Solt, R. Cameron, B. Laishes, K. Ogawa, and A. Medline. 1977. Newer insights into the pathogenesis of liver cancer. Am. J. Pathol. 89:477–482.

Miller, J. A., and E. C. Miller. 1977. Ultimate chemical carcinogens as reactive mutagenic electro-philes, *in* Cold Spring Harbor Conferences on Cell Proliferation, H. H. Hiatt, J. D. Watson, and J. A. Winsten, eds., Vol. 4. Cold Spring Harbor Laboratory, Cold Spring Harbor, New York, pp. 605–629.

Peraino, C., R. J. M. Fry, and E. Staffeldt. 1977. Effects of varying the onset and duration of exposure to phenobarbital on its enhancement of 2-acetylaminofluorene-induced hepatic tumori-genesis. Cancer Res. 37:3623–3627.

Roberts, J. J. 1976. DNA repair and carcinogenesis, *in* Scientific Foundations in Oncology, T. Symington and R. L. Carter, eds., Year Book Medical Publishers, Inc., Chicago, pp. 319–333.

Stout, D., and F. F. Becker. 1978. Alteration of the ability of liver microsomes to activate N-2-FAA to a mutagen of *Salmonella typhimurium* during haepatocarcinogenesis. Cancer Res. 38:2274–2278.

Teebor, G. W., and F. F. Becker. 1971. Regression and persistence of hyperplastic nodules induced by N-2-flourenylacetamide and their relationship to hepatocarcinogenesis. Cancer Res. 31:1–3.

Teebor, G. W., N. J. Duker, and F. F. Becker. 1977. Normal endonuclease activities for damaged DNA during hepatocarcinogenesis. Biochim. Biophys. Acta 477(2):125–131.

Uriel, J. 1976. Cancer, retrodifferentiation and the myth of Faust. Cancer Res. 36:4269–4275.

Wolman, S. R., R. F. Phillips, and F. F. Becker. 1972. Fluorescent banding patterns of rat chromo-somes in normal cells and primary hepatocellular carcinomas and hepatic nodules. Science 175:1267–1269.

Zimmerman, M. R. 1977. An experimental study of mummification pertinent to the antiquity of cancer. Cancer 40:1358–1362.

The Ernst W. Bertner Memorial
Award Lectures

Carcinogens: Identification and Mechanisms
of Action, edited by A. Clark Griffin and
Charles R. Shaw. Raven Press, New York © 1979.

Introduction of the Ernst W. Bertner Memorial Award Recipients

R. Lee Clark

The University of Texas System Cancer Center M. D. Anderson Hospital and Tumor Institute, Houston, Texas 77030

DR. ISAAC BERENBLUM

Dr. Isaac Berenblum had extensive training in the areas of experimental pathology and chemical carcinogenesis. During most of his distinguished career, he has been affiliated with Oxford University in England and The Weizmann Institute of Science in Israel.

We wish to congratulate Dr. Berenblum on the 50th anniversary of the first of his many significant publications—his first paper was published in 1928. Very significantly, in 1929 he published a paper entitled, "The *Modifying Influence of Dichloroethyl Sulfide (Otherwise Known as Mustard Gas) on the Induction of Tumors in Mice by Tar*," in the *Journal of Pathology and Bacteriology*. In subsequent studies Dr. Berenblum was looking for other substances that would modify carcinogenesis. He inadvertently employed croton oil and observed the opposite effect—that the croton oil actually enhanced or promoted carcinogenesis. Thus the earliest beginnings of the important two-stage concept of carcinogenesis were initiated.

In 1941, Dr. Berenblum began to repeat experimental results, which led to the development of the theory of cocarcinogenesis, utilizing, as his experimental agent, croton resin. This work suggested a multistage mechanism underlying the effect of croton oil in the development of epidermal neoplasms. With Dr. Philippe Shubik, he later confirmed this two-stage cocarcinogenesis hypothesis and instigated the concept of separate initiating and promoting agents. This concept, which brought to the attention of experimentalists the sequential nature of the carcinogenic process, raised the possibility that noncarcinogenic agents might participate in malignant evolution. This concept became one of the foundations of modern investigations for defining chemical carcinogenesis.

Many important findings were reported early in his career relating to the carcinogenic properties of coal tars and the constituent hydrocarbons. While much of the early work establishing the multistage aspects of carcinogenesis was concerned with the skin, Dr. Berenblum and co-workers have extended these findings on the promoting action of phorbol structures (the active components of croton oils) to liver, lung, and mammary carcinogenesis. More recently, he has studied the leukemogenic action of phorbol and made fundamental contributions relating to radiation leukemogenesis.

The significance of the multistage concept of the origin of tumors, as developed by Drs. Berenblum and Shubik, becomes more apparent with the increasing numbers of important publications in almost every issue of cancer journals. For instance, Dr. Boutwell, one of the associates of the Millers at Wisconsin, recently reported that the sulfur mustard (the "war gas," bis-[2-chloroethyl]-sulfide) will inactivate or block the transformation of skin cells initiated by the potent hydrocarbon, dimethyl benzanthracine. These investigators are able to study the biochemical events within the promotion or progression of the development of tumors.

Dr. Boutwell, as well as Dr. Sporn, whose presentation is included in this Symposium, have shown that the retinoids, analogues of vitamin A, compounds that are now classified as chemopreventive agents for cancer, block specific events or stages of the promotional phase of carcinogenesis.

These reports represent some major advances in the elucidation of the precise mechanisms of carcinogenesis and provide new insights into possible means for the prevention of environmental or chemical carcinogenesis.

These investigations, as well as most of the presentations of this Symposium, have been greatly influenced by the contributions of Drs. Berenblum and Shubik.

DR. PHILIPPE SHUBIK

Dr. Philippe Shubik received his medical training at Oxford University and London Hospital in England. He then served from 1944 to 1947 in the British Army Medical Corps. From 1947 until the present, Dr. Shubik has been directly involved in many activities and investigations relating to chemical carcinogenesis.

One of the most important concepts in carcinogenesis, that of the multistage origin of tumors, was developed by Dr. Isaac Berenblum and Dr. Shubik, and the original articles were published by these eminent scientists in the *British Journal of Cancer* from 1947 to 1949.

Another of Dr. Shubik's investigations, in collaboration with Dr. Byron Riegel at Northwestern University, contributed significantly to the subsequent development of the concepts of microsomal oxidation of chemical agents into inactive metabolites and to the identification of compounds now recognized as proximate or ultimate carcinogens.

Dr. Shubik was Professor of Oncology and Director of the Chicago Medical Institute for Medical Research from 1953 to 1968. During this period, he and his collaborators continued to make outstanding contributions toward defining the mechanisms involved in skin carcinogenesis, the role of hyperplasia, dose-effect and age relationships, the role of burns and other injuries in carcinogenesis, the induction of melanotic, bladder, and hepatic tumors, lymphomas, and tracheobronchial carcinomas with a wide spectrum of chemicals.

In collaboration with Drs. W. Lijinsky, Saffiotti and others, important contributions were made to the discovery of carcinogens in cooked and smoked food and to the environmental aspects of lung cancer induction.

During 1968, Dr. Shubik and many of his collaborators moved to Omaha, Nebraska, to establish the Eppley Institute for Research in Cancer. Dr. Shubik has served as Professor of Pathology and Director of this institute since 1968. The scientific world has finally caught up with Dr. Shubik's and a few other investigators' long-standing, unwavering conviction of the importance of chemicals as the major causative factors in human cancer. Dr. Shubik and his collaborators have established one of the outstanding centers for the study of experimental carcinogenesis, designing and testing procedures for the detection of environmental carcinogens, and conducting many other studies related to the roles of occupational exposure, drugs, food additives, airborne particulates, and water contaminants in the causation of human cancer.

Dr. Shubik is a member of a number of national and international organizations and committees, including: The Committee on Cancer Prevention of the International Union Against Cancer (UICC), Chairman of the Committee on the Quantitative Aspects of Environmental Carcinogenesis of the UICC, Consultant to the Director of the National Cancer Institute, the Committee for Environmental Carcinogenesis, the American Association for Cancer Research, the Advisory Committee on Environmental Carcinogenesis of the International Agency for Research on Cancer of the World Health Organization, and Chairman of the Subcommittee on Environmental Carcinogens of the National Cancer Advisory Board.

Carcinogens: Identification and Mechanisms of
Action, edited by A. Clark Griffin and
Charles R. Shaw. Raven Press, New York © 1979.

The Ernst W. Bertner Memorial Award Lecture

Theoretical and Practical Aspects of the Two-Stage Mechanism of Carcinogenesis

Isaac Berenblum

The Weizmann Institute of Science, Rehovot, Israel

To be invited to deliver the Bertner Memorial Award Lecture for 1978 is indeed an honor and, at the same time, a challenging assignment in light of the high standards set by those chosen for it in previous years. I feel greatly privileged on both counts.

I propose to deal with Theoretical and Practical Aspects of the Two-Stage Mechanism of Carcinogenesis—the postulated system of tumor induction that was first adumbrated 37 years ago (Rous and Kidd 1941, Berenblum 1941 [see also Friedewald and Rous 1944, Berenblum and Shubik 1947]), and which has recently acquired a new lease of life. I should like to discuss the reasons for this revival of interest and, more particularly, to consider some of its implications, in practical terms, for man.

I can safely bypass any detailed description of the two-stage, initiation-promotion system of carcinogenesis, with so many comprehensive reviews available that cover the field, e.g., by Steinbäck, Garcia and Shubik (1974), Berenblum (1975, 1978), Van Duuren (1976), to quote only the most recent publications on the subject. I shall, therefore, have little to say about the past and shall concentrate on the present with an eye to the future.

The renewed interest in the two-stage mechanism of carcinogenesis stems from growing support in favor of a mutational change in the genome as the most likely mechanism of *initiating* action and the current, intensive researches into the mechanism of *promoting* action, rendered possible by the isolation of the active principle of croton oil (Hecker 1968, Van Duuren 1969). There is, however, a third, overriding factor—the realization of a possible role of initiation-promotion in human carcinogenesis.

I propose to deal briefly with the two theoretical aspects and allow myself more time to speculate on the impact of these academic studies on new concepts of cancer prevention in man.

THE ROLE OF INITIATION IN CARCINOGENESIS

The somatic cell mutation theory of cancer, in its original formulation of 50 years ago by Bauer (1928), was based on theoretical considerations only, but it did have some highly attractive features: It could, for instance, account for (1) the irreversible nature of neoplastic transformation, (2) the almost unlimited variety of tumors, whether arising spontaneously or induced artificially, and (3) the tendency for each individual tumor to "breed true to type." It had, however, a serious defect or limitation: A mutational change in the genome of a cell is a very rapid process and could hardly account for the long latent period of carcinogenesis, which in man might be up to 30 years, or even more. (Attempts to allow for the long latent period of carcinogenesis by postulating a sequence of random mutations [Charles and Luce-Clausen 1942, Fisher and Hollomon 1951, Nordling 1953, De Waard 1964] are rendered invalid by the experimental finding that carcinogenesis by the two-stage technique does not operate when the initiating and promoting actions are applied in reverse order [Berenblum 1941, Berenblum and Haran 1955], as would have been expected to function if the two had identical modes of action.)

In its modern version, the mutation theory of tumor induction is considered to apply to the initiating phase only, which happens to be very rapid in action (Mottram 1944, Berenblum 1954)—in fact, known to be completed within a matter of hours (Ball and McCarter 1960, Gelboin et al. 1965, Berenblum and Armuth 1977)—and which is also irreversible, in the sense that the resulting dormant tumor cells can be quantitatively activated by promoting action after very long intervals (Berenblum and Shubik 1949, Van Duuren 1969). The promoting phase, on the other hand, is almost certainly epigenetic in mode of action (see section on The Role of Promotion in Carcinogenesis).

The underlying principle of a mutational change as an essential factor in carcinogenesis has received much support from the biochemical evidence of covalent binding with DNA by the different classes of "complete" carcinogens, especially in the organs in which they act carcinogenically (Magee and Farber 1962, Wheeler 1962, Brookes and Lawley 1964, Goshman and Heidelberger 1967, Matsumoto and Terayama 1970, Lijinsky et al. 1972, Lawson and Pound 1973; see also reviews by Van Duuren 1969, Miller 1970, Sarma et al. 1975, Lawley 1976), and more particularly by the metabolically activated proximate or ultimate carcinogenic derivatives (Dingman and Sporn 1967, Warwick 1969, Jackson and Irving 1970, Kriek 1971, Coombs et al. 1975, Weinstein et al. 1976, Yang et al. 1977), also by initiators alone (Boutwell et al. 1969, Nietert et al. 1974, Pound and Lawson 1976) but not, apparently, by promoting agents (Helmes et al. 1974, McCann et al. 1975). This, then, is the practical support for what was initially a speculative concept but limited now to the initiating component only.

The fairly close correlation that exists between mutagens and carcinogens (see reviews by Fishbein et al. 1970, Knudson 1973, Brookes and De Serres

1976), and more particularly in connection with proximate and ultimate carcinogens (McCann *et al.* 1975, Purchase *et al.* 1976), is, of course, added support for a mutational change being involved in carcinogenesis.

The fact that induced mutations may undergo repair (see review by Trosko and Chu 1975) naturally introduces certain complications in the interpretation of results, but this does not necessarily invalidate the idea of a mutational change as the most likely basis for initiating action

THE ROLE OF PROMOTION IN CARCINOGENESIS

The situation regarding the promoting phase of carcinogenesis is by no means as clear. It is manifestly epigenetic in mode of action (Berenblum and Shubik 1949, Knudson 1973, Chu *et al.* 1977). One is thus faced with a dual problem: (1) its actual mechanism of action, and (2) how its effect, the "awakening" of dormant tumor cells, resulting in progressively growing tumors, eventually becomes self-perpetuating (i.e., without the need for further promoting action). The problem, in short, is how epigenetic action could produce the irreversible change exemplified by the promoting phase of carcinogenesis.

In general terms, one could postulate several different ways whereby the awakening process might be achieved: e.g., (1) as a consequence of deficient or aberrant differentiation (Sherbet 1970, Farber 1973, Iversen 1973, Pierce 1974), or (2) as a consequence of excessive cell proliferation, resulting in a kind of "adaptive ontogenesis" (Nery 1976), or (3) by a disturbance in the chalone mechanism of cell division (Bullough 1965, Elgjo 1976), or (4) by immunological effects (Burnet 1959, Lappé 1971, Prehn 1971, Muller and Sutherland 1971, Cairns 1975), or (5) by modification of the genetic control mechanism at the gene level (Pitot and Heidelberger 1963, based on Jacob and Monod's model, 1961), i.e., not strictly epigenetic but nonmutational all the same.

All these suggested mechanisms are essentially speculative in approach. I do not mean it in a disparaging sense but merely wish to indicate that they are based on indirect evidence and do not readily lend themselves to direct experimental verification. This does not mean necessarily that they are wrong, but they cannot all be right. An alternative lead would be to argue that since carcinogens are known to bind with proteins as well as with nucleic acids (Miller and Miller 1947, Heidelberger and Moldenhauer 1956, Beije and Hultin 1971, Carruthers *et al.* 1976), the mechanism of promoting action might somehow be related to the deletion of a specific protein, as originally postulated for liver carcinogenesis with azo dyes (Sorof *et al.* 1951). Except for the characterization of the protein in question (Sorof *et al.* 1974, Sarrif *et al.* 1975), little progress seems to have been made in following up this lead.

A more positive approach to the problem of the mechanism of promoting action is the study of biological and biochemical side effects of promoting agents, including chemically related, weakly acting and inactive compounds, in the hope of discovering a correlation between potency of promoting action and one or another of the side effects among the group of compounds tested. There has been considerable activity lately into this type of enquiry (see Slaga *et al.* 1978), using TPA (12-0-tetradecanoyl-phorbol-13-acetate—the active principle of croton oil) and related compounds, tested in mouse skin. (The subject was dealt with in some detail at last year's Gatlinburg Symposium, the proceedings of which have been published [see Slaga *et al.* 1978].)

Some of the side effects that correlated fairly well with promoting activity included certain morphological changes in the skin (Setälä 1960, Major 1970, Janoff *et al.* 1970, Bach and Goerttler 1971, Raick 1973, Slaga *et al.* 1976), modified patterns in tritiated thymidine incorporation (Paul 1969, Baird *et al.* 1971, Krieg *et al.* 1974, Yuspa *et al.* 1976), changes in cellular metabolism (Rohrschneider and Boutwell 1973, Balmain and Hecker 1974, Colburn *et al.* 1975), notably an increase in induction of ornithine decarboxylase (O'Brien 1976), possible changes in hormonal responses in the skin (Belman and Troll 1972), and biochemical alterations in cell surface membrane function (Rohrschneider and Boutwell 1973, Grimm and Marks 1974, Belman and Troll 1974, Verma *et al.* 1976).

One of the limitations of such comparative studies is that correlations based on small numbers of compounds may merely reflect chance associations. To overcome this difficulty, it has been suggested (Berenblum 1978) that the comparisons be extended to include the skin of other species (rat, rabbit, guinea pig, etc.) in which croton oil fails to act as promoting agent (Shubik 1950). If the side effects were observed in these species as well, they would hardly have relevance to promoting action. In this way, the number of *meaningful* correlations could be decreased considerably.

TWO-STAGE CARCINOGENESIS IN TISSUES OTHER THAN SKIN

Before turning to the problem of initiation-promotion in human carcinogenesis, it is necessary to examine how widely applicable the two-stage system is for different tissues in the body.

The fact that the most detailed information we possess about the two-stage system of carcinogenesis is derived from experimental studies in mouse skin is due partly to the fact that croton oil—the first effective promoting agent— happened to have been most active for that tissue and partly because the demonstration of two-stage carcinogenesis in other organs has proved to be rather difficult for technical reasons. Yet, there are now many examples of initiation-promotion operating in other organs, such as in the thyroid (Hall 1948, Christov 1975), the liver (Glinos *et al.* 1951, Armuth and Berenblum 1972, Kimura *et al.* 1976), the mammary gland (Jull 1954, Dao and Sunderland 1959, Cassell *et al.* 1971, Armuth and Berenblum 1974), the forestomach (Berenblum and Haran 1955, Peirce 1961), the thymus (Berenblum and Trainin 1960), the subcutaneous tissues (Haran-Ghera *et al.* 1962), the kidney (Rosen and Cole 1962), the lungs (Armuth and Berenblum 1972, Nettesheim and Schreiber 1975), the colon (Narisawa *et al.* 1974, Reddy *et al.* 1977), the pancreas (Konishi *et al.* 1976), and also in cells grown in tissue culture (Mondal *et al.* 1976, Lasne *et al.* 1977).

Although not all of these experimental models can be accepted as conforming strictly to the initiation-promotion system (some being possibly manifestations of other kinds of cocarcinogenic action [see Berenblum 1969]), there is no doubt that in the broad sense of "precipitating factors," of which promoting action is only one example, such modifying influences undoubtedly play an important role in many forms of carcinogenesis in animals, and presumably so in man.

PATTERNS OF ENVIRONMENTAL CANCER IN MAN

It has long been recognized that environmental factors play a major role in human cancer (WHO Technical Report, 1964) and that the theoretical possibilities for cancer prevention may be as high as 90 percent (Higginson 1968). That does not mean that all the causative agents are known for 90 percent of human cancers. In fact, most of the evidence of environmental influences in man is derived indirectly, from epidemiological studies, pointing to striking differences in distribution of cancer for organ site according to geographical location, yet not attributable to racial differences (see reviews by Higginson and Muir 1976, Doll 1977).

One could actually make a rough distinction between three categories of human cancer: (1) in cases in which environmental carcinogens are known with certainty to be responsible for the majority of cancers, e.g., skin, mouth, lungs, liver, urinary bladder, and possibly acute leukemia, (2) in cases in which there is scant evidence of specific carcinogens acting from outside the body, yet where environmental factors are known to influence tumor incidence, e.g., in the breast, uterus, ovaries, prostate, thyroid, pancreas, larynx, esophagus, stomach, colon and rectum, and (3) in cases in which there is no evidence of any kind about outside influences, which must provisionally be classed as nonenvironmental in origin.

The second category, in which environmental factors are not clearly identified, is the most intriguing one, especially since it accounts for up to 50 percent of all human cancers. The question here is whether the failure to attribute specific carcinogens for these organs is because of inadequate information, or whether one is dealing here with a more complicated set-up, possibly involving a two-stage mechanism, with both initiator and promoter acting independently from outside; or, more likely, with the initiating stimulus being inherited or arising as a spontaneous mutation or induced by a vertically transmitted virus or by some other *intrinsic* factor, while the *environmental* determinant for the tumor to manifest itself is a promoting agent acting from outside the body.

Let us deal with these two contingencies separately. With both the initiating stimulus and the co-factor operating from outside the body, the prospects of recognizing the dual system by epidemiological surveys are reasonably good.

This was found, for instance, in connection with the study of lung cancer among asbestos workers in relation to cigarette smoking. The incidence of the disease, among those exposed to both factors, was far greater than that which could have been expected from either alone or from a simple additive effect, thus pointing to some form of synergism (Selikoff *et al.* 1968), possibly to the operation of an initiation-promotion system. There are many other reported examples of multiple environmental factors involved in human carcinogenesis, though the distinction between simple additive action and involvement of promoting or other forms of cocarcinogenic action is not clear in most cases.

Where the initiating stimulus is *intrinsic* in origin (or, at any rate, unrecognized), the involvement of a specific environmental "precipitating factor" may still be discovered by epidemiological analyses, but the identification of the responsible factor is likely to prove much more difficult in such cases, since the conventional procedures for identification—whether by routine testing for "complete" carcinogenesis in animals or with the use of the "Ames test" based on mutagenesis (Ames *et al.* 1975, McCann *et al.* 1975)—are not applicable to promoting action.

Thus, we are faced with a new problem in connection with cancer prevention in man, or at least with one that has received insufficient attention in the past, namely, the search for promoting factors in man's environment. One can safely predict a shift in emphasis from a main concern with "complete" carcinogens in man's environment to more and more preoccupation with cocarcinogens in general and promoting factors in particular. Here again, both epidemiological studies and laboratory testing will have to play their part (Selikoff 1976) but with a new orientation in connection with epidemiological studies and the introduction of radically new methods in connection with laboratory testing for promoting factors.

METHODS OF CANCER PREVENTION IN MAN

Assuming that all the carcinogenic agents and all the co-factors involved in carcinogenesis in man were ultimately discovered, how would one exploit the information and thus prevent the postulated 90 percent of human cancer attributable to the environment from arising in the first place? As a first approximation, the answer would be to eliminate all the incriminating factors from man's environment. But this is difficult enough to execute in practice in the case of "complete" carcinogens, as we know from experience; it would be more difficult still in connection with promoting agents and other cocarcinogenic factors. Cancer prevention in man *by elimination procedures* could, therefore, be no more than a partial solution.

There is fortunately another potential approach, which takes the form of *interference* with the carcinogenic process during the long latent period, as distinct from *elimination* of the causative factors. We now know of many examples of anticarcinogenic action, demonstrated experimentally in animals, by chemical agents (Berenblum 1929, Crabtree 1941, Wattenberg 1977), by hormonal action (Houssay *et al.* 1951, Shay *et al.* 1960, Meisels 1966, Belman and Troll 1972, Kledzik *et al.* 1974, Hamilton *et al.* 1975), by vitamins (Saffiotti *et al.* 1967, Sporn *et al.* 1977), as well as by caloric restriction (Tannenbaum and Silverstone 1953). (For reviews of anticarcinogenic action, see Crabtree 1947, Morris 1952, Tannenbaum and Silverstone 1953, Van Duuren and Melchionne 1969, Falk 1971, Homburger 1974, Van Duuren 1976, Wattenberg 1978). Many of the experimental models seem to be operating as blocking agents during the latent period of carcinogenesis and are, therefore, essentially antipromoting agents, but some act on the inciting agents themselves rather than on the responding tissues (Wattenberg 1978).

Though the phenomenon of anticarcinogenesis has been known for so long a time, there is much yet to be elucidated at the experimental level before the information can be applied to man. Yet in principle, it should eventually serve as an important method of cancer prevention. In short, the prospects are good, although the goal is still far ahead.

ACKNOWLEDGMENT

The work of the author was supported in part by Grant 1 RO1 CA 21088-01 of the National Cancer Institute, USPHS.

REFERENCES

Ames, B. N., J. McCann, and E. Yamasaki. 1975. Methods for detecting carcinogens and mutagens with the *Salmonella*/mammalian microsome mutagenicity test. Mutat. Res. 31:347–364.

Armuth, V., and I. Berenblum. 1972. Promoting action of phorbol in liver and lung carcinogenesis in AKR mice. Cancer Res. 32:2259–2262.

Armuth, V., and I. Berenblum. 1974. Promotion of mammary carcinogenesis and leukemogenic action by phorbol in virgin female Wistar rats. Cancer Res. 34:2704–2707.

Bach, H., and K. Goerttler. 1971. Morphologische Untersuchungen zur hyperplastogenen Wirkung des biologisch aktiven Phorbolesters A$_1$. Virchow's Archive, Abt. B. Zellpath. 8:196–205.

Baird, W. M., J. A. Sedgwick, and R. K. Boutwell. 1971. Effects of phorbol and four diesters of phorbol on the incorporation of tritiated precursors into DNA, RNA and protein in mouse epidermis. Cancer Res. 31:1434–1439.

Ball, J. K., and J. A. McCarter. 1960. A study of dose and effect in initiation of skin tumours by a carcinogenic hydrocarbon. Br. J. Cancer 14:577–590.

Balmain, A., and E. Hecker. 1974. On the biochemical mechanism of tumorigenesis in mouse skin. VI. Early effects of growth-stimulating phorbol esters on phosphate transport and phospholipid synthesis in mouse epidermis. Biochim. Biophys. Acta 362:457–468.

Bauer, K. H. 1928. Mutationstheorie der Geschwulst-Entstehung. Übergang von Körperzellen in Geschwulstzellen durch Gen-änderung. Julius Springer, Berlin.

Beije, B., and T. Hultin. 1971. Oxidation and protein binding of aromatic amines by rat liver microsomes. Chem. Biol. Interact. 3:321–336.

Belman, S., and W. Troll. 1972. The inhibition of croton oil-promoted mouse skin tumorigenesis by steroid hormones. Cancer Res. 32:450–454.

Belman, S., and W. Troll. 1974. Phorbol-12-myristate-13-acetate effect on cyclic adenosine 3′, 5′-monophosphate levels in mouse skin and inhibition of phorbol-myristate-acetate-promoted tumorigenesis by theophylline. Cancer Res. 34:3446–3455.

Berenblum, I. 1929. The modifying influence of dichloro-ethyl sulphide on the induction of tumours in mice by tar. J. Pathol. Bacteriol. 32:425–434.

Berenblum, I. 1941. The mechanism of carcinogenesis: A study of the significance of cocarcinogenic action and related phenomena. Cancer Res. 1:807–814.

Berenblum, I. 1954. A speculative review: The probable nature of promoting action and its significance in the understanding of the mechanism of carcinogenesis. Cancer Res. 14:471–477.

Berenblum, I. 1969. A re-evaluation of the concept of cocarcinogenesis. Prog. Exp. Tumor Res. 11:21–30.

Berenblum, I. 1975. Sequential aspects of chemical carcinogenesis: Skin, in Cancer: A Comprehensive Treatise. Vol. 1. F. F. Becker, ed., Plenum Press, New York, pp. 323–344.

Berenblum, I. 1978. Historical perspective, in Mechanisms of Tumor Promotion and Cocarcinogenesis. Vol. 2. T. J. Slaga, A. Sivak, and R. K. Boutwell, eds., Carcinogenesis: A Comprehensive Survey. Raven Press, New York, pp. 1–10.

Berenblum, I., and V. Armuth. 1977. Effect of colchicine injection prior to initiating phase of two-stage skin carcinogenesis in mice. Br. J. Cancer 35:615–620.

Berenblum, I., and N. Haran. 1955. The influence of croton oil and of polyethylene glycol-400 on carcinogenesis in the forestomach of the mouse. Cancer Res. 15:510–516.

Berenblum, I., and P. Shubik. 1947. A new, quantitative approach to the study of the stages of chemical carcinogenesis in the mouse's skin. Br. J. Cancer 1:383–391.

Berenblum, I., and P. Shubik. 1949. An experimental study of the initiating stage of carcinogenesis, and a re-examination of the somatic cell mutation theory of cancer. Br. J. Cancer 3:109–118.

Berenblum, I., and N. Trainin. 1960. Possible two-stage mechanism of experimental leukemogenesis. Science 132:40–41.

Boutwell, R. K., N. H. Colburn, and C. C. Muckerman. 1969. In vivo reactions of β-propiolactone. Ann. NY Acad. Sci. 163:751–764.

Brookes, P., and P. D. Lawley. 1964. Reaction of some mutagenic and carcinogenic compounds with nucleic acids. J. Cell Comp. Physiol. 64(Suppl.1):111–128.

Brookes, P., and F. J. DeSerres. 1976. Report on the workshop on the mutagenicity of chemical carcinogens. Mutat. Res. 38:155–160.

Bullough, W. S. 1965. Mitotic and functional homeostasis: A speculative review. Cancer Res. 25:1683–1727.

Burnet, F. M. 1959. The Clonal Selection Theory of Acquired Immunity. Cambridge University Press, Cambridge.

Cairns, J. 1975. Review article: Mutation selection and the natural history of cancer. Nature 255:197–200.

Carruthers, C., A. Baumler, A. Neilson, and D. Pressman. 1976. Detection of liver-bound metabolites of azocarcinogens by the use of anti-hapten antibodies. Cancer Res. 36:1568–1572.

Cassell, E. E., J. Meites, and C. W. Welsch. 1971. Effects of ergocornine and ergocryptine on growth of 7,12-dimethylbenzanthracene-induced mammary tumors in rats. Cancer Res. 31:1051–1053.

Charles, D. R., and E. M. Luce-Clausen. 1942. The kinetics of papilloma formation in benzpyrene-treated mice. Cancer Res. 2:261–263.

Christov, K. 1975. Thyroid cell proliferation in rats and induction of tumors by x-rays. Cancer Res. 35:1256–1262.

Chu, E. H. Y., J. E. Trosko, and C.-C. Chang. 1977. Mutational approaches to the study of carcinogenesis. J. Toxicol. Environ. Health 2:1317–1334.

Colburn, N. H., S. Lau, and R. Head. 1975. Decrease of epidermal histidase activity by tumor-promoting phorbol esters. Cancer Res. 35:3154–3159.

Coombs, M. M., T. S. Bhatt, and C. W. Vose. 1975. The relationship between metabolism, DNA binding, and carcinogenicity of 15,16-dihydro-11-methylcyclo-penta(a)phenanthren-17-one in the presence of a microsomal enzyme inhibitor. Cancer Res. 35:305–309.

Crabtree, H. G. 1941. Retardation of the rate of tumor induction by hydrolyzing chlor-compounds. Cancer Res. 1:39–43.

Crabtree, H. G. 1947. Anti-carcinogenesis. Br. Med. Bull. 4:345–347.

Dao, T. L., and H. Sunderland. 1959. Mammary carcinogenesis by 3-methylcholanthrene. I. Hormonal aspects in tumor induction and growth. J. Nat. Cancer Inst. 23:567–585.

De Waard, R. H. 1964. Coincidence of mutations as a possible cause of malignancy. Int. J. Radiat. Biol. 8:381–387.

Dingman, C. W., and M. B. Sporn. 1967. The binding of metabolites of aminoazo dyes to rat liver DNA in vivo. Cancer Res. 27:938–944.

Doll, 1977. Strategy for detection of cancer hazards to man. Nature 265:589–596.

Elgjo, K. 1976. Epidermal chalone in experimental skin carcinogenesis, *in* Chalones, J. C. Houck, ed., North-Holland Publishing Co. and American Elsevier Co., Inc., Amsterdam & New York, pp. 229–245.

Falk, H. L. 1971. Anticarcinogenesis—An alternative. Prog. Exp. Tumor Res. 14:105–137.

Farber, E. 1973. Carcinogenesis—Cellular evolution as a unifying thread: Presidential address. Cancer Res. 33:2537–2550.

Fishbein, L., W. G. Flamm, and H. L. Falk. 1970. Chemical Mutagens: Environmental Effects on Biological Systems. Academic Press, New York and London.

Fisher, J. C., and J. H. Hollomon. 1951. A hypothesis for the origin of cancer foci. Cancer 4:916–918.

Friedewald, W. F., and P. Rous. 1944. The initiating and promoting elements in tumor production. An analysis of the effects of tar, benzpyrene, and methylcholanthrene on rabbit skin. J. Exp. Med. 80:101–126.

Gelboin, H. V., M. Klein, and R. R. Bates. 1965. Inhibition of mouse skin tumorigenesis by actinomycin D. Proc. Nat. Acad. Sci. USA 53:1353–1360.

Glinos, A. D., N. L. R. Bucher, and J. C. Aub. 1951. The effect of liver regeneration on tumor formation in rats fed 4-dimethylaminoazobenzene. J. Exp. Med. 93:313–324.

Goshman, L. M., and C. Heidelberger. 1967. Binding of tritium-labeled polycyclic hydrocarbons to DNA of mouse skin. Cancer Res. 27:1678–1688.

Grimm, W., and F. Marks. 1974. Effect of tumor-promoting phorbol esters on the normal and the isoproterenol-elevated level of adenosine $3',5'$-cyclic monophosphate in mouse epidermis *in vivo*. Cancer Res. 34:3128–3134.

Hall, W. H. 1948. The role of initiating and promoting factors in the pathogenesis of tumours of the thyroid. Br. J. Cancer 2:273–280.

Hamilton, J. M., A. Flaks, P. G. Saluja, and S. Maguire. 1975. Hormonally induced renal neoplasia in the male Syrian hamster and the inhibitory effect of 2-bromo-α-ergocryptine methanesulfonate. J. Natl. Cancer Inst. 54:1385–1400.

Haran-Ghera, N., N. Trainin, L. Fiore-Donate, and I. Berenblum. 1962. A possible two-stage mechanism in rhabdomyosarcoma induction in rats. Br. J. Cancer 16:653–664.

Hecker, E. 1968. Cocarcinogenic principles from the seed oil of *Croton tiglium* and from other Euphorbiaceae. Cancer Res. 28:2338–2349.

Heidelberger, C., and M. G. Moldenhauer. 1956. The interaction of carcinogenic hydrocarbons with tissue constituents. IV. A quantitative study of the binding to skin proteins of several C^{14}-labeled hydrocarbons. Cancer Res. 16:442–449.

Helmes, C. T., T. Hillesund, and R. K. Boutwell. 1974. The binding of tritium-labeled phorbol esters to the macromolecular constituents of mouse epidermis. Cancer Res. 34:1360–1365.

Higginson, J. 1968. Present trends in cancer epidemiology, *in* Canadian Cancer Conference, Pergamon of Canada, Ltd., pp. 40–75.

Higginson, J., and C. S. Muir. 1976. The role of epidemiology in elucidating the importance of environmental factors in human cancer. Cancer Detection and Prevention, 1:79–105.

Homburger, F. 1974. Modifiers of carcinogenesis, *in* The Physiopathology of Cancer. Vol. 1. P. Shubik, ed., S. Karger, Basel. pp. 110–154.

Houssay, A., G. M. Higgins, and W. A. Bennett. 1951. The influence exerted by desoxycorticosterone acetate upon the production of adrenal tumors in gonadectomized mice. Cancer Res. 11:297–300.

Iversen, O. H. 1973. Cell proliferation kinetics and carcinogenesis: A review, *in* Proceedings of the Fifth International Symposium on the Biological Characterization of Human Tumours. Excerpta Medica, Amsterdam, pp. 21–29.

Jackson, C. D., and C. C. Irving. 1970. The binding of N-hydroxy-2-acetylaminofluorene to replicating and nonreplicating DNA in rat liver. Chem. Biol. Interact. 2:261–265.

Jacob, F., and J. Monod. 1961. On the regulation of gene activity. Cold Spring Harbor Symp. Quant. Biol. 26:193–211.

Jacobs, M. M., B. Jansson, and A. C. Griffin. 1977. Inhibitory effects of selenium on 1,2-dimethylhydrazine and methylazoxymethanol acetate induction of colon tumors. Cancer Lett. 2:133–138.

Janoff, A., A. Klassen, and W. Troll. 1970. Local vascular changes induced by the cocarcinogen, phorbol myristate acetate. Cancer Res. 30:2568–2571.

Jull, J. W. 1954. The effect of oestrogens and progesterone on the chemical induction of mammary cancer in mice of the IF strain. J. Pathol. Bacteriol. 68:547–559.

Kimura, N. T., T. Kanematsu, and T. Baba. 1976. Polychlorinated biphenyl(s) as a promotor in experimental hepatocarcinogenesis in rats. *Zeitschrift für Krebsforschung* 87:257–266.

Kledzik, G. S., C. J. Brandley, and J. Meites. 1974. Reduction of carcinogen-induced mammary cancer incidence in rats by early treatment with hormones or drugs. Cancer Res. 34:2953–2956.

Knudson, A. G. Jr. 1973. Mutation and human cancer. Adv. Cancer Res. 17:317–352.

Konishi, Y., A. Denda, Y. Miyata, and H. Kawabata. 1976. Enhancement of pancreatic tumorigenesis by 4-hydroxyaminoquinoline 1-oxide by ethionine in rats. Gann 67:91–95.

Krieg, L., I. Kühlmann, and F. Marks. 1974. Effect of tumor-promoting phorbol esters and of acetic acid on mechanisms controlling DNA synthesis and mitosis (chalones) and on the biosynthesis of histidine-rich protein in mouse epidermis. Cancer Res. 34:3135–3146.

Kriek, E. 1971. On the mechanism of action of carcinogenic aromatic amines. II. Binding of N-hydroxy-N-acetyl-4-aminobiphenyl to rat-liver nucleic acids *in vitro*. Chem. Biol. Interact. 3:19–28.

Lappé, M. A. 1971. Evidence for immunological surveillance during skin carcinogenesis. Isr. J. Med. Sci. 7:52–65.

Lasne, C., A. Gentil, and I. Chouroulinkov. 1977. Two-stage carcinogenesis with rat embryo cells in tissue culture. Br. J. Cancer 35:722–729.

Lawley, P. D. 1976. Carcinogenesis by alkylating agents, *in* Chemical Carcinogens. C. E. Searle, ed., American Cancer Society Monograph 173, American Chemical Society, Washington, pp. 83–244.

Lawson, T. A., and A. W. Pound. 1973. The interaction of carbon-14-labelled alkyl carbamates, labelled in the alkyl and carbonyl positions, with DNA *in vivo*. Chem. Biol. Interact. 6:99–105.

Lijinsky, W., H. Garcia, L. Keefer, J. Loo, and A. E. Ross. 1972. Carcinogenesis and alkylation of rat liver nucleic acids by nitrosomethylurea and nitrosoethylurea administered by intraportal injection. Cancer Res. 32:893–897.

Magee, P. N., and E. Farber. 1962. Toxic liver injury and carcinogenesis. Methylation of rat liver nucleic acid by dimethylnitrosamine *in vivo*. Biochem. J. 83:114–124.

Major, I. R. 1970. Correlation of initial changes in the mouse epidermal cell population with two stage carcinogenesis—a quantitative study. Br. J. Cancer 24:149–163.

Matsumoto, M., and H. Terayama. 1970. The fate of N-alkyl groups in the course of binding of metabolites of several N-alkyl amino azo dyes to rat-liver proteins. Chem. Biol. Interact. 2:41–45.

McCann, J., E. Choi, E. Yamasaki, and B. N. Ames. 1975. Detection of carcinogens as mutagens in the *Salmonella*/microsome test: Assay of 300 chemicals. Proc. Nat. Acad. Sci. USA 72:5135–5139.

Meisels, A. 1966. Effect of sex hormones on the carcinogenic action of dimethylbenzanthracene on the uterus of intact and castrated mice. Cancer Res. 26:757–764.

Miller, E. C., and J. A. Miller. 1947. The presence and significance of bound aminoazo dyes in the livers of rats fed p-dimethylaminoazobenzene. Cancer Res. 7:468–480

Miller, J. A. 1970. Carcinogenesis by chemicals: An Overview—G. H. A. Clowes Memorial Lecture. Cancer Res. 30:559–576.

Mondal, S., D. W. Brankow, and C. Heidelberger. 1976. Two-stage chemical oncogenesis in cultures of C3H/10T1/2 cells. Cancer Res. 36:2254–2260.

Morris, H. P. 1952. Nutritional and hormonal interrelationships in the development of experimental cancer. Texas Rep. Biol. Med. 10:1028–1054.

Mottram, J. C. 1944. A sensitizing factor in experimental blastogenesis. J. Pathol. Bacteriol. 56:391–402.

Muller, H. K., and R. C. Sutherland. 1971. Epidermal antigens in cutaneous dysplasia and neoplasia. Nature. 230:384–385.

Narisawa, T., N. E. Magadia, J. H. Weisburger, and E. L. Wynder. 1974. Promoting effect of bile acids on colon carcinogenesis after intrarectal instillation of N-methyl-N'-nitro-N-nitroso-guanidine in rats. J. Nat. Cancer Inst. 53:1093–1097.

Nery, R. 1976. Carcinogenic mechanisms: A critical review and a suggestion that oncogenesis may be adaptive ontogenesis. Chem. Biol. Interact. 12:145–169.

Nettesheim, P., and H. Schreiber. 1975. Advances in experimental lung cancer research, *in Handbuch der allgemeinen Pathologie.* Vol. 6. Springer-Verlag, Berlin, Heidelberg, New York, pp. 603–691.

Nietert, W. C., L. M. Kellicutt, and H. Kubinski. 1974. DNA-protein complexes produced by a carcinogen, β-propiolactone. Cancer Res. 34:859–864.

Nordling, C. O. 1953. A new theory on the cancer-inducing mechanisms. Br. J. Cancer 7:68–72.

O'Brien, T. G. 1976. The induction of ornithine decarboxylase as an early, possibly obligatory, event in mouse skin carcinogenesis. Cancer Res. 36:2644–2653.

Paul, D. 1969. Effects of carcinogenic, noncarcinogenic, and cocarcinogenic agents on the biosynthesis of nucleic acids in mouse skin. Cancer Res. 29:1218–1225.

Peirce, W. E. H. 1961. Tumour-promotion by lime oil in the mouse forestomach. nature 189:497–498.

Pierce, G. B. 1974. Neoplasms, differentiation and mutations. Am. J. Pathol. 77:103–118.

Pitot, H. C., and C. Heidelberger. 1963. Metabolic regulatory circuits and carcinogenesis. Cancer Res. 23:1694–1700.

Pound, A. W., and T. A. Lawson. 1976. Carcinogenesis by carbamic acid esters and their binding to DNA. Cancer Res. 36:1101–1107.

Prehn, R. T. 1971. Immunosurveillance, regeneration and oncogenesis. Prog. Exp. Tumor Res. 14:1–24.

Purchase, I. F. H., E. Lonstaff, J. Ashby, J. A. Styles, D. Anderson, P. A. Lefevre, and F. R. Westwood. 1976. Evaluation of six short term tests for detecting organic chemical carcinogens and recommendations for their use. Nature 264:624–627.

Raick, A. N. 1973. Ultrastructural, histological, and biochemical alterations produced by 12-O-tetradecanoyl-phorbol-13-acetate on mouse epidermis and their relevance to skin tumor promotion. Cancer Res. 33:269–286.

Reddy, B. S., K. Watanabe, J. H. Weisburger, and E. L. Wynder. 1977. Promoting effect of bile acids in colon carcinogenesis in germ-free and conventional F344 rats. Cancer Res. 37:3238–3242.

Rohrschneider, L. R., and R. K. Boutwell. 1973. The early stimulation of phospholipid metabolism by 12-O-tetradecanoyl-phorbol-13-acetate and its specificity for tumor promotion. Cancer Res. 33:1945–1952.

Rosen, V. J., and L. J. Cole. 1962. Accelerated induction of kidney neoplasms in mice after X radiation (690 rad) and unilateral nephrectomy. J. Nat. Cancer Inst. 28:1031–1041.

Rous, P., and J. G. Kidd. 1941. Conditional neoplasms and subthreshold neoplastic states. J. Exp. Med. 73:365–390.

Saffiotti, U., R. Montesano, A. R. Sellakumar, and S. A. Borg. 1967. Experimental cancer of the lung. Inhibition by vitamin A of the induction of tracheobronchial squamous metaplasia and squamous cell tumors. Cancer 20:857–864.

Sarma, D. S. R., S. Rajalakshmi, and E. Farber. 1975. Chemical carcinogenesis: Interactions of carcinogens with nucleic acids. in Cancer: A Comprehensive Treatise. Vol. 1. F. F. Becker, ed., Plenum Press, New York and London. pp. 235–287.

Sarrif, A. M., J. S. Bertram, M. Kamarck, and C. Heidelberger. 1975. The isolation and characterization of polycyclic hydrocarbon-binding proteins from mouse liver and skin cytosols. Cancer Res. 35:816–834.

Selikoff, I. J. 1976. The search for carcinogenic environmental agents: The role of the physician. Cancer Detection and Prevention 1:7–41.

Selikoff, I. J., E. C. Hammond, and J. Churg. 1968. Asbestos exposure, smoking and neoplasia. J. A. M. A. 204:106–112.

Setälä, K. 1960. Progress in carcinogenesis, tumor-enhancing factors. A bioassay of skin tumor formation, in Experimental Tumor Research, Vol. 1. F. Homburger, ed., S. Karger, Basel. pp. 225–278

Shay, H., C. Harris, and M. Gruenstein. 1960. Further studies in prevention of experimentally induced breast cancer in the rat. Some endocrine aspects. Acta Union Internationale contre le Cancer 16(1):225–232.

Sherbet, G. V. 1970. Epigenetic processes and their relevance to the study of neoplasia. Adv. Cancer Res. 13:97–167.

Shubik, P. 1950. Studies on the promoting phase in the stages of carcinogenesis in mice, rats, rabbits and guinea pigs. Cancer Res. 10:13–17.

Slaga, T. J., J. D. Scribner, S. Thompson, and A. Viaje. 1976. Epidermal cell proliferation and promoting ability of phorbol esters. J. Nat. Cancer Inst. 57:1145–1149.

Slaga, T. J., A. Sivak, and R. K. Boutwell, eds. 1978. Mechanisms of Tumor Promotion and Cocarcinogenesis, Vol. 2. Carcinogenesis: A Comprehensive Survey. Raven Press, New York.

Sorof, S., P. P. Cohen, E. C. Miller, and J. A. Miller. 1951. Electrophoretic studies on the soluble proteins from livers of rats fed aminoazo dyes. Cancer Res. 11:383–387.

Sorof, S., B. P. Sani, V. M. Kish, and H. P. Meloche. 1974. The isolation and properties of the principal protein conjugate of a hepatic carcinogen. Biochemistry 13:2612–2620.

Sporn, M. B., R. A. Squire, C. C. Brown, J. M. Smith, M. L. Wenk, and S. Springer. 1977. 13-cis-retinoic acid: Inhibition of bladder carcinogenesis in the rat. Science 195:487–489.

Steinbäck, F., H. Garcia, and P. Shubik. 1974. Present status of the concept of promoting action and cocarcinogenesis in skin, in The Physiopathology of Cancer, Vol. 1. P. Shubik, ed., S. Karger, Basel. pp. 155–225.

Tannenbaum, A., and H. Silverstone. 1953. Nutrition in relation to cancer. Adv. Cancer Res. 1:451–501.

Trosko, J. E., and E. H. Y. Chu. 1975. The role of DNA repair and somatic mutation in carcinogenesis. Adv. Cancer Res. 21:391–425.

Van Duuren, B. L. 1969. Tumor-promoting agents in two-stage carcinogenesis. Prog. Exp. Tumor Res. 11:31–68.

Van Duuren, B. L. 1976. Tumor-promoting and co-carcinogenic agents in chemical carcinogenesis, in Chemical Carcinogens. C. E. Searle, ed., American Cancer Society Monograph 173, American Chemical Society, Washington, pp. 24–51.

Van Duuren, B. L., and S. Melchionne. 1969. Inhibition of tumorigenesis. Prog. Exp. Tumor Res. 12:55–94.

Verma, A. K., M. Froscio, and A. W. Murray. 1976. Croton-oil and benzo(a)pyrene-induced changes in cyclic adenosine 3′:5′-monophosphate and cyclic guanosine 3′:5′-monophosphate phosphodiesterase activities in mouse epidermis. Cancer Res. 36:81–87.

Warwick, G. P. 1969. The covalent binding of metabolites of 4-dimethylaminoazobenzene to liver nucleic acids in vitro, in Physico-Chemical Mechanisms of Carcinogenesis, Vol. 1. E. D. Bergmann and B. Pullman, eds., Israel Academy of Sciences and Humanities, Jerusalem. pp. 218–225.

Wattenberg, L. W. 1977. Inhibition of carcinogenic effects of polycyclic hydrocarbons by benzyl isothiocyanate and related compounds. J. Nat. Cancer Inst. 58:395–398.

Wattenberg, L. W. 1978. Guest editorial: Inhibition of chemical carcinogenesis. J. Natl. Cancer Inst. 60:11–18.

Weinstein, I. B., A. M. Jeffrey, K. W. Jennette, S. H. Blobstein, R. G. Harvey, C. Harris, H. Autrup, H. Kasai, and K. Nakanishi. 1976. Benzo(a)pyrene diol epoxides as intermediates in nucleic acid binding in vitro and in vivo. Science 193:592–595.

Wheeler, G. P. 1962. Studies related to the mechanisms of action of cytotoxic alkylating agents. A review. Cancer Res. 22:651–688.

World Health Organization Technical Report Series No. 276. 1964. Prevention of Cancer. World Health Organization, Geneva.

Yang, S. K., H. V. Gelboin, B. F. Trump, H. Autrup, and C. C. Harris. 1977. Metabolic activation of benzo(a)pyrene and binding to DNA in cultured human bronchus. Cancer Res. 37:1210–1215.

Yuspa, S. H., T. Ben, E. Patterson, D. Michael, K. Elgjo, and H. Hennings. 1976. Stimulated DNA synthesis in mouse epidermal cell cultures treated with 12-0-tetradecanoyl-phorbol-13-acetate. Cancer Res. 36:4062–4068.

Carcinogens: Identification and Mechanisms of Action, edited by A. Clark Griffin and Charles R. Shaw. Raven Press, New York © 1979.

The Ernst W. Bertner Memorial Award Lecture

Identification of Environmental Carcinogens: Animal Test Models

Philippe Shubik

Eppley Institute for Research in Cancer, University of Nebraska Medical Center, Omaha, Nebraska 68105

Animal test methods used in chemical carcinogenesis and the interpretation of these tests are under closer scrutiny than ever before, except perhaps for the time of the first induction of skin cancer in the rabbit (Yamagiwa and Itchikawa 1918). It is not surprising that there was a great deal of concern and skepticism at that time about the nature of the lesions, since cancer in an animal had not previously been induced chemically.

Studies in chemical carcinogenesis before 1940 can be divided into essentially two groups. The larger of the two consisted of experimental studies concerned with elucidating mechanisms of carcinogenesis; the other group of studies concerned the attempted induction of cancer in animals with materials that, as a result of epidemiological observations, were suspected of causing cancer in humans. The latter experiments provided the primary basis for recent developments in the field of environmental cancer.

There was a division of opinion during the 1930's when the major effort in research was confined to a comparison of polycyclic aromatic hydrocarbons (PAH). Parallel studies were carried out in the United Kingdom and the United States. In the United Kingdom, mouse skin painting was used as the primary test method, and in the more practical, labor-saving United States, subcutaneous injection was used. Both used random mice for the studies. If one looks back, one can see no major reason for preferring one method over the other. Both benign and malignant tumors were induced, and the significance of the induction of the benign papilloma was never really elucidated.

There were many polycyclic hydrocarbon studies in which only a few papillomas were induced. They obviously meant something, but the results were ignored. It is now obvious that papillomas in some of those early studies were caused by impurities (Donahue *et al.* 1978). Misleading results occurred with such studies, which can perhaps be explained by physical factors.

These partially understood biological data were used as a basis for chemical theories. Numerous efforts were made (and some continue) to arrange PAH

37

in the "order of their potency" and to correlate this range of activity with variations in chemical structure that might be associated with reactivity. The studies of the Pullmans (1955) were among the best of these, but all the studies had two or more inherent defects that were conveniently ignored. First, "potency" varied with the route of administration used (relative potencies, of course, differ among species); second, the inaccuracy of these studies and the number of unknown variables made quantitative comparisons (except of a gross kind) quite illusory.

The simplistic cause and effect relationship that was assumed at that time had an impact on future thinking. One treated an animal and caused a tumor to appear; ergo, the substance was a carcinogen. However, even in the early days of cancer research it was known that when one painted the skin of a mouse with coal tar, pulmonary adenomas were induced in addition to the local tumors (Murphy and Sturm 1925). It became clear that in many cases both a systemic and a local component to carcinogenesis existed. With perhaps some minor exceptions, it is difficult to be sure that a compound has only a local or only a systemic effect rather than both. The main problem is that varying the species and other parameters of carcinogenesis experiments often introduces new positive findings. A negative is never as convincing as a positive. However it would seem reasonable to believe that isoniazid producing only lung adenomas, for example, has only a systemic "enhancing" effect, whereas carbon tetrachloride producing only hepatomas has only a local effect—superficially different but, nonetheless, perhaps the same mechanisms. Is this "enhancing effect" the same, for example, as the induction of a skin cancer in treated animals when no skin cancer appears in the controls? Our good friend Dr. Michael Shimkin (Shimkin and Stoner 1975, Shimkin et al. 1966) has maintained for some years that the enhancement of lung adenomas in a high-tumor incidence strain of mice (Strain A) can be done in a six-month experiment and has proposed this method for the rapid screening of carcinogenic chemicals. Unfortunately, the test has not been widely used. There is a high correlation between those compounds inducing lung adenomas and those inducing tumors in other locations. Obviously one must know the mechanism in order to understand the matter. It is unlikely that no major difference exists between the mechanisms involved in lung adenoma induction and the "direct" induction of a tumor not otherwise present. No precise counterpart of the mouse lung adenoma exists in humans, but it certainly is a neoplasm. It is thought by some to be always malignant, and it is certainly accepted as a tumor that eventuates in malignancy. The cause of the lung adenoma in the untreated mouse is unknown. Many have thought it probably viral, but this theory has not been substantiated, in spite of many efforts to do so. It is the theory most appealing to me.

Even if the lung adenoma proved to be viral in origin, our problem would not be completely solved. I draw your attention to some data generated in our laboratory. In one study (Toth and Shubik 1967) the effects of two well-known carcinogenic chemicals, benzo[a]pyrene (B[a]P) and dimethylnitrosamine

(DMN), were studied in the AKR mouse (a strain with an almost 100% incidence of lymphoma associated with an established virus). The carcinogens had no apparent effect on the viral lymphoma incidence. There were early lymphomas induced by B(a)P. However these were stem lymphomas similar to those induced by B(a)P in many other mouse strains and histologically distinguishable from the lymphocytic lymphomas developing in the AKR mice. These may be similar in origin to the AKR lymphomas and histologically different only as a result of their earlier development, but this prospect must be investigated. In any event, B(a)P induced the same tumors (lung adenomas and lymphomas of the stem cell variety) as in experiments using other strains of mice. In the AKR mice, leukemias occurred as well. The DMN did nothing unusual. Hepatomas occurred, but no effect on lymphoma incidence was observed. Apparently the chemical and the virus can act quite independently of one another in the same mouse; interestingly enough, lung tumors occurred in the test animals although there were none in the control.

Without question, different responses occur in animal model systems that clearly imply different mechanisms. However, our present state of knowledge does not permit more precise statements about these differences.

The experimentalist moved along rapidly during the 1930's, and after the discovery of the PAH, a variety of systemically acting carcinogens was found. Among them were the azo dyes, giving rise to hepatomas in rats and mice following ingestion, and subsequently acetylaminofluorene, causing a variety of cancers in many organs in various species, with the notable exception of the refractory guinea pig. This latter observation was exploited in the brilliant studies of Miller *et al.* (1964) who demonstrated that N-hydroxylation was essential to the development of the proximate carcinogen and that the necessary enzyme was not present in the guinea pig. It would be ideal if the rules governing extrapolation from one species to another could always be so well understood; however, there are no other examples in which extrapolation between species can be understood properly at the biochemical level.

Since biochemistry in the 1930's and 1940's was essentially the science of investigating the changes of chemical-biological significance in the rat liver, the induction of hepatomas in rats became, for a while, the center point of cancer research. The pathology of these lesions was accepted without much questioning. Occasionally a pathologist might be heard to moan quietly in a corner that much biochemistry was being undertaken using liver lesions not properly diagnosed by a pathologist and that perhaps a certain number of "tumors" on which complex biochemical studies had been made were merely regenerative nodules. When hepatomas were first induced a few decades ago, their pathological characteristics did not arouse much interest.

Another induced lesion of interest to the experimentalist was the bladder tumor. The reason for this was the fact that bladder tumors occurred in humans occupationally exposed to aromatic amines. Hueper *et al.* (1938) induced bladder tumors, similar to those seen in the dye workers, by feeding 2-naphthylamine to dogs. A rigid approach ensued suggesting that to investigate potential bladder carcinogens it was essential to use dogs in these experiments, and an experiment lasting seven years was barely adequate. My colleagues (Tomatis *et al.* 1961) demonstrated that *o*-aminoazotoluene caused a high incidence of bladder tumors in the Syrian hamster. As a result of that study, 2-naphthylamine was tested in the hamster, and bladder tumors were induced (Sellakumar *et al.* 1969). Studies were mounted by several groups to determine if a metabolite of these compounds, which was a "proximate carcinogen," could be isolated from the urine. Among the techniques introduced was implantation of pelleted test material into the urinary bladder. This technique resulted in the induction of many tumors, but unfortunately the vehicles used for the pellet (cholesterol, paraffin wax, etc.) gave rise to large numbers of age-dependent tumors in the control series (Bonser *et al.* 1953) and made the determination of activity difficult. In addition, although the technique was fundamentally introduced to determine the carcinogenicity of metabolites, it was subsequently used to test compounds that would be administered orally to humans, and a variety of problems resulted.

At about the time the bladder implantation technique was introduced, some studies were undertaken on subcutaneous carcinogenesis (Oppenheimer *et al.* 1948). These investigators demonstrated that certain materials (plastics) could result in the induction of sarcomas at the site of an implant by virtue of their physical rather than chemical characteristics. Later, these observations were expanded to demonstrate similar behavior by metals and various other materials (Oppenheimer *et al.* 1956). Once again, the mechanism is unknown, although elegant hypotheses have been adduced to explain the findings. Clearly, observations of this kind cast doubt on some of the previous work using subcutaneous injection techniques.

The study of genetic factors overlapped much of the work. In particular, a variety of inbred mouse strains became available with specific tumor incidences; the classic studies of L. C. Strong (1940, 1944, 1945) investigated the interrelationship between genetic susceptibility and localization of tumors. The mechanisms were not explained and still remain to be elucidated. The only exceptions are those tumors resulting from vertically transmitted oncogenic viruses.

I have little time or need to expound on two-stage mechanisms but will point out that skin carcinogenesis can be clearly shown to involve an initiation and promotion sequence (Berenblum and Shubik 1949, Shubik 1950). This demonstration leads to various possible approaches to studies of mechanisms in the experimental setting and to the interpretation of possible causes of human cancers. Efforts have been made to extend this concept to other animal models, including the liver and the bladder, but none of the model systems are as clear cut as the skin. They do, however, lend credence to the view that the two-stage mechanism is likely to be a general one.

The second stage of the animal test that I have separated arbitrarily concerns the use of these systems in toxicology. Until around 1940, few, if any, routine toxicological tests were designed specifically to test for carcinogenicity. Major credit must be given to the United States Department of Agriculture and the United States Food and Drug Administration (FDA) for introducing such procedures. The landmark study was that of Wilson *et al.* (1941) in which the pesticide 2-acetylaminofluorene (AAF) was found to be a potent carcinogen. Consequently, it was not introduced for general use. Investigators at the FDA subsequently studied many compounds in the long-term test, i.e., the "two-year rat study" (Lehman *et al.* 1955) that became standard with the toxicologist in the post-World War II era. There was some debate about the utility of this expensive procedure, which by current standards is considered far from an adequate test for carcinogenicity. The leading British toxicologist, the late John Barnes, felt that it should not be necessary to test compounds for this long period and that anything toxic could be detected in short-term tests (Barnes and Denz 1954)—this is, of course, counter to the philosophy of the cancer researcher who believes that many carcinogens can only be detected in long-term tests and that, indeed, many are notable for their lack of general toxicity.

Since 1955, various reviews and committee reports have addressed themselves to the requirements for testing potentially carcinogenic compounds, and the nature of these tests is a subject of continuing debate. I shall not belabor the whole question of what should and should not be tested and how selection of test materials might be made. I shall merely say that I believe, with many others, that all proposed food additives (many old ones, too) and many naturally occurring contaminants and components should be tested for chronic effects, as should drugs, household products, and environmental contaminants.

I believe that a primary requirement before embarking on a program in this area is to ascertain the practicability of any recommendations. Who is available with adequate training to do the tests properly and thoroughly? Can these procedures be mechanized? I am sure that they cannot be mechanized, and we should hesitate to impose programs upon ourselves that cannot be done properly.

The use of the animal test for toxicological purposes has resulted in the acquisition of a great deal of data that is extremely difficult to interpret in practical terms. Almost all the problems that have arisen could easily have been predicted from a contemplation of the data accrued when these procedures were used for research. Some of the problems have, of course, been laid to rest already, and I am sure that if we are just patient, the remaining absurdities will be eliminated.

Many food dyes were originally tested by the subcutaneous route. It became obvious following the work of the Oppenheimers (Oppenheimer *et al.* 1948, 1956) that subcutaneous tests were not necessarily indicative of toxicity for orally administered materials. It is now generally accepted that the subcutaneous route can provide misleading results, and it is not often used except to test materials administered subcutaneously to humans. One should not ignore results obtained in this way, but they should not be used in isolation. Additional information must be taken into account. Few researchers now accept the finding of carcinogenicity following implantation of a material in the urinary bladder as final proof that that material administered orally might be carcinogenic.

There are, therefore, some clear examples of responses in experimental carcinogenesis that cannot be extrapolated to man by the toxicologist. The question before us, then, is how appropriate and adequate are the other procedures in common use and what problems are outstanding.

The problems that are commonly discussed fall into two categories. First, there are matters that concern the design of the experiments; second, there is the matter of the interpretation of certain results.

In the design of experiments for carcinogenesis there are a series of obvious problems that I shall touch on, but I will clearly be unable to cover the whole area and will present some personal views.

It is universally agreed that toxicological studies should approximate conditions of practical use as closely as possible with the proviso that a safety margin be employed involving exaggerated dosage as a primary protection. How high this dose should be is a matter of considerable concern. Should the dose be the "maximal tolerated dose" (MTD), and how does one define the MTD? I am sure that the dose should be high; I am equally sure that an arbitrary MTD makes no sense at all. In some cases this might be 20% of an animal's diet and would introduce a totally unrealistic physiological background to an experiment. Perhaps this could be solved by redefining MTD, and efforts to do this are underway.

Conditions of use primarily involve the route of administration, and it would seem only reasonable to use the same route of administration in the experimental situation as occurs in the actual situation. I believe this should rarely, if ever, be departed from. I believe that one should use at least two species and perhaps more if possible. I believe that one should always attempt to have at least three dose levels in these studies, since the finding of a dose response is quite the most impressive of all end points.

Should a two-generation study be routine (if indeed any of this can be made routine)? Work on transplacental carcinogenesis is of major importance in the elucidation of mechanisms and certainly indicates that many childhood cancers are most likely to have been due to exposure in utero. The occurrence of Wilm's tumors (Miller 1968) and neoplasms of the central nervous system (Miller *et al.* 1968) in such studies cannot be interpreted otherwise.

The use of the transplacental model system by the toxicologist, the use of the newborn mouse, and the study of factors transmitted in milk must be considered too. We are, in my view, far from a situation in which we can recommend a single model system, such as the F_0-F_1 study about to be used on a wide scale by the FDA. Few materials have been studied this way, and I believe— old-fashioned though it might be—that it might be a good idea to validate and investigate all new methods before they become toxicological "requirements." Indeed, an excellent example of what not to do, which could likely have been surmised from a contemplation of mechanisms, was attempting to use *as a new rapid test* the discovery by Pietra *et al.* (1959) that the newborn mouse appeared particularly sensitive to some carcinogens. It was apparent to us at once that compounds such as AAF, requiring metabolism to proximate carcinogens, would not be detected and that, anyhow, the newborn is probably not more sensitive and that, as with transplacental carcinogenesis, different types of tumors are induced. Transplacental systems can give rise to different tumors, but so far, all compounds found carcinogenic in this way are also carcinogenic in the adult (Rice 1973).

The most distressing of all aspects of these procedures, to me, concerns the use of commercial diets for experiments of this sort. These diets, with their various contaminants, introduce such obvious complications that common sense alone points to the confusion that can be caused. In fact, many studies using this crude method may eventually have to be scrapped.

The most controversial of current problems include:

1) The relevance of hepatomas
2) The induction of bladder tumors in rodents and calculus formation
3) Problems of hormonal carcinogenesis
4) The possible difference between induction and enhancement
5) Quantitative differences between carcinogens
6) The importance of benign neoplasms.

A great deal has been written and said about the significance of hepatomas, particularly in the mouse and particularly in studies involving chlorinated hydrocarbons. I do not wish to take a categorical stand on either side of this controversy, and I believe that considerable additional work is required to clarify the situation. There can be no question that the induction of hepatomas in the mouse by DDT with no corresponding tumors observed in adequate experiments in the rat and the hamster needs explanation (IARC 1974). The first explanation that comes to mind is that metabolism to the proximate carcinogen may be different. We have found differences between the hamster and the mouse, but this does not solve the problem. The fungicide hexachlorobenzene is, conversely, carcinogenic in the hamster (Cabral *et al.* 1977) but not in rat liver.

There are other examples of compounds carcinogenic to the liver in a limited manner, including carbon tetrachloride, chloroform (also carcinogenic to the kidney), other pesticides, griseofulvin (also carcinogenic to the thyroid), and phenobarbital (IARC 1972, 1974, 1976, 1977). None of these compounds appears to enhance tumor incidence in other organs in test animals in the same way as does, for example, acetylaminofluorene. Their action seems local and is preceded by pathological changes, although I always hesitate to use categorical, negative statements such as *no* systemic effect will ever by found. Whatever else, it is clear that there is great difference between aflatoxin and these compounds or even between dimethylnitrosamine (DMN) and these agents. Many people would feel extremely worried about DMN added in low levels to the diet, but as much as a ppm of DDT would not cause worry. I am among those. It is possible that some of the recent studies (Peraino *et al.* 1971, Pitot 1977) on the possible role of phenobarbital as a promoting agent may explain some of these discrepancies. Unquestionably the most inconsistent of many inconsistent attitudes concerns the hepatomas induced by synthetic estrogens of the types used in oral contraceptive preparations. Several of these compounds induced hepatomas in rodents, and I believe that there is unequivocal evidence that oral contraceptives are responsible for a certain number of hepatomas in young women (Mahboubi and Shubik 1976). It is a major deficiency in chronic toxicity testing that compounds (including oral contraceptives) that are known to interfere with liver function and could, therefore, easily increase susceptibility to toxic substances are not evaluated. We must face facts and not merely classify all these agents together to simplify classification.

The induction of bladder tumors represents one of those paradoxical situations that seems to recur. In the 1930's, when efforts were underway to elucidate occupational bladder carcinogenesis, it was a major achievement to induce cancers of the bladder. This year it would seem almost impossible NOT to induce bladder tumors. One of the great "causes" of the moment is the potential carinogenicity of cyclamate and saccharin. In the case of saccharin a series of bladder tumors have been induced in two-generation studies in rats in which 5% or more saccharin was added to the diet (unpublished data from the FDA, Canadian Health Protection Board, and Wisconsin Alumni Research Foundation). These studies require explanation. This result may be due to the presence of an impurity; it may be due to the presence in the urine of microcrystals that scour the bladder. More recently, several other substances have been found to induce bladder tumors in an unexpected manner; the sweetener xylitol causes calculi and bladder tumors in mice at 10% in the diet (unpublished data from the Huntingdon Research Centre); an important industrial chemical, terephthalic acid, does the same (unpublished data from the U.S. Department of Agriculture); there are more. Clearly, the mechanisms of action need to be studied, and in each instance a reasoned explanation determined and recommended action taken.

The occurrence of bladder tumors in rodents in response to calculus formation is an interesting problem that should have received more attention. Much work is now planned in the area; are the calculi primary or secondary factors? There have been suggestions from studies begun by Hicks (Hicks *et al.* 1975) that the two-stage mechanism may apply in the case of the bladder, but more studies are needed before this can be substantiated.

There are numerous examples of animal studies in which induced tumors have, to some extent, a hormonal origin. The tumors of the thyroid that appear in various carcinogenesis studies would seem usually to be related to initial hormonal stimulation (Doniach 1958). It is possible that at least some of the hormone-associated tumors result from a two-stage mechanism, but this has not been demonstrated. It is clear that a tumor induction situation that requires long, continued stimulation by relatively high levels of a chemical is probably different from situations in which a single dose at low levels can have a demonstrable effect.

It would seem unequivocal that there must be a fundamental difference in mechanism in experiments in which the only manifestation is an early appearance of tumors occurring in equal or almost equal incidence in experimental and control animals. If one observes some examples of carcinogenesis that may have practical importance, there are clear instances in which common sense has prevailed. The immensely valuable drug isoniazid enhanced lung adenoma induction in mice but did not induce or enhance tumors in rats or hamsters (Peacock and Peacock 1966). I draw your attention briefly to another study in which we investigated the effects of isoniazid in the C3H mouse (Toth and Shubik 1966); while isoniazid induced a small number of lung adenomas even in this strain, the primary effect of the compound was to almost abolish the "spontaneous" mammary cancers. This study has not, as far as I am aware, been followed up epidemiologically. Isoniazid is still used in the therapy of tuberculosis; I believe that if isoniazid were to be discovered tomorrow, rather than 30 years ago, it would not see the light of day.

The matter of quantitative differences among chemical carcinogens has been of interest to many people during the past several years. Using any data it is obvious that carcinogens represent a range of potency of at least 10^7. Efforts have been made to arrange a series of carcinogens in order of potency and compare their potency under various conditions. Recent efforts in this direction by Ames and various collaborators (Ames *et al.* 1972a,b, McCann *et al.* 1975) range the potency of carcinogenic chemicals tested in animal systems for comparison with their potency in a bacterial mutagenesis assay system. They have recognized the fact that one must have a set of animal experiments using comparable routes of administration. Obviously one must do something like this, but at the same time the limitations of the exercise—again similar to the problems that confronted the Pullmans (Pullman and Pullman 1955)—must be recognized.

The in-depth study of benign neoplasms in carcinogenesis studies has been overlooked by most investigators. Clearly the sequence of events in the skin from hyperplasia through a variety of benign tumors to malignancy must be understood in order to understand the basic nature of neoplasia. I have studied the problem myself for many years and have published some conclusions (Shubik 1977). The fine studies of Becker (1973) have concentrated on the same problem in the liver tumor system.

Insofar as benign lesions are concerned, a great deal has been said recently by various groups interested in their toxicological interpretation. The current consensus is that the occurrence of benign tumors in an experiment only cannot be taken as demonstration of carcinogenicity; such a finding should indicate that additional studies are necessary.

I have attempted to outline some of the features of animal tests to determine carcinogenicity of chemicals, both from the standpoint of the research worker and from the standpoint of the toxicologist. It must be obvious that these methods leave a great deal to be desired, and perhaps our current striving for perfection will result in basic discoveries. For the moment, such tests can, I believe, help us avoid the introduction of potent carcinogens into our environment. The tests can also be grossly over-interpreted, as I believe has been done in recent years. It would be a shame to "throw the baby out with the bath water," but I fear that continued emotional pressure about carcinogens may soon result in a reaction that may have this result. It is most important that good scientists continue to investigate these systems as projects in research side by side with the toxicological studies. I do not believe that the stage has come in which studies can be considered routine.

REFERENCES

Ames, B. N., E. G. Gurney, J. A. Miller, and H. Bartsch. 1972a. Carcinogens as frameshift mutagens: Metabolites and derivatives of acetylaminofluorene and other aromatic amine carcinogens. Proc. Natl. Acad. Sci. USA 69:3128–3132.

Barnes, J. M., and F. A. Denz. 1954. Experimental methods used in determining chronic toxicity. A critical review. Pharmacol. Rev. 6:191–242.

Ames, B. N., P. Sims, and P. L. Grover. 1972b. Epoxides of carcinogenic polycyclic hydrocarbons are frameshift mutagens. Science 176:47–49.

Becker, F. F. 1973. Hepatoma—nature's model tumor. A review. Am. J. Pathol. 74:179–200.

Berenblum, I., and P. Shubik. 1949. An experimental study of the initiating state of carcinogenesis, and a re-examination of the somatic cell theory of cancer. Br. J. Cancer 3:109–118.

Bonser, G. M., D. B. Clayson, J. W. Jull, and L. N. Pyrah. 1953. The induction of tumours of the bladder epithelium in rats by the implantation of paraffin wax pellets. Br. J. Cancer 7:456–459.

Cabral, J. R. P., P. Shubik, T. Mollner, and F. Raitano. 1977. Carcinogenic activity of hexachlorobenzene in hamsters. Nature 269:510–511.

Donahue, E. V., J. McCann, and B. N. Ames. 1978. Detection of mutagenic impurities in carcinogens and noncarcinogens by high-pressure liquid chromatography and the Salmonella/microsome test. Cancer Res. 38:431–438.

Doniach, I. 1958. Experimental induction of tumours of the thyroid by radiation. Br. Med. Bull. 14:181–183.

Hicks, R. M., J. St. J. Wakefield, and J. Chowanicek. 1975. Evaluation of a new model to detect bladder carcinogens or co-carcinogens: Results with saccharin, cyclamate and cyclophosphamide. Chem.-Biol. Interact. 11:225–233.

Hueper, W. C., F. H. Wiley, H. D. Wolfe, K. E. Ranta, M. F. Leming, and F. R. Blood. 1938. Experimental production of bladder tumors in dogs by administration of β-naphthylamine. Journal of Industrial Hygiene and Toxicology 20:46–84.

IARC. 1972. Chlorinated hydrocarbons, in IARC Monographs on the Evaluation of Carcinogenic Risk of Chemicals to Man. Vol. 1. International Agency for Research on Cancer, Lyon, pp. 53–65.

IARC. 1974. DDT and associated substances, in IARC Monographs on the Evaluation of Carcinogenic Risk of Chemicals to Man. Vol. 5. International Agency for Research on Cancer, Lyon, pp. 83–124.

IARC. 1976. Griseofulvin, in IARC Monographs on the Evaluation of Carcinogenic Risk of Chemicals to Man. Vol. 10. International Agency for Research on Cancer, Lyon, pp. 153–158.

IARC. 1977. Phenobarbital and phenobarbital sodium, in IARC Monographs on the Evaluation of Carcinogenic Risk of Chemicals to Man. Vol. 13. International Agency for Research on Cancer, Lyon, pp. 157–173.

Lehman, A. J., W. I. Patterson, B. Davidow, E. C. Hagan, G. Woodard, E. P. Laug, J. P. Frawley, O. G. Fitzhugh, A. R. Bourke, J. H. Draize, A. A. Nelson, and B. J. Vos. 1955. Procedures for the appraisal of the toxicity of chemicals in foods, drugs and cosmetics. Food Drug Cosmetic Law Journal 10:679–748.

Mahboubi, E., and P. Shubik. 1976. Benign liver cell adenomas in women using oral contraceptives. Cancer Letters 1:331–338.

McCann, J., E. Choi, E. Yamasaki, and B. N. Ames. 1975. Detection of carcinogens as mutagens in the *Salmonella*/microsome test: Assay of 300 chemicals. Proc. Natl. Acad. Sci. USA 72:5135–5139.

Miller, E. C., J. A. Miller, and M. Enomoto. 1964. The comparative carcinogenicities of 2-acetyla-minofluorene and its *N*-hydroxy metabolite in mice, hamsters, and guinea pigs. Cancer Res. 24: 2018–2026.

Miller, R. W. 1968. Relation between cancer and congenital defects: An epidemiologic evaluation. J. Natl. Cancer Inst. 40:1079–1085.

Miller, R. W., J. F. Fraumeni, Jr., and J. A. Hill. 1968. Neuroblastoma: Epidemiologic approach to its origin. Am. J. Dis. Child. 115:253–261.

Murphy, J. B., and E. Sturm. 1925. Primary lung tumors in mice following the cutaneous application of coal tar. J. Exp. Med. 42:693.

Oppenheimer, B. S., E. T. Oppenheimer, and A. P. Stout. 1948. Sarcomas induced in rats by implanting cellophane. Proc. Soc. Exp. Med. 67:33–34.

Oppenheimer, B. S., E. T. Oppenheimer, I. Danishefsky, and A. P. Stout. 1956. Carcinogenic effect of metals in rodents. Cancer Res. 16:439–441.

Peacock, A., and P. R. Peacock. 1966. The results of prolonged administration of isoniazid to mice, rats and hamsters. Br. J. Cancer 20:307–325.

Peraino, C., M. R. J. Fry, and E. Staffeldt. 1971. Reduction and enhancement by phenobarbital of hepatogenesis induced in the rat by 2-acetylaminofluorene. Cancer Res. 31:1506–1512.

Pietra, G., K. Spencer, and P. Shubik. 1959. The response of newborn mice to a chemical carcinogen. Nature 183:1689.

Pitot, H. C. 1977. The natural history of neoplasia: Newer insights into an old problem. Am. J. Pathol. 89:401–412.

Pullman, A., and B. Pullman. 1955. Electronic structure and carcinogenic activity of aromatic molecules, *in* Advances in Cancer Research, Vol. III. J. P. Greenstein, and A. Haddow, eds., Academic Press, New York, pp. 117–169.

Rice, J. M. 1973. The biological behavior of transplacentally induced tumours in mice, *in* Transplacental Carcinogenesis (IARC Scientific Publications No. 4), International Agency for Research on Cancer, Lyon, pp. 71–83.

Sellakumar, A. R., R. Montesano, and U. Saffiotti. 1969. Aromatic amines carcinogenicity in hamster. Proc. Am. Assoc. Cancer Res. 10:78.

Shimkin, M. B., J. H. Weisburger, E. K. Weisburger, N. Gubareff, and V. Suntzeff. 1966. Bioassay of 29 alkylating chemicals by the pulmonary-tumor response in strain A mice. J. Natl. Cancer Inst. 36:915–935.

Shimkin, M. B., and G. D. Stoner. 1975. Lung tumors in mice: Application to carcinogenesis bioassay. Adv. Cancer Res. 21:1–58.

Shubik, P. 1950. Studies on the promoting phase in the stages of carcinogenesis in mice, rats, rabbits and guinea pigs. Cancer Res. 10:13–17.

Shubik, P. 1977. The implications of multiple tumor induction in rodent skin for the biologic nature of neoplasia. Cancer 40:1821–1824.

Strong, L. C. 1940. A genetic analysis of the induction of tumors by methylcholanthrene, with a note in the origin of the NH strain of mice. Am. J. Cancer 39:347–349.

Strong, L. C. 1944. Genetic nature of the constitutional states of cancer susceptibility and resistance in mice and men. Yale J. Biol. Med. 17:289–299.

Strong, L. C. 1945. Genetic analysis of the induction of tumors by methylcholanthrene. IX. Induced and spontaneous adenocarcinomas of the stomach in mice. J. Natl. Cancer Inst. 5:339–362.

Tomatis, L., G. Della Porta, and P. Shubik. 1961. Urinary bladder and liver cell tumors induced in hamsters with *o*-aminoazotoluene. Cancer Res. 21:1513–1517.

Toth, B., and P. Shubik. 1966. Mammary tumor inhibition and lung adenoma induction by isonicotinic acid hydrazide. Science 152:1376–1377.

Toth, B., and P. Shubik. 1967. Carcinogenesis in AKR mice injected at birth with benzo(a)pyrene and dimethylnitrosamine. Cancer Res. 27:43–51.

Wilson, R. H., F. DeEds, and A. J. Cox, Jr. 1941. The toxicity and carcinogenic activity of 2-acetaminofluorene. Cancer Res. 1:595–608.

Yamagiwa, K., and K. Itchikawa. 1918. Experimental study of the pathogenesis of carcinoma. J. Cancer Res. 3:1–21.

Identification of Environmental Carcinogens

Carcinogens: Identification and Mechanisms of Action, edited by A. Clark Griffin and Charles R. Shaw. Raven Press, New York © 1979.

Epidemiological Studies of Cancer

Joseph F. Fraumeni, Jr.

Environmental Epidemiology Branch, National Cancer Institute, Bethesda, Maryland 20014

Over the years the epidemiological approach has contributed substantially to our knowledge of the causes of cancer in man. The pace of this research has recently quickened, particularly in efforts to identify environmental factors, which are generally held responsible for a large proportion of cancers in the population. Less obvious are genetic factors, although these may be more difficult to detect and not less important. This paper reviews some recent developments in cancer epidemiology, including clues generated by a geographic analysis of cancer in the United States.

DEMOGRAPHIC LEADS

International Patterns

It has been reported that up to 90% of all cancer is related to environmental influences (Higginson 1976). These estimates are based primarily on calculations derived from the international variation in cancer incidence, in which rates for the countries at lowest risk are subtracted from the rates prevailing in the United States (Higginson and Muir 1973). The resulting difference is attributed to environmental causes, and the lowest risk is assumed to represent the base line level for tumors that develop "spontaneously" and therefore cannot be prevented. Around the world the reported age-adjusted incidence rates for total cancer vary by a factor of about three, while the range of rates for certain anatomic sites (i.e., the esophagus and liver) is greater than 100-fold (Muir 1975). Even the risks for the common tumors in western countries differ by factors of about 8 to 40. Some of this variation is likely to have a genetic basis, but the major contribution of environmental factors is illustrated by the statistics involving migrant populations, such as the Japanese who have moved to Hawaii and California (Haenszel and Kurihara 1968). In general, as migrant groups have adopted customs of the new land, their risk of various cancers has shifted away from the rate prevailing in the country of origin to approximate that of the host country.

Time Trends

Variation in cancer risk over time may reflect the activity of environmental factors, although some fluctuations can be anticipated by changing medical practices and reporting procedures. In examining trends over several decades, one depends on mortality data that have shown, most notably, an increase in lung cancer and a decrease in stomach cancer in the U.S. (Devesa and Silverman 1978).

Over the short term, variations in risk can be gauged with greater sensitivity by incidence data from cancer registries or surveys (Devesa and Silverman 1978). Table 1 shows the percent change in cancer incidence among U.S. whites from the Second National Cancer Survey conducted in 1947–1948 to the Third Survey in 1969–1971. For all cancers combined, there was a 9% increase in men and a 16% decrease in women. The upward trends for some cancers, such as multiple myeloma, are at least partly explained by improvements in diagnosis and reporting. This interpretation is less likely for tumors that are readily diagnosed, such as testicular cancer, although the factors responsible for this increase are unclear. More is known about the factors contributing to the rising trend for other tumors, such as x-ray exposures to the head and neck in childhood (thyroid cancer), changing clothing habits and recreational exposures to sunlight (melanoma), and treatments with menopausal estrogen (endometrial cancer). Pronounced decreases in incidence have involved not only stomach cancer but also cancers of the liver and cervix. In the black population, the rates have risen 46% in men and declined 15% in women (Table 2). The rise has been especially sharp for cancers of the lung, esophagus, prostate, and pancreas, and for myeloma, so that these tumors are now considerably more common in blacks than whites.

TABLE 1. *Changing incidence rates for selected cancers in U.S. whites (National Cancer Surveys, 1947–1948 to 1969–1971)*

	% Change	
Type of cancer	Males	Females
Myeloma	+183	+229
Thyroid	+100	+50
Lung	+131	+122
Melanoma	+85	+42
Kidney	+58	+31
Testis	+38	—
Endometrium	—	+36
Prostate	+21	—
Pancreas	+20	+16
Liver	−43	−71
Stomach	−63	−68
Cervix	—	−61
Total	+9	−16

TABLE 2. *Changing incidence rates for selected cancers in U.S.*
non-whites (National Cancer Surveys, 1947–1948 to 1969–1971)

Type of Cancer	% Change	
	Males	Females
Myeloma	+473	+245
Lung	+234	+176
Esophagus	+116	+126
Bladder	+104	−38
Intestines	+68	+99
Prostate	+57	—
Kidney	+44	+32
Pancreas	+42	+100
Oropharynx	+38	−17
Stomach	−52	−58
Cervix	—	−58
Total	+46	−15

Cancer Maps

Many of the best leads to cancer etiology have been supplied by alert clinicians who felt they were seeing an excessive number of patients with the same tumor and called attention to a particular etiologic factor. These clinical discoveries were usually possible because the "case clusters" involved rare tumors in the general population (e.g., vaginal adenocarcinoma, liver angiosarcoma, mesothelioma). It is difficult for a clinician to recognize clustering of a common tumor, but opportunities are available through the analysis of population-based cancer statistics. Although variations in cancer within nations are not as great as those seen internationally, the mapping of U.S. mortality statistics on a county level has revealed patterns that are not readily explained by diagnostic and statistical biases and seem likely to reflect high-risk environments (Blot *et al.* 1977c, Fraumeni 1977).

At the National Cancer Institute, we have developed a step-wise approach to these studies. First, an atlas of cancer mortality was published for the white population (Mason *et al.* 1975), followed by a companion atlas for the nonwhite population (Mason *et al.* 1976). Nearing completion are maps of nonneoplastic diseases, emphasizing conditions that may predispose to cancer or those that share common etiologic factors. Second, to seek explanations for the geographic variation in cancer across the country, correlation studies are used to relate the county mortality for a particular form of cancer to demographic and environmental data available at the county level. These analyses are designed to raise etiologic questions, not resolve them, and need to be used cautiously, with an understanding of their limitations. In some studies the starting point is a particular environmental exposure, which is then correlated with the risk of various forms of cancer. For example, in counties where the chemical industry is concentrated, the rates are significantly high for various cancers, particularly of the lung, bladder, and liver (Hoover and Fraumeni 1975). In counties where the petroleum industry is located, high rates are seen for cancers of the lung, nasal cavity, and skin, including melanoma (Blot et al. 1977a). In counties with furniture industries, the risk is greatest for cancer of the nasal cavity, a relationship previously reported in Europe but not studied in the U.S. (Brinton et al. 1976). This correlation approach may also help to evaluate exposures that affect the general community. For example, in counties where the water is naturally or artificially fluoridated, no excess risk of cancer is found, despite continued reports of a hazard by anti-fluoridationists (Hoover et al. 1976b). On the other hand, recent studies suggest that certain tumors, particularly of the bladder, may be related to the level of trihalomethanes in drinking water (Cantor et al., in press).

The third and crucial phase of our program is the testing of specific hypotheses by analytic investigations, mainly case-control interview studies in the high-risk communities. A number of such field studies are underway around the country, but as a preliminary measure we often look at the death certificates in counties with high rates for a particular cancer or with a special exposure. For example, after finding high rates of nasal cancer in furniture-industry counties, an examination was made of the death certificates for patients dying with this tumor in North Carolina, where the industry is heavily concentrated. Although such records have their limitations, a fourfold risk among furniture workers and a threefold risk associated with any occupational exposure to wood was seen (Brinton et al. 1977).

CAUSES OF CANCER

Tobacco

Much remains to be learned about the factors responsible for the variations in cancer around the country and around the world, yet a number of carcinogenic exposures have been identified to date through epidemiological studies. The principal hazard is the use of tobacco (cigarettes, cigars, or pipes), which produces cancers of the mouth, pharynx, esophagus, larynx, lung, bladder, and pancreas. It has been estimated that in men smoking accounts for nearly 90% of lung cancer and 40% of all cancers (Doll 1977). The risk of lung cancer has declined in persons who stopped smoking or switched to filter tips and low-tar brands, though remaining well above the risk for people who never smoked regularly. Tobacco chews in the form of snuff-dipping may account for the excessive rates for oral cancer among women in rural southern counties of the U.S. (Blot and Fraumeni 1977). In these areas, snuff use has been reported in over 75% of women with cancer of the gingival-buccal fold, where snuff is in closest contact with the oral mucosa. In other parts of the world the rates for oral cancer are unusually high in people with heavy exposures to various tobacco chews (e.g., *khaini* in India, *nass* in the Soviet Union, and *betal quid* in Asia), although in these situations the tobacco is often mixed with lime and other agents that may contribute to the exceptional risks.

Alcohol

Alcohol potentiates the effects of tobacco smoke (and perhaps other agents) on cancers of the mouth, pharynx, esophagus, and larynx, and, by inducing cirrhosis, it appears to increase the risk of liver cancer (Rothman 1975). It is difficult to estimate the contribution of alcohol to cancer risk, but by a combined effect with tobacco smoking it may account for 75% of mouth cancers and about 5% of all cancers in men. The mechanisms by which alcohol promotes carcinogenesis are not clear, but they may involve the promotion of nutritional deficiencies or some as yet unidentified cocarcinogens in alcoholic beverages. Further clues may come from studies of esophageal cancer in several high-risk areas of the world, including the excessive rates seen in American blacks living in the cities and in a belt of rural counties extending along the coastline from Charleston, South Carolina, into northern Florida (Fraumeni and Blot 1977).

Radiation

Ultraviolet radiation from sunlight is the major cause of skin cancers, including melanoma, and accounts for a high incidence in the southern part of the U.S. (Mason *et al.* 1975) and for the predisposition of fair-complexioned individuals. In a recent study of seven melanoma-prone families, susceptibility was related to the presence of a heritable precursor syndrome consisting of multiple, large, variably pigmented moles that are prone to malignant change, particularly in areas of sunlight exposure (Reimer *et al.* 1978). These lesions represent a distinctive clinical marker helping to identify high-risk individuals who should avoid sunlight exposure and be monitored closely for changes suggesting early stage melanoma.

Ionizing radiation, including natural background radiation, would appear to account for no more than 2 to 3% of all cancers, although a sizable fraction of thyroid cancer has been linked to therapeutic exposures in childhood. Table 3 lists some tumors that have been attributed to radiation, usually following excessive irradiation, as from the atomic bomb and from occupational or iatrogenic exposures (Jablon 1975). As evidence accumulates, however, it appears that virtually no site of the body is spared and that even low doses may have a carcinogenic potential in susceptible individuals.

Because of concern over the possible hazards of mammography, there has been special interest recently in the risk of breast cancer following various exposures, particularly from the atomic bomb (McGregor *et al.* 1977) and fluoroscopy in the management of tuberculosis patients treated with artificial pneumothorax

TABLE 3. *Radiogenic cancers*

Site	Exposure
Leukemia	Atomic bombs, radiotherapy for ankylosing spondylitis, radioactive materials
Thyroid	Radiotherapy for thymic enlargement
Breast	Atomic bombs, repeated chest fluoroscopy, radiotherapy for postpartum mastitis
Brain	Epilation of scalp for ringworm
Liver	Thorotrast
Bone	Radium and mesothorium
Intestines and uterus	Radiotherapy for metropathia hemorrhagica
Childhood cancers	Pelvimetry in prenatal life

(Boice and Monson 1977). These studies have shown a reasonably linear dose-response curve, with an effect evident at doses as low as 17 rads in the A-bomb survivors. A consistent finding is the predisposition of young women to radiation effects. In the fluoroscopy study, the effects were most pronounced when exposure occurred at menarche or during pregnancy—times when the breast tissue is actively proliferating. In the various studies, the intervals from exposure to diagnosis extend from 5 to at least 40 years. However, the latency period appears to be unaffected by dose levels, so that the age distribution of cases after radiation resembles that seen for "spontaneous" breast cancer. This suggests that age-related risk factors influence the development of radiogenic tumors of the breast. In the A-bomb study, a similar pattern was seen for lung cancer, whereas radiogenic leukemia occurred much earlier than the distribution of "spontaneous" cases and displayed a "wave" of increased incidence following exposure. It has been suggested that the basic mechanisms involved in the induction of leukemia may be different from those responsible for carcinomas such as those involving the breast and lung.

Occupational Chemicals

Industrial exposures have been reported to account for less than 5% of all cancers in men (Wynder and Gori 1977), but the percentage is much higher for certain tumors (e.g., bladder, nasal cavity) and is likely to rise as new hazards are recognized. Most of the discoveries shown in Table 4 were made by clinical and epidemiological observations (Cole and Goldman 1975), with subsequent confirmation by laboratory studies, although risk from arsenic and benzene exposure still lacks experimental evidence. In the case of mustard gas and vinyl chloride the risks were detected in man after the substances had been shown to induce tumors in laboratory animals, although little attention was given to the experimental studies when first reported. Some agents are known to be carcinogenic (asbestos, radon), yet their effects are greatly potentiated by tobacco

TABLE 4. *Occupational cancers*

Agent	Site
Ionizing radiation	Bronchus, Skin, Bone, Marrow
Mustard gas	Respiratory tract
Asbestos	Bronchus, Pleura, Peritoneum
Polycyclic hydrocarbons	Bronchus, Skin
Bis-chloromethyl ether	Bronchus
Nickel	Bronchus, Nasal sinuses
Chromium	Bronchus
Arsenic	Bronchus, Skin, Liver
Furniture industry*	Nasal sinuses
Leather industry*	Nasal sinuses
Isopropyl oil	Nasal sinuses
Aromatic amines	Bladder
Vinyl chloride	Liver, Lung(?), Brain(?)
Benzene	Marrow

* Specific agents unidentified

smoke (Selikoff and Hammond 1975). There is clearly a need for more epidemiological studies that are designed to measure these kinds of interactions.

Occupational hazards have implications beyond the workforce, since many agents are not confined to the plant but may spread into the general environment (Fraumeni 1975). In this way large populations may be at increased risk of cancer from such agents as asbestos, arsenic, polycyclic hydrocarbons, radioactive materials, and vinyl chloride. The extent of the hazard resulting from environmental pollution, however, remains uncertain. Still, the best opportunities for identifying chemical carcinogens probably continues to be the study of occupational groups, which may be regarded as sentinels in evaluating hazards to the general population.

In addition to clinical and experimental observations, clues to occupational carcinogens may come from the geographic peculiarities of cancer in the U.S. For example, the highest rates for lung cancer in men are clustered in rural counties along the Gulf of Mexico and along the southeast Atlantic coast (Blot and Fraumeni 1976). Through correlation analyses that adjust for demographic influences, we have found elevated mortality in counties with paper, chemical, petroleum, and shipbuilding industries. Based on preliminary data from a case-control interview study in coastal Georgia, it would appear that at least some of the clustering of lung cancer in this area may be traced to asbestos exposures in shipyards that operated during World War II and were then closed.

The rates for bladder cancer in men are especially high in New Jersey and other sections of the Northeast, in urban areas around the Great Lakes, in southern Louisiana, and in rural areas of New York and New England (Hoover *et al.* 1975). This distribution appears influenced, to some extent, by the location of chemical and probably other industries. To clarify the role of occupational exposures, smoking habits, pollutants in drinking water, artificial sweeteners, and other possible risk factors, a case-control study of bladder cancer is underway in several parts of the country including some high-risk and some low-risk areas.

Drugs

It may be that medicinal chemicals pose a greater hazard than previously thought (Table 5). Although current knowledge suggests that these agents account for about 2 to 3% of all cancers, estimates may rise as the risks of hormonally induced tumors are clarified. A major development was the report in 1971 indicating that synthetic estrogens given during pregnancy may cross the placenta to produce adenocarcinomas of the vagina and cervix years later in exposed daughters (Herbst *et al.* 1971). This first demonstration of transplacental carcinogenesis in man drew attention to the potential importance of prenatal and early life exposures and stimulated further investigation into the carcinogenic potential of estrogens. A series of case-control studies then linked endometrial cancer to the use of conjugated estrogens for menopausal symptoms (McDonald *et al.* 1977). A recent follow-up study of 1,891 women receiving menopausal estrogens suggests that the risk of other tumors may be increased. Breast cancer showed a 30% excess overall, which increased with the duration of follow-up and reached twofold after 10 years (Hoover *et al.* 1976a), while ovarian cancer occurred two to three times more often than expected, with the excess limited to a small group of women also using stilbestrol (Hoover *et al.* 1977).

Another problem under study is the hazard of acute leukemia among patients treated with certain cytotoxic drugs. In a recent study of 5,455 patients with ovarian cancer, mostly receiving alkylating agents, the risk of acute nonlymphocytic leukemia was 36 times the expected value, rising to 171 for those surviving two years (Reimer *et al.* 1977). This potential for causing leukemia may be acceptable when the agents are effective in treating conditions with a poor prognosis, such as breast cancer with axillary node involvement. However, the risks should be taken into account when the agents are used for conditions with a more favorable survival rate.

The 32-fold risk of non-Hodgkin's lymphoma in renal transplant recipients has indicated the potential hazard of immunosuppressive agents (Hoover and Fraumeni 1973), although the risk following treatment of other disorders has not been defined. The rapid onset of lymphoma within a few weeks of transplantation suggests a breakdown of immune surveillance with loss of control over cells already initiated and transformed. For other tumors, the excess risk is about twofold and begins to appear two years after transplantation. It has not affected all tumors across the board, as might be predicted by the immunosurveillance hypothesis. Whatever the mechanisms, there does appear to be an increased risk of cancers of the liver, bile duct, and bladder, plus lung adenocarcinoma, leukemia, soft-tissue sarcoma, and skin cancers, including melanoma (Hoover 1977).

TABLE 5. *Drug-induced cancers*

Agent	Site
Radioisotopes	Marrow, Bone, Liver
Alkylating agents	Marrow, Bladder
Immunosuppressants	Lymphoma
Coal tar ointments	Skin
Phenacetin	Renal pelvis
Arsenic	Skin, Liver
Diphenylhydantoin	Lymphoma
Stilbestrol	Genital tract
Conjugated estrogens	Endometrium, Breast(?)
Steroid contraceptives	Liver, Endometrium(?)
Androgenic anabolic steroids	Liver

Oncogenic Viruses

Viruses have not been causally tied to the origins of any human cancer, but the search continues on several fronts (Heath *et al.* 1975). The epidemiological patterns of cervical cancer have long suggested venereal transmission of an oncogenic agent, and herpes virus (type 2) now seems a strong candidate. Another agent, the Epstein-Barr (EB) virus, has been associated with nasopharyngeal carcinoma (NPC) and Burkitt's lymphoma, while hepatitis-B infection has been linked with hepatoma in endemic zones. There is little evidence that any form of cancer is transmitted from one case to another, although in some (but not other) studies of Hodgkin's disease, the cases seemed linked by close interpersonal contact (Grufferman 1977). It may be that some viruses are oncogenic only when combined with other factors. In this manner, the EB virus may require certain histocompatibility antigens to induce the high rate of NPC in Chinese populations, may interact with malarial infection to induce community clusters of Burkitt's lymphoma in Africa, or may combine with a genetic immunodeficiency trait to cause family clusters of lymphoma (Purtilo *et al.* 1977). It is not possible to estimate the fraction of human cancer caused by viruses, but it may be small. In animal models the production of immunodeficiency enhances viral carcinogenesis, so that the narrow range of tumors complicating immunodeficiency states of man would suggest that viruses play only a limited role. Their influence, however, should be carefully sought among the tumors that develop excessively in immunodeficiency states.

Dietary Factors

It seems almost a certainty that some aspects of the Western diet are at least partly responsible for the substantial geographic variation in colon cancer.

Correlational and case-control studies have suggested the influence of high dietary fat and meat consumption and the possible protective effect of high fiber intake (Berg 1975). These hypotheses are under study, but the mechanisms appear to be complex. One suggestion is that excess dietary fat increases the concentration of bile acids in the bowel, which are then metabolized by bacterial flora into carcinogens or cocarcinogens (Wynder and Reddy 1975). As in the case of viral studies, the epidemiologist needs to collaborate with the experimentalist in order to make headway. Further clues may come from international and migrant studies to identify the dietary and metabolic factors responsible for the risk differentials from one country to another. Opportunities may also exist in the U.S., since rates for colon cancer in the urban Northeast are two times higher than in the rural Southeast (Blot *et al.* 1976). The relatively low rates in the South include even areas with a concentration of residents who moved from the North, suggesting the possibility of a "migrant effect." Another lead may be provided by an outlier from the usual geographic pattern of colon cancer, namely, the clustering of elevated rates in rural farming communities in southeastern Nebraska. A case-control study has been started in this area.

Dietary factors may also influence the development of breast cancer, as suggested by the international correlations with colon cancer and with fat consumption (Armstrong and Doll 1975). Within the U.S., the pattern for breast cancer parallels that for colon cancer, with high rates in the Northeast, other urban areas throughout the country, and upper income groups; but only limited nutritional data are available to make correlations (Blot *et al.* 1977b). When breast cancer is analyzed by age group, the variation within the U.S. is primarily among postmenopausal women, who would appear most affected by dietary and other environmental influences. The more uniform distribution of premenopausal breast cancer is consistent with evidence from family studies relating genetic factors to early-onset tumors (Anderson 1977). Again, multidisciplinary studies should help to identify and tease apart the nutritional mechanisms, reproductive and hormonal factors, and genetic components that appear to contribute to this tumor. The role of nutrition, through dietary fat and caloric excess, seems even stronger for endometrial cancer. It has been suggested that this kind of diet stimulates endometrial proliferation by enhancing estrogen production and may account for the associated manifestations of obesity, diabetes, and hypertension (Armstrong 1977).

Despite the substantial international variation and the declining incidence in the U.S., the causes of stomach cancer remain uncertain. In studies of Japanese moving to the U.S., the tumor has been linked to a deficiency of various Western vegetables and an excess of pickled vegetables and dried or salted fish in the diet (Haenszel *et al.* 1972). Among Norwegian immigrants in the U.S., the tumor has been related to a low intake of vegetables and fruits containing ascorbic acid, a substance that may inhibit the production of carcinogenic nitrosamines in the stomach (Bjelke 1974). It appears that ethnic factors are primarily responsible for the clustering of stomach cancer in the North Central and Southwest regions of the U.S. (Hoover *et al.* 1975), so that further studies of Scandinavian descendants and Spanish-Americans may be indicated.

CONCLUSIONS

In summary, many causes of cancer have been identified, but these still account for only a minority of cases. Despite the large gaps in knowledge, circumstantial evidence suggests that the bulk of human cancer is related to environmental exposures that should succumb in time to epidemiological and experimental research. All promising leads and approaches should be pursued, including efforts to uncover host as well as environmental determinants. Opportunities for study are provided not only by the international peculiarities in cancer risk but also by the delineation of high-risk communities in the U.S. where particular exposures may be more conspicuous than usual. It seems very likely that a number of hazards (e.g., nutritional factors, oncogenic viruses, genetic susceptibility) act through complex and subtle mechanisms that will be clarified only through the joint efforts of epidemiologists and laboratory investigators.

REFERENCES

Anderson, D. 1977. Breast cancer in families. Cancer 40:1855–1860.

Armstrong, B., and R. Doll. 1975. Environmental factors and cancer incidence and mortality in different countries, with special reference to dietary practices. Int. J. Cancer 15:617–631.

Armstrong, B. K. 1977. The role of diet in human carcinogenesis with special reference to endometrial cancer, *in* Origins of Human Cancer: Book A, Incidence of Cancer in Humans, H. H. Hiatt, J. D. Watson, and J. A. Winsten, eds., Cold Spring Harbor Laboratory, Cold Spring Harbor, New York, pp. 557–565.

Berg, J. W. 1975. Diet, *in* Persons at High Risk of Cancer: An Approach to Cancer Etiology and Control, J. F. Fraumeni, Jr., ed., Academic Press, New York, pp. 201–224.

Bjelke, E. 1974. Epidemiologic studies of cancer of the stomach, colon, and rectum; with special reference on the role of diet. Scand. J. Gastroenterol. 9 (Suppl. 31): 1–235.

Blot, W. J., L. A. Brinton, J. F. Fraumeni, Jr., and B. J. Stone. 1977a. Cancer mortality in U.S. counties with petroleum industries. Science 198:51–53.

Blot, W. J., and J. F. Fraumeni, Jr. 1976. Geographic patterns of lung cancer: Industrial correlations. Am. J. Epidemiol. 103:539–550.

Blot, W. J., and J. F. Fraumeni, Jr. 1977. Geographic patterns of oral cancer in the United States: Etiologic implications. J. Chron. Dis. 30:745–757.

Blot, W. J., J. F. Fraumeni, Jr., and B. J. Stone. 1977b. Geographic patterns of breast cancer in the United States. J. Natl. Cancer Inst. 59:1407–1411.

Blot, W. J., J. F. Fraumeni, Jr., B. J. Stone, and F. W. McKay. 1976. Geographic patterns of large bowel cancer in the United States. J. Natl. Cancer Inst. 57:1225–1231.

Blot, W. J., T. J. Mason, R. Hoover, and J. F. Fraumeni, Jr. 1977c. Cancer by county: Etiologic implications, *in* Origins of Human Cancer: Book A, Incidence of Cancer in Humans, H. H. Hiatt, J. D. Watson, and J. A. Winsten, eds., Cold Spring Harbor Laboratory, Cold Spring Harbor, New York, pp. 21–32.

Boice, J. D., Jr., and R. R. Monson. 1977. Breast cancer in women after repeated fluoroscopic examinations of the chest. J. Natl. Cancer Inst. 59:823–832.

Brinton, L. A., W. J. Blot, B. J. Stone, and J. F. Fraumeni, Jr. 1977. A death certificate analysis of nasal cancer among furniture workers in North Carolina. Cancer Res. 37:3473–3474.

Brinton, L. A., B. J. Stone, W. J. Blot, and J. F. Fraumeni, Jr. 1976. Nasal cancer in U.S. furniture industry counties. Lancet 2:628.

Cantor, K. P., R. Hoover, T. J. Mason, and L. J. McCabe. 1978. Association of halomethanes in drinking water with cancer mortality. J. Natl. Cancer Inst. (In press).

Cole, P., and M. B. Goldman. 1975. Occupation, *in* Persons at High Risk of Cancer: An Approach to Cancer Etiology and Control, J. F. Fraumeni, Jr., ed., Academic Press, New York, pp. 167–184.

Devesa, S. S., and D. T. Silverman. 1978. Cancer incidence and mortality trends in the United States: 1935–74. J. Natl. Cancer Inst. 60:545–571.

Doll, R. 1977. The prevention of cancer. J. R. Coll. Physicians Lond. 11:125–140.

Fraumeni, J. F., Jr. 1975. Respiratory carcinogenesis: An epidemiologic appraisal. J. Natl. Cancer Inst. 55:1039–1046.

Fraumeni, J. F., Jr. 1977. Geographic clues to high-risk groups in cancer. The Cancer Bulletin 29:191–194.

Fraumeni, J. F., Jr., and W. J. Blot. 1977. Geographic variation in esophageal cancer mortality in the United States. J. Chron. Dis. 30:759–767.

Grufferman, S. 1977. Clustering and aggregation of exposures in Hodgkin's disease. Cancer 39:1829–1833.

Haenszel, W., and M. Kurihara. 1968. Studies of Japanese migrants. I. Mortality from cancer and other diseases among Japanese in the United States. J. Natl. Cancer Inst. 40:43–68.

Haenszel, W., M. Kurihara, M. Segi, and R. K. C. Lee. 1972. Stomach cancer among Japanese in Hawaii. J. Natl. Cancer Inst. 49:969–988.

Heath, C. W., Jr., G. G. Caldwell, and P. C. Feorino. 1975. Viruses and other microbes, *in* Persons at High Risk of Cancer: An Approach to Cancer Etiology and Control, J. F. Fraumeni, Jr., ed., Academic Press, New York, pp. 241–265.

Herbst, A. L., H. Ulfelder, and D. C. Poskanzer. 1971. Adenocarcinoma of the vagina: Association of maternal stilbestrol therapy with tumor appearance in young women. N. Engl. J. Med. 284:878–881.

Higginson, J., and C. S. Muir. 1973. Epidemiology, *in* Cancer Medicine, J. F. Holland and E. Frei, III, eds., Lea and Febiger, Philadelphia, pp. 241–306.

Higginson, J. 1976. A hazardous society? Individual versus community responsibility in cancer prevention. Am. J. Public Health 66:359–366.

Hoover, R. 1977. Effects of drugs—immunosuppression, *in* Origins of Human Cancer: Book A, Incidence of Cancer in Humans, H. H. Hiatt, J. D. Watson, and J. A. Winsten, eds., Cold Spring Harbor Laboratory, Cold Spring Harbor, New York, pp. 369–379.

Hoover, R., and J. F. Fraumeni, Jr. 1973. Risk of cancer in renal-transplant recipients. Lancet 2:55–57.

Hoover, R., and J. F. Fraumeni, Jr. 1975. Cancer mortality in U.S. counties with chemical industries. Environ. Res. 9:196–207.

Hoover, R., L. A. Gray, Sr., P. Cole, and B. MacMahon. 1976a. Menopausal estrogens and breast cancer. N. Engl. J. Med. 295:401–405.

Hoover, R., L. A. Gray, Sr., and J. F. Fraumeni, Jr. 1977. Stilboesterol (diethylstilbestrol) and the risk of ovarian cancer. Lancet 2:533–534.

Hoover, R., T. J. Mason, F. W. McKay, and J. F. Fraumeni, Jr. 1975. Cancer by county: New resource for etiologic clues. Science 189:1005–1007.

Hoover, R. N., F. W. McKay, and J. F. Fraumeni, Jr. 1976b. Fluoridated drinking water and the occurrence of cancer. J. Natl. Cancer Inst. 57:757–768.

Jablon, S. 1975. Radiation, *in* Persons at High Risk of Cancer: An Approach to Cancer Etiology and Control, J. F. Fraumeni, Jr., ed., Academic Press, New York, pp. 151–165.

Mason, T. J., F. W. McKay, R. Hoover, W. J. Blot, and J. F. Fraumeni, Jr. 1975. Atlas of Cancer Mortality for U.S. Counties: 1950–1969. Government Printing Office, DHEW Publ. No. (NIH) 75–780, Washington, D.C.

Mason, T. J., F. W. McKay, R. Hoover, W. J. Blot, and J. F. Fraumeni, Jr. 1976. Atlas of Cancer Mortality among U.S. Nonwhites: 1950–1969. Government Printing Office, DHEW Publ. No. (NIH) 76–1204, Washington, D.C.

McDonald, T. W., J. F. Annegers, W. M. O'Fallon, M. B. Dockerty, G. D. Malkasian, and L. T. Kurland. 1977. Exogenous estrogen and endometrial carcinoma: Case-control and incidence study. Am. J. Obstet. Gynecol. 127:572–580.

McGregor, D. H., C. E. Land, K. Choi, S. Tokuoka, P. I. Liu, T. Wakabayashi, and G. W. Beebe. 1977. Breast cancer incidence among atomic bomb survivors, Hiroshima and Nagasaki, 1950–69. J. Natl. Cancer Inst. 59:799–811.

Muir, C. S. 1975. International variation in high-risk populations, *in* Persons at High Risk of Cancer: An Approach to Cancer Etiology and Control, J. F. Fraumeni, Jr., ed., Academic Press, New York, pp. 293–305.

Purtilo, D. T., D. DeFlorio, L. M. Hutt, J. Bhawan, J. P. S. Yang, R. Otto, and W. Edwards. 1977. Variable phenotypic expression of an X-linked recessive lymphoproliferative syndrome. N. Engl. J. Med. 297:1077–1081.

Reimer, R. R., W. H. Clark, M. H. Greene, A. M. Ainsworth, and J. F. Fraumeni, Jr. 1978. Precursor lesions in familial melanoma: A new genetic preneoplastic syndrome. J.A.M.A. 239:744–746.

Reimer, R. R., R. Hoover, J. F. Fraumeni, Jr., and R. C. Young. 1977. Acute leukemia after alkylating-agent therapy of ovarian cancer. N. Engl. J. Med. 297:177–181.

Rothman, K. J. 1975. Alcohol, *in* Persons at High Risk of Cancer: An Approach to Cancer Etiology and Control, J. F. Fraumeni, Jr., ed., Academic Press, New York, pp. 139–150.

Selikoff, I. J., and E. C. Hammond. 1975. Multiple risk factors in environmental cancer, *in* Persons at High Risk of Cancer: An Approach to Cancer Etiology and Control, J. F. Fraumeni, Jr., ed., Academic Press, New York, pp. 467–483.

Wynder, E. L., and B. S. Reddy. 1975. Dietary fat and colon cancer. J. Natl. Cancer Inst. 54: 7–10.

Wynder, E. L., and G. B. Gori. 1977. Contribution of the environment to cancer incidence: An epidemiologic exercise. J. Natl. Cancer Inst. 58:825–832.

Carcinogens: Identification and Mechanisms
of Action, edited by A. Clark Griffin and
Charles R. Shaw. Raven Press, New York © 1979.

Carcinogenesis Studies on Organ Cultures of Animal and Human Respiratory Tissues

Umberto Saffiotti and Curtis C. Harris

Experimental Pathology Branch, Carcinogenesis Research Program, Division of Cancer Cause and Prevention, National Cancer Institute, Bethesda, Maryland 20014

The identification of environmental carcinogens has been traditionally based on long-term bioassays in experimental animals and, whenever possible, on epidemiological studies of exposed human populations. The critical evaluation of both epidemiological and experimental data provides a basis for classification of substances in relation to carcinogenicity, as recently defined (Saffiotti 1977b). Some substances will be classified as positive, others as negative under the conditions of test, and a third group as inconclusive because of inadequate evidence.

In addition to the traditional methods for long-term tests in mammalian species, new short-term methods have been developed to detect certain effects of carcinogens that may be good indicators of their carcinogenic activity. These test methods are designed to measure molecular level effects of carcinogens (such as DNA damage and repair), the induction of genetic damage (as expressed by mutations), and the induction of neoplastic transformation of cells in culture. It is now possible to use several of these methods, preferably as a battery of tests, to supplement animal level studies on the effect of carcinogens.

In the development of an effective strategy toward cancer prevention in our society, a major problem is represented by the choice of criteria that can be used to predict human cancer hazards due to environmental carcinogens on the basis of experimental tests. While mathematical dose-response extrapolation methods are applicable within one biological system, other criteria are needed for an evaluation of species differences and other biological variations (Saffiotti 1978).

A general qualitative similarity has been well demonstrated between the carcinogenic response of humans and that of experimental mammalian species. In fact, work of the last twenty years, particularly of the last decade, has led to the development, by chemical induction, of animal models for most major forms of human cancers, including models for cancers of the bronchus and lung, larynx, esophagus, glandular stomach, large bowel, pancreas, kidney, bladder, and breast. Their histopathogenesis has been found quite similar to that in their human counterpart. This correlation can be considered as strong supportive evidence for a chemical origin of a large proportion of human cancers (Saffiotti 1977b).

Thus, the *qualitative* similarity of the response to carcinogens in humans and in experimental mammalian species has been well established. We now face the difficult problem of determining if a reliable *quantitative* methodology can be developed for a selective and precise estimate of the human risk in relation to given carcinogenic exposures. No reliable procedure has yet been found for a direct quantitative extrapolation of the results of carcinogenic studies from one or more experimental species to another species (particularly the human). Carcinogenic effects in different species may be greatly affected by specific variables in the host species. Marked differences in the response to a carcinogen, in different species and in different individual members of a population, indicate that a careful evaluation of these variables should be taken into account when attempting to correlate effects in different biological systems.

While much attention has been given to this problem in the last decade, no methodology has been established to provide an adequate and reliable quantitative assessment of human risk simply on the basis of experimental animal findings.

If we want to assess the specific effects of carcinogens on humans, we need to define by accurate methods the metabolic requirements for activation of carcinogens, the localization and interaction of carcinogens in the target cells, and the induced changes as they occur in the human tissues. In other words, we have to bring the experimental method to the study of the human response to carcinogens. Naturally we cannot experiment with carcinogens on people, for obvious ethical reasons. But in our environment, human exposure to carcinogens occurs continuously and often in uncontrolled conditions. Human population groups at high risk for cancer have been identified and studied in several instances. Their neoplastic and preneoplastic response can be critically compared with that in controlled experimental models.

An effective methodological approach to the direct study of the response to carcinogens in humans is based on the use of organ culture systems that make it possible to maintain human target tissues in well-controlled conditions, removed from the body and thus available for experimentation. The recent developments in this area will be reviewed below.

SEQUENTIAL STUDY OF IN VIVO AND IN VITRO MODELS OF CARCINOGENESIS IN TARGET TISSUES

The general approach considered here involves a step-by-step development of methods at different levels of observation, centered on the target cells from which a given type of cancer arises. This approach is summarized in Figure 1.

One starts with the observational study of human disease, i.e., epidemiology and pathology, obtaining evidence on the natural history, environmental associa-

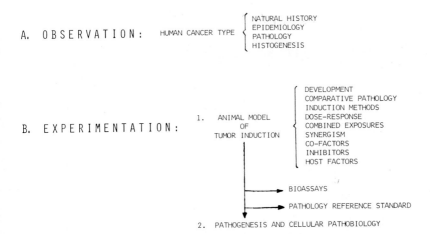

A. OBSERVATION: HUMAN CANCER TYPE
- NATURAL HISTORY
- EPIDEMIOLOGY
- PATHOLOGY
- HISTOGENESIS

B. EXPERIMENTATION:

1. ANIMAL MODEL
   OF
   TUMOR INDUCTION
- DEVELOPMENT
- COMPARATIVE PATHOLOGY
- INDUCTION METHODS
- DOSE–RESPONSE
- COMBINED EXPOSURES
- SYNERGISM
- CO–FACTORS
- INHIBITORS
- HOST FACTORS

BIOASSAYS

PATHOLOGY REFERENCE STANDARD

2. PATHOGENESIS AND CELLULAR PATHOBIOLOGY

FIG. 1. Sequential study of in vivo and in vitro models of carcinogenesis in target tissues.

tions, morphology, and histogenesis of the given cancer type. The next step is that of experimental studies, first aimed at the development of animal models in which the human type of cancer can be reproduced with good comparability of the tissue and cellular response by induction with carcinogens. Conditions of experimental exposure to carcinogens in the animal model can then be made to correlate as closely as possible to known or potential human exposures associated with the type of cancer under study. The animal model can often be further refined and used to study dose-response patterns with various carcinogens. Combined exposures to carcinogens and/or cofactors in the induction of the given cancer type can be explored, particularly in relation to those factors that are especially relevant to the organ or tissue under study. The animal model will also be useful in the study of host- or tissue-specific susceptibility factors.

When an animal model is well established, it becomes available as a research tool, chiefly for the following purposes: (1) carcinogenesis bioassays, particularly for those materials that relate in a special way to the target site, (2) as a pathology reference standard for morphological characterization and diagnosis in bioassays as well as in research, (3) as a model for mechanism studies on pathogenesis and cellular pathobiology.

The main value of the experimental animal models of carcinogenesis is their availability for investigating and identifying pathogenetic mechanisms in the target tissues and cells and their correlation with human disease. A systematic analysis of the constituent parts of an animal model will reveal a great deal of its mechanisms.

Sequential studies on the histogenesis of the induced tumor response in the animal model, at the optical, ultrastructural, and histochemical level, can lead to the identification of the specific types of cells from which the neoplastic response originates. A careful comparison with the observation of the early stages of preneoplastic and neoplastic changes in human pathology can throw much new light on both human and animal level studies.

The identification of the cells of origin of a cancer type is of considerable importance in the further analysis of pathogenetic mechanisms, for example in assessing the relevance of studies on carcinogen localization and binding or in the understanding of inhibitory mechanisms. One can therefore indicate cellular pathogenesis as an important sequence to histogenesis, in which not only the cells of origin are identified, but their sequential structural changes are recognized as a component of the carcinogenic response. Early changes in both tissues and cells can be identified by morphological as well as biochemical methods, and these changes can become useful markers of the early response to carcinogens in the target organ (NCI 1976).

The methods needed for a coordinated morphological and biochemical study of the target tissues depend, of course, on the nature and special characteristics of the tissue itself.

Animal Models of Respiratory Carcinogenesis

Our main research interest has been focused on the study of epithelial lining tissues, from which the vast majority of human cancers derive, such as the laryngo-bronchial epithelium, the mucosa of the large bowel and of the stomach, the pancreatic duct, the esophagus, the uterine cervix, and the bladder. Much of our laboratory work has been devoted to studies of the respiratory epithelium, and the present review will be mostly limited to this tissue.

The development of an effective animal model of respiratory carcinogenesis was stimulated by previous studies on particulate materials administered by intratracheal instillation, their penetration and their effects on respiratory tissues (Saffiotti and Tommasini Degna 1958, Saffiotti 1960, 1962, Saffiotti *et al.* 1960). The choice of animal species was based on studies on the responsiveness of the Syrian golden hamster to chemical carcinogens (Shubik *et al.* 1962) and on the observation that the hamster was particularly suitable for intratracheal administration of carcinogens and was resistant to respiratory infections (Della Porta *et al.* 1958, Saffiotti *et al.* 1964).

A methodology was developed for the intratracheal administration of aqueous suspensions of a finely particulated carcinogen such as benzo[*a*]pyrene (BP) attached to fine carrier particles of a nonfibrogenic material such as ferric oxide. These methods for administering carcinogens directly into the respiratory tract proved highly effective and induced high incidences of bronchogenic carcinomas, morphologically similar to those observed in human pathology. The hamster proved to be a species of choice for its susceptibility to several respiratory carcinogens, for its lack of respiratory tumors in untreated or vehicle-treated controls, and for its resistance to respiratory infections (Saffiotti *et al.* 1964, 1965, 1966, 1967, 1968, Saffiotti 1969a, 1970a, b).

This model was used for a wide range of studies in our laboratories and by other investigators. Dose-response studies were first undertaken varying the dose of carcinogen in single or repeated administrations, the frequency of the administrations and the dose, and physical characteristics of the carrier particles (Saffiotti 1970a, Montesano *et al.* 1970, Saffiotti *et al.* 1972a, b, Sellakumar *et al.* 1973). The characteristics and functions of carrier particles were also investigated (Saffiotti *et al.* 1964, 1965, Saffiotti 1970a, Henry and Kaufman 1973, Henry *et al.* 1974, Farrell and Davis 1974). Combined and synergistic effects of different carcinogens were demonstrated using intratracheal BP and ferric oxide administrations combined with the systemic administration of diethylnitrosamine (Montesano *et al.* 1970, 1974) or with the intratracheal administration of *N*-methyl-*N*-nitrosourea (Kaufman and Madison 1974). The histogenesis and cellular pathogenesis of the respiratory epithelial response was examined in this experimental animal model at the light and electron microscopic levels (Harris *et al.* 1972a, b, 1973a, b, c, 1974b, Saffiotti and Kaufman 1975). Autoradiographic studies were used to identify the cellular localization of the carcinogen and the cellular targets in the epithelial response (Harris *et al.* 1973a).

Extensive subsequent studies on this model, using combined techniques of light and electron transmission microscopy, scanning microscopy, and histochemistry have recently resulted in the elucidation of the cells of origin in the pathogenesis of bronchogenic carcinoma and its precursor lesions in the animal model (Becci *et al.* 1978a, b, c in press) and in the demonstration of a close similarity in the histogenesis observed in the animal model and in human pathology studies (McDowell *et al.* 1978a, b, in press, Trump *et al.*, in press).

The cytokinetics of the respiratory epithelium have been studied using this animal model (Boren and Paradise 1978, Paradise and Boren 1978).

Factors capable of modulating the carcinogenic response were identified in this system. Notable among them was the role of vitamin A in inhibiting epithelial squamous metaplasia, as well as carcinogenesis (Saffiotti *et al.* 1967, Saffiotti 1969b).

Work on respiratory carcinogenesis, based on the use of this experimental animal model, has developed extensively in several laboratories and has been reviewed periodically in the last decade (Saffiotti 1969a, Hanna *et al.* 1970, Nettesheim *et al.* 1970, Karbe and Park 1974, Harris 1978).

ORGAN CULTURE METHODS IN CARCINOGENESIS

As the next step in the sequence from the whole animal to the cellular and molecular level, one can consider the investigation of the pathogenesis and cellular pathobiology of the process of tumor induction in the tissue under study (Figure 2).

The penetration, localization, and metabolic fate of carcinogens affecting the tissue can be studied to elucidate the specific pathways required for metabolic activation and for carcinogen interaction with critical macromolecular targets.

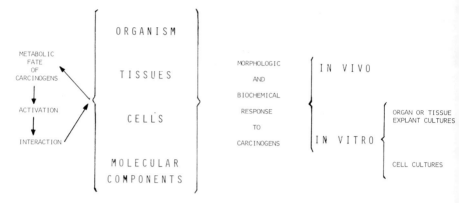

FIG. 2. Pathogenesis and cellular pathobiology.

Such analytical investigations can be conducted in a coordinated manner at different levels of biological organization, studying the effects of carcinogens on the whole organism, on a selected organ, on its constituent tissues, on their target cells, and on their molecular components.

Coordination of morphological and biochemical methods makes it possible to focus on the fundamental lesions and their functional significance. Two levels of experimentation can be usefully integrated, in vivo and in vitro. The latter includes methods using organ or tissue explant cultures and methods using cell cultures.

In developing a coordinated research effort for the Carcinogenesis Program of the National Cancer Institute, it was considered important to build a direct bridge between carcinogenesis studies conducted in animals and those in humans, by using in vitro organ cultures of the target tissues obtained both from the in vivo animal models and from humans (Saffiotti 1972).

A considerable amount of work has been devoted to this subject in our laboratory and also in an expanding number of other laboratories. The progress derived from this effort already suggests that a substantial contribution to the understanding of human cancer risks can be obtained using this approach, as indicated by a recent state-of-the-art review meeting on "Carcinogenesis Studies in Human Cells and Tissues" (Harris *et al.* 1978d).

The role of organ culture methods in carcinogenesis research can be viewed as being a central one, which can be used for studies of the target tissues obtained from the animal models as well as from human sources. It can be further extended to studies of the cellular constituents in vitro and to their analysis using morphological and biochemical techniques as well as biological methods that define growth characteristics in cell culture and after transplantation into suitable recipient animals (Figure 3). A wide range of experimental designs can be developed to investigate the effects of carcinogens, procarcinogens, metabolic activators

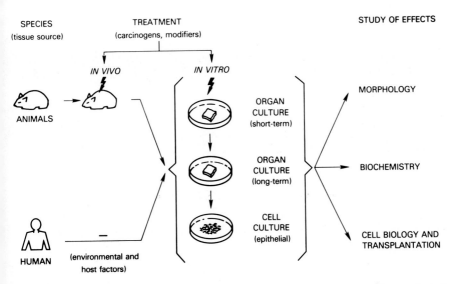

FIG. 3. Comparative studies on tissues from animal and human sources can be conducted by culture methods. Carcinogens and/or modifiers (enzyme inducers and inhibitors, cocarcinogens and anticarcinogens) can be administered in vivo in the animal models and in vitro in both animal and human systems. Different combinations of experimental treatment can therefore be designed. Cell cultures can be derived from previously established organ cultures. Each level of organization can be analyzed concurrently by morphological and biochemical techniques and by observation of cellular properties and growth characteristics in culture, as well as after transplantation into immunocompatible animals.

and inhibitors, anticarcinogens, and other modifying factors that can be applied in vivo or in vitro in different sequences.

The advantages of working with target tissues maintained as organ cultures for carcinogenesis studies are manifold:

1) The tissues can be kept for extended periods of time (weeks to months) with good morphological and functional integrity.

2) The epithelium maintains its differentiated state and its intercellular as well as epithelial-stromal relationships.

3) The tissue can be studied experimentally, e.g., in its response to carcinogens, as a single unit, removed from organismic influences but retaining its internal structural complexity so that its various cell types can be studied concurrently.

4) As a biological unit the tissue explant represents a highly manageable experimental system that offers good control conditions of its milieu and is particularly efficient for work with small quantities of radioactively labeled carcinogens or biochemical reagents.

5) Carcinogens can be metabolically detoxified and activated in epithelial tissue explants, and their interaction with cellular macromolecules can be local-

ized at the cellular level by autoradiography and at the molecular level by biochemical and biophysical techniques.

6) The effects of carcinogens can be studied at different levels: the whole tissue, the epithelium, the individual epithelial cell types, and their organelles and molecular components.

7) As opposed to the case of cell cultures, organ cultures show histological reactions, such as hyperplasia, metaplasia, and dysplasia, which correlate well with those observed in animal models and in human pathology.

8) The tissues, after in vitro manipulation, can be transplanted into suitable recipient animals for further observation in vivo of neoplastic properties.

9) The tissue explants can be used to start cell monolayer cultures.

10) Last, but not least, the organ culture methods can be used with human tissues, thereby allowing direct human experimentation with carcinogens, as well as controlled comparisons between animal and human tissue responses and between experimentally treated human tissues and their counterpart in human pathology.

There are, of course, certain limitations to organ culture methods for carcinogenesis studies, primarily the need to "extrapolate" back to the whole organism in evaluating the overall effects of carcinogens. Exposure of the explanted tissues to a given carcinogen may not closely mimic the in vivo conditions of exposure of the same tissue in either experimental animals or humans. The interactions taking place during the penetration and distribution of a carcinogen in the organism and the effects of different organs on its metabolic fate may determine conditions of exposure and cellular response which are not reproduced in the culture. Experimental procedures can be devised to compensate for some of these limitations, but this problem needs to be always considered in the evaluation of carcinogenesis studies in culture systems.

ORGAN CULTURE STUDIES IN RESPIRATORY TISSUES FROM EXPERIMENTAL ANIMALS

The development of organ culture methods for respiratory tissues and their use in carcinogenesis studies traces its origins to early work in several laboratories, which has been recently reviewed (Karbe and Park 1974, Lane 1978).

Studies on human tissues in culture exposed to chemical carcinogens were pioneered by Lasnitzki (1956, 1958, 1968) who observed the induction of cell proliferation and squamous metaplasia in human fetal lung explants treated with polynuclear aromatic hydrocarbons and/or cigarette smoke condensates. Crocker and co-workers developed organ culture methods for tracheal segments from several species for carcinogenesis studies (Crocker *et al.* 1965, Crocker 1969, Crocker and Neilsen 1967, Crocker and Sanders 1970) and extended this technique to studies of bronchial organ cultures from primates and humans

(Crocker 1970). A technique using rat tracheal rings in culture was also developed (Palekar *et al.* 1978). These methods gave an early indication of the research potential offered by such an approach.

In the Carcinogenesis Program laboratories at the National Cancer Institute the organ culture method was first selected to analyze the tissue response to respiratory carcinogens in the previously established hamster model. Using hamster tracheobronchial mucosa, methods were developed for the separation of the epithelium from the connective tissue and for the dissociation of individual epithelial cells (Smith *et al.* 1971). Short-term organ culture methods were used to determine the integrity of the tissue and to assess the feasibility of measuring cellular properties that are representative of the functional state of the tissue with appropriate micromethods (Kaufman *et al.* 1972).

In vitro incubation methods were developed for the study of the incorporation of precursors into DNA, RNA, and proteins using both autoradiographic and biochemical techniques. The cellular composition of the epithelium and the functional activity of the different cell types were determined (Kaufman *et al.* 1972).

The patterns of high molecular weight RNA synthesis and maturation were studied in the epithelial cells (Kaufman *et al.* 1972). Highly purified DNA was isolated from the epithelial cells, and the binding of ^{3}H-labeled benzo[*a*]pyrene (BP) to DNA following incubation in vitro with the organ cultures was determined. In vivo pretreatment with the same polycyclic hydrocarbon, acting as an enzyme inducer, enhanced the in vitro binding to DNA. This response was inhibited by incubation either in the presence of 7,8-benzoflavone, an inhibitor of aryl hydrocarbon hydroxylase activity, or at near 0°C (Kaufman *et al.* 1973).

In the same organ culture system, quantitative light microscopic autoradiography showed the in vitro binding of ^{3}H-BP to both nuclear and cytoplasmic sites in mucous, ciliated, and basal cells and its inhibition by incubation either with 7,8-benzoflavone or at near 0°C. By electron microscopy, the nuclear localization of bound ^{3}H-BP was found to be primarily in the heterochromatin (Harris *et al.* 1973a).

The binding levels of BP to tracheal DNA in cultures from the experimental hamster model were found to vary among different strains of hamsters and also to be higher in weanling hamsters than in animals at progressively older ages (Kaufman *et al.* 1974).

Studies on the role of vitamin A in the inhibition of epithelial respiratory carcinogenesis begun in the animal model in vivo (Saffiotti *et al.* 1967, Harris *et al.* 1972b) were extended using the organ culture model. A state of vitamin A deficiency was found to enhance markedly the level of ^{3}H-BP binding to epithelial cells' DNA in organ cultures of hamster tracheas from vitamin A-deficient animals in comparison with those from pair-fed normal controls (Genta *et al.* 1974). Keratinized squamous metaplasia, induced by vitamin A deficiency in vivo, could be reversed in organ cultures of hamster tracheas by several retinoids, indicating that the organ culture system can be a valuable model for studies on the inhibitory mechanisms of carcinogenesis (Clamon *et al.* 1974, Sporn *et al.* 1974, 1975).

A number of other carcinogenesis studies on respiratory epithelial tissues in organ cultures were reported from several other laboratories and recently reviewed (Karbe and Park 1974, Lane 1978, Nettesheim and Griesemer 1978).

The neoplastic transformation in vitro of respiratory epithelium was recently obtained by exposure of rat tracheal organ cultures to *N*-methyl-*N'*-nitro-*N*-nitrosoguanidine followed by subculture of the epithelial cell outgrowths (Steele *et al.* 1977).

ORGAN CULTURE STUDIES IN HUMAN RESPIRATORY TISSUES

After establishing in vivo animal models and organ culture models for the target animal tissue, the next step was to apply the organ culture technique to the development of culture methods for the analogous human tissues. A particular effort was made to establish adequate methods for long-term maintenance of the human tissues in culture. The ability of human bronchial epithelium to metabolize procarcinogens into reactive forms that tightly bind to target cell macromolecules was initially studied using biochemical and autoradiographic techniques (Harris *et al.* 1974a).

The methods adopted for the organ culture of human bronchus included the following procedures. Human specimens are collected under aseptic conditions at surgery or at "immediate autopsy" (Trump *et al.* 1974) and immersed in Leibowitz medium L-15 at 0-4° C for transport to the culture laboratory. The tissues are then trimmed and cut into 1-2 sq. cm. pieces of bronchus and placed into 60 mm plastic Petri dishes with the epithelium facing upward. The medium used is CMRL 1066 (Grand Island Biological Co., Grand Island, NY) supplemented with insulin (1.0 μg/ml), hydrocortisone hemisuccinate (0.1 μg/ml), retinyl acetate (0.1 μg/ml), and antibiotics. For long-term cultures (up to six months), 5% heat-inactivated fetal calf serum is added, while for short-term studies (up to four weeks) no serum addition to the chemically defined medium is necessary. The cultures are incubated in an atmosphere of 50% O_2, 45% N_2, and 5% CO_2 in an airtight chamber kept on a rocking platform (10 cycles/minute). The culture conditions are described in detail elsewhere (Trump *et al.* 1974, Barrett *et al.* 1976, Harris 1976).

The interactions between chemical carcinogens and the target respiratory epithelium were examined using several complementary experimental approaches, which made it possible to study—directly at the level of human pathology—the patterns of carcinogen localization, metabolic activation mechanisms, interactions of carcinogens with target cells and cellular components, as well as the cellular and tissue responses. Morphological changes induced by chemical carcinogens directly applied to human tissue explants in culture can be studied by light microscopy, histochemistry, transmission and scanning electron microscopy, and autoradiography.

Studies are presently under way to identify the morphological response of human bronchial tissue directly exposed to carcinogens in culture; preliminary observations indicate that preneoplastic epithelial lesions are induced in vitro (Stoner *et al.,* unpublished observations).

An additional methodology which allows for the long-term maintenance of human tissues is that of xenotransplantation into athymic nude mice. By this technique it was possible to maintain adult human bronchial explants and tubular subsegmental bronchi as xenotransplants for over 14 months; hyperplastic and squamous metaplastic lesions were induced in this system with pellets containing 7,12-dimethylbenz[a]-anthracene (DMBA) (Harris *et al.* 1978b, Valerio *et al.,* unpublished results).

Autoradiographic techniques were used to determine the functional state of the various cell populations in the human respiratory epithelium by measurements of the incorporation and localization of radioactively labeled thymidine, uridine, and leucine (Barrett *et al.* 1976) and also to study the binding of labeled carcinogens in cultured human bronchus (Harris *et al.* 1976b). The latter method was used for determining the cellular distribution of bound ^{3}H-BP in the different cell types of the human bronchial epithelium. Binding levels were found to be fourfold higher in epithelial cells (basal, mucous, and ciliated) than they were in the fibroblasts.

Biochemical studies were conducted in human respiratory tissues cultured in a chemically defined medium to remove the biological variability associated with serum supplementation. Several classes of chemical procarcinogens were found to be enzymatically activated by human tissues to electrophilic metabolites that bind to DNA, including the following compounds: the polynuclear aromatic hydrocarbons, BP, DMBA, 3-methylcholanthrene, and dibenz[a,h]anthracene (Harris *et al.* 1974a, 1976a, b, 1977c, Yang *et al.* 1977); the *N*-nitrosamines, *N*-nitrosodimethylamine, *N*-nitrosodiethylamine, *N,N'*-dinitrosopiperazine, *N*-nitrosopyrrolidine, and *N*-nitrospiperidine (Harris *et al.* 1977a, b); a substituted hydrazine, 1,2-dimethylhydrazine (Harris *et al.* 1977b); and a mycotoxin, aflatoxin B_1 (Autrup *et al.,* unpublished results).

The carcinogen-DNA interaction is quantitatively controlled by the enzymatic systems required for the metabolic activation of the procarcinogens to the reactive form that binds to DNA. This mechanism was confirmed for BP in the cultured human tissues by modifying carcinogen-DNA binding levels with agents that respectively inhibit or enhance the carcinogen's metabolic activation (Harris *et al.* 1976b, 1977c, and in press).

The adducts formed between the ultimate metabolites of carcinogens and nucleic acids in the human tissues were isolated and directly identified. The structures of BP adducts with DNA and RNA, formed in human bronchial explants exposed to the carcinogen in culture, were identified (Jeffrey *et al.* 1977) and found to be similar to those that were isolated from the tissues of animal species, e.g., bovine bronchus (Weinstein *et al.* 1976), mouse epidermis (Moore *et al.* 1977), and cultured mouse and hamster cells (Shinohara and Cerutti 1977).

The experimental evidence developed in the last few years on the interaction of carcinogens with human tissues suggests a close *qualitative* similarity of response to carcinogens in experimental animals and in humans. From the *quantitative* point of view, however, marked differences in the metabolic activation and binding of carcinogens to target cells were found among different individuals in human studies, as well as among different strains and species in experimental animals. The human population is highly heterogeneous both from the genetic and the environmental point of view, as shown by human pharmacogenetic studies on xenobiotics (Vesell 1977). It may therefore be expected that the interindividual variations in the response to carcinogens may be analogous to those that could be found among a range of different animal species and strains. In the human organ culture system, a marked interindividual variation was found in the binding levels of both BP and DMBA to human bronchial DNA (Harris *et al.* 1976a, 1977c). This marked variation was confirmed also in studies with other human tissues in culture (Harris *et al., in press*). In studying the process of carcinogenesis in the human population from a public health point of view, we must be particularly concerned with the most susceptible individuals in a population, since they are the ones that have the highest risk for developing a neoplastic disease.

The metabolic conversion of procarcinogens to their reactive forms in human tissues is the basis for the trigger interaction that leads to self-replicating molecular injury, i.e., the type of toxic injury that requires cell replication for its expression, as in mutagenic or carcinogenic events. This type of toxicity is clearly distinct from the terminal type of toxicity leading to cell degeneration and death (Saffiotti 1977a).

The genetic damage inflicted to somatic cells by the interaction of substances that are both mutagenic and carcinogenic can only be detected if the target mammalian cells can replicate and show the phenotypic expression of their genetic damage. Somatic mammalian cell systems that are good indicators of mutagenesis may not have the enzymatic activity required for carcinogen activation, but this activation can be provided by adjacent cells having metabolic competence. Such a combined process involving two cell types has been clearly demonstrated in animal cells by Huberman and Sachs (1976) by cocultivating Chinese hamster V-79 cells (in which mutations can be detected using either ouabain or 8-azaguanine resistance as a marker) together with metabolically active cells (Syrian golden hamster embryo cells).

A human tissue-mediated mutagenesis system has now been developed by cocultivation of V-79 cells together with human bronchial explants, blood monocytes, or pulmonary macrophages (Hsu *et al.* 1978a, b, Harris *et al.* 1978b); V-79 cells do not effectively metabolize BP or its metabolite (−)r7,t8-dihydroxy-7,8-dihydrobenzo*[a]*pyrene (7,8-diol-BP) to ultimate mutagens and are not mutated by these compounds. However, when V-79 cells and human bronchial explants were cocultivated and exposed to either BP or its 7,8-diol, an increase in frequencies of ouabain-resistant mutations (2- to 60-fold) and in sister chromatid exchanges (2- to 3-fold) in the V-79 cells was observed. In this system, the mutagenic response was found to be proportional to the amount of human tissue in the cultures; a marked quantitative interindividual variation was observed. The metabolic activation in the human tissues was decreased by enzyme inhibitors leading to a decreased mutation frequency in V-79 cells (Hsu *et al.* 1978a, b).

This direct demonstration of mutagenic activity, obtained by metabolic activation of procarcinogens in human tissues, provides a new probe for the assessment of the responsiveness of human target tissues to environmental chemicals and may provide a valuable approach toward a quantitation of the susceptibility to carcinogens in humans. The wide-ranging interindividual variations in the response of human tissues to carcinogens may provide a basis for identifying individuals at high risk.

Additional work on the culture of human tissues for carcinogenesis studies has shown the metabolic activation of carcinogens by pulmonary alveolar macrophages (Autrup *et al.* 1978b). Several other studies, similar to those described above for human bronchi, have been conducted for human colon (Autrup *et al.* 1977, and in press), pancreatic duct (Harris *et al.* 1977c, Jones *et al.* 1977), and peripheral lung (Stoner *et al.,* in press). Work is under way to attempt to establish human epithelial cell cultures derived from these tissue explants (Stoner *et al.,* unpublished observations).

The development of these research methods is expected to provide an entirely new, experimentally controlled and quantifiable approach to the old problem of how to correlate animal and human observations in carcinogenesis (Saffiotti 1978) and to represent a focal point of observation in the correlations of carcinogenic effects at various levels of biological organization, from whole organisms to organs and tissues and from these to the cells and their molecular components.

ACKNOWLEDGMENTS

Work on the organ culture of respiratory tissues was conducted in the laboratories of the National Cancer Institute's Carcinogenesis Program, initially in the Lung Cancer Unit, Office of the Associate Director for Carcinogenesis (U. Saffiotti, M. B. Sporn, C. C. Harris, D. G. Kaufman, V. Genta) and subsequently in the Lung Cancer Branch (M. B. Sporn, C. C. Harris, D. G. Kaufman, V. Genta, G. H. Clamon) and in the Experimental Pathology Branch (U. Saffiotti, C. C. Harris, H. Autrup, I-C. Hsu, Y. Katoh, and G. Stoner); the human tissue studies were developed with the collaboration of the Department of Pathology, University of Maryland School of Medicine (B. F. Trump, L. A. Barrett, and E. M. McDowell) and the Department of Surgery, Veterans Administration Hospital, Washington, D.C. (P. Schafer). To all these, and to their co-workers, the authors wish to acknowledge their gratitude.

REFERENCES

Autrup, H., L. A. Barrett, F. E. Jackson, M. L. Jesudason, G. Stoner, P. Phelps, B. F. Trump, and C. C. Harris. 1978a. Explant culture of human colon. Gastroenterology (In press).

Autrup, H. N., C. C. Harris, G. D. Stoner, M. L. Jesudason, and B. F. Trump. 1977. Binding of chemical carcinogens to macromolecules in cultured human colon. J. Natl. Cancer Inst. 59:351–355.

Autrup, H., C. Harris, G. Stoner, J. Selkirk, P. Schafer, and B. Trump. 1978b. Metabolism of ^{3}H-benzo[a]pyrene by cultured human pulmonary alveolar macrophages. Lab. Invest. 38:217–223.

Barrett, L. A., E. M. McDowell, A. L. Frank, C. C. Harris, and B. F. Trump. 1976. Long-term organ culture of human bronchial epithelium. Cancer Res. 36:1003–1010.

Becci, P. J., E. M. McDowell, and B. F. Trump. 1978a. Studies of respiratory epithelium. II. Hamster trachea, bronchus and bronchioles. J. Natl. Cancer Inst. (In press).

Becci, P. J., E. M. McDowell, and B. F. Trump. 1978b. Studies of respiratory epithelium. IV. Histogenesis of epidermal metaplasia and carcinoma *in situ* in the hamster. J. Natl. Cancer Inst. (In press).

Becci, P. J., E. M. McDowell, and B. F. Trump. 1978c. Studies of respiratory epithelium. VI. Histogenesis of lung tumors induced by benzo[a]pyrene-ferric oxide in the hamster. J. Natl. Cancer Inst. (In press).

Boren, H. G., and L. J. Paradise. 1978. Cytokinetics of lung, *in* Pathogenesis and Therapy of Lung Cancer, C. C. Harris, ed., Marcel Dekker, New York, pp. 369–418.

Clamon, G., M. Sporn, J. Smith, and U. Saffiotti. 1974. α- and β-retinyl acetate reverse metaplasias of vitamin A deficiency in hamster trachea in organ culture. Nature 250:64–66.

Crocker, T. 1969. Effect of benzo[a]pyrene on hamster, rat, dog and monkey respiratory epithelia in organ culture, *in* Inhalation Carcinogenesis, M. G. Hanna, P. Nettesheim, and J. R. Gilbert, eds., AEC Symposium Series No. 18 (Conf-691001). Oak Ridge, Tennessee, U.S. Atomic Energy Commission, Division of Technical Information Extension, pp. 433–443.

Crocker, T. T. 1970. Bronchial mucosa of monkey and man in organ culture. Application to the study of bronchial carcinogenesis. Am. Rev. Resp. Dis. 101:443–445.

Crocker, T. T., and B. I. Neilsen. 1967. Effect of carcinogenic hydrocarbons on suckling rat trachea in living animals and in organ culture, *in* Lung Tumours in Animals, L. Severi, ed., Division of Cancer Research, University of Perugia, Perugia, Italy, pp. 765–787.

Crocker, T. T., B. I. Neilsen, and I. Lasnitzki. 1965. Carcinogenic hydrocarbons; effect on suckling rat trachea in organ culture. Arch. Environ. Health 10:240–250.

Crocker, T. T., and L. L. Sanders. 1970. Influence of vitamin A and 3,7-dimethyl-2,6-octadienal (Citral) on the effect of benzo[a]pyrene on hamster trachea in organ culture. Cancer Res. 30:1312–1318.

Della Porta, G., L. Kolb, and P. Shubik. 1958. Induction of tracheobronchial carcinomas in the Syrian golden hamster. Cancer Res. 18:592–597.

Farrell, R. L., and G. W. Davis. 1974. Effect of particulate benzo(a)-pyrene carrier on carcinogenesis in the respiratory tract of hamsters, *in* Experimental Lung Cancer. Carcinogenesis and Bioassays, E. Karbe and J. F. Park, eds., Springer-Verlag, Berlin, Heidelberg, New York, pp. 186–198.

Genta, V. M., D. G. Kaufman, C. C. Harris, J. M. Smith, M. B. Sporn, and U. Saffiotti. 1974. Vitamin A deficiency enhances binding of benzo[a]pyrene to tracheal epithelial DNA. Nature 247:48–49.

Hanna, M. G., Jr., P. Nettesheim, and J. R. Gilbert, eds. 1970. Inhalation Carcinogenesis. Atomic Energy Commission Symposium Series No. 18 (Conf-691001). Oak Ridge, Tennessee, U.S. Atomic Energy Commission, Division of Technical Extension, 524 pp.

Harris, C. 1976. Chemical carcinogenesis and experimental models using human tissues. Beitr. Path. 158:389–404.

Harris, C. C., ed. 1978. Pathogenesis and Therapy of Lung Cancer. Marcel Dekker, New York.

Harris, C. C., H. Autrup, R. Connor, L. A. Barrett, E. M. McDowell, and B. F. Trump. 1976a. Interindividual variation in binding of benzo[a]pyrene to DNA in cultured human bronchi. Science 194:1067–1069.

Harris, C. C., H. Autrup, and G. Stoner. 1978a. Metabolism of benzo[a]pyrene in cultured human tissues and cells, *in* Polycyclic Hydrocarbons and Cancer: Chemistry, Molecular Biology and Environment, P. O. P. Ts'o and H. V. Gelboin, eds., Academic Press, New York (In press).

Harris, C. C., H. Autrup, G. Stoner, E. M. McDowell, B. F. Trump, and P. Schafer. 1977a. Metabolism of acyclic and cyclic N-nitrosamines in cultured human bronchi. J. Natl. Cancer Inst. 59:1401–1406.

Harris, C. C., H. Autrup, G. Stoner, E. M. McDowell, B. F. Trump, and P. Schafer. 1977b. Metabolism of dimethylnitrosamine and 1,2-dimethylhydrazine in cultured human bronchi. Cancer Res. 37:2309–2311.

Harris, C. C., H. Autrup, G. D. Stoner, M. Valerio, E. Fineman, P. W. Schafer, L. A. Barrett, E. M. McDowell, and B. F. Trump. 1978b. Explant culture and xenotransplantation of human bronchi, *in* In Vivo Carcinogenesis. Guide to the Literature, Recent Advances and Laboratory Procedures, U. Saffiotti and H. Autrup, eds., National Cancer Institute Carcinogenesis Technical Report Series No. 44. Department of Health, Education and Welfare Publication No. (NIH) 78–844, Washington, D.C., pp. 144–151.

Harris, C. C., H. Autrup, G. Stoner, S. K. Yang, J. C. Leutz, H. V. Gelboin, J. K. Selkirk, R. J. Connor, L. A. Barrett, R. T. Jones, E. McDowell, and B. F. Trump. 1977c. Metabolism of benzo*[a]*pyrene and 7,12-dimethylbenz*[a]*anthracene in cultured human bronchus and pancreatic duct. Cancer Res. 37:3349–3355.

Harris, C. C., A. L. Frank, C. van Haaften, D. G. Kaufman, R. Connor, F. Jackson, L. A. Barrett, E. McDowell, and B. F. Trump. 1976b. Binding of [³H]benzo*[a]*pyrene to DNA in cultured human bronchus. Cancer Res. 36:1011–1018.

Harris, C., V. Genta, A. Frank, D. Kaufman, L. Barrett, E. McDowell, and B. Trump. 1974a. Carcinogenic polynuclear hydrocarbons bind to macromolecules in cultured human bronchi. Nature 252:68–69.

Harris, C. C., I. C. Hsu, G. D. Stoner, B. F. Trump, and J. K. Selkirk. 1978c. Human pulmonary alveolar macrophages metabolize benzo*[a]*pyrene to proximate and ultimate mutagens. Nature 272:633–634.

Harris, C. C., D. G. Kaufman, F. Jackson, J. M. Smith, P. Dedick, and U. Saffiotti. 1974b. Atypical cilia in the tracheobronchial epithelium of the hamster during respiratory carcinogenesis. J. Pathol. 114:17–19.

Harris, C. C., D. G. Kaufman, M. B. Sporn, H. Boren, F. Jackson, J. M. Smith, J. Pauley, P. Dedick, and U. Saffiotti. 1973a. Localization of benzo*[a]*pyrene-³H and alterations in nuclear chromatin caused by benzo*[a]*pyrene-ferric oxide in the hamster respiratory epithelium. Cancer Res. 33:2842–2848.

Harris, C. C., D. G. Kaufman, M. B. Sporn, and U. Saffiotti. 1973b. Histogenesis of squamous metaplasia and squamous cell carcinoma of the respiratory epithelium in an animal model. Cancer Chemother. Rep. 4:43–54.

Harris, C. C., D. G. Kaufman, M. B. Sporn, J. M. Smith, F. Jackson, and U. Saffiotti. 1973c. Ultrastructural effects of N-methyl-nitrosurea on the tracheobronchial epithelium of the Syrian golden hamster. Int. J. Cancer 12:259–269.

Harris, C. C., U. Saffiotti, and B. F. Trump. 1978d. Meeting report. Carcinogenesis studies in human cells and tissues. Cancer Res. 38:474–475.

Harris, C. C., M. B. Sporn, D. G. Kaufman, J. M. Smith, M. S. Baker, and U. Saffiotti. 1972a. Acute ultrastructural effects of benzo*[a]*pyrene and ferric oxide on the hamster tracheobronchial epithelium. Cancer Res. 31:1977–1981.

Harris, C. C., M. B. Sporn, D. G. Kaufman, J. M. Smith, F. E. Jackson, and U. Saffiotti. 1972b. Histogenesis of squamous metaplasia in the hamster tracheal epithelium caused by vitamin A deficiency or benzo*[a]*pyrene-ferric oxide. J. Natl. Cancer Inst. 48:743–761.

Henry, M. C., and D. G. Kaufman. 1973. Clearance of benzo*[a]*pyrene from hamster lungs after administration on coated particles. J. Natl. Cancer Inst. 51:1961–1964.

Henry, M. C., C. D. Port, and D. G. Kaufman. 1974. Role of particles in respiratory carcinogenesis bioassay, *in* Experimental Lung Cancer. Carcinogenesis and Bioassays, E. Karbe and J. F. Park, eds., Springer-Verlag, Berlin, Heidelberg, New York, pp. 173–185.

Hsu, I. C., H. Autrup, G. Stoner, B. F. Trump, and C. C. Harris. 1978a. Human blood monocytes and pulmonary alveolar macrophages metabolize benzo*[a]*pyrene to proximate and ultimate mutagens. Proceedings of the Environmental Mutagen Society, p. 54.

Hsu, I. C., H. Autrup, G. D. Stoner, B. F. Trump, J. K. Selkirk, and C. C. Harris. 1978b. Human bronchus-mediated mutagenesis of mammalian cells by carcinogenic polynuclear aromatic hydrocarbons. Proc. Natl. Acad. Sci. USA 75:2003–2007.

Huberman, E., and L. Sachs. 1976. Mutability of different genetic loci in mammalian cells by metabolically activated carcinogenic polycyclic hydrocarbons. Proc. Natl. Acad. Sci. USA pp. 188–192.

Jeffrey, A. M., I. B. Weinstein, K. W. Jennette, K. Grzeskowiak, K. Nakanishi, R. G. Harvey, H. Autrup, and C. Harris. 1977. Structures of benzo[a]pyrene-nucleic acid adducts formed in human and bovine bronchial explants. Nature 269:348–350.

Jones, R., L. Barrett, C. van Haaften, C. Harris, and B. Trump. 1977. Long-term organ culture of bovine and human pancreatic ducts. J. Natl. Cancer Inst. 58:557–565.

Karbe, E., and J. F. Park, eds. 1974. Experimental Lung Cancer. Carcinogenesis and Bioassays. Springer-Verlag, Berlin, Heidelberg, New York, 611 pp.

Kaufman, D. G., M. S. Baker, C. C. Harris, J. M. Smith, H. Boren, M. B. Sporn, and U. Saffiotti. 1972. Coordinated biochemical and morphologic examination of hamster tracheal epithelium. J. Natl. Cancer Inst. 49:783–792.

Kaufman, D. G., V. M. Genta, and C. C. Harris. 1974. Studies on carcinogen binding *in vitro* in isolated hamster tracheas, *in* Experimental Lung Cancer, E. Karbe and J. F. Park, eds., Springer-Verlag, Berlin, Heidelberg, New York, pp. 564–574.

Kaufman, D. G., V. M. Genta, C. C. Harris, J. M. Smith, M. B. Sporn, and U. Saffiotti. 1973. Binding of ^{3}H-labeled-benzo[a]pyrene to DNA in hamster tracheal epithelial cells. Cancer Res. 33:2837–2841.

Kaufman, D. G., and R. M. Madison. 1974. Synergistic effects of benzo[a]pyrene and N-methyl-N-nitrosourea on respiratory carcinogenesis in Syrian golden hamsters, *in* Experimental Lung Cancer. Carcinogenesis and Bioassays, E. Karbe and J. F. Park, eds., Springer-Verlag, Berlin, Heidelberg, New York, pp. 207–218.

Lane, B. P. 1978. In vitro studies, *in* Pathogenesis and Therapy of Lung Cancer, C. C. Harris, ed., Marcel Dekker, New York, pp. 419–444.

Lasnitzki, I. 1956. The effect of 3-4-benzpyrene on human foetal lung grown *in vitro*. Br. J. Cancer 10:510–516.

Lasnitzki, I. 1958. Observations on the effects of condensates from cigarette smoke on human foetal lung *in vitro*. Br. J. Cancer 12:547–552.

Lasnitzki, I. 1968. The effect of hydrocarbon-enriched fraction of cigarette smoke condensate on human fetal lung grown *in vitro*. Cancer Res. 28:510–516.

McDowell, E. M., L. A. Barrett, F. Glavin, C. C. Harris, and B. F. Trump. 1978a. Studies of respiratory epithelium. I. Human bronchus. J. Natl. Cancer Inst. (In press).

McDowell, E. M., J. S. McLaughlin, D. K. Merenyl, R. F. Kieffer, C. C. Harris, and B. F. Trump. 1978b. Studies of respiratory epithelium. V. Histogenesis of lung carcinomas in the human. J. Natl. Cancer Inst. (In press).

Montesano, R., U. Saffiotti, A. Ferrero, and D. G. Kaufman. 1974. Brief communication: Synergistic effects of benzo[a]pyrene and diethylnitrosamine on respiratory carcinogenesis in hamster. J. Natl. Cancer Inst. 53:1395–1397.

Montesano, R., U. Saffiotti, and P. Shubik. 1970. The role of topical and systemic factors in experimental respiratory carcinogenesis, *in* Inhalation Carcinogenesis, P. Nettesheim and J. R. Gilbert, eds., Atomic Energy Commission Symposium Series No. 18 (Conf-691001), Oak Ridge, Tennessee, U.S. Atomic Energy Commission, Division of Technical Information Extension, pp. 353–371.

Moore, P. D., M. Koreda, P. G. Wislocki, W. Levin, A. H. Conney, H. Yagi, and D. M. Jerina. 1977. In vitro reactions of the diastereomeric 9,10-expoxides of (+) and (−)-trans-7,8-dihydroxy-7,8-dihydrobenzo[a]pyrene with polyguanylic acid and evidence for formation of an enantiomer of each diastereomeric 9,10-epoxide from benzo[a]pyrene in mouse skin, *in* Drug Metabolism Concepts, D. M. Jerina, ed., ACS Symposium Series No. 44, American Chemical Society, pp. 127–154.

National Cancer Institute. 1976. Early lesions and the development of epithelial cancer. (Symposium sponsored by the Division of Cancer Cause and Prevention, National Cancer Institute, 1975). Cancer Res. 36:2475–2706.

Nettesheim, P., and R. A. Griesemer. 1978. Experimental models for studies of respiratory tract carcinogenesis, *in* Pathogenesis and Therapy of Lung Cancer, C. C. Harris, ed., Marcel Dekker, New York, pp. 75–188.

Nettesheim, P., M. G. Hanna, Jr., and J. W. Deatherage, Jr., eds. 1970. Morphology of Experimental Respiratory Carcinogenesis. Atomic Energy Commission Symposium Series No. 21 (Conf-700501), Oak Ridge, Tennessee, U.S. Atomic Energy Commission, Division of Technical Information Extension, 483 pp.

alekar, L., M. Kuschner, and S. Laskin. 1968. Effect of 3-methylcholanthrene on rat trachea in organ culture. Cancer Res. 28:2098–2104.

aradise, L. J., and H. G. Boren. 1978. Tumorigenesis and cytokinetics of hamster tracheal epithelium after exposure to *N*-methyl-*N*-nitrosourea (MNU). (Abstract) Proc. Am. Assoc. Cancer Res. 19:136.

affiotti, U. 1960. The histogenesis of experimental silicosis. I. Methods for the histological evaluation of experimentally induced dust lesions. Med. Lav. 51:10–17.

affiotti, U. 1962. The histogenesis of experimental silicosis. III. Early cellular reactions and the role of necrosis. Med. Lav. 53:5–18.

affiotti, U. 1969a. Experimental respiratory tract carcinogenesis, *in* Progress in Experimental Tumor Research, Vol. 11, F. Homburger, ed., Basel/New York, S. Karger, 1969, pp. 302–333.

affiotti, U. 1969b. Role of vitamin A in carcinogenesis. Am. J. Clin. Nutr. 8:1088.

affiotti, U. 1970a. Experimental respiratory tract carcinogenesis and its relations to inhalation exposures, *in* Inhalation Carcinogenesis, M. G. Hanna, Jr., P. Nettesheim, and J. R. Gilbert, eds., Atomic Energy Commission Symposium Series No. 18 (Conf-691001), Oak Ridge, Tennessee, U.S. Atomic Energy Commission, Division of Technical Information Extension, pp. 27–54.

affiotti, U. 1970b. Morphology of respiratory tumors induced in Syrian golden hamsters, *in* Morphology of Experimental Respiratory Carcinogenesis, P. Nettesheim, M. G. Hanna, Jr., and J. W. Deatherage, Jr., eds., Atomic Energy Commission Symposium Series No. 21 (Conf-700501), Oak Ridge, Tennessee, U.S. Atomic Energy Commission, Division of Technical Information Extension, pp. 245–254.

affiotti, U. 1972. The laboratory approach to the identification of environmental carcinogens, *in* Proceedings of the Ninth Canadian Cancer Research Conference, P. J. Scholenfield, ed., University of Toronto Press, Toronto, pp. 23–36.

affiotti, U. 1977a. Scientific bases of environmental carcinogenesis and cancer prevention: Developing an interdisciplinary science and facing its ethical implications. J. Toxicol. Environ. Health 2:1435–1447.

affiotti, U. 1977b. Identifying and defining chemical carcinogens, *in* Origins of Human Cancer, H. Hiatt, J. D. Watson, and J. Winsten, eds., Cold Spring Harbor Conference on Cell Proliferation, Vol. 4. Cold Spring Harbor Laboratory, Cold Spring Harbor, New York, pp. 1311–1326.

affiotti, U. 1978. Experimental identification of chemical carcinogens, risk evaluation and animal-to-human correlations. Environ. Health Perspect. 22:107–113.

affiotti, U., S. A. Borg, M. I. Grote, and D. B. Karp. 1964. Retention rates of particulate carcinogens in the lungs. Studies in an experimental model for lung cancer induction. Chicago Medical School Quarterly 24:10–17.

affiotti, U., F. Cefis, and L. H. Kolb. 1968. A method for the experimental induction of bronchogenic carcinoma. Cancer Res. 28:104–124.

affiotti, U., F. Cefis, L. H. Kolb, and P. Shubik. 1965. Experimental studies of the conditions of exposure to carcinogens for lung cancer induction. J. Air Pollut. Contr. Assoc. 15:23–25.

Saffiotti, U., F. Cefis, and P. Shubik. 1966. Histopathology and histogenesis of lung cancer induced in hamsters by carcinogens carried by dust particles, *in* Lung Tumours in Animals, L. Severi, ed., Division of Cancer Research, University of Perugia, Perugia, Italy, pp. 537–546.

Saffiotti, U., and D. G. Kaufman. 1975. Carcinogenesis of laryngeal carcinoma. Laryngoscope 85:454–467.

Saffiotti, U., R. Montesano, A. R. Sellakumar, and S. A. Borg. 1967. Studies on experimental lung cancer: Inhibition by vitamin A of the induction of tracheobronchial squamous metaplasia and squamous cell tumors. Cancer 20:857–864.

Saffiotti, U., R. Montesano, A. R. Sellakumar, F. Cefis, and D. G. Kaufman. 1972a. Respiratory tract carcinogenesis in hamsters induced by different numbers of administrations of benzo*[a]*pyrene and ferric oxide. Cancer Res. 32:1073–1081.

Saffiotti, U., R. Montesano, A. R. Sellakumar, and D. G. Kaufman. 1972b. Respiratory tract carcinogenesis induced in hamsters by different dose levels of benzo*[a]*pyrene and ferric oxide. J.Natl. Cancer Inst. 49:1199–1204.

Saffiotti, U., and A. Tommasini Degna. 1958. Studi sulla silicosi sperimentale da materiali referattari. I-Attività silicotigena di polveri di mattoni refrattari usati nei forni Martin. Med. Lav. 49:347–367.

Saffiotti, U., A. Tommasini Degna, and L. Mayer. 1960. The histogenesis of experimental silicosis. II-Cellular and tissue reactions in the histogenesis of pulmonary lesions. Med. Lav. 51:518–552.

Sellakumar, A. R., R. Montesano, U. Saffiotti, and D. G. Kaufman. 1973. Hamster respiratory carcinogenesis induced by benzo[a]pyrene and different dose levels of ferric oxide. J. Natl. Cancer Inst. 50:507–510.

Shinohara, K., and P. A. Cerutti. 1977. Excision repair of benzo[a]-deoxyguanosine adducts in baby hamster kidney 21/C93 cells and in secondary mouse embryo fibroblasts C57B1/6J. Proc. Natl. Acad. Sci. USA 74:979–983.

Shubik, P., G. Della Porta, G. Pietra, L. Tomatis, H. Rappaport, U. Saffiotti, and B. Toth. 1962. Factors determining the neoplastic response induced by carcinogens, in Biological Interactions in Normal and Neoplastic Growth, M. B. Brennan and W. L. Simpson, eds., Little, Brown, and Co., Boston, pp. 285–297.

Smith, J. M., M. B. Sporn, D. M. Berkowitz, T. Kakefuda, E. Callan, and U. Saffiotti. 1971. Isolation of enzymatically active nuclei from epithelial cells of the trachea. Cancer Res. 31:199–202.

Sporn, M. B., G. H. Clamon, N. M. Dunlop, D. L. Newton, J. M. Smith, and U. Saffiotti. 1975. Activity of vitamin A analogues in cell cultures of mouse epidermis and organ cultures of hamster trachea. Nature 253:47–50.

Sporn, M. B., G. H. Clamon, J. M. Smith, N. M. Dunlop, D. L. Newton, and U. Saffiotti. 1974. The reversal of keratinized squamous metaplastic lesions of vitamin A deficiency in tracheobronchial epithelium by vitamin A analogs in organ culture: A model system for anti-carcinogenesis studies, in Experimental Lung Cancer. Carcinogenesis and Bioassays, E. Karbe and J. F. Park, eds., Springer-Verlag, Berlin, Heidelberg, New York, pp. 575–582.

Steele, V. E., A. C. Marchok, and P. Nettesheim. 1977. Transformation of tracheal epithelium exposed in vitro to N-methyl-N'-nitro-N-nitrosoguanidine (MNNG). Int. J. Cancer 20:234–238.

Stoner, G. D., C. C. Harris, H. Autrup, B. F. Trump, W. W. Kingsbury, and G. Meyers. 1978. Explant culture of human peripheral lung tissue. I. Metabolism of benzo[a]pyrene. Lab. Invest. (In press).

Trump, B. F., E. McDowell, L. A. Barrett, A. L. Frank, and C. C. Harris. 1974. Studies of ultrastructure, cytochemistry, and organ culture of human bronchial epithelium, in Experimental Lung Cancer. Carcinogenesis and Bioassays, E. Karbe and J. F. Park, eds., Springer-Verlag, Berlin, Heidelberg, New York, pp. 548–563.

Trump, B. F., E. M. McDowell, F. Glavin, L. A. Barrett, P. J. Becci, W. Schurch, H. E. Kaiser, and C. C. Harris. 1978. Studies of respiratory carcinogenesis. III. Histogenesis of epidermoid metaplasia and carcinoma in situ in the human. J. Natl. Cancer Inst. (In press).

Vesell, E. S. 1977. Genetic and environmental factors affecting drug disposition in man. Clin. Pharmacol. Ther. 22:659–679.

Weinstein, I. B., A. M. Jeffrey, K. W. Jennette, S. H. Blobstein, R. G. Harvey, C. Harris, H. Kasai, and K. Nakanishi. 1976. Benzo[a]pyrene diol epoxides as intermediates in nucleic acid binding in vitro and in vivo. Science 193:592–595.

Yang, S. K., H. V. Gelboin, B. F. Trump, H. Autrup, and C. C. Harris. 1977. Metabolic activation of benzo[a]pyrene and binding to DNA in cultured human bronchus. Cancer Res. 37:1210–1215.

Carcinogens: Identification and Mechanisms of Action, edited by A. Clark Griffin and Charles R. Shaw. Raven Press, New York © 1979.

In Vitro Chemical Carcinogenesis

Charles Heidelberger and Sukdeb Mondal

University of Southern California Comprehensive Cancer Center, Los Angeles, California 90033

Dr. Frederick Becker's keynote address that opened this Symposium was erudite, elegant, and eloquent. He forgot, however, to mention a ninth TAM (thou art mortal), namely, that rat liver in vivo is much too complicated! Those of us who are not intellectually and technically able to cope with such formidable complexity have resorted to the development of simplified model systems that employ cell cultures for studying chemical carcinogenesis. These systems, and there are many, deal with relatively homogeneous cell populations cultured under reasonably defined conditions, away from the nutritional, physiological, and immunological complexities of the host animal. With such systems one can keep track of cell numbers, do bookkeeping, and come up with quantitative data. In most of these systems, cells that are not oncogenic and have a highly developed respect for each others' territory are treated with chemical carcinogens and give rise to populations or clones of cells with altered social behavior involving lack of respect for their neighbors' turf and that give rise to tumors on inoculation into syngeneic hosts; this latter property is the ultimate criterion of oncogenic transformation or in vitro carcinogenesis.

The title of this Symposium is "Carcinogens: Identification and Mechanisms of Action." The systems for in vitro carcinogenesis are useful both for identification and studies of mechanism, at the cellular and molecular levels.

In this presentation we will attempt to give some facts as to what can be done with such cell culture systems and not deal with the latest data from our laboratory, which will be published elsewhere in due course. Rather, we will present an incomplete review of the field. We have written more complete reviews than this one of carcinogenesis in vitro (Heidelberger 1973, 1975, 1977). This topic has also been reviewed by Casto and DiPaolo (1973), Mishra and DiMayorca (1974), and Freeman et al. (1975).

The first success in the transformation of cells with chemical carcinogens was achieved by Berwald and Sachs (1963, 1965) using primary or secondary cultures of Syrian hamster embryo cells and polycyclic hydrocarbons. This system has been used extensively by DiPaolo et al. (1969, 1971), Mager et al. (1977), and Pienta et al. (1977). This system is described elsewhere in this Symposium by Dr. Pienta, who has obtained an excellent correlation between the transformation frequency in these cells and the carcinogenic activity in vivo of a large number of compounds. The advantages of this system are that the cells are diploid, transformation can be scored in about 10 days, and there is essentially no spontaneous transformation. In our opinion some disadvantages are that there is considerable variability in response from one embryo to another, the cell population is heterogeneous, and the cloning efficiency is very low in the absence of a feeder layer.

The other type of system used for studies of carcinogenesis in vitro involves the use of permanent lines of cells from various species. These lines are generally aneuploid and take several weeks to score for transformation. However, they do have advantages in that they clone with high efficiency in the absence of a feeder layer, and multiple-transformed clones can be obtained in large quantities from a single nontransformed clone and used for critical comparisons of morphological, structural, antigenic, enzymatic, and metabolic properties. Such systems have been developed from C3H mouse prostate fibroblasts (Chen and Heidelberger 1969, Marquardt *et al.* 1974), C3H/10T1/2 mouse embryo fibroblasts (Reznikoff *et al.* 1973a,b), BALB/3T3 clones (DiPaolo *et al.* 1972, Kakunaga 1973), high passage rat embryo cells (Freeman *et al.* 1975), mouse embryo cells infected with leukemia virus (Rhim *et al.* 1974), rat embryo cells expressing an endogenous oncornavirus (Rasheed *et al.* 1976), hamster BHK21 cells (Mishra and DiMayorca 1974, Styles 1977), and guinea pig embryo cells (Evans and DiPaolo 1975). We are aware of only one report of the chemical transformation of human diploid cells, which was accomplished by Kakunaga (1977), with 4-nitroquinoline-N-oxide (NQO) and N-methyl-N'-nitro-N-nitrosoguanidine (MNNG).

All of the systems mentioned above involve fibroblasts. Consequently, the tumors induced by inoculation of transformed cells into syngeneic hosts are sarcomas. There have been efforts to develop quantitative systems for the chemical transformation of epithelial cells that would give rise to carcinomas in suitable hosts. Such systems would be relevant to the quantitatively more numerous carcinomas in human malignancy. The effort has been devoted primarily to cultured rat hepatocytes, and although there are reports of chemical transformation of such cultures (Williams *et al.* 1973, Montesano *et al.* 1973, 1975, Yamaguchi and Weinstein 1975, Borenfreund *et al.* 1975), in general the results could not be quantitated; sometimes undifferentiated sarcomas were induced, and no demonstration of the production of hepatomas on inoculation of the transformed liver cells has appeared. Similarly, although epithelial cell cultures have been obtained from mouse skin (Elias *et al.* 1974, Fusenig and Worst 1974), they have not been transformed consistently by chemical carcinogens. Hashimoto and Kitagawa (1974) have demonstrated the neoplastic transformation by nitrosamines of cultured rat urinary bladder epithelial cells. Clearly, more effort is needed to provide suitable epithelial cell transformation systems, and such work is ongoing in our laboratory and others.

Since this review is not intended to be complete, we will illustrate the usefulness and applications of the use of permanent cell lines for studies of carcinogenesis in vitro primarily with examples chosen from our own research.

The C3H/10T1/2 mouse embryo fibroblast system represents our example of a cloned permanent cell line derived from C3H mouse embryos. It is tetraploid, has a low saturation density, has a very low incidence of spontaneous transformation when properly cared for, and does not give rise to tumors when 10^7 cells are inoculated into irradiated C3H mice (Reznikoff *et al.* 1973b). On treatment with polycyclic hydrocarbons, the cells lose their density-dependent inhibition of replication and pile-up, after a confluent monolayer is reached, to give foci of transformed cells that give rise to fibrosarcomas on inoculation into immuno-suppressed C3H mice (Reznikoff *et al.* 1973a). They also exhibit several other characteristics of the transformed fibroblast phenotype (Jones *et al.* 1976b). There was a close correlation between the number of transformed foci produced and the carcinogenic activity of a series of polycyclic hydrocarbons. However, it is not possible at present to determine accurately the transformation frequency, because there is an inverse relationship between the number of cells plated and the number of transformed colonies produced (Reznikoff *et al.* 1973a, Haber *et al.* 1977). In spite of this, the system has been used in a number of laboratories, and in addition to polycyclic hydrocarbons, the cells have been transformed by X-rays (Terzaghi and Little 1976), ultraviolet light (Chan and Little 1976), cancer chemotherapeutic agents (Jones *et al.* 1976a, Benedict *et al.* 1977), cigarette smoke condensates (Benedict *et al.* 1975), hair dyes (Benedict 1976), and alkylating agents (Bertram and Heidelberger 1974). In this system, decreasing the concentration of fetal calf serum in the medium somewhat increases the transformation frequency (Bertram 1977).

In our laboratory we have devoted our major attention to the use of these systems for the elucidation of cellular and molecular mechanisms of chemical carcinogenesis. One area of particular interest has been metabolic activation of polycyclic aromatic hydrocarbons (PAH). The pioneering metabolic investigations by Boyland led him to postulate (1950) that epoxides were the intermediates in the metabolism of these hydrocarbons. Subsequent work by Sims and Grover (reviewed 1974) suggested that epoxides could be the ultimately carcinogenic form of PAH. In collaboration with these researchers, we showed (Grover *et al.* 1971) that in mouse prostate cells the K-region epoxides (more correctly termed arene oxides) were more active than the parent hydrocarbons and the corresponding phenols and dihydrodiols at producing oncogenic transformation (Marquardt *et al.* 1972), in being covalently bound to DNA, RNA, and proteins (Kuroki *et al.* 1971), in producing mutations to 8-azaguanine resistance in Chinese hamster cells (Huberman *et al.* 1971), and in transforming hamster embryo cells (Huberman *et al.* 1972). Moreover, in the mouse prostate cells, inhibition of mixed-function oxidase activity by 7,8-benzoflavone (BF) abolished, and induction by benz[a]anthracene increased, the transformation produced by 3-methylcholanthrene (MCA) (Marquardt and Heidelberger 1972). Those findings lent strong support to the hypothesis that the cytochrome P_{450} mixed-function oxidases produced the activation of MCA. Subsequently, further evidence came from the studies in C3H/10T1/2 cells by Nesnow and Heidelberger (1976), who repeated the previous observations and correlated them with total metabolism of MCA to water-soluble products and determination of aryl hydrocarbon hydroxylase. Furthermore, inhibition of epoxide hydrase increased transformation by MCA, indicating that that enzyme was functioning primarily to detoxify the intermediate epoxide. More recently, the monumental progress in determining that the ultimate metabolically active form of benzo[a]pyrene is the anti-7,8-dihydroxy-7,8-dihydro-9,10-epoxide is reviewed elsewhere in the Symposium (see pages 399 to 418, this volume, Weinstein 1979). This diol epoxide is very active at transforming Syrian hamster embryo cells (Huberman et al. 1977), and the non-K-region diol epoxide of 7-methylbenz[a]anthracene is active in transforming mouse prostate fibroblasts (Marquardt et al. 1977).

Turning to a more biological problem, Bertram and Heidelberger (1974) showed that the transformation of synchronized C3H/10T1/2 cells by the short-acting carcinogen that does not require metabolic activation, i.e., MNNG, was highly phase specific. The highest transformation frequency was obtained if the MNNG was added about three hours prior to the onset of DNA synthesis. MNNG was a powerful inducer of alkali-labile lesions in the cellular DNA, which were subsequently repaired (Peterson et al. 1974a), but in synchronized cells, this damage and repair was not correlated with the phase-specific transformation (Peterson et al. 1974b). The transformation of these same synchronized cells by the cancer chemotherapeutic agent, arabinosylcytosine, was also phase specific; however, with this compound, the S phase was the most sensitive (Jones et al. 1977).

With respect to the cellular mechanisms of chemical carcinogenesis, one of the most important general questions is whether carcinogens transform normal cells into cancer cells, as most commonly assumed, or whether the carcinogen somehow selects for preexisting cancer cells. There was no way to approach this question in whole animals. However, in the mouse prostate system, Mondal and Heidelberger (1970) found that single cells in individual dishes were transformed by MCA such that every treated cell gave rise to transformed clones. This extraordinarily high transformation frequency eliminates the selection hypothesis and establishes that the chemical does transform these cells directly. Similar conclusions have subsequently been reached in several other systems.

Another hierarchical question is whether the carcinogen transforms cells by itself or accomplishes the transformation indirectly by "switching-on" a "latent" C-type RNA tumor virus (oncornavirus), as has been suggested in the "oncogene" hypothesis of Huebner and Todaro (1969). This hypothesis was carefully examined by Rapp et al. (1975), who found that in over 20 clones of C3H/10T1/2 cells transformed to malignancy by various carcinogens there was no detectable production of infectious murine leukemia-sarcoma virus as detected by the XC test, no detectable P_{30} group-specific antigen, and no detectable reverse transcriptase. Thus, there was no "switch-on" of infectious oncornaviruses or their cores during the transformation of these cells. However, it was possible to obtain contact-inhibited, nonmalignant cells from AKR mice and to transform these to malignancy with carcinogens. All such clones, whether or not transformed, produced infectious virus, viral antigens, and reverse transcriptase (Rapp *et al.* 1975). From these experiments it can be concluded that in this system the genome of the cell, and not the transformed phenotype, determines the expression of endogenous virus. The treatment of nontransformed and transformed C3H/10T1/2 cells with iododeoxyuridine (IUdR) caused the sequential expression of reverse transcriptase, P_{30} antigen, and infectious virus; hence, the proviral information is present in the genome of these C3H cells (Rapp *et al.* 1975). However, its expression is irrelevant to transformation, since the endogenous virus so elicited is not transforming, and IUdR does not transform these cells. If the "switch-on" of endogenous viruses were important in the process of chemical carcinogenesis, IUdR should be a potent carcinogen in vivo, which it is not. Similar lack of involvement of an oncornavirus in the chemical transformation of Syrian hamster embryo cells has been found by Reitz *et al.* (1977). Thus, there is no "switch-on" of endogenous oncornaviruses or their cores during the chemical transformation of C3H/10T1/2 or hamster embryo cells.

What about the "switch-on" of the transcription of oncornavirus-specific RNA? Getz *et al.* (1978) found, using a DNA probe complementary to the entire murine leukemia virus genome, in both nontransformed and transformed C3H/10T1/2 cells that there was transcription of about 25% of the RNA sequences from the proviral DNA. This result is difficult to interpret, but whatever the explanation, it is clearly unrelated to chemical transformation. A more critical experiment asked whether there was any transcription of RNA complementary to the *src* gene of the murine sarcoma virus, and in appropriate molecular hybridization experiments no such transcription was detected in transformed C3H/10T1/2 cells (E. M. Scolnick, personal communication). Thus, it seems reasonably safe to conclude that in this model *system,* the carcinogen "does its own thing" without the intermediacy of an endogenous oncornavirus, its core, or its *src*-specific RNA.

One of the major characteristics of PAH-induced sarcomas in vivo is that they have individual, noncross-reacting, tumor-specific transplantation antigens (TSTA) (Prehn 1962). Since this is a sophisticated and poorly understood phenomenon, it seemed appropriate to check the validity of our cell culture models with respect to this property. It was soon found (Mondal *et al.* 1970) that individual clones of mouse prostate fibroblasts that had undergone malignant transformation with MCA had TSTA's detectable by classical tumor transplantation rejection techniques. Moreover, pairs of transformed clones derived from the same dishes were not cross-reactive, in analogy with the in vivo results. Nontransformed clones were not detectably antigenic nor were the majority of a few spontaneously transformed clones that were examined. Using the more rapid and quantitative techniques of indirect immunofluorescence and lympho-cyte-mediated cytotoxicity, Embleton and Heidelberger (1972) found, in carefully cloned nontransformed cells, that multiple, chemically induced transformants had individual TSTA's. This shows that these antigens are produced on the cell membrane during the process of transformation and were not selected from preexisting antigens on a mixed population of nontransformed cells. We also found (Mondal *et al.* 1971) that revertants selected from transformed mouse prostate fibroblasts lost their TSTA's. The C3H/10T1/2 cells were then tested in a similar series of experiments, and it was found (Embleton and Heidelberger 1975) that transformed clones also expressed individual TSTA's on their surface membranes. However, it was found that transformed clones expressed a common embryonic antigen, which was not detected in the nontransformed cells, even though they were embryonic in origin. It is clear that there are many advantages in using cell cultures to study the origin and possible relevance to transformation of TSTA's, rather than in whole animals where immunoselection can operate, and such work is now in progress in our and other laboratories.

The relationship between mutagenesis and carcinogenesis is a vitally important subject for study, and the enormous activity in this field is beyond the scope of this presentation. Suffice it to say that in our laboratory we are attempting to develop methods whereby mutation and transformation frequencies can be measured simultaneously in C3H/10T1/2 cells treated with various carcinogens. Such a study would doubtless be a more relevant comparison than between those two parameters measured in different phyla.

The Bertner award at this Symposium is very justly being awarded to Drs. I. Berenblum and P. Shubik for their pioneering research on the two-stage process of chemical carcinogenesis in mouse skin (Berenblum and Shubik 1947). This field was greatly advanced by Hecker (1971), who isolated and determined the structure of the active promoting constituents of croton oil to be phorbol esters. We have now established the two-stage transformation of C3H/10T1/2 cells (Mondal *et al.* 1976). This process can be demonstrated by using a subeffec-tive dose of a PAH, which does not transform the cells, followed after five days with continual addition to the medium of 12-0-tetradecanoyl-phorbol-13-acetate (TPA), the most active constituent of croton oil, which by itself does not transform the cells. However, in the above sequence, the compounds pro-duced a high level of transformation. In analogy with mouse skin, treatment in the reverse order did not lead to enhanced transformation; there was a close correlation between the promoting activities of a series of phorbol esters in vivo and in the cultures, and other promoting agents such as anthralin are also effective in the C3H/10T1/2 cells. In our hands (Mondal and Heidelberger 1976) ultraviolet light acts as a pure initiator. Moreover, TPA enhances the X-ray-induced transformation of these cells (Kennedy *et al.* 1978).

The establishment of two-stage transformation in cell culture provides us with the opportunity for studying the cellular and molecular mechanisms of initiation and promotion separately. In looking at the effects of TPA on DNA synthesis in these cells, we discovered that there was no stimulation of thymidine incorporation or an increase in the saturation density (Peterson *et al.* 1977), which is unlike the massive hyperplasia produced by these compounds on mouse skin. We are now investigating other aspects of promoter action, as is Dr. Weinstein (see pages 399 to 418, this volume).

In this brief and thus incomplete review we have tried to illustrate the general utility of studies of carcinogenesis in vitro by citing a few examples from our own research. Such systems have already demonstrated their utility in studies of the cellular and molecular mechanisms of chemical carcinogenesis, where they appear to be valid models for in vivo carcinogenesis. Moreover, with the great societal and political pressures to screen for a large number of environmental carcinogens, these systems have a great potential for acting as highly relevant systems (of malignant transformation) for prescreening large numbers of compounds. Such systems are considerably more expensive and time consuming than the Ames test in *Salmonella typhimurium* (Ames *et al.* 1975). Nevertheless, they are much faster and less expensive than the in vivo tests that require that hundreds of rodents be treated throughout their lifetimes. And the studies of Pienta (1977, 1979, see pages 123 to 143, this volume) show clearly that the transformation of hamster embryo cells correlates very closely with in vivo carcinogenic activities of a large series of compounds. We are currently working toward this end with the C3H/10T1/2 cell system, in which additional metabolic activation must be provided for certain classes of carcinogens. On the other hand, since promoting agents do not appear to require metabolic activation, the C3H/10T1/2 cell system may prove more useful for the prescreening of promoters than for complete carcinogens, and there is every reason to believe that promoting agents in the environment represent a severe health hazard, perhaps as great as some complete carcinogens.

REFERENCES

Ames, B. N., J. McCann, and E. Yamasaki. 1975. Methods for detecting carcinogens and mutagens with the *Salmonella*/mammalian-microsome mutagenicity test. Mutat. Res. 31:347–368.

Benedict, W. F. 1976. Morphological transformation and chromosomal aberrations produced by two hair dye components. Nature 260:368–369.

Benedict, W. F., A. Banerjee, A. Gardner, and P. A. Jones. 1977. Induction of morphological transformation in mouse C3H/10T1/2 Clone 8 cells and chromosomal damage in hamster $A(T_1)$ CL-3 cells by cancer chemotherapeutic agents. Cancer Res. 37:2202–2208.

Benedict, W. F., N. Rucker, J. Faust, and R. E. Kouri. 1975. Malignant transformation of mouse cells by cigarette smoke condensate. Cancer Res. 35:857–860.

Berenblum, I., and P. Shubik. 1947. A new quantitative approach to the study of the stages of chemical carcinogenesis in the mouse's skin. Br. J. Cancer 1:383–391.

Bertram, J. S. 1977. Effects of serum concentration on the expression of carcinogen-induced transformation in the C3H/10T1/2 Cl 8 cell line. Cancer Res. 37:514–523.

Bertram, J. S., and C. Heidelberger. 1974. Cell cycle dependency of oncogenic transformation induced by N-methyl-N′-nitro-N-nitrosoguanidine in culture. Cancer Res. 34:526–537.

Berwald, Y., and L. Sachs. 1963. In vitro transformation with chemical carcinogens. Nature 200:1182–1184.

Berwald, Y., and L. Sachs. 1965. In vitro transformation of normal cells to tumor cells by carcinogenic hydrocarbons. J. Natl. Cancer Inst. 35:641–661.

Borenfreund, E., P. J. Higgins, M. Steinglass, and A. Bendich. 1975. Properties and malignant transformation of established rat liver parenchymal cells in culture. J. Natl. Cancer Inst. 55:375–384.

Boyland, E. 1950. The biological significance of metabolism of polycyclic compounds. Symp. Biochem. Soc. 5:40–54.

Casto, B. C., and J. A. DiPaolo. 1973. Virus, chemicals, and cancer. Prog. Med. Virol. 16:1–47.

Chan, G. L., and J. B. Little. 1976. Induction of oncogenic transformation in vitro by ultraviolet light. Nature 264:442–444.

Chen, T. T., and C. Heidelberger. 1969. Quantitative studies on the malignant transformation in vitro of cells derived from adult C3H mouse ventral prostate. Int. J. Cancer 4:166–178.

DiPaolo, J. A., P. Donovan, and R. L. Nelson. 1969. Quantitative studies of in vitro transformation by chemical carcinogens. J. Natl. Cancer Inst. 42:867–874.

DiPaolo, J. A., R. L. Nelson, and P. J. Donovan. 1971. Morphological, oncogenic, and karyological characteristics of Syrian hamster embryo cells transformed in vitro by carcinogenic polycyclic hydrocarbons. Cancer Res. 31:1118–1127.

DiPaolo, J. A., K. Takano, and N. C. Popescu. 1972. Quantitation of chemically induced neoplastic transformation of BALB/3T3 cloned cell lines. Cancer Res. 32:2686–2695.

Elias, P. M., S. H. Yuspa, M. Gullino, D. L. Morgan, R. R. Bates, and M. A. Lutzner. 1974. In vitro neoplastic transformation of mouse skin cells: Morphology and ultrastructure of cells and tumors. J. Invest. Dermatol. 62:569–581.

Embleton, M. J., and C. Heidelberger. 1972. Antigenicity of clones of mouse prostate cells transformed in vitro. Int. J. Cancer 9:8–18.

Embleton, M. J., and C. Heidelberger. 1975. Neoantigens on chemically transformed cloned C3H mouse embryo cells. Cancer Res. 35:2049–2055.

Evans, C. H., and J. A. DiPaolo. 1975. Neoplastic transformation of guinea pig fetal cells in culture induced by chemical carcinogens. Cancer Res. 35:1035–1044.

Freeman, A. E., H. J. Igel, and P. J. Price. 1975. Carcinogenesis in vitro. 1. In vitro transformation of rat embryo cells: Correlation with the known tumorigenic activities of chemicals in rodents. In Vitro 11:107–115.

Fusenig, N. E., and P. K. M. Worst. 1974. Mouse epidermal cell cultures. 1. Isolation and cultivation of epidermal cells from adult mouse skin. J. Invest. Dermatol. 63:187–193.

Getz, M. J., P. K. Elder, and H. L. Moses. 1978. Equivalent expression of endogenous murine leukemia virus-related genes in C3H/10T1/2 cells and chemically transformed derivative cells. Cancer Res. 38:566–569.

Grover, P. L., P. Sims, E. Huberman, H. Marquardt, T. Kuroki, and C. Heidelberger. 1971. In vitro transformation of rodent cells by K-region derivatives of polycyclic hydrocarbons. Proc. Natl. Acad. Sci. USA 68:1098–1101.

Haber, D. A., D. A. Fox, W. S. Dynan, and W. G. Thilly. 1977. Cell density dependence of focus formation in the C3H/10T1/2 transformation assay. Cancer Res. 37:1644–1648.

Hashimoto, Y., and H. S. Kitagawa. 1974. In vitro neoplastic transformation of epithelial cells of rat urinary bladder by nitrosamines. Nature 252:497–499.

Hecker, E. 1971. Isolation and characterization of the cocarcinogenic principles from croton oil. Methods Cancer Res. 6:439–484.

Heidelberger, C. 1973. Chemical oncogenesis in culture. Adv. Cancer Res. 18:317–366.

Heidelberger, C. 1975. Chemical carcinogenesis. Ann. Rev. Biochem. 44:79–121.

Heidelberger, C. 1977. Oncogenic transformation of rodent cell lines by chemical carcinogens, *in* Origins of Human Cancer, H. H. Hiatt, J. D. Watson, and J. A. Winsten, eds., Cold Spring Harbor Laboratory, Cold Spring Harbor, New York, pp. 1513–1520.

Huberman, E., L. Aspiras, C. Heidelberger, P. L. Grover, and P. Sims. 1971. Mutagenicity to mammalian cells of epoxides and other derivatives of polycyclic hydrocarbons. Proc. Natl. Acad. Sci. USA 68:3195–3199.

Huberman, E., T. Kuroki, H. Marquardt, J. K. Selkirk, C. Heidelberger, P. L. Grover, and P. Sims. 1972. Transformation of hamster embryo cells by epoxides and other derivatives of polycyclic hydrocarbons. Cancer Res. 32:1391–1396.

Huebner, R. J., and G. J. Todaro. 1969. Oncogenes of RNA tumor viruses as determinants of cancer. Proc. Natl. Acad. Sci. USA 64:1087–1094.

Jones, P. A., M. S. Baker, J. S. Bertram, and W. F. Benedict. 1977. Cell cycle-specific oncogenic transformation of C3H/10T1/2 clone 8 mouse embryo cells by 1-β-D-arabinofuranosylcytosine. Cancer Res. 37:2214–2217.

Jones, P. A., W. F. Benedict, M. S. Baker, S. Mondal, U. Rapp, and C. Heidelberger. 1976a. Oncogenic transformation of C3H/10T1/2 clone 8 mouse embryo cells by halogenated pyrimidine nucleosides. Cancer Res. 36:101–107.

Jones, P. A., W. E. Laug, A. Gardner, C. A. Nye, L. M. Fink, and W. F. Benedict. 1976b. In vitro correlates of transformation in C3H/10T1/2 clone 8 mouse cells. Cancer Res. 36:2863–2867.

Kakunaga, T. 1973. Quantitative system for assay of malignant transformation by chemical carcinogens using a clone derived from BALB/3T3. Int. J. Cancer 12:463–473.

Kakunaga, T. 1977. The transformation of human diploid cells by chemical carcinogens, in Origins of Human Cancer, H. H. Hiatt, J. D. Watson, and J. A. Winsten, eds., Cold Spring Harbor Laboratory, Cold Spring Harbor, New York, pp. 1537–1548.

Kennedy, A. R., S. Mondal, C. Heidelberger, and J. B. Little. 1978. Enhancement of X-ray transformation by 12-0-tetradecanoyl-phorbol-13-acetate in a cloned line of C3H mouse embryo cells. Cancer Res. 38:439–443.

Kuroki, T., E. Huberman, H. Marquardt, J. K. Selkirk, C. Heidelberger, P. L. Grover, and P. Sims. 1971. Binding of K-region epoxides and other derivatives of benz[a]anthracene and dibenz[a,h]anthracene to DNA, RNA, and proteins of transformable cells. Chem.-Biol. Interact. 4:389–397.

Mager, R., E. Huberman, S. K. Yang, H. V. Gelboin, and L. Sachs. 1977. Transformation of normal hamster cells by benzo[a]pyrene diol-epoxide. Int. J. Cancer 19:814–817.

Marquardt, H., and C. Heidelberger. 1972. Influence of "feeder cells" and inducers and inhibitors of microsomal mixed-function oxidases on hydrocarbon-induced malignant transformation of cells derived from C3H mouse prostate. Cancer Res. 32:721–725.

Marquardt, H., S. Baker, B. Tierney, P. L. Grover, and P. Sims. 1977. The metabolic activation of 7-methylbenz[a]anthracene: The induction of malignant transformation and mutation in mammalian cells by non-K-region dihydrodiols. Int. J. Cancer 19:828–833.

Marquardt, H., T. Kuroki, E. Huberman, J. K. Selkirk, C. Heidelberger, P. L. Grover, and P. Sims. 1972. Malignant transformation of cells derived from mouse prostate by epoxides and other derivatives of polycyclic hydrocarbons. Cancer Res. 32:716–720.

Marquardt, H., T. E. Sodergren, P. Sims, and P. L. Grover. 1974. Malignant transformation in vitro of mouse fibroblasts by 7,12-dimethylbenz[a]-anthracene and by their K-region derivatives. Int. J. Cancer 13:304–310.

Mishra, N. K., and G. DiMayorca. 1974. In vitro malignant transformation of cells by chemical carcinogens. Biochim. Biophys. Acta 355:205–219.

Mondal, S., and C. Heidelberger. 1970. In vitro malignant transformation by methylcholanthrene of the progeny of single cells derived from C3H mouse prostate. Proc. Natl. Acad. Sci. USA 65:219–225.

Mondal, S., and C. Heidelberger. 1976. Transformation of 10T1/2 Cl 8 mouse embryo fibroblasts by ultraviolet irradiation and a phorbol ester. Nature 260:710–711.

Mondal, S., D. W. Brankow, and C. Heidelberger. 1976. Two-stage chemical oncogenesis in cultures of 10T1/2 cells. Cancer Res. 36:2254–2260.

Mondal, S., M. J. Embleton, H. Marquardt, and C. Heidelberger. 1971. Production of variants of decreased malignancy and antigenicity from clones transformed in vitro by methylcholanthrene. Int. J. Cancer 8:410–420.

Mondal, S., P. T. Iype, L. M. Griesbach, and C. Heidelberger. 1970. Antigenicity of cells derived from mouse prostate cells after malignant transformation in vitro by carcinogenic hydrocarbons. Cancer Res. 30:1593–1597.

Montesano, R., L. Saint Vincent, and L. Tomatis. 1973. Malignant transformation in vitro of rat liver cells by dimethylnitrosamine and N-methyl-N'-nitro-N-nitrosoguanidine. Br. J. Cancer 28:215–220.

Montesano, R., L. Saint Vincent, C. Drevon, and L. Tomatis. 1975. Production of epithelial and mesenchymal tumours with rat liver cells transformed in vitro. Int. J. Cancer 16:550–558.

Nesnow, S., and C. Heidelberger. 1976. The effect of modifiers of microsomal enzymes on chemical oncogenesis in cultures of C3H mouse cell lines. Cancer Res. 36:1801–1808.

Peterson, A. R., J. S. Bertram, and C. Heidelberger. 1974a. DNA damage and its repair in transformable mouse fibroblasts treated with N-methyl-N'-nitro-N-nitrosoguanidine. Cancer Res. 34:1592–1599.

Peterson, A. R., J. S. Bertram, and C. Heidelberger. 1974b. Cell cycle dependency of DNA damage and its repair in transformable mouse fibroblasts treated with N-methyl-N'-nitro-N-nitrosoguanidine. Cancer Res. 34:1600–1607.

Peterson, A. R., S. Mondal, D. W. Brankow, W. Thon, and C. Heidelberger. 1977. Effects of promoters on DNA synthesis in 10T1/2 mouse fibroblasts. Cancer Res. 37:3223–3227.

Pienta, R. J. 1979. A hamster embryo cell model system for identifying carcinogens, *in* Carcinogens: Identification and Mechanisms of Action (The University of Texas System Cancer Center 31st Annual Symposium on Fundamental Cancer Research, 1978), A. C. Griffin and C. R. Shaw, eds., Raven Press, pp. 123–143.

Pienta, R. J., J. A. Poiley, and W. B. Lebherz. 1977. Morphological transformation of early passage golden Syrian hamster embryo cells derived from cryopreserved primary cultures as a reliable in vitro bioassay for identifying diverse carcinogens. Int. J. Cancer 19:642–655.

Prehn, R. T. 1962. Specific isoantigenicities among chemically induced tumors. Ann. N.Y. Acad. Sci. 101:107–113.

Rapp, U. R., R. C. Nowinski, C. A. Reznikoff, and C. Heidelberger. 1975. The role of endogenous oncornaviruses in chemically induced transformation. 1. Transformation independent of virus production. Virology 65:392–409.

Rasheed, S., A. E. Freeman, M. B. Gardner, and R. J. Huebner. 1976. Acceleration of transformation of rat embryo cells by rat type C virus. J. Virol. 18:776–782.

Reitz, M. S., W. C. Saxinger, R. C. Ting, R. C. Gallo, and J. A. DiPaolo. 1977. Lack of expression of type C hamster virus after neoplastic transformation of hamster embryo fibroblasts by benzo*[a]*pyrene. Cancer Res. 37:3585–3589.

Reznikoff, C. A., J. S. Bertram, D. W. Brankow, and C. Heidelberger. 1973a. Quantitative and qualitative studies of chemical transformation of cloned C3H mouse embryo cells sensitive to postconfluence inhibition of cell division. Cancer Res. 33:3239–3249.

Reznikoff, C. A., D. W. Brankow, and C. Heidelberger. 1973b. Establishment and characterization of a cloned line of C3H mouse embryo cells sensitive to postconfluence inhibition of division. Cancer Res. 33:3231–3238.

Rhim, J. S., D. K. Park, E. K. Weisburger, and J. A. Weisburger. 1974. Evaluation of an in vitro assay system for carcinogens based on prior infection of rodent cells with nontransforming RNA tumor virus. J. Natl. Cancer Inst. 52:1167–1173.

Sims, P., and P. L. Grover. 1974. Epoxides in polycyclic aromatic hydrocarbon metabolism and carcinogenesis. Adv. Cancer Res. 20:166–274.

Styles, J. A. 1977. A method for detecting carcinogenic organic chemicals using mammalian cells in culture. Br. J. Cancer 36:558–563.

Terzaghi, M., and J. B. Little. 1976. X-radiation-induced transformation in a C3H mouse embryo-derived cell line. Cancer Res. 36:1367–1374.

Weinstein, I. B. 1979. Markers of transformation and the action of promoting agents, *in* Carcinogens: Identification and Mechanisms of Action (The University of Texas System Cancer Center 31st Annual Symposium of Fundamental Cancer Research, 1978), A. C. Griffin and C. R. Shaw, eds., Raven Press, New York, pp. 399–418.

Williams, G. M., J. M. Elliott, and J. H. Weisburger. 1973. Carcinoma after malignant conversion in vitro of epithelial-like cells from rat liver following exposure to chemical carcinogens. Cancer Res. 33:606–612.

Yamaguchi, N., and I. B. Weinstein. 1975. Temperature-sensitive mutants of chemically transformed epithelial cells. Proc. Natl. Acad. Sci. USA 72:214–218.

Carcinogens: Identification and Mechanisms
of Action, edited by A. Clark Griffin and
Charles R. Shaw. Raven Press, New York © 1979.

Bacterial Mutagenesis and Its Role in the Identification of Potential Animal Carcinogens

David Brusick

Department of Molecular Toxicology, Litton Bionetics, Inc., Kensington, Maryland 20795

Interest in establishing short-term test procedures for the identification of chemical carcinogens has increased during the past several years as a result of a realization that the list of potential chemical carcinogens is growing faster than our capacity to test the materials (Stolz *et al.* 1974, Bridges 1976). The accepted procedures of lifetime feeding studies in mice or rats present a number of problems, including the length of time required from initiation of testing until the final report (2 to 4 years), limitations imposed on the sensitivity of the system because of small treatment populations (50 males and 50 females per dose), and problems in extrapolating the data obtained from these studies to humans. If the problem of environmental carcinogenesis is to be controlled, greater numbers of potentially hazardous compounds must be screened and placed into a priority system for further testing. This appears to be the primary role of short-term carcinogenicity tests. For these tests to be meaningful, they must not only be faster, easier to interpret, more sensitive, and less expensive than the standard feeding studies, but they must also be reliable and relevant to the in vivo assay upon which they are modeled.

The development of microbial mutagenesis systems with the intention of looking for chemicals having carcinogenic potential began in the 1950s. Demerec *et al.* (1951) and Hemmerly and Demerec (1955) postulated that the identification of chemical mutagens with bacteria might be a technique for identifying potential anticancer agents, since many chemicals that possessed mutagenic activity were both carcinogenic and carcinostatic in animal model systems. This approach was further explored by Szybalski (1958) in a series of studies in which the plate assay technique was introduced. This assay procedure was developed by Iyer and Szybalski (1958) to rapidly evaluate large numbers of chemicals for the identification of potential antineoplastic chemicals. These procedures employed *Escherichia coli* (Streptomycin dependent) as the indicator organism, which was screened for reversion of Strep-dependence to Strep-independence. A summary of the data from tests with 431 substances produced 22 (5.1%) mutagens (Szybalski 1958). The majority of the mutagens identified in this early study was alkylating compounds that were directly mutagenic. Although this approach did not provide an effective screen for identifying antineoplastic drugs, it did establish the utility of microbial plate assays for screening large numbers of chemicals for mutagenic activity.

Plate tests were later used by Whitfield *et al.* (1966) and Brammer *et al.* (1967) to study the reversion patterns of chemical mutagens in *E. coli* and *Salmonella typhimurium* mutants to classify the agents as base-substitution or frameshift agents. Through the development of bacterial mutants with known molecular lesions in their DNA, chemicals could not only be tested for mutagenicity but could also be presumptively classified according to the type of DNA alterations they induced. Similar types of plate test assays were developed using other microbial indicator cells (Mayer *et al.* 1969, Pittman and Brusick 1971, Zimmermann 1971). In 1971, Ames reported mutagenicity data from tests on a large number of chemicals using a series of histidine-requiring mutants of *S. typhimurium*. This set of mutants responded to most of the mutagens examined, and it was proposed that screening for chemical carcinogens might be possible using his assay procedures, since many, if not all, of the mutagens identified using the *Salmonella* assay were also rodent carcinogens. In that same year, Slater *et al.* (1971) introduced an *E. coli* DNA repair test to identify potential carcinogens.

The role of mammalian metabolism in producing active metabolites from biologically inactive molecules stimulated modifications in the microbial plate assay (Ames 1973a). Liver microsomal enzyme fractions and certain cofactors have been coupled with the mutagenesis procedure to add an activation system capable of generating the ultimate mutagen during incubation on the plate. This critical modification, as well as the introduction of mutations in the *Salmonella* indicator organisms eliminating excision repair and the lipopolysaccharide coat, have significantly enhanced the sensitivity of this assay to a wide range of chemical classes (Ames *et al.* 1975). R-plasmids affecting additional repair systems have been introduced into two of these strains, increasing their sensitivity to an even broader range of chemicals (McCann *et al.* 1975b).

The Ames *Salmonella* tester strains have been used to screen large numbers of carcinogens for mutagenic activity (McCann *et al.* 1975a, Teranishi *et al.* 1975, Purchase *et al.* 1976). The results showed a positive correlation of 90% between mutagenicity and carcinogenicity. The likelihood of generating "false-positive" results appears to be low, indicating that this assay may have a high level of reliability in reproducing qualitative results from in vivo studies.

Although a great deal of developmental emphasis has been placed on the *Salmonella*/microsome assay (Ames *et al.* 1975), other plate assays using *E. coli* indicator cells have also been studied. A series of tryptophan-requiring mutants (WP$_2$ series) has been developed by Bridges (1972); microbial DNA repair tests have been developed using two *E. coli* strains, one capable of carrying out excision repair and the other a mutant for excision repair enzymes (Slater *et al.* 1971), and two strains of *Bacillus subtilus* have been developed by Kada and co-workers (1972). The latter three systems have not been examined as extensively for their ability to correlate with carcinogenicity, although many carcinogens are active in these assays (Longnecker *et al.* 1974, McCalla and Voutsinos 1974, Yahagi *et al.* 1974, Kada 1975, Green and Muriel 1976).

During the past few years, several modifications of the plate assay technique for screening chemicals have demonstrated the flexibility inherent in microbial assays. One approach, which was developed early, was the host-mediated assay technique reported by Gabridge and Legator (1969). The method combined in vivo and in vitro techniques. Durston and Ames (1974) later developed a method by which urine of treated animals could be screened in the *Salmonella* assay. Subsequently, this method was adapted to human urine (Yamasaki 1977). Another combined in vivo/in vitro approach utilizing microbial mutation systems employs bacteria or other microorganisms which are injected intravenously into the host mammal (usually a mouse). Following this procedure, the animal is dosed with a test chemical, killed, and the microbial cells are then removed from sites in various organs, such as the liver, lungs, and spleen (Arni *et al.* 1977). These host-mediated methods permit a comparison of in vitro with in vivo metabolism. Some chemicals that are not mutagenic following evaluation in the "standard" plate assays are active in the combined host-mediated-type approaches. One such compound is dimethylnitrosamine (DMN). DMN is not mutagenic when tested in the standard Ames *Salmonella*/microsomal assay, but it is active in the host-mediated methods, as well as in another modification

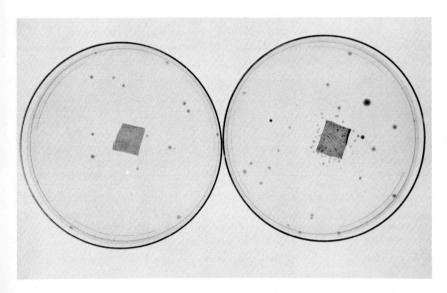

FIG. 1. A demonstration of the flexibility of microbial plate tests. A small section of commercial children's sleepwear treated with the flame retardant chemical tris 2,3 (dibromopropyl) phosphate is evaluated for mutagenicity with *S. typhimurium* TA-1535. The plate on the left contains S9 mix plus cells in the overlay. The plate on the right contains only cells in the overlay.

designated the "preincubation technique" (Gabridge and Legator 1969, Arni et al. 1977). The preincubation method includes a short preincubation period for the chemical, S9 mixture, and bacteria prior to the addition of the molten overlay agar. Volatile liquids can also be evaluated using the preincubation method. Highly volatile liquids and gases, however, must be tested in closed systems. Jagannath (personal communication) has recently evaluated the mutagenic properties of a series of chlorofluorocarbon gases using the Ames *Salmonella*/microsome assay. Even fabric material can be successfully tested using modified plate assays. Figure 1 illustrates the use of the plate assay to measure the mutagenic activity of Tris metabolites leached from pretreated fabric.

Thus, an economical, rapid, and flexible series of bacterial assays is available to screen large numbers of diverse chemicals for their carcinogenic potential. The systems appear to be highly predictive, and Meselson and Russell (1977) have suggested that carcinogenic potency might be determined using the Ames technique. This approach to predicting carcinogenic potency from mutagenic potency has also been supported by Clive (1977) and McCann and Ames (1977).

MOLECULAR BASIS FOR THE MUTAGENIC/CARCINOGENIC RELATIONSHIP

If bacterial assays are capable of identifying chemicals with carcinogenic potential for mammals, there must be an intimate relationship between genetic alterations and the production of malignant cells. Logically, this relationship would appear evident in the etiology of neoplastic diseases. The following points all contribute to the logic trail leading to the proposed link between mutation and transformation.

1) Tumors appear to be clonal in origin (Gould et al. 1978). This leads to the assumption that a single cell event is involved in tumor initiation.
2) Transformed cells are phenotypically different from their nontransformed precursor cells, and they transmit this new phenotype to all daughter cells. This is evidence that a genotypic alteration has been induced in the DNA of the original transformed cells.
3) Tumorigenic properties are associated directly with the affected cell, since transformed cells transplanted into a healthy syngeneic animal will develop into a tumor.
4) Most chemical carcinogens are also mutagens (Magee 1977).
5) Cells that are more sensitive to mutagenic lesions are also more sensitive to malignant transformation. This phenomenon is clearly demonstrated in the human disease xeroderma pigmentosum (Cleaver and Bootsma 1975).

Other types of indirect evidence support the assumption that DNA alterations provide the substrate for the processes involved in malignant transformation. Data correlating metabolic activation potential with tumor susceptibility among a series of procarcinogens and mutagens indicate that the mutagenic metabolite and the ultimate carcinogen are the same moiety (Nebert and Felton 1975, Huberman et al. 1972). Sex and age etiologic parameters associated with tumor susceptibilities can be replicated using in vitro metabolic activation systems prepared from organs of animals of different sexes and ages (Brusick et al. 1976). A concordance between the formation of the mutagen and the ultimate carcinogen would be mandatory if mutation is a critical cellular step leading to the malignant state.

Thus, a careful analysis of the properties of malignant and normal cells strongly suggests a mutation etiology. Data from bacteria correlative studies and in vitro metabolism investigations support the mutagenesis model.

The "Bacteria Bioassay"

The dilemma of carcinogen detection and control cannot be completely solved by more and larger rodent lifetime carcinogenicity bioassays. The time and expense involved would be too prohibitive, even if the results of such tests could always be relied on as accurate indicators of human risk or safety. The need for rapid answers to the multitude of questions raised concerning chemical safety has introduced the concept of short-term predictive tests, and the Ames Salmonella/microsome assay has placed us into the era of the "bacteria bioassay." The results of this test certainly have serious political, if not necessarily scientific, implications. The hair coloring, chemical flame retardant, and pesticide industries have all felt the political impact of the Ames test, and the procedure must be considered a factor to deal with whenever chemical safety evaluations are made. Because of its political and scientific implications, a closer inspection of the Ames assay may be of value. The following sections will attempt to define the assays, the type of data generated, and the significance of the data in terms of carcinogen identification.

The Ames Salmonella/Microsome Assay

The series of histidine-requiring mutants typically employed in the Ames assay has evolved from mutants isolated during studies centered on the elucidation of the histidine biosynthesis pathway in S. typhimurium. The development of the TA-1535, TA-1537, and TA-1538 series of mutant strains has been described by Ames et al. (1973b), and the development of the TA-98 and TA-100 set of strains containing plasmid pkM101 has been described by McCann et al. (1975b).

The underlying rationale for this system is that a battery of tester strains constructed to permit the minimum amount of interference to a reaction between an active mutagen and the target molecule (DNA) will provide an extremely sensitive assay procedure. The carefully engineered alterations of S. typhimurium LT_2 into the typhimurium Ames (TA) set of mutant strains have not altered the biological significance of the mutations that are induced in the cells but have been used to reduce the threshold for activity (Figure 2). Thus, chemicals

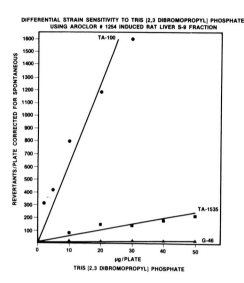

DIFFERENTIAL STRAIN SENSITIVITY TO TRIS [2,3 DIBROMOPROPYL] PHOSPHATE
USING AROCLOR # 1254 INDUCED RAT LIVER S-9 FRACTION

FIG. 2. An illustration, using known mutagens, of the effect on sensitivity introduced by the strain modification in *S. typhimurium* G-46; G-46 is *his⁻*; TA-1535 is *his⁻*, *uvr*B⁻, *rfa⁻*; and TA-100 is *his⁻*, *uvr*B⁻, *rfa⁻*, and contains the plasmid pKM101.

that are bacterial mutagens but do not register in *S. typhimurium* strain G-46 because insufficient concentrations of the active chemicals are able to reach the target molecule are active in the modified strain TA-1535. Not only are the strains derived more susceptible to compound-induced mutation, but the spontaneous background mutation rate also increases with the level of sensitivity (Figure 3).

Descriptions of the *Salmonella* strains as "crippled" or "sick" are not accurate. Certainly, the *Salmonella* mutants are engineered to optimum sensitivity while retaining the qualities of biological systems, but they cannot be considered "sick." The only question that can be answered by the Ames technique is whether the chemical under test can damage DNA. If not, the chemical is unlikely to

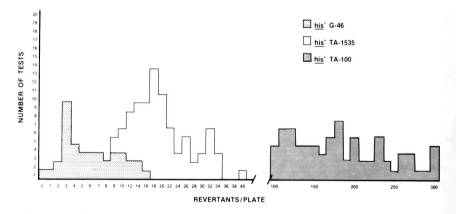

FIG. 3. The range of spontaneous mutation is shown for G-46 and the two strains derived from G-46. As the strains were modified to increase their sensitivity to detect induced mutation, they also demonstrated increased spontaneous levels of mutation.

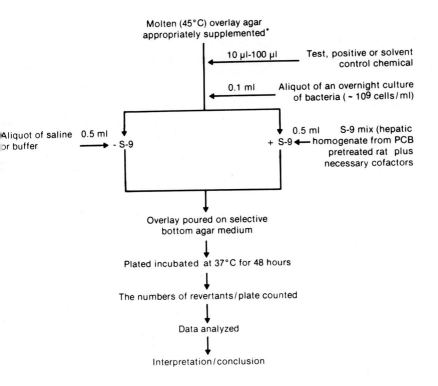

*A modification of this test called the "Preincubation Modification" consists of a 15-20 minute preincubation of the cells, chemical and S-9 at 37°C before the overlay is added. Certain agents not active in the standard method will be positive in this modification.

FIG. 4. Reverse mutation assay (agar incorporation method).

be mutagenic or carcinogenic in any less sensitive bioassay system. There are some notable exceptions to this latter assumption. False-negatives are known for certain chemicals in the Ames test (McCann *et al.* 1975a, McCann and Ames 1977). Some types of chemicals cannot be adequately evaluated in microbial assays because they have activities that will only be manifested in animal cells (Clive 1977). It is also possible that the specificity of a chemical for DNA nucleotide sequences is not found among the available mutant nucleotide sequences in *his* G-46, *his* C3076, or *his* D3052.

The design of the Ames test is shown in Figure 4. A recommended protocol outlining the preparation of the components of this test has been published by Ames *et al.* (1975). Modifications of the method have been developed by numerous investigators (Gabridge and Legator 1969, Mohn and Ellenberger 1973 Nebert and Felton 1975, Batzinger *et al.* 1977). Some of the modifications have, as previously mentioned for DMN, been useful in demonstrating mutagenic activity in chemicals not active in the standard test.

There has been some suggestion that chemicals demonstrated to have mutagenic activity in a modification of the recommended procedure do not carry the implications for carcinogenesis associated with substances active in the standard or recommended procedure. Since the implications for carcinogenesis rest only with the demonstration of genetic activity and not with methodological manipulations, the ability of the chemical to clearly mutate DNA should be the only criterion used in developing the carcinogen/mutagen correlation. All bioassay systems must undergo modification if adequate evaluation of certain chemicals is to be made. This is especially true for gases, highly volatile liquids, and chemical mixtures.

The use of modified procedures has created, however, a certain sense of uncertainty about negative findings in the standard test. The possibility always exists that a modified version of the test will generate a response. A controversy has recently developed with the publication of a paper by Batzinger *et al.* (1977) reporting the mutagenicity of saccharin using modifications of the Ames test. Saccharin is not mutagenic when tested by the procedure outlined by Ames. Concern has been expressed that with sufficient adjustments, most chemicals demonstrate mutagenic effects in the *Salmonella* mutants. Without consensus as to what constitutes a reasonable attempt to demonstrate mutagenicity in the Ames test, there will be no alleviation of this concern. The development of a defined protocol that can be expected to give confidence that an adequate test has been conducted is both reasonable and necessary if the Ames test is to be useful.

INTERPRETATION OF RESULTS AND CONCLUSIONS

If the problem of protocol consistency is the greatest concern associated with the use of the bacteria bioassay, then the next most serious problem is how to analyze and interpret the results obtained in the test. This serious problem is not unique to the Ames test. All in vivo chronic toxicity bioassays are confronted with debates on how to analyze and interpret the data. Data analysis and data interpretation are subtopics of "test result evaluation," and they often become confused.

Data analysis is the procedure by which data are organized and studied to determine if an effect has been generated and whether such an effect is significantly different from what has been obtained in a control test. Data interpretation is an attempt to put the test results into perspective with respect to the data base already established for the test procedure and to attempt to outline the consequences implied by the test results.

Analysis of Ames test data has been predicated primarily on experience and intuition. No generally accepted procedures have been formalized or validated. The majority of chemicals comprising the validation data base for the Ames test has been clearly negative or positive. The number of agents left open to debate is few. Most currently available statistical analyses for use in the Ames

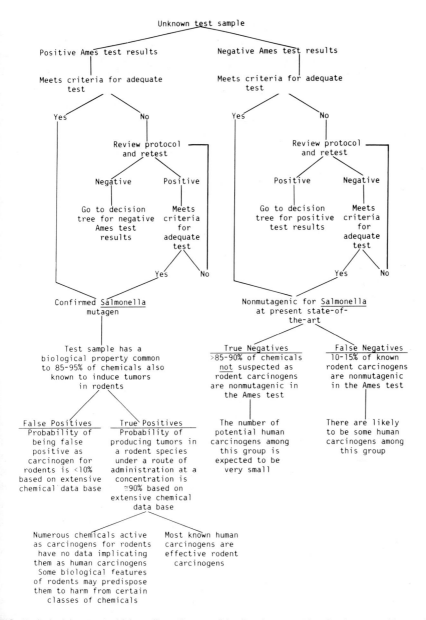

FIG. 5. A decision tree which outlines the possible data interpretation for Ames positive and Ames negative compounds. The criteria for adequate test determinations are given on page 104.

test would probably be of little value in resolving the responses of the controversial agents.

Interpretation of Ames test results has ranged from a belief that they are of no predictive value for carcinogen identification to the concept that the Ames test is a definitive test for chemical carcinogens. Attempting to take as many of the parameters as possible into consideration, an "interpretation decision tree" has been outlined in Figure 5. The interpretation decision tree is not a guide for data analysis but rather an attempt to define what positive or negative Ames test data mean with respect to carcinogen identification once a confirmed positive or negative effect is obtained. While this decision tree does not present all the possible interpretations of Ames test results, it probably represents a consensus of published opinion.

Criteria for *positive* test data

1. A positive response must be directly attributable to a genetic lesion at the DNA level.
2. A positive response must be significantly different from a well-defined spontaneous background.
3. A positive response should be dose related and shown to be reproducible in chronologically independent tests using the same procedure.
4. A positive response must be established as compound induced and not an artifact of the test conditions.
5. The genetically active chemical must be similar in nature to the form of the chemical found in vivo.
6. The compound is not closely related to chemicals known to produce false-positive responses.

Criteria for *negative* test data

1. The lack of a positive response must be reproducible in chronologically independent tests using the same procedure.
2. The test material must be examined under test conditions demonstrating some evidence of biological activity such as cytotoxicity.
3. If the compound is known to be metabolized in vivo, an in vitro activation system must be employed in the evaluation. Mutagenic evaluation of any known mammalian metabolites in conjunction with the in vitro metabolism is recommended.
4. The compound should not be closely related to chemicals known to produce false-negative responses.
5. The test data should not differ significantly from a well-defined spontaneous mutation range.

The bacteria bioassay is a potentially valuable tool. However, it must be used with care and forethought. It clearly is useful in identifying chemicals that have carcinogenic potential. Confirmation of that potential still requires in vivo investigation. Verification of the predictive power of the test, however, could render the desire to confirm carcinogenic potential with long and expensive rodent bioassays a luxury reserved for chemicals with widespread human exposure or significant economic importance.

REFERENCES

Ames, B. N. 1971. The detection of chemical mutagens with enteric bacteria, *in* Chemical Mutagens: Principles and Methods for Their Detection, A. Hollaender, ed., Vol. 1. Plenum Press, New York–London, pp. 267–282.

Ames, B. N., W. E. Durston, E. Yamasaki, and F. D. Lee. 1973a. Carcinogens are mutagens: A simple test system combining liver homogenates for activation and bacteria for detection. Proc. Natl. Acad. Sci. USA 70(8):2281–2285.

Ames, B. N., F. D. Lee, and W. E. Durston. 1973b. An improved bacterial test system for the detection and classification of mutagens and carcinogens. Proc. Natl. Acad. Sci. USA 70:782–786.

Ames, B. N., J. McCann, and E. Yamasaki. 1975. Methods for detecting carcinogens and mutagens with the *Salmonella*/mammalian-microsome mutagenicity test. Mutat. Res. 31(6):347–364.

Arni, P., Th. Mantel, E. Deparade, and D. Müller. 1977. Intrasanguine host-mediated assay with *Salmonella typhimurium*. Mutat. Res. 45(3):291–307.

Batzinger, R., S. Y. Ou, and E. Bueding. 1977. Saccharin and other sweeteners: Mutagenic properties. Science 198:944–946.

Brammer, W. H., H. Berger, and C. Yanofsky. 1967. Altered amino acid sequences produced by reversion of frameshift mutants of tryptophane synthetase A gene of *E. coli.* Proc. Natl. Acad. Sci. USA 58:1499.

Bridges, B. A. 1972. Simple bacterial systems for detecting mutagenic agents. Lab. Pract. 21:413.

Bridges, B. A. 1976. Short term screening tests for carcinogens. Review article. Nature 261:195–200.

Brusick, D., D. Jagannath, and U. Weekes. 1976. The utilization of in vitro mutagenesis techniques to explain strain, age and sex related differences in dimethylnitrosamine tumor susceptibilities in mice. Mutat. Res. 41:51–60.

Cleaver, J. E., and D. Bootsma. 1975. Xeroderma pigmentosum: Biochemical and genetic characteristics, *in* Annual Review of Genetics, H. L. Roman, ed., Annual Reviews, Inc., Palo Alto, California, pp. 19–38.

Clive, D. 1977. A linear relationship between tumorigenic potency in vivo and mutagenic potency at the heterozygous thymidine kinase (TK$^{+/-}$) locus of L5178Y mouse lymphoma cells coupled with mammalian metabolism, *in* Progress in Genetic Toxicology, D. Scott, B. A. Bridges, and F. H. Sobels, eds., Elsevier/North-Holland Biomedical Press, Amsterdam, pp. 241–247.

Demerec, M., G. Bertani, and J. Flint. 1951. A survey of chemicals for mutagenic action on *E. coli.* American Naturalist 85:119–136.

Durston, W. E., and B. N. Ames. 1974. A simple method for the detection of mutagens in urine: Studies with the carcinogen 2-acetylaminofluorene. Proc. Natl. Acad. Sci. USA 71:737–741.

Frantz, C. N., and H. V. Malling. 1975. The quantitative microsomal mutagenesis assay method. Mutat. Res. 31(6):365–380.

Gabridge, M. G., and M. S. Legator. 1969. A host-mediated microbial assay for the detection of mutagenic compounds. Proc. Soc. Exp. Biol. Med. 130:831.

Gould, M. N., R. Jirtle, J. Crowley, and K. H. Clifton. 1978. Reevaluation of the number of cells involved in the neutron induction of mammary neoplasms. Cancer Res. 38:189–192.

Green, M. H. L., and W. J. Muriel. 1976. Mutagen testing using *trp*$^+$ reversion in *Escherichia coli.* Mutat. Res. 38:3–32.

Hemmerly, J., and M. Demerec. 1955. Test of chemicals for mutagenicity. Cancer Res. (Suppl. No. 3):69–75.

Huberman, E., P. J. Donovan, and J. A. DiPaolo. 1972. Mutation and transformation of cultured mammalian cells by N-acetoxy-N-2-fluorenylacetamide. Brief communication. J. Natl. Cancer Inst. 48:837–840.

Iyer, V. N., and W. Szybalski. 1958. Two simple methods for the detection of chemical mutagens. Appl. Microbiol. 6:23–29.

Kada, T. 1975. Mutagenicity and carcinogenicity screening of food additives by the rec-assay and reversion procedures. IARC Scientific Publication No. 12:105–115.

Kada, T., K. Tutikawa, and Y. Sadaie. 1972. In vitro and host-mediated "rec-assay" procedures for screening chemical mutagens; and phloxine, a mutagenic red dye detected. Mutat. Res. 16:165–174.

Longnecker, D. S., T. J. Curphey, S. T. James, D. S. Daniel, and N. J. Jacobs. 1974. Trial of a bacterial screening system for rapid detection of mutagens and carcinogens. Cancer Res. 34:1658–1663.

Magee, P. N. 1977. The relationship between mutagenesis, carcinogenesis and teratogenesis, *in* Progress in Genetic Toxicology, D. Scott, B. A. Bridges, and F. H. Sobels, eds., Vol. 2. Elsevier/North-Holland Biomedical Press, Amsterdam, pp. 15–27.

Mayer, V. W., M. G. Gabridge, and E. J. Oswald. 1969. Rapid plate test for evaluating phage induction capacity. Appl. Microbiol. 18(4):697–698.

McCalla, D. R., and D. Voutsinos. 1974. On the mutagenicity of nitrofurans. Mutat. Res. 26(1):3–16.

McCann, J., and B. N. Ames. 1977. The *Salmonella*/microsome mutagenicity test: Predictive value for animal carcinogenicity, *in* Origins of Human Cancer, H. H. Hiatt, J. D. Watson, and J. A. Winsten, eds., Vol. 4. Cold Spring Harbor Laboratory, Cold Spring Harbor, New York, pp. 1431–1450.

McCann, J., E. Choi, E. Yamasaki, and B. N. Ames. 1975a. Detection of carcinogens as mutagens in the *Salmonella*/microsome test: Assay of 300 chemicals. Proc. Natl. Acad. Sci. USA 72(12):5135–5139.

McCann, J., N. Spingarn, J. Kobori, and B. N. Ames. 1975b. The detection of carcinogens as mutagens: Bacterial tester strains with R factor plasmids. Proc. Natl. Acad. Sci. USA 72:979–983.

McCoy, E. C., W. T. Speck, and H. S. Rosenkranz. 1977. Activation of a procarcinogen to a mutagen by cell-free extracts of anaerobic bacteria. Mutat. Res. 46(4):261–264.

Meselson, M., and K. Russell. 1977. Comparisons of carcinogenic and mutagenic potency, *in* Origins of Human Cancer, H. H. Hiatt, J. D. Watson, and J. A. Winsten, eds., Vol. 4. Cold Spring Harbor Laboratory, Cold Spring Harbor, New York, pp. 1473–1481.

Mohn, G., and J. Ellenberger. 1973. Mammalian blood-mediated mutagenicity tests using a multipurpose strain of *Escherichia coli* K-12. Short communication. Mutat. Res. 19(2):257–260.

Nebert, D. W., and J. S. Felton. 1975. Evidence for the activation of 3-methylcholanthrene as a carcinogen in vivo and as a mutagen in vitro by P_1-450 from inbred strains of mice, *in* Cytochromes P-450 and b_5, D. Y. Cooper, O. Rosenthal, R. Snyder, and C. Witmer, eds., Plenum Press, New York, pp. 127–149.

Pittman, D., and D. Brusick. 1971. Detection of presumptive base-pair substitution and frameshift mutations in *Saccharomyces cerevisiae*. Molec. Gen. Genet. 111:352.

Purchase, I. F. H., E. Longstaff, J. Ashby, J. A. Styles, D. Anderson, P. A. Lefevre, and F. R. Westwood. 1976. Evaluation of six short term tests for detecting organic chemical carcinogens and recommendations for their use. Nature 264:624–627.

Slater, E. E., M. D. Anderson, and H. S. Rosenkranz. 1971. Rapid detection of mutagens and carcinogens. Cancer Res. 31:970–973.

Stolz, D. R., L. A. Poirier, C. C. Irving, H. F. Stich, J. H. Weisburger, and H. C. Grice. 1974. Evaluation of short-term tests for carcinogenicity. Toxicol. Appl. Pharmacol. 29(2):157–180.

Szybalski, W. 1958. Special microbial systems. II. Observations on chemical mutagenesis in microorganisms. Ann. NY Acad. Sci. 75:475.

Teranishi, K., K. Hamada, and H. Watanabe. 1975. Quantitative relationship between carcinogenicity and mutagenicity of polyaromatic hydrocarbons in *Salmonella typhimurium* mutants. Mutat. Res. 31(2):97–102.

Whitfield, H. J., R. G. Martin, and B. N. Ames. 1966. Classification of aminotransferase (C gene) mutants in the histidine operon. J. Mol. Biol. 21:335.

Yahagi, T., M. Nagao, K. Hara, T. Matsushima, T. Sugimura, and G. T. Bryan. 1974. Relationships between the carcinogenic and mutagenic or DNA-modifying effects of nitrofuran derivatives, including 2-(2-furyl)-3-(5-nitro-2-furyl)acrylamide, a food additive. Cancer Res. 34:2266–2273.

Yamasaki, E., and B. N. Ames. 1977. Concentration of mutagens from urine by adsorption with the nonpolar resin XAD-2: Cigarette smokers have mutagenic urine. Proc. Natl. Acad. Sci. USA 74:3555–3559.

Zimmermann, F. K. 1971. Induction of mitotic gene conversion by mutagens. Mutat. Res. 11:327.

Carcinogens: Identification and Mechanisms of Action, edited by A. Clark Griffin and Charles R. Shaw. Raven Press, New York © 1979.

Molecular Test Systems for Identification of DNA-Reactive Agents

Roger R. Hewitt,* Julie Harless,* R. Stephen Lloyd,† Jack Love,* and Donald L. Robberson†

Section of Environmental Biology, Department of Biology, and † Section of Molecular Biology, Department of Biology, The University of Texas System Cancer Center M. D. Anderson Hospital and Tumor Institute, Houston, Texas 77030

Reactivity with deoxyribonucleic acid (DNA) is a commonly encountered characteristic of genetically toxic physical and chemical agents. In the case of carcinogens, the production of mutagenic DNA lesions is a likely initiating molecular event leading to a cancerous state. Many research efforts in the areas of mechanisms of carcinogenesis and carcinogen identification presume DNA reactivity in the model cellular systems utilized and in the experimental approaches taken in their study. In view of these considerations, we have assumed that the development of sensitive, rapid, and inexpensive methods with which to identify DNA-reactive chemicals and to classify their reaction products would be beneficial. The approach we have taken in the development or application of appropriately sensitive methods of detection is to employ covalently closed circular DNA (ccDNA) as a target molecule in cell-free reactions with potentially damaging physical and chemical agents.

In order to evaluate the utility of this approach, we present a summary of the major classes of DNA damage produced by physical and chemical agents and the general approaches taken to detect these lesions, as well as a review of the characteristics of ccDNA that can be exploited in sensitive measurements of DNA structure damage. Several applications are described that indicate future trends for development of cell-free testing systems that employ ccDNA, homogeneous in size and sequence content, as reactant with the physical or chemical agent.

GENERAL APPROACHES TO THE DETECTION OF DNA STRUCTURE DAMAGE

The most commonly encountered DNA structural damage resulting from interactions with radiation or chemicals is a *single-strand break* that is caused by interrupting the phosphodiester backbone of a DNA strand (Figure 1). When breaks occur in both complementary strands within about sixteen base pairs

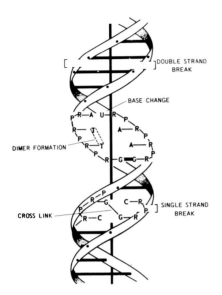

FIG. 1. Diagrammatic model of double-stranded DNA helix illustrating nature of possible lesions that damage or alter the helical structure.

of one another (at 37°C and ionic strength of 0.01), a *double-strand break* will result from dissociation of the intervening base pairs (Freifelder *et al.* 1977). Also, *base damage* can occur by chemical modifications of individual purines or pyrimidines and can involve more than one base, as in the case of *pyrimidine dimer* formation produced by ultraviolet light (Figure 1). Covalent *cross-links* between bases in complementary DNA strands can also be produced by bifunctional alkylating agents, for example.

A variety of direct physical or chemical methods are available to detect the presence of certain of these DNA structure damages. Some types of base damage, such as pyrimidine dimers (Kato and Fraser 1973), can cause distortions in the helical conformation of the DNA molecule, which in turn can be measured by physical methods that detect this altered helicity of the modified DNA molecules. In the case of sufficiently large distortions of the helix that produce localized regions of denaturation, endodeoxyribonucleases (endoDNases) that recognize single-stranded DNA as a substrate will introduce single-strand breaks into the distorted regions. These latter types of helix distortion can thus be detected as single-strand breaks after treatment with the appropriate endoDNases. EndoDNases specific for pyrimidine dimers (Friedburg and King 1971), apurinic or apyrimidinic sites (Ljungquist and Lindahl 1974), and glycosylase activities directed at certain methylated or unusual DNA bases (Lindahl 1976) have been described. The presence of these types of base damage in duplex DNA can thus be indicated by virtue of their susceptibility to appropriate enzymes, which transform the damaged sites to measurable numbers of single-strand breaks. In addition, certain chemical modifications of bases such as methylations at the N7 of guanine or N3 of adenine can lead to depurination, and

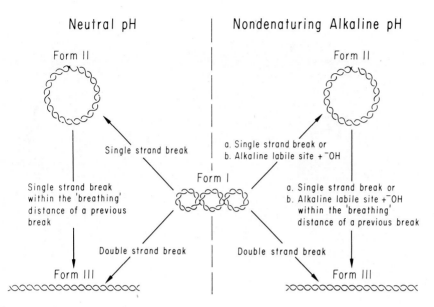

FIG. 2. Conversions of covalently closed circular (form I) DNA to nicked circular (form II) and linear duplex (form III) DNAs under neutral or nondenaturing alkaline conditions as a result of exposure to DNA-reactive agents.

with subsequent hydrolysis of the phosphodiester backbone, single-strand breaks will occur under alkaline conditions. Such *alkali-labile base damage* would also be expressed as single-strand breaks after alkali treatment.

It is apparent that many types of mutagenic or carcinogenic modifications of duplex DNA can be manipulated under neutral and alkaline conditions to cause their expression as single-strand or double-strand scissions of the phosphodiester backbone. Maximum sensitivity for the detection of these single-strand or double-strand scissions in any testing system can be obtained with the use of a covalently closed circular duplex DNA of moderately large molecular weight which can be converted by appropriate reaction conditions to nicked circular and linear duplex forms, as diagrammatically illustrated in Figure 2.

THE EXPLOITABLE PROPERTIES OF COVALENTLY CLOSED CIRCULAR PM2 DNA

The marine bacteriophage PM2 contains a covalently closed circular DNA (Espejo and Canelo 1968) with a molecular weight of about 6.0×10^6 daltons (Espejo *et al.* 1969), corresponding to approximately 10,250 nucleotide pairs (D. L. Robberson, unpublished observation). The DNA can be produced and purified in sufficiently large quantities to make feasible its use as a substrate in assays with DNA-reactive agents. The utility of this DNA derives from the dramatically different physical-chemical properties associated with ccDNA

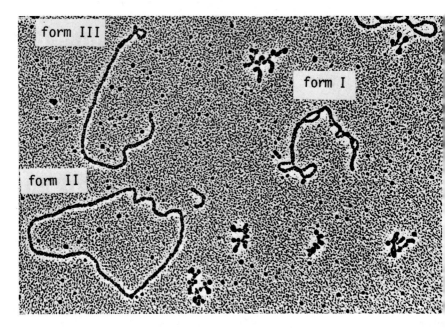

FIG. 3. Electron micrograph of the three topological forms of duplex PM2 DNA. The particula topological form is indicated above each molecule. Also included in this micrograph are exam ples of the appearance of single-stranded DNA which occur as collapsed "bushes." The sample was prepared by the aqueous basis protein (Kleinschmidt) technique of Davis *et a*l (1971), as applied by Robberson *et al.* (1971). Grids were rotary shadowed with Pt:Pd (80:20) and examined in a Philips 300 electron microscope. Magnification is indicated by the contou length of form II PM2 DNA, containing 10,250± 200 base-pairs.

(form I) compared to the properties of nicked circular DNA (ncDNA, forn II) and linear duplex DNA (form III). Electron micrographs of these differen topological forms of PM2 DNA are shown in Figure 3. Form I PM2 DNA possesses a highly twisted conformation with approximately 113 negative super helical turns. When a single-strand break is introduced into form I DNA, ar open circular conformation of form II DNA is achieved by relaxation of the superhelical turns (see Figure 2).

The compact conformation of ccDNA (Figure 3) allows it to be distinguishec from either nicked circular or linear duplex molecules in velocity sedimentation and gel electrophoretic analyses. Furthermore, the covalent continuity of each strand in a native ccDNA molecule prohibits complete physical separation o the strands under mild denaturation conditions, and this latter property o ccDNA results in greater stability to denaturing treatments such as heat o alkali than its breakage products.

Velocity sedimentation in sucrose or CsCl gradients reveals that the highly twisted form I DNA sediments more rapidly than either form II or form II DNA molecules (Figure 4). In alkaline medium, form I DNA assumes a highly

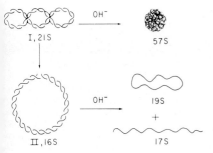

FIG. 4. Observed sedimentation coefficients of covalently closed circular (I) and nicked circular (II) PM2 DNA at neutral pH (at left) and in denaturing alkaline medium (at right). Under denaturing alkaline conditions, form I DNA is converted to a highly collapsed coil, while form II DNA is strand separated to give mixtures of single-stranded circular and linear forms. The sedimentation coefficients corrected to 20°C in water at infinite dilution ($S°_{20.w}$) are 27.0 S (form 1) and 20.4S (form II) (Ostrander *et al.* 1974).

collapsed structure in which each of the circular strands remain topologically bound and associated. The strands of both forms II and III DNAs are separated upon denaturation in alkali and assume a somewhat extended conformation. As expected, the denatured form I DNA sediments much more rapidly than the single strands arising from denaturation of forms II and III DNAs (Figure 4).

Using velocity sedimentation analyses, a number of studies have been conducted to examine endoDNase activity on ccDNA treated with DNA-reactive agents. These sedimentation studies utilize either neutral or alkaline sucrose or CsCl gradients to determine the fraction of ccDNA remaining after reaction with the active agent. While sedimentation analyses have been successfully applied in a variety of studies, this procedure has limited application for assays involving the very large number of samples as would be required for the screening of suspected DNA-reactive compounds.

Another approach employing ccDNA that is currently being developed can, in principle, accommodate this requirement for the large number of samples to be screened as DNA-reactive compounds. This approach is outlined in Figure 5. In this assay, ccDNA is reacted with a DNA breakage agent and incubated at pH 12.1 in phosphate buffer. This alkaline condition is shown to selectively denature form II and III DNAs, but not ccDNA, which retains approximately 80% of its initial duplex structure as measured by fluorescence enhancement with ethidium bromide. Ethidium bromide is a phenanthridium dye that intercalates between base-pairs in duplex DNA or duplex segments of single-stranded DNA (LePecq and Paoletti 1967). Intercalation of the dye results in an approximate 25-fold increase in the quantum efficiency of fluorescence. Therefore, the fluorescence of PM2 DNA reaction mixtures after exposure to DNA-breaking agents and the addition of pH 12.1 buffer and ethidium bromide can provide a direct measure of the proportion of ccDNA molecules surviving treatment with the DNA-reactive agents.

This solution fluorescence assay measures the loss of ccDNA during treatment with DNA-reactive agents. However, it cannot provide a classification of the individual types of damage produced by the agents. This derives from the fact that single-strand and double-strand breaks as well as alkali-labile base damage

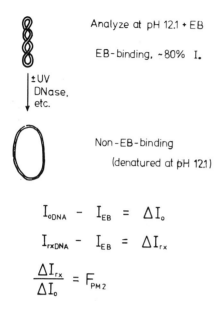

Analyze at pH 12.1 + EB

EB-binding, ~80% $I_.$

±UV
DNase,
etc.

Non-EB-binding

(denatured at pH 12.1)

$$I_{oDNA} - I_{EB} = \Delta I_o$$

$$I_{rxDNA} - I_{EB} = \Delta I_{rx}$$

$$\frac{\Delta I_{rx}}{\Delta I_o} = F_{PM2}$$

FIG. 5. Diagrammatic illustration of solution fluorescence assay of PM2 DNA to estimate fraction of covalently closed circular DNA present in reaction mixture. Samples are analyzed at pH 12.1 in the presence of ethidium bromide (EB) in which form II DNA is strand separated and does not intercalate the dye while form I DNA remains strand associated and exhibits 80% of the fluorescence intensity (I) at neutral pH. The fraction of form I DNA present in the reaction is determined from the ratio of differences of fluorescence intensity before (ΔIo) and after (ΔIrx) reaction with DNA-reactive agents such as UV and then treatment with a specific endoDNase. For treatments with DNA-reactive agents that lead directly to single-strand or double-strand breaks, the subsequent treatment with specific endoDNases would not be required.

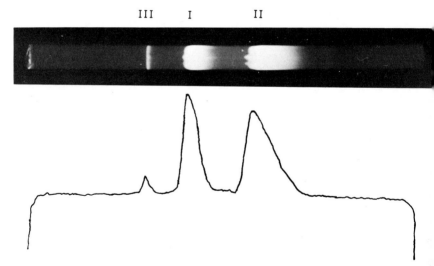

III   I   II

FIG. 6. Electrophoresis of PM2 DNA in 1.4% agarose gels. A mixture of forms I, II, and III PM2 DNAs were subjected to electrophoresis in 1.4% agarose tube gels at 100 V, 2.5 mamps/tube for 5.5 hours at 23°C. The gel was stained with ethidium bromide (0.5 μg/ml) and then scanned in an Aminco-Bowman spectrofluorometer as described (Grdina *et al.* 1973). The photograph at top depicts the gel positions of forms I, II, and III (as indicated), and the trace at the bottom depicts the relative amounts of each of these topological forms in the gels.

have the net effect of reducing the fraction of ccDNA in the reaction mixture, which is the only parameter measured in the assay. The primary value of a solution assay of this type is that large numbers of samples can be rapidly analyzed. Once DNA-reactive agents are identified, the damage which is produced as either single-strand or double-strand breaks can be determined by other methods that permit product identification.

The most powerful method that has been developed recently to resolve these breakage products is gel electrophoresis in a medium such as agarose (Sharp et al. 1973). As illustrated in Figure 6, in 1.4% agarose gels, form III PM2 DNA migrates more rapidly than form I PM2 DNA, which in turn migrates more rapidly than form II PM2 DNA; and each of these respective topological forms of DNA are exceedingly well resolved. The positions of each of these forms of DNA in the gel can be localized by staining the gel with ethidium bromide and the relative mass fraction of each topological form determined by scanning spectrofluorometry (Figure 6). Alternatively, if the PM2 DNA had been radioactively labeled, quantitation of the different forms could be achieved by slicing of the gel and by scintillation spectrometry.

These different methods of analyses have been employed singly or in combination with specific endonucleases to assay damage produced by physical and chemical agents to different topological forms of PM2 DNA. Several examples to illustrate these applications are presented in the following section.

UTILIZATION OF COVALENTLY CLOSED CIRCULAR PM2 DNA IN ASSAYS OF STRUCTURE-DAMAGING AGENTS

Several types of DNA damage may not directly lead to single-strand or double-strand scissions but provide substrates for specific endoDNases whose biological function involves the recognition of such DNA damage and introduction of single-strand breaks in the vicinity of the damage. This recognition and breakage comprise initial events in DNA-repair reactions. Ultraviolet-induced pyrimidine dimers or regions of base loss, which can be introduced into ccDNA without interrupting the continuity of either strand, fall into this category of DNA damage and can be recognized by treating the DNA with damage-specific endoDNases. For example, exposure of DNA to ultraviolet light (254 nm) produces pyrimidine dimers that are substrates for an endoDNase purified from T4 bacteriophage-infected Escherichia coli (Friedburg and King 1973). This activity, which is traditionally referred to as the T4 UV endoDNase, can be used as a probe for pyrimidine dimers because it introduces an incision near the site of each dimer. Figure 7 includes an analysis of dimer production in PM2 DNA using T4 UV endoDNase. The loss of ccDNA after enzyme treatment of DNA exposed to varying UV fluences was measured using the solution fluorescence assay described earlier. The irradiated DNA is not broken at the low UV fluences employed in this case unless it is treated with UV endoDNase.

Ultraviolet lesions in DNA are also known to alter the helicity of native

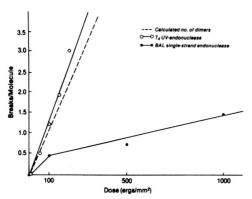

Fig. 7. Dose-response of PM2 DNA exposed to ultraviolet light and treated with either T4 UV-endonuclease (open circles) or the BAL single-strand specific endonuclease (solid circles). The number of breaks per molecule of PM2 DNA introduced by the two respective enzymes after irradiation was estimated from the fraction of form I DNA remaining, as assayed by solution alkaline fluorescence as in Figure 5.

DNA such that localized regions of base-pair denaturation occur with unwinding of the helix. These regions are potential substrates for single-strand specific endoDNases. An enzyme of this type has been reported by Gray *et al.* (1975) and is produced by *Pseudomonas,* strain BAL 31, the natural bacterial host for PM2 bacteriophage. This enzyme, which is purified from the extracellular growth medium, degrades single-stranded DNA and also cleaves superhelical ccDNA, presumably in response to weakly hydrogen-bonded regions within the supercoiled ccDNA. Thus, in order to utilize the BAL enzyme to probe localized regions of denaturation in damaged DNA, it is essential to remove the superhelical turns while preserving covalent, closed circularity. This is readily feasible by using any of several nicking-closing (NC) enzymes, which, when reacted with native PM2 DNA, relax the negative superhelical turns. The resultant relaxed covalently closed circular DNA has, on the average, zero superhelical turns (Figure 8A). Since the BAL enzyme does not cleave ccDNA from which the superhelical turns have been removed (Gray *et al.* 1975), it is feasible to use this form I° DNA as reactant for structure-damaging agents. Subsequent treatment with the enzyme probes for single-strand regions that are produced by the agent. The rationale for this approach is summarized in Figure 10, and the results of one such study are presented in Figure 7 for ultraviolet-irradiated

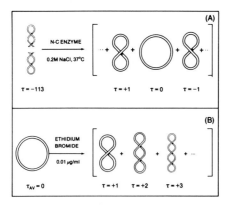

FIG. 8. Diagrammatic illustration of the effect of treating native PM2 DNA containing 11 negative superhelical turns (Upholt 1977) with nicking-closing (NC) enzyme (A). The population of covalently closed circular DNAs resulting from this treatment have an average of zero superhelical turns but are converted to a population of positive superhelical turns by the addition of ethidium bromide (B).

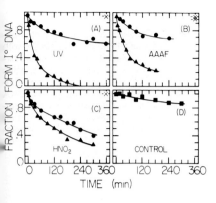

FIG. 9. Time-course of BAL nuclease digestion of PM2 form I° DNAs exposed to ultraviolet (UV) irradiation (A), reacted with AAAF (B), or HNO₂ (C), with control (D). The fraction of form I° DNA was monitored by band sedimentation for experiments in A and B and by gel electrophoresis for experiments presented in C and D. Δ, the more extensive treatment or reaction; X, samples that were incubated with buffer alone. Irradiated samples contained 7.2 and 48 pyrimidine dimers, respectively; AAAF reacted samples contained 35 and 68 fluorenylated dGuo residues, respectively; HNO₂ reacted samples contained 1.0 and 2.1 interstrand cross-links, respectively. (Reproduced from Legerski *et al.* (1977), with permission of J. Biol. Chem.)

DNA. At increasing UV fluences, the irradiated DNA becomes susceptible to attack by the BAL enzyme. Since UV-irradiated molecules are much less susceptible to the BAL enzyme than to the T4 UV endoDNase (see Figure 7), it is clear that *single* pyrimidine dimer sites are insufficient substrates for the BAL enzyme. It is probable that the distortions which are recognized represent either small regions in which several dimers are produced or base damage distortions produced at a much lower frequency than dimers or conformational distortions that occur throughout the molecule in response to accumulation of several damage types.

The same rationale for assay of ultraviolet damage to form I° DNA depicted in Figure 7 can be applied to monitor other DNA-reactive agents. The results of one such study by Legerski *et al.* (1977) are reproduced in Figure 9 for reaction of form I° PM2 DNA with N-acetoxy-N-2-acetylaminofluorene (AAAF) and nitrous acid, Panels B and C, respectively. For comparison, the results obtained for the DNA irradiated with ultraviolet light are shown in Panel A of Figure 9. After treatment with these agents and digestion with the BAL enzyme, the fraction of form I° DNA remaining was determined by either velocity sedimentation or gel electrophoresis rather than by the alkali ethidium bromide fluorescence described in Figure 10. Although the general utility of the BAL enzyme is illustrated by these experiments, it is also clear from the studies by Legerski *et al.* (1977) that a single pyrimidine dimer (UV) or modified guanine residue (AAAF) is not recognized by the enzyme. A single interstrand cross-link produced by reaction with nitrous acid does appear, however, to provide sufficient helix distortion to provide a substrate for the BAL enzyme.

In contrast to the indirect endoDNase assays that recognize damage in DNA structure, electrophoresis of modified form I° DNA permits a direct assessment of damage that alters the duplex helix structure. This type of analysis starts with form I° DNA usually prepared by application of a nicking-closing enzyme (see Figure 8A). Thermal fluctuations in the pitch of the DNA helix that have occurred at the time of closure of the phosphodiester bond where the NC enzyme is acting will result in a population of molecules that differ by integral numbers

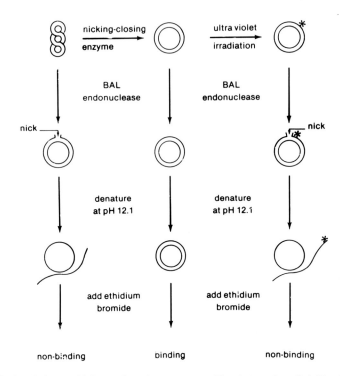

FIG. 10. Rationale for combining endonuclease assays with substrate form I° (without superhel ical turns) PM2 DNA form I. PM2 DNA is cleaved by the BAL endonuclease and denatured at pH 12.1 to give single-strand circles and linears that do not intercalate ethidium bromide under these conditions (shown at left). Application of nicking-closing enzyme gives covalently closed circular DNA without superhelical turns which are resistant to cleavage by the BAL enzyme and which are incompletely denatured at pH 12.1 and therefore bind ethidium bromide (shown in center). Irradiation of form I° DNA or treatment with DNA-reactive chemicals can produce helix disruptions recognized and cleaved by the BAL enzyme. Subsequent denaturation of the DNA leads to strand separation and lack of binding of ethidium bromide to single strand circles and linears (shown at right). The fraction of form I° DNA that resists denaturation is typically estimated by solution fluorescence assay (see Figure 5).

of superhelical turns. These individual subpopulations can be resolved by agarose gel electrophoresis in the presence of ethidium bromide (Figure 8B). A low concentration of ethidium bromide converts the population of form I° DNA initially with negative and positive superhelical turns (on the average zero) to a population in which the molecules have different integral numbers of positive superhelical turns (Figure 8B). These different species of DNA are then resolved by agarose gel electrophoresis as discrete bands distributed about an average positive superhelical value (Figure 11A). If form I° DNA is reacted with an agent that produces structure damage resulting in unwinding or winding of the helix by a fraction of one turn, subsequent addition of ethidium bromide and electrophoresis reveals that the populations lose their discrete character. This is illustrated for ultraviolet irradiation of PM2 DNA shown in Figure

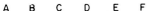

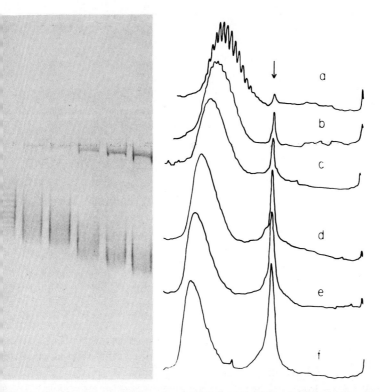

IG. 11. Agarose gel electrophoresis of PM2 form I° DNAs irradiated with ultraviolet light
ɔr 0 (A), 9 (B), 18 (C), 45 (D), 67.5 (E), and 90 seconds (F). The slab gel was stained with
thidium bromide and photographed in ultraviolet light (254 nm). Optical density scans (a to
of corresponding electrophoretic patterns in photographs (A to F) are shown *at right* with
ɔsition of PM2 form II marker DNA indicated by arrow. Direction of electrophoretic migration
ɾas from top to bottom. (Reproduced from Legerski *et al.* 1977, with permission of J. Biol.
ːhem.)

1. Formation of the pyrimidine dimer results in unwinding of the duplex helix
ɓy 12° (Legerski *et al.* 1977), and with increasing fluences of irradiation, the
ɗistribution of superhelical turns among the population of form I° DNAs be-
omes continuous (Figure 11B-F). The population is seen to progressively migrate
ɱore rapidly. The increased migration rate results from an increased average
ɲumber of positive superhelical turns producing more compact superhelical
ᴑNAs (Figure 8).

Finally, the same approach can be applied to assess the DNA structural
ɗamage produced by a chemical agent. This is illustrated for reaction of form
° DNA with AAAF. Modification of guanine by AAAF results in unwinding
ɒf the helix by 36° (Legerski *et al.* 1977), and when the population of closed-
ircular DNA is subjected to electrophoresis in the presence of ethidium bromide,

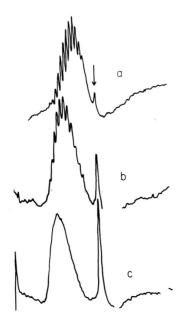

FIG. 12. Optical density scans of photographs of agarose gels containing PM2 form I° DNA reacted with AAAF at 0 (a), 1 (b), and 10 (c) molecules of AAAF per molecule of deoxyguanosine residue. Position of form II marker DNA is indicated by arrow. (Reproduced from Legerski et al. (1977), with permission of J. Biol. Chem.)

the discrete populations are converted to populations with continuous distributions of positive superhelical turns (Figure 12). These populations contain closed circular molecules with increasing numbers of positive superhelical turns on the average and migrate more rapidly. Measurement of the average position migrated and knowledge of the unwinding angle for a single lesion make it possible to calculate the average number of lesions introduced by the particular agent under consideration. The dependence of the distance migrated on the number of positive superhelical turns is inherently determined from control experiments with the discrete populations in which positive superhelical molecules differ by integral numbers of turns.

DISCUSSION

There are many factors that must be considered in establishing an appropriate and practical cell-free assay for DNA-reactive agents of a suspected carcinogenic nature. Consideration of the sensitivity of the assay must be weighed with respect to the economy of performing a large number of tests on different chemical or physical agents. As we have illustrated in this presentation, a variety of methodologies with differing degrees of damage resolution are readily applied to reactant DNA of covalently closed circular structure. The sensitivity of detecting DNA structural damage is maximized by the use of covalently closed circular DNA, since hydrolysis of a single phosphodiester bond results in conversion of the superhelical molecule to a nicked circular molecule with an open conforma tion possessing dramatically different hydrodynamic and physical-chemical properties. It is important in this regard to select a covalently closed circular DNA that has a sufficiently large molecular weight to provide detection of minimal number of bases damaged. However, the molecule should not be so large in molecular weight that adventitious nicking, which could occur in the course of analysis, becomes a serious limitation. The covalently closed circular DNA chosen must also be available in large quantities and be relatively inexpensive to prepare. All of these criteria are satisfied in the choice of PM2 DNA, which, as we have illustrated, has been the choice for initial evaluations of cell-free test systems. We fully anticipate that the use of PM2 DNA for these purposes will be expanded with development of additional assay methodologies.

It is also apparent that several powerful physical techniques are currently available to examine different aspects of DNA structural damage when the covalently closed circular DNA is used as reactant. Alterations in strand continuity, alkaline lability, and helix pitch are all readily assessed by one or another of the techniques that have been presented here. A concerted application of several of these procedures can lead to a thorough description of DNA structural damage produced by a given agent. In addition, a few of these procedures, while not providing complete information in themselves, are easily adapted to survey efficiently a very large number of compounds suspected of being DNA structure-damaging agents.

In summary, we anticipate that the use of appropriate covalently closed circular DNA, such as PM2 DNA, homogeneous in size and sequence content in conjunction with sedimentation, electrophoretic, and alkali-fluorescence assays, will provide highly proficient molecular screening systems for suspected DNA-reactive carcinogens.

ACKNOWLEDGMENTS

We wish to express our gratitude to our colleagues Drs. H. B. Gray, Jr., Charles W. Haidle, and James Strong for continued interest and support in development of certain methodologies described in this review. We are especially grateful to Diane Hicks for her excellent help in preparation of this manuscript. Portions of this research were supported by grants from the National Cancer Institute, CA-16527 (D. L. Robberson) and CA-4484 (R. R. Hewitt), from the National Pancreatic Cancer Project of the National Cancer Institute, CA-20142 (R. R. Hewitt), Institutional Biomedical Research Support Grant, RR-5511-15, Allotment No. BR-18 (D. L. Robberson), and by a Rosalie B. Hite Fellowship in Cancer Research (J. Harless).

REFERENCES

Davis, R. W., M. Simon, and N. Davidson. 1971. Electron microscope heteroduplex methods for mapping regions of base sequence homology in nucleic acids, *in* Methods in Enzymology XXI, L. Grossman and K. Moldave, eds., Academic Press, New York, pp. 413–428.

Espejo, R. T., and E. S. Canelo. 1968. Properties of bacteriophage PM2: A lipid-containing bacterial virus. Virology 34:738–747.

Espejo, R. T., E. S. Canelo, and R. L. Sinsheimer. 1969. DNA of bacteriophage PM2: A closed circular double-stranded molecule. Proc. Natl. Acad. Sci. USA 63:1164–1168.

Freifelder, D., A. Baran, and N. Bromlow. 1977. Positions of single-strand breaks in DNA. Biochim. Biophys. Acta 474:44–48.

Friedburg, E. C., and J. J. King. 1971. Dark repair of ultraviolet-irradiated deoxyribonucleic acid by bacteriophage T4: Purification and characterization of a dimer-specific phage-induced endonuclease. J. Bacteriol. 106:500–507.

Gray, H. B., Jr., D. A. Ostrander, J. L. Hodnett, R. J. Legerski, and D. L. Robberson. 1975. Extracellular nucleases of *Pseudomonas* BAL 31. I. Characterization of single strand-specific deoxyribonucleases and double-strand deoxyribonuclease activities. Nucleic Acid Res. 2:1459–1492.

Grdina, D. J., P. H. M. Lohman, and R. R. Hewitt. 1973. A fluorometric method for the detection of endodeoxyribonuclease on DNA-polyacrylamide gels. Anal. Biochem. 51:255–264.

Kato, A. C., and M. J. Fraser. 1973. Action of single-strand specific *Neurospora crassa* endonuclease on ultraviolet light-irradiated native DNA. Biochim. Biophys. Acta 312:645–655.

Legerski, R. J., H. Gray, Jr., and D. L. Robberson. 1977. A sensitive endonuclease probe for lesions in deoxyribonucleic acid helix stucture produced by carcinogenic or mutagenic agents. J. Biol. Chem. 252:8740–8746.

LePecq, J. B., and C. Paoletti. 1967. A fluorescent complex between ethidium bromide and nucleic acids. J. Mol. Biol. 27:87–106.

Lindahl, T. 1976. New class of enzymes acting on damaged DNA. Nature 259:64–66.

Ljungquist, S. and T. Lindahl. 1974. A mammalian endonuclease specific for apurinic sites in double-stranded deoxyribonucleic acid. J. Biol. Chem. 249:1530–1535.

Lloyd, R. S., C. W. Haidle, and R. R. Hewitt. 1978. Bleomycin-induced alkaline-labile damage and direct strand breakage of PM2 DNA. Cancer Res. (In press).

Ostrander, D. A., H. B. Gray, Jr., and D. L. Robberson. 1974. Catenanes of closed circular intracellular PM2 phage DNA. Biochim. Biophys. Acta 349:296–304.

Robberson, D., Y. Aloni, and G. Attardi. 1971. Electron microscopic visualization of mitochondrial RNA-DNA hybrids. J. Mol. Biol. 55:267–270.

Sharp, P. A., B. Sugden, and J. Sambrook. 1973. Detection of two restriction endonuclease activities in *Haemophilus parainfluenzae* using analytical agarose-ethidium bromide electrophoresis. Biochemistry 12:3055–3063.

Upholt, W. B. 1977. Superhelix densities of circular DNA's. A generalized equation for their determination by the buoyant method. Science 195:891.

Carcinogens: Identification and Mechanisms of Action, edited by A. Clark Griffin and Charles R. Shaw. Raven Press, New York © 1979.

A Hamster Embryo Cell Model System for Identifying Carcinogens

Roman J. Pienta

Chemical Carcinogenesis Program, Frederick Cancer Research Center, Frederick, Maryland 21701

Chemicals in the environment are considered to be a major contributing factor for causing cancer in man. Therefore, one of the major goals of cancer research today is the identification of potential carcinogens to which humans may be exposed so that these agents can be eliminated or prevented from entering the environment. A recent survey summarized by Maugh (1978) (Table 1) indicated that there are approximately 63,000 chemicals in everyday use, as estimated by the Environmental Protection Agency (EPA) and the Food and Drug Administration (FDA). These include active ingredients in pesticides and drugs as well as excipients added to drugs and other substances added to food for flavoring and nutrition or to extend shelf life of the products. In addition to the chemicals already in use, it has been estimated that several thousand new chemicals are placed into the environment yearly. For practical reasons, only several hundred of these can be bioassayed for carcinogenicity in conventional animal exposure tests, which require several years and can currently cost as much as $250,000 for each chemical. A simple calculation will show that the existing chemicals alone would require over 100 years of testing at the expense of several billion dollars. Therefore, there is an obvious need for short-term tests that can be used for prescreening and setting priorities for chemicals requiring further evaluation in the long-term animal studies.

CELL CULTURE SYSTEMS AVAILABLE FOR STUDYING CARCINOGENESIS

A number of model systems for studying the malignant transformation of mammalian cells in culture have been described in recent years. These have been extensively reviewed (Casto and Di Paolo 1973, Di Paolo 1974, Di Paolo and Casto 1976, 1977, Heidelberger 1973a,b, 1975a,b, Heidelberger and Boshell 1975). These systems primarily involve the use of fibroblast cultures of either early passage diploid strains or established lines of various rodent cells (Table 2). Either mass cultures or small numbers of cells are treated with chemicals. The formation of foci of altered cells on a monolayer or altered discrete colonies

TABLE 1. *Chemicals in common use*

Chemicals in everyday use	50,000*
In addition to active ingredients in:	
Pesticides	1,500†
Drugs	4,000†
Excipients (stabilizers, bacteriostats, etc.)	2,000†
Food additives (flavoring, nutrition, etc.)	2,500†
Additives to promote product life	3,000†
Total	63,000

* Estimate of the Environmental Protection Agency.
† Estimate of the Food and Drug Administration.
Data are summarized from Maugh 1978.

on a feeder layer correlates with malignancy and can be used as a reliable indicator of carcinogenicity. In another cell system, diverse carcinogens have been reported to either enhance or inhibit the morphological transformation of hamster cells by a tumor virus (Casto *et al.* 1973, 1974, Casto and Di Paolo 1973). Di Mayorca *et al.* (1973) demonstrated the chemical transformation of baby hamster kidney cells by the ability of these cells to grow in semisolid agar following treatment with carcinogenic nitrosamines. The increase in the frequency of growth of transformed cells in semisolid agar has been used to

TABLE 2. *In vitro carcinogenesis systems employing morphological endpoints for activity*

System	Chemicals examined*	References
Rat embryo fibroblasts infected with oncornavirus	35	Freeman *et al.* 1970, 1973, 1975, Price *et al.* 1971
Rat embryo fibroblasts	4	Rhim and Huebner 1973, Gordon *et al.* 1973
Syrian hamster embryo cells, direct assay	28	Berwald and Sachs 1963, 1965, Di Paolo *et al.* 1969, 1972
Syrian hamster embryo cells, host-mediated assay	9	Di Paolo *et al.* 1973
Syrian hamster embryo cells, mass culture focus assay	8	Casto *et al.* 1977
Swiss mouse embryo cells infected with oncornavirus	26	Rhim *et al.* 1971, 1974
C3H mouse prostrate cells	29	Chen and Heidelberger 1969, Marquardt 1974, 1976, Marquardt *et al.* 1974, 1976
C3H/10T½ mouse embryo cells	26	Reznikoff *et al.* 1973, Heidelberger 1972, 1975a,b, Benedict *et al.* 1975, 1977, Jones *et al.* 1972, 1976
BALB/3T3 mouse embryo cells	13	Di Paolo *et al.* 1972, Kakunaga 1973
Strain 2 guinea pig fetal cells	9	Evans and Di Paolo 1975

* From a list of approximately 90 carcinogens and noncarcinogens surveyed.

identify carcinogenic organic chemicals (Purchase *et al.* 1976, Styles 1977). This nonmorphological endpoint, when used in their study designed to predict the carcinogenic activity of 120 chemicals, accurately identified 91% of the carcinogens and 97% of the noncarcinogens.

In the cell systems employing morphological transformation, almost 100 chemicals with known or unknown carcinogenic activity have been examined (see Table 2). In general, the results between the reported in vivo carcinogenicity of the chemicals and their ability to transform cells in vitro correlated well, especially with the polycyclic hydrocarbons or other classes of chemicals not requiring additional metabolic activation by liver enzymes. False-negative results were observed in only a few cases and were attributed to spontaneous transformation sometimes seen with the systems employed (Freeman *et al.* 1973, Rhim *et al.* 1974). The range of carcinogens that can be identified by these systems is difficult to assess because only a limited number of chemical classes have been investigated in any one of the systems. From the entire list of chemicals, only N-methyl-N'-nitro-N-nitrosoguanidine, aflatoxin B_1, and seven polycyclic hydrocarbons, namely, pyrene, benzo[*a*]pyrene, 3-methylcholanthrene, anthracene, dibenz[*a,h*]anthracene, 7,12-dimethyl-benz[*a*]anthracene, and phenanthrene were tested in five or more of the systems listed in Table 2. Forty-five of the chemicals were tested in only one or another of the systems.

In these systems, endpoints are indicated by morphologically transformed colonies when target cells are planted at low densities or by foci of transformed cells when higher densities of cells or mass cultures are used and monolayers are formed. Each of the systems has its advantages and disadvantages. For example, although it is possible to identify transformed colonies after only eight to ten days in the hamster cell system, it is difficult to clone and subculture normal diploid hamster cells so that their characteristics can be compared in parallel with transformed cells.

On the other hand, several weeks are required before transformed foci are detected when aneuploid mouse cells are used, but normal cells at comparable passage levels are available for comparative studies of normal and transformed properties. However, the incidence of spontaneous transformation of these cell lines is higher under certain culture conditions and can pose problems by masking induced transformation by the chemical when used in bioassay systems.

Although transformation has been demonstrated with all these systems, most have not been standardized to the extent that they can be used routinely for prescreening chemicals with unknown carcinogenic activities; however, recently, several of these have been selected for further evaluation and validation in a coordinated program sponsored by the National Cancer Institute (Dunkel 1976).

HAMSTER EMBRYO CELL CARCINOGENESIS BIOASSAY

The use of in vitro model systems for studying chemical carcinogenesis is a relatively new field. The effects of 3-methylcholanthrene on cells from C3H and other established mouse cell lines were first studied more than three decades ago (Earle 1943, Earle and Nettleship 1943). However, it was concluded that cultured mouse cells spontaneously transformed and, therefore, were unsuitable for studying chemical carcinogenesis in culture. Nevertheless, after a hiatus of more than two decades, several cell culture systems have been described for quantitative studies of in vitro carcinogenesis. The studies by Berwald and Sachs (1963, 1965) reporting the transformation of Syrian hamster cells were further expanded by other investigators (Huberman and Sachs 1966, Di Paolo *et al.* 1969, 1971a,b, 1972), who were able to demonstrate the transformation of early passage diploid hamster cells by a number of diverse carcinogens. Their studies showed that morphological criteria for transformation correlated with malignancy and could be used as endpoints for detecting carcinogenicity of chemicals. Transformation was determined to be a one-hit dose-dependent phenomenon of induction and not the selection of preexisting cancer cells. Transformation was not due to toxicity, and these could be separated as unrelated events. Repeated unsuccessful attempts to induce or isolate oncogenic viruses from chemically transformed cells suggest that the carcinogens acted directly and did not depend on the activation of latent endogenous tumor viruses.

Because of these considerations and the general absence of spontaneous transformation with this species, we chose early passage Syrian hamster cells in our efforts to standardize a reliable in vitro carcinogenesis bioassay that could be used routinely for prescreening large numbers of chemicals or for identifying carcinogens directly. Historically, the bioassay employing hamster cells is based on the formation of morphologically altered discrete colonies. Since the cloning efficiency of primary or secondary cultures of diploid hamster fibroblast cells is very low, X-irradiated feeder cells are used to provide growth factors needed to support adequate numbers of colonies when small numbers of cells are planted. In the experiments described by the various investigators, the cultures were treated with chemicals for times varying from several hours to eight days, after which the cells were fixed, stained, and examined for transformation. Although procedures for studying in vitro carcinogenesis varied with the investigators using the cell system, the criteria for assessing morphologically transformed hamster cells have been well defined (Di Paolo *et al.* 1971b). Fibroblast cells in transformed colonies lose their polarity and grow in randomly disoriented patterns. The cells exhibit three-dimensional growth with extensive crossing-over so that the transformed colonies present a ragged edged periphery when stained. Transformed cells generally are more basophilic, vary in size, and have a decreased ratio of cytoplasm to nucleus (Sandford 1974). Fibroblasts in normal colonies are usually polar oriented and exhibit orderly growth in parallel arrays radiating from the center of the colony. They are less basophilic, less variable in size, have small cytoplasm to nucleus ratios, and usually grow as monolayer colonies with smooth edges. Typical transformed colonies are shown in Figure 1.

In all of the previous studies with Syrian hamster cells, primary cultures

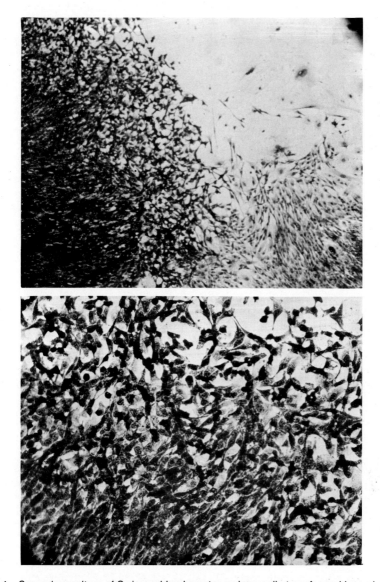

FIG. 1. Secondary culture of Syrian golden hamster embryo cells transformed by a chemical carcinogen. Cells fixed and stained with Giemsa. A, Note portion of a normal colony to the right of the transformed colony ($\times$ 40); B, randomly oriented cells at the periphery of a transformed colony ($\times$ 100).

were prepared from pooled hamster embryos as they were needed for each new experiment. Although we had limited success, our initial efforts to standardize the bioassay were hindered by the variation in response we observed among different batches when freshly prepared cultures were used as target cells (Pienta *et al.* 1977a, 1978, in press). At least half of the secondary cultures were completely refractory to transformation when treated with several doses of known carcinogens. Interestingly, recent studies show that, as with cells prepared from pooled embryos, variations in susceptibility to transformation also may occur in cultures prepared from individual embryos of a single litter (Table 3). This may be explained by the fact that randomly bred hamsters are used as the source of target cells, and susceptibility to transformation may be genetically controlled. Huberman and Sachs (1973) showed that cells from individual human embryos differed markedly in their ability to metabolize a carcinogenic hydrocarbon, although cells from organs of the same embryo responded equally well. Similar variations in the metabolism or binding of carcinogens by individuals have been reported.

Since such variability in response precluded the use of the system as a routine prescreen, attempts were made to identify susceptible target cultures that were consistently responsive after storage in liquid nitrogen. Therefore, a number of primary cultures were prepared from the pooled 12- to 13-day old embryos of individual litters of the LVG/LAK strain of Syrian golden hamsters (Pienta *et al.* 1977a). The cultures were disaggregated by trypsin, divided into aliquot samples, and stored in liquid nitrogen. Each litter provided about 50 ampules of cells. Representative samples from each pool of cells were then thawed, cultured, and tested for susceptibility to transformation by a known reference carcinogen. Cultures that did not respond were either discarded or used for other purposes. Feeder cell cultures were generally prepared from 14-day-old embryos and also were stored in liquid nitrogen as aliquot samples. Cultures that were positive in the original test generally responded to a panel of carcinogens and

TABLE 3. *Transformation responses of cell cultures prepared from individual embryos*

Litter	Percent transformation of cells from embryo:[*]									Positive/Total
	1	2	3	4	5	6	7	8	9	
1	0.31	1.10	0	0	0.41	0	—	—	—	3/6
2	0	0	0	0	—	—	—	—	—	0/4
3	0	0	0	0	0	0.49	0	0.42	0.19	3/9
4	0	0	0	0	0	—	—	—	—	0/5
5	0.26	0.27	0	0	0	—	—	—	—	2/5
6	0.24	0	0	0	0.32	0.09	—	—	—	3/6
7	0.47	0.21	0.30	0	0	0	—	—	—	3/6
						Total responsive embryos				14/41(34%)

* Embryos were obtained from LVG/LAK Syrian hamsters during the 13th day of gestation. Secondary culture cells were treated for eight days with a transforming dose of 3-methylcholanthrene, stained, and scored for transformation.

served as the source of target cells in a number of experiments. One such pool of cells consistently responded to transformation by 3-methylcholanthrene in 20 consecutive experiments (Pienta *et al.* 1977a). Recently, the Ela/ENG strain of hamster was surveyed and provided a number of responsive batches of cells that were used in the standard bioassay and in studies with mass cultures of cells.

During the course of our studies we observed that several other factors affected the reproducibility of the bioassay. To avoid aberrant morphological responses and to prevent interference with responses of cells that might be isolated and further characterized, fetal calf serum and other animal-derived reagents were routinely monitored to ensure the absence of mycoplasma or other adventitious agents. Not all samples of fetal calf serum supported the growth of newly transformed cells. Each batch of plastic dishes and culture medium had to be tested for the optimum growth of small numbers of cells. Prolonged storage of culture medium affected transformation frequency. When preparing primary cultures for use as candidate target cells, the cultures had to be seeded densely because the cells became less sensitive to transformation if too many population doublings had occurred before the cells were collected and frozen. The nonresponsiveness of cells used beyond the second subculture appears to parallel the loss of or low levels of certain endogenous enzymes and is being further investigated. When these factors are considered, a reliable bioassay can be established.

Standard Bioassay Procedure

The standard procedure used for bioassay of the reference chemicals is modified from the basic procedures described previously (Huberman and Sachs 1966, Di Paolo *et al.* 1969). Important modifications include the use of selected target cell cultures, fetal calf serum, culture medium, and plasticware. Special attention must be given to the logistics for the husbandry of the cells and the performance of the bioassays. For each bioassay an aliquot sample of cryopreserved feeder cells is grown to about 80% confluence. The cells are then X-irradiated with 5000R, plated at 60 to 80×10^3 cells per 60 mm dish. In the meantime, an aliquot sample of target cells will have been thawed and grown to no more than 80 to 90% confluence, so they can be trypsinized and seeded at 500 cells per dish onto feeder cells plated 24 hours previously. Target cells grown to confluence appear to be less sensitive to transformation. The cultures are then treated with graded doses of candidate chemical or appropriate control solutions and incubated for eight days without disturbing. The cultures are then fixed and stained and examined under low power magnification for transformation.

All test and control chemicals were coded prior to bioassay. Stock solutions were prepared on the day of use. To minimize exposure of personnel to potentially hazardous materials, plastic gloves were worn, and all manipulations with test chemicals, such as weighing and preparation of stock solutions, were done in appropriate fume hoods or safety cabinets. Cell culturing was performed in

TABLE 4. *Transformation of secondary cultures of Syrian hamster embryo cells by selected chemical carcinogens*

Chemical	Dose (μg/ml)	Surviving colonies*	Transformed colonies	Percent transformation
1,2,3,4-diepoxybutane	0	791	0	0
	0.05	751	1	0.13
	0.10	643	3	0.46
	0.5	462	4	0.86
	1.0	122	0	0
benzo[a]pyrene	0	343	0	0
	1.0	244	1	0.41
	2.5	289	2	0.69
	5.0	298	3	1.01
	10.0	387	8	2.07
	20.0	303	0	0
3-methylcholanthrene	0	491	0	0
	0.1	327	2	0.61
	0.5	199	4	2.01
	1.0	213	7	3.28
N-methyl-N'-nitro-N-nitrosoguanidine	0	471	0	
	0.05	364	1	0.27
	0.10	404	2	0.50
	0.50	403	7	1.74
	1.00	373	9	2.41
	5.00	111	2	1.80
N-hydroxy-2-acetylaminofluorene	0	461	0	0
	0.1	489	0	0
	1.0	534	1	0.18
	5.0	424	5	1.17
	10.0	300	2	0.66

* Each of six dishes containing 6×10^4 feeder cells was seeded with approximately 500 target cells. Cells were treated with chemical for eight days.

vented laminar flow cabinets. Spent culture medium was collected on absorbent material and incinerated. To avoid chemical contamination from recycled glassware, disposable glass or plastic labware was incinerated after use. Cell culture incubators were vented to the air exhaust system to prevent contamination of the laboratory. Table 4 summarizes data from several representative bioassays illustrating the collection of data. In earlier bioassays, six to nine dishes were used for each dose group. Recent bioassays employ 12 to 15 dishes.

RESULTS FROM THE STANDARD HAMSTER EMBRYO CELL TRANSFORMATION SYSTEM

The validity of any short-term carcinogenesis bioassay is based on the extent of correlation of the in vitro responses with the reported activities obtained from long-term tests in experimental animals. The animal tests must have been adequately performed and their results accepted. Only on this basis can attempts be made to validate the short-term bioassays. The study reported here concerns the validation of the hamster cell system by extending the data base to establish the range and limitations of the bioassay performed under standardized conditions. A large number of reference chemicals with known carcinogenic activities were obtained from the Carcinogenesis Standard Reference Compound Bank of the National Cancer Institute. A few were obtained directly from commercial sources. They included carcinogenic and noncarcinogenic analogues of direct-acting alkylating agents, polycyclic aromatic hydrocarbons, nitrosamines, nitrosamides and other nitro compounds, aromatic amines and aminoazo dyes, several metal carcinogens, and a number of miscellaneous chemicals. Included among these were several chemicals known or suspected as human carcinogens, namely, benzidine, 2-naphthylamine, 4-nitrobiphenyl, and the aflatoxins B_1 and B_2.

Mammalian cell transformation systems measure carcinogenicity directly since cultures derived from transformed cells are malignant. Primarily because of the extensive work done with the *Salmonella*/microsome mutagenesis system (Ames *et al.* 1973a,b, McCann *et al.* 1975, McCann and Ames 1977), it is generally accepted that many carcinogens can be detected as mutagens. The correlation of mutagenic activity with carcinogenesis is about 90% (McCann and Ames 1977). McCann and Ames (1977) reported that 157 of 175 carcinogens were mutagenic, and 94 of 108 noncarcinogens were nonmutagenic in the bacterial system. Results summarizing the mutagenic activities of the chemicals tested in the hamster cell bioassay are included in Table 5 to compare responses obtained in both systems.

TABLE 5. *Transformation of golden Syrian hamster cells by diverse classes of chemicals*

Chemicals tested	Reported activity	Hamster cell transformation	Bacterial mutagenesis*
Direct Alkylating Agents			
ε-Caprolactone	Noncarcinogen	0	0
Glycidol	Carcinogen	+	+
1,4-butane sultone	Carcinogen	+	+
1,3-propane sultone	Carcinogen	+	+
Methyl iodide	Carcinogen	+	+
Dimethylcarbamyl chloride	Carcinogen	+	+
Benzyl chloride	Carcinogen	+	+
Glycidaldehyde	Carcinogen	+	+
Ethyl-p-toluenesulfonate	Carcinogen	+	+
1,2,3,4-diepoxybutane	Carcinogen	+	+
Propyleneimine	Carcinogen	+	+
Polycyclic Aromatic Hydrocarbons and Derivatives			
Pyrene	Noncarcinogen	0	0
Benzo[a]pyrene	Carcinogen	+	+
Benzo[e]pyrene	Noncarcinogen	0	+
Phenanthrene	Noncarcinogen	0	0
3-methylcholanthrene	Carcinogen	+	+
Anthracene	Noncarcinogen	0	0
Benz[a]anthracene	Carcinogen	+	+
7,12-dimethylbenzanthracene	Carcinogen	+	+

TABLE 5. Continued

Chemicals tested	Reported activity	Hamster cell transformation	Bacterial mutagenesis*
Polycyclic Aromatic Hydrocarbons and Derivatives (Continued)			
1,2,3,4-dibenzanthracene	Carcinogen	+	+
1,2,5,6-dibenzanthracene	Carcinogen	+	+
Chrysene	Carcinogen	+	+
1,8,9-trihydroxyanthracene	Promoter	0	?
Nitrosamines and Nitrosamides			
N-nitrosodiethylamine	Carcinogen	0	+
N-nitrosodimethylamine	Carcinogen	+	+
N-nitrosoethylurea	Carcinogen	+	+
N-nitrosopiperidine	Carcinogen	+	+
N-nitrosodiphenylamine	Noncarcinogen	0	?
N-methyl-N'-nitro-N-nitrosoguanidine	Carcinogen	+	+
Methylazoxymethanol acetate	Carcinogen	+	+
Aromatic Amines, Aminoazo Dyes, and Nitro Compounds			
1-naphthylamine	Noncarcinogen	0	+
2-naphthylamine	Carcinogen	+	+
1-anthramine	Noncarcinogen	0	+
2-anthramine	Carcinogen	+	+
Benzidine	Carcinogen	+	+
2,4-toluenediamine	Carcinogen	+	+
2-nitro-*p*-phenylenediamine	Carcinogen	+	+
4-nitro-o-phenylenediamine	Undetermined	+	+
m-phenylenediamine	Undetermined	+	+
4-methoxy-m-phenylenediamine	Carcinogen	+	+
4-aminoazobenzene	Carcinogen	0	+
4-dimethylaminoazobenzene	Carcinogen	+	+
3-methoxy-4-aminoazobenzene	Carcinogen	0†	+
2-methyl-4-dimethylaminoazobenzene	Noncarcinogen	0	0
3'-methyl-4-dimethylaminoazobenzene	Carcinogen	+	+
7,9-dimethylbenz[*c*]acridine	Carcinogen	+	+
Acridine orange	Carcinogen	+	+
Aniline	Noncarcinogen	0	0
o-chloroaniline	Noncarcinogen	0	0
p-chloroaniline	Noncarcinogen	0	0
p-rosaniline	Carcinogen	0†	0
4-(*o*-tolylazo)-*o*-toluidine	Carcinogen	+	+
Azaserine	Carcinogen	+	+
2-aminobiphenyl	Noncarcinogen	0	0
4-aminobiphenyl	Carcinogen	+	+
2,3'-dimethyl-4-aminobiphenyl · HCi	Carcinogen	+	+
4-nitrobiphenyl	Carcinogen	+	+
2-nitronaphthalene	Carcinogen	+	+
2-nitrofluorene	Carcinogen	0†	+
4-nitroquinoline-1-oxide	Carcinogen	+	+
4-hydroxylaminoquinoline-1-oxide	Carcinogen	+	+
2-fluorenamine	Carcinogen	+	+
N-4-acetylaminofluorene	Noncarcinogen	0	0
N-2-acetylaminofluorene	Carcinogen	+	+
N-hydroxy-2-acetylaminofluorene	Carcinogen	+	+
N-acetoxy-2-acetylaminofluorene	Carcinogen	+	+
Bis(p-dimethylamino)-diphenylmethane	Carcinogen	+	0

TABLE 5. Continued

Chemicals tested	Reported activity	Hamster cell transformation	Bacterial mutagenesis*
Heavy Metal Salts			
Lead acetate	Carcinogen	+	?
Beryllium sulfate · 4H$_2$O	Carcinogen	+	?
Titanocene dichloride	Carcinogen	+	?
Nickel sulfate hexahydrate	Carcinogen	+	?
Solvents			
Acetone	Noncarcinogen	0	0
Ethyl alcohol	Noncarcinogen	0	0
Methyl alcohol	Noncarcinogen	0	0
Dimethyl sulfoxide	Noncarcinogen	0	0
Dimethyl formamide	Noncarcinogen	0	0
1,2-propanediol	Noncarcinogen	0	?
Miscellaneous Classes			
Acetamide	Carcinogen	+	0
Thioacetamide	Carcinogen	+	0
Thiourea	Carcinogen	+	0
5-iododeoxyuridine	Noncarcinogen	0	0
5-bromodeoxyuridine	Noncarcingoen	0	0
5-fluorodeoxyuridine	Noncarcinogen	0	0
Bromobenzene	Noncarcinogen	0	0
Hydrazine sulfate	Carcinogen	+	0
1,2-dimethylhydrazine	Carcinogen	+	0
Safrole	Carcinogen	+	0
Aflatoxin B$_1$	Carcinogen	+	+
Aflatoxin B$_2$	Carcinogen	+	+
N-[4-(5-nitro-2-furyl)-thiazolyl]-formamide	Carcinogen	+	+
2-(2-furyl)-3-(5-nitro-2-furyl)-acrylamide	Carcinogen	+	+
α-naphthylisothiocyanate	Noncarcinogen	0	0
Saccharin	Carcinogen	0	0
Methyl carbamate	Noncarcinogen	0	0
Ethyl carbamate (Urethan)	Carcinogen	0†	0
Succinic anhydride	Carcinogen	+	0
Auramine	Carcinogen	0†	0
Ethionine	Carcinogen	+	0
3-amino-1,2,4-triazole	Carcinogen	+	0
1-phenyl-3,3-dimethyltriazene	Carcinogen	+	+
Natulan · HCl (Procarbazine)	Carcinogen	0†	0
12-O-tetradecanoyl-phorbol-13-acetate	Promoter	0	0
Aroclor 1254	Noncarcinogen	0	?
Limonene	Promoter	0	?
Caffeine	Noncarcinogen	0	0
Methotrexate	Noncarcinogen	0	0
Hycanthone methanesulfonate	Carcinogen	+	+
Sodium nitrite	Noncarcinogen	0	+
Hydroxylamine · HCl	Noncarcinogen	0	0
Methoxychlor	Noncarcinogen	0	?

* Data summarized from McCann *et al.* 1975.

† These chemicals transformed cells when hamster liver S-9 homogenate was added to the system.

The reported carcinogenic activities of most of the chemicals used in this study were taken from publications of the International Agency for Research on Cancer (IARC) (1972–1976) and the United States Public Health Service (USPHS) (1972–1973). In view of the voluminous amount of data that would have to be presented, results of the bioassay of the large number of chemicals summarized in Table 5 are presented merely as plus or minus values because most of the data is presented elsewhere (Pienta *et al.* 1977a, 1978, in press). It should be noted that throughout these studies, spontaneous morphological transformation was never observed in any of the control groups that were treated with either the solvent used for dissolving water-insoluble compounds or cell culture medium. In addition to the negative controls, each bioassay experiment included a known carcinogen, usually 3-methylcholanthrene, as a positive control.

As mentioned earlier, the standardized protocol was used throughout this study. However, as batches of culture medium, fetal calf serum, or target and feeder cells were consumed, they were replaced by reagents selected to support transformation.

Direct-Acting Alkylating Agents

These agents do not require metabolic activation and react directly with cellular macromolecules. Hamster cells were not transformed by the noncarcinogen ε-caprolactone. The remaining carcinogenic alkylating agents induced morphological transformation and correlated completely with results obtained in bacterial mutagenesis assays. When tested against leukemia virus-infected rat cells (Freeman *et al.* 1973, 1975) and hamster cells in the transplacental host-mediated assay (Di Paolo *et al.* 1973), 1,3-propane sultone also gave positive results.

Polycyclic Aromatic Hydrocarbons

Polycyclic aromatic hydrocarbons constitute the class of carcinogens most extensively studied in cell culture systems. Although they must be metabolized to the active form, most fibroblast systems appear to have the required mixed function oxidase enzymes, as evidenced by the excellent correlation between in vitro and in vivo activities in most of the cell systems studied. These systems have been used to identify a number of active metabolites.

In the modified hamster cell system, complete correlation was observed when seven carcinogens and four noncarcinogens were tested. It is interesting to note that the promoter 1,8,9-trihydroxyanthracene did not transform hamster cells. According to the authors, toxicity prevented adequate testing of it in the mutagenicity test. None of the promoters tested in this study could transform hamster cells directly. Benzo[*e*]pyrene, which did not transform cryopreserved hamster cells, was positive in the Ames test and was reported to transform freshly prepared hamster cells (Di Paolo *et al.* 1969) but not BALB/3T3 cells (Sivak, personal communication).

Nitrosamines and Nitrosamides

We report here on the activities of only seven nitrosamines and nitrosamides although a larger number are presently being investigated in the presence or absence of exogenous metabolic activation to determine the range of nitrosamines that can be detected as carcinogens. Those results will be reported elsewhere. There was close correlation in the limited number of compounds tested. However, N-nitrosodiethylamine (DEN) was negative, obviously because of the need for metabolic activation not provided by the fibroblast cells of the hamster embryo culture. DEN was also negative when tested against early passage hamster cells (Di Paolo *et al.* 1972) but was positive in the host-mediated hamster cell system (Di Paolo *et al.* 1973). As discussed later, we observed transformation when DEN was tested in the presence of hamster liver microsomal enzymes.

Aromatic Amines, Aminoazo Dyes, and Nitro Compounds

These groups of chemicals contained several carcinogenic and noncarcinogenic pairs whose activity could be differentiated by the modified hamster cell bioassay. These include 2-naphthylamine and 1-naphthylamine, 4-aminobiphenyl and 2-aminobiphenyl, 3'-methyl-4-dimethylaminoazobenzene and 2-methyl-4-dimethylaminoazobenzene, N-2-acetylaminofluorene and N-4-acetylaminofluorene.

The system was also able to detect 2,4-toluenediamine, a carcinogenic hair dye component which has been removed from the market. Several other hair dye components, *m*-phenylenediamine sulfate, 4-nitro-*o*-phenylenediamine sulfate, 2-nitro-*p*-phenylenediamine, and 4-nitro-*o*-phenylenediamine gave positive results. The latter two compounds also transformed C3H/10T 1/2 clone 8 cells (Benedict 1976). All of these hair dye components were positive in the *Salmonella*/microsome test (Ames *et al.* 1975).

The carcinogenicity of the aminoazo dyes, 4-aminoazobenzene and 3-methyl-4-dimethylaminoazobenzene, and the aromatic amines, 2-nitrofluorene and *p*-rosaniline, was not detected in the standard test. However, as described later, all of these compounds could be activated, and they transformed cells when either hamster liver microsome enzymes or intact hepatocytes were added to the system.

In earlier phases of this study, N-2-acetylaminofluorene (AAF) consistently failed to transform certain batches of target cells that apparently lacked adequate levels of activating enzymes. However, these cells could be transformed by the active intermediate metabolites hydroxy-AAF and acetoxy-AAF. Similar results were observed with rat cells (Freeman *et al.* 1973). Other selected cell cultures of mixed embryo cells could be transformed by AAF, indicating the variable or low levels of endogenous enzymes in different batches of cells.

Miscellaneous Classes of Chemicals

When 41 compounds, including several metal carcinogens and solvents that did not fit into the previous classes, were bioassayed to further determine the range of chemicals detectable by their ability to transform hamster cells, most of the carcinogens with the exception of natulan, auramine, and urethan gave positive results. Urethan also failed to transform hamster cells directly (Di Paolo 1972) but transformed hamster cells in the host-mediated system (Di Paolo et al. 1973). A number of compounds of particular interest were detected in the standard bioassay. These included the nitrofuran, 2-(2-furyl)-3-(5-nitro-2-furyl)-acrylamide (AF-2), which consistently transformed cells in several bioassays. Cells transformed by AF-2 formed sarcomas when inoculated into suckling hamsters (Pienta et al., unpublished observations). This compound was used extensively in Japan for a number of years before its mutagenic and carcinogenic properties were revealed by various investigators. The standard bioassay was also able to detect some carcinogens that are natural products such as aflatoxin B_1 and B_2 and safrole. All of the solvents tested were negative. During this study dimethylsulfoxide was used as the solvent control at concentrations up to 0.2%. No transformed colonies were observed when several thousand dishes were examined.

Correlation of Transformation and Reported Carcinogenicity

The data summarized in Table 6 show that in the standardized hamster cell bioassay that is run without the addition of an exogenous activation system there was complete correlation between the in vitro morphological transforming ability and the reported in vivo carcinogenic activity of the direct-acting alkylating agents and polycyclic hydrocarbons. The correlation with the other classes of chemicals was good but not complete since eight compounds apparently requiring further metabolic activation were not detected. These included several aromatic amines, aminoazo dyes, a nitrosamine, and a few other miscellaneous

TABLE 6. *Correlation of in vitro transformation of hamster embryo cells in the standard bioassay with reported in vivo, carcinogenic activities of reference chemicals*

Chemical class	Reported activity	Number tested	Concurrence	False-negatives	False-positives
Direct alkylating agents	Carcinogen	10	10/10	0	—
	Noncarcinogen	1	1/1	—	0
Polycyclic hydrocarbons	Carcinogen	7	7/7	0	—
and derivatives	Noncarcinogen	5	5/5	—	0
Nitrosamines and amides	Carcinogen	6	5/6	1	—
	Noncarcinogen	1	1/1	—	0
Aromatic amines and	Carcinogen	27	22/27	5	—
aminoazo dyes	Noncarcinogen	8	8/8	—	0
Metal salts	Carcinogen	4	4/4	0	—
Solvents	Noncarcinogen	6	6/6	—	0
Miscellaneous compounds	Carcinogens	18	16/18	3	—
	Noncarcinogen	13	13/13	—	0
Totals	Carcinogens	72		9	
			97/106 (92%)		
	Noncarcinogens	34			0

chemicals. Saccharin, which may be a very weak carcinogen, also did not transform cells in the standard bioassay. No transformation was observed with any of the noncarcinogens.

Metabolic Activation

The failure of certain classes of carcinogens to transform fibroblast cultures has been observed with several of the model systems currently in use and indicates that, in general, these cells lack functional enzyme systems required for metabolizing some procarcinogens to an active form. In the bacterial mutagenesis systems these enzymes are provided by the addition of rat liver homogenates (Ames et al. 1973). As mentioned previously, certain target cell cultures were not transformed directly by AAF. However, these same cells were readily transformed when the assay was further modified to incorporate liver microsomal enzymes (S-9) prepared according to the method of Ames et al. (1973) but from phenobarbital-treated hamsters rather than rats. When target cells were treated simultaneously with AAF and hamster liver S-9, the cells were readily transformed. These results are summarized in Table 7. Similarly, in preliminary experiments, when eight of the carcinogens that gave false-negative results in the standard bioassay were retested in the presence of hamster liver homogenates and cofactors, seven of the carcinogens induced transformation but at low frequencies of response (Table 8).

These observations indicate that liver homogenates can provide microsomal enzymes needed to activate certain carcinogens. Our efforts to standardize the use of liver homogenates have been hindered by inherent cytotoxicity often observed with some of the preparations. An alternative is to use intact cells from early passage cultures of hepatocytes.

TABLE 7. *Metabolic activation of N-2-acetylaminofluorene (AAF) by hamster liver microsomal enzymes*

		Transformed colonies per survivors*			
			Final concentration of liver microsomal protein		
Chemical	Dose μg/ml	0	1.31 mg/ml	0.66 mg/ml	0.33 mg/ml	0.17 mg/ml
Control		0/1532	0/711	0/910	0/1417	0/529
AAF	5	0/1742	5/591	16/735	5/886	1/410
AAF	10	0/1669	11/686	3/503	7/916	8/468
Hydroxy-AAF	5	7/1030				
Hydroxy-AAF	10	9/240				
Acetoxy-AAF	5	5/1289				
Acetoxy-AAF	10	2/126				

* Composite values from two experiments. S-9 mix with cofactors was added immediately after chemicals were added to target cell culture 75–370. Cultures were incubated for eight days, stained, and scored for transformation.

TABLE 8. *Metabolic activation of carcinogens by the addition of hamster liver homogenates to the standard hamster cell bioassay*

Carcinogen	Transforming dose (μg/ml)	Transformed colonies per survivors
Diethylnitrosamine	1,250	1/182
Urethan	2,500	1/91
Auramine	2	2/543
2-nitrofluorene	50	1/68
3-methoxy-4-aminoazobenzene	25	1/348
	50	1/347
p-Rosaniline	2	1/673
Natulan	100	1/713
	200	1/827
4-Aminoazobenzene	5	0/735
	10	0/657

Leffert *et al.* (1977) described a method for perfusing rat livers in situ. We have modified the procedure for culturing hamster hepatocytes that retain high enzymatic activities for at least two days (Table 9). When either hamster embryo fibroblasts or hepatocytes obtained from juvenile hamsters were incubated for six hours with AAF-(9-^{14}C), hepatocytes metabolized AAF to N-hydroxy-AAF at rates 60 to 90 times greater than the hamster embryo fibroblasts. The formation of 2-aminofluorene was 350 to 500 times greater with hepatocytes than with the fibroblasts. This low rate of metabolism of AAF to N-hydroxy-AAF, the active metabolite, by the fibroblasts correlates with lack of transformation of these cells by the carcinogen.

The high rate of enzyme activity of the cultured hepatocytes suggested that these cells can activate a broad spectrum of carcinogens and may serve as effective feeder cells. In preliminary experiments with DEN, 2-nitrofluorene, and 4-aminoazobenzene, this appears to be so. These carcinogens, which gave false-negative results in the standard bioassay, were able to transform the hamster embryo target cells when hepatocytes were incorporated into the bioassay (Table 10).

TABLE 9. *Metabolism of AAF to N-hydroxy-AAF and AF by cultures of hamster embryo cells or hamster hepatocytes*

Cells	pMoles formed per 10^6 cells* N-hydroxy-AAF	AF	pMoles AAF metabolized per 10^6 cells
Hamster embryo cells	8 ± 0.1†	307 ± 28†	339 ±3†
Hamster hepatocytes			
1 day in culture	691	153,000	161,000
2 days in culture	472	110,000	114,000

* Cells were treated with 4.8 μg/ml of AAF-(9-^{14}C) and incubated for six hours at 37°C.
† Values are from triplicate samples.

TABLE 10. *Metabolic activation of carcinogens by hamster hepatocytes*

Group	Dose µg/ml	Total colonies per dishes seeded	Percent cloning efficiency	Transformed colonies	Percent transformation
		Experiment 1			
Dimethyl sulfoxide	0.2%	839/9	18.6	0	0
Benzo[a]pyrene	2.5	758/12	12.6	7	0.92
	7.8	733/12	12.2	1	0.14
Diethylnitrosamine	625	1071/12	17.8	1	0.09
	1250	1093/12	18.2	1	0.09
	2500	893/12	14.9	3	0.34
2-Nitrofluorene	5	979/12	16.3	0	0
	10	981/12	16.4	0	0
	20	765/12	12.8	7	0.92
		Experiment 2			
Dimethyl sulfoxide	0.2%	811/11	14.7	0	0
4-Aminoazobenzene	3.2	232/3	15.4	0	0
	10.0	992/12	16.8	0	0
	32	826/12	13.8	3	0.36

Approximately 500 secondary culture target cells were seeded into each dish containing feeder cells. Primary cultures of liver cells were added just prior to carcinogens. Cultures were incubated for eight days, then scored for transformation.

Efforts are being made to standardize the procedure so that it can be used routinely to minimize or eliminate false-negative results with this short-term bioassay.

IDENTIFICATION OF CARCINOGENS— TIER VERSUS BATTERY SYSTEMS

Short-term tests can be used in either of two ways as prescreens for identifying carcinogens. In a tier system, chemicals are subjected to a relatively simple test that is easily run. Positive compounds are then subjected progressively to more biologically complex tests until they are either finally eliminated or selected for evaluation in long-term conventional animal systems. In a battery system, chemicals are simultaneously subjected to several tests of varying complexity. The battery approach should be more reliable in identifying carcinogens because all short-term tests yield a portion of false-negative and false-positive results, and, therefore, no single test is reliable enough to be used alone. A potent carcinogen might not be detected if tested in a tier system that gave a false-negative response. For example, Table 11 shows that the spectrum of false-negative responses differs markedly in the standard hamster cell transformation system and the bacterial mutagenic system. The inability to detect several carcinogens by both of the systems further points out the need for a larger panel of tests when using the battery approach and the increased risk of relying on any one test in a tier approach.

TABLE 11. *False-negative responses*

Hamster cell transformation without activation	Bacterial mutagenesis with activation
4-aminoazobenzene*	
3-methoxy-4-aminoazobenzene†	
2-nitrofluorene*†	
Diethylnitrosamine*†	
p-rosaniline*	p-rosaniline
Natulan*	Natulan
Urethan*	Urethan
Auramine*	Auramine
Saccharin‡	Saccharin
	Acetamide
	Thiourea
	1,2-dimethylhydrazine
	Ethionine
	Succinic anhydride
	Safrole
	3-Amino-1,2,4-triazole
	Bis(p-dimethylamino)diphenylmethane

* Positive with hamster liver microsomal preparations.
† Positive with hamster hepatocytes.
‡ Saccharin was not tested in the presence of hamster liver microsome enzymes or hepatocytes.

CONCLUSIONS

A hamster embryo cell in vitro carcinogenesis bioassay has been modified and standardized by the use of cryopreserved aliquot samples of preselected responsive cultures as the source target cells. The standard bioassay, run without added metabolic activation, was able to identify 64/72 (89%) of the carcinogens and 34/34 (100%) of the noncarcinogens. There were no false-positive results with the noncarcinogens. When exogenous metabolic activation was incorporated by the addition of liver microsomal enzymes or intact hamster hepatocytes, all of the carcinogens that gave false-negative results in the standard bioassay were able to transform the cells in preliminary experiments. These observations suggest the utility of the system as a reliable prescreen for identifying carcinogens.

ACKNOWLEDGMENTS

The author extends his appreciation to his colleague William B. Lebherz III, for his efforts concerning the standardization of the hamster embryo cell transformation system, and to Judith A. Poiley and Ronald Raineri for their work concerning the metabolism of carcinogens.

This study was sponsored by the National Cancer Institute, Department of

Health, Education and Welfare, under contracts N01-C0-25423 and N01-C0-75380 with Litton Bionetics, Inc.

REFERENCES

Ames, B. N., W. E. Durston, E. Yamasaki, and F. D. Lee. 1973a. Carcinogens are mutagens: A simple test system combining liver homogenates for activation and bacteria for detection. Proc. Natl. Acad. Sci. USA 70:2281–2285.

Ames, B. N., H. O. Kammen, and E. Yamasaki. 1975. Hair dyes are mutagenic: Identification of a variety of mutagenic agents. Proc. Natl. Acad. Sci. USA 72:2423–2427.

Ames, B. N., F. D. Lee, and W. E. Durston. 1973b. An improved bacterial test system for the detection and classification of mutagens and carcinogens. Proc. Natl. Acad. Sci. USA 70:782–786.

Benedict, W. F. 1976. Morphological transformation and chromosome aberrations produced by two hair dye components. Nature 260:368–369.

Benedict, W. F., A. Banerjee, A. Gardner, and P. A. Jones. 1977. Induction of morphological transformation in mouse C3H/10T1/2 clone 8 cells and chromosomal damage in hamster $A(T_1)C1$-3 cells by cancer chemotherapeutic agents. Cancer Res. 37:2202–2208.

Benedict, W. F., N. Rucker, J. Faust, and R. E. Kouri. 1975. Malignant transformation of mouse cells by cigarette smoke condensate. Cancer Res. 35:857–860.

Berwald, Y., and L. Sachs. 1963. In vitro transformation with chemical carcinogens. Nature 200:1182–1184.

Berwald, Y., and L. Sachs. 1965. In vitro transformation of normal cells to tumor cells by carcinogenic hydrocarbons. J. Natl. Cancer Inst. 35:641–657.

Casto, B. C., and J. A. Di Paolo. 1973. Virus, chemicals and cancer. Prog. Med. Virol. 16:1–47.

Casto, B. C., N. Janosko, and J. A. Di Paolo. 1977. Development of a focus assay model for transformation of hamster cells in vitro by chemical carcinogens. J. Natl. Cancer Inst. 37:3508–3515.

Casto, B. C., W. J. Pieczynski, and J. A. Di Paolo. 1973. Enhancement of adenovirus transformation by pretreatment of hamster cells with carcinogenic polycyclic hydrocarbons. Cancer Res. 33:819–824.

Casto, B. C., W. J. Pieczynski, and J. A. Di Paolo. 1974. Enhancement of adenovirus transformation by treatment of hamster embryo cells with diverse chemical carcinogens. Cancer Res. 34:72–78.

Chen, T. T., and C. Heidelberger. 1969. Quantitative studies on the malignant transformation of mouse prostate cells by carcinogenic hydrocarbons in vitro. Int. J. Cancer 4:166–178.

Di Mayorca, G., M. Greenblatt, T. Trauthen, A. Soller, and R. Giordano. 1973. Malignant transformation of BHK_{21} clone 13 cells in vitro by nitrosamines—A conditioned state. Proc. Natl. Acad. Sci. USA 70:46–49.

Di Paolo, J. A. 1974. Quantitative aspects of in vitro chemical carcinogenesis, in Chemical Carcinogenesis, Part B, P. O. P. T'so, J. A. Di Paolo, eds., Marcel Dekker, Inc., New York, pp. 443–455.

Di Paolo, J. A., and B. C. Casto. 1976. In vitro transformation: Interaction of chemical carcinogens with viruses and physical agents, in Screening Tests in Chemical Carcinogenesis, R. Montesano, H. Bartsch, and L. Tomatis, eds., Vol. 12. International Agency for Research on Cancer Scientific Publications, Lyon, France, pp. 415–431.

Di Paolo, J. A., and B. C. Casto. 1977. Chemical Carcinogenesis, in Recent Advances in Cancer Research: Cell Biology, Molecular Biology, and Tumor Virology, R. C. Gallo, ed., CRC Press, Inc., Cleveland, Ohio, pp. 17–47.

Di Paolo, J. A., P. J. Donovan, and R. L. Nelson. 1969. Quantitative studies of in vitro transformation by chemical carcinogens. J. Natl. Cancer Inst. 42:867–876.

Di Paolo, J. A., P. J. Donovan, and R. L. Nelson. 1971a. In vitro transformation of hamster cells by polycyclic hydrocarbons: Factors influencing the number of cells transformed. Nature 230:240–242.

Di Paolo, J. A., R. L. Nelson, and P. J. Donovan. 1971b. Morphological, oncogenic, and karyological characteristics of Syrian hamster embryo cells transformed in vitro by carcinogenic polycyclic hydrocarbons. Cancer Res. 31:1118–1127.

Di Paolo, J. A., R. L. Nelson, and P. J. Donovan. 1972. *In vitro* transformation of Syrian hamster embryo cells by diverse chemical carcinogens. Nature 235:278–280.

Di Paolo, J. A., R. L. Nelson, P. J. Donovan, and C. H. Evans. 1973. Host-mediated *in vivo-in vitro* assay for chemical carcinogenesis. Arch. Pathol. 95:380–385.

Di Paolo, J. A., K. Takano, and N. C. Popescu. 1972. Quantitation of chemically induced neoplastic transformation of BALB/3T3 cloned cell lines. Cancer Res. 32:2686–2695.

Dunkel, V. C. 1976. In vitro carcinogenesis: A National Cancer Institute coordinated program, *in* Screening Tests in Chemical Carcinogenesis, R. Montesano, H. Bartsch, and L. Tomatis, eds., IARC Scientific Publication No. 12, International Agency for Research on Cancer, Lyon, France, pp. 25–28.

Earle, W. R. 1943. Production of malignancy *in vitro*. IV. The mouse fibroblast cultures and changes seen in living cells. J. Natl. Cancer Inst. 4:165–212.

Earle, W. R., and A. Nettleship. 1943. Production of malignancy *in vitro*. V. Results of injections of cultures into mice. J. Natl. Cancer Inst. 4:213–227.

Evans, C. H., and J. A. Di Paolo. 1975. Neoplastic transformation of guinea pig fetal cells in culture induced by chemical carcinogens. Cancer Res. 35:1035–1044.

Freeman, A. E., H. J. Igel, and P. J. Price. 1975. Carcinogenesis *in vitro*. I. *In vitro* transformation of rat embryo cells: Correlations with the known tumorigenic activities of chemicals in rodents. In Vitro 11:107–116.

Freeman, A. E., P. J. Price, H. J. Igel, J. C. Young, J. M. Maryak, and R. J. Huebner. 1970. Morphological transformation of rat embryo cells induced by diethylnitrosamine and murine leukemia viruses. J. Natl. Cancer Inst. 44:65–78.

Freeman, A. E., E. K. Weisburger, J. H. Weisburger, R. G. Wolford, J. M. Maryak, and R. J. Huebner. 1973. Transformation of cell cultures as an indication of the carcinogenic potential of chemicals. J. Natl. Cancer Inst. 51:799–808.

Gordon, R. J., R. J. Bryan, J. S. Rhim, C. Demoise, R. G. Wolford, A. E. Freeman, and R. J. Huebner. 1973. Transformation of rat and mouse embryo cells by a new class of carcinogenic compounds isolated from particles in city air. Int. J. Cancer 12:223–232.

Heidelberger, C. 1972. *In vitro* studies on the role of epoxides on carcinogenic hydrocarbon activation, *in* Topics in Chemical Carcinogenesis, W. Nakahara, S. Takayama, T. Sugimura, and S. Odashima, eds., University Park Press, Baltimore, pp. 371–388.

Heidelberger, C. 1973a. Current trends in chemical carcinogenesis. Fed. Proc. 32:2154–2161.

Heidelberger, C. 1973b. Chemical oncogenesis in culture. Adv. Cancer Res. 18:317–366.

Heidelberger, C. 1975a. Chemical carcinogenesis. Ann. Rev. Biochem. 44:79–121.

Heidelberger, C. 1975b. Studies on the cellular mechanisms of chemical oncogenesis in culture, *in* Fundamental Aspects of Neoplasia, A. A. Gottlieb, O. J. Plescia, and D. H. L. Bishop, eds., Springer-Verlag, New York, pp. 357–363.

Heidelberger, C. 1977. Oncogenic transformation of rodent cell lines by chemical carcinogens, *in* Origins of Human Cancer, Book C, Human Risk Assessment, H. H. Hiatt, J. D. Watson, and J. A. Winston, eds., Cold Spring Harbor Conferences on Cell Proliferation, Vol. 4, Cold Spring Harbor Laboratory, Cold Spring Harbor, New York, pp. 1513–1520.

Heidelberger, C., and P. F. Boshell. 1975. Chemical oncogenesis in cultures. Gann Monogr. Cancer Res. 17:39–58.

Huberman, E., and L. Sachs. 1966. Cell susceptibility to transformation and cytotoxicity by the carcinogenic hydrocarbon benzo[*a*]pyrene. Proc. Natl. Acad. Sci. USA 56:1123–1129.

Huberman, E., and L. Sachs. 1973. Metabolism of the carcinogenic hydrocarbon benzo[*a*]pyrene in human fibroblast and epithelial cells. Int. J. Cancer 11:412–418.

IARC Monograph on the Evaluation of Carcinogenic Risk of Chemicals to Man. 1972–1976. Vols. 1–10, International Agency for Research on Cancer, Lyon.

Jones, P. A., W. F. Benedict, M. S. Baker, S. Mondal, U. Rapp, and C. Heidelberger. 1976. Oncogenic transformation of C3H/10T 1/2 CL8 mouse embryo cells by halogenated pyrimidine nucleosides. Cancer Res. 36:101–107.

Jones, P. A., J. V. Taderera, and A. O. Hawtrey. 1972. Transformation of hamster cells *in vitro* by 1-β-D-arabinofuranosylcytosine, 5-fluorodeoxyuridine and hydroxyurea. Eur. J. Cancer. 8:595–599.

Kakunaga, T. 1973. A quantitative system for assay of malignant transformation by chemical carcinogens using a clone derived from BALB/3T3. Int. J. Cancer 12:463–473.

Leffert, H. L., T. Moran, R. Boorstein, and K. S. Koch. 1977. Procarcinogen activation and hormonal control of cell proliferation in differentiated primary adult rat liver cell cultures. Nature 267:58–61.

Marquardt, H. 1974. Cell cycle dependence of chemically induced malignant transformation. Cancer Res. 34:1612–1615.

Marquardt, H. 1976. Malignant transformation *in vitro:* A model system to study mechanisms of action of chemical carcinogens and to evaluate the oncogenic potential of environmental chemicals, *in* Screening Tests in Chemical Carcinogenesis, IARC Scientific Publications No. 12, International Agency for Research on Cancer, Lyon, pp. 389–410.

Marquardt, H., P. L. Grover, and P. Sims. 1976. *In vitro* malignant transformation of mouse fibroblasts by non-K-region dihydrodiols derived from 7-methylbenz[*a*]anthracene, 7,12-dimethylbenz[*a*]-anthracene, and benzo[*a*]pyrene. Cancer Res. 36:2059–2064.

Marquardt, H., J. E. Sodergren, P. Sims, and P. L. Grover. 1974. Malignant transformation *in vitro* of mouse fibroblasts by 7,12-dimethylbenz[*a*]anthracene and 7-hydroxymethylbenz[*a*]-anthracene and by their K-region derivatives. Int. J. Cancer 13:304–310.

Maugh, T. H., II. 1978. Chemicals: How many are there? Science 199:162.

McCann, J. E., and B. N. Ames. 1977. The *Salmonella*/microsome mutagenicity test: Predictive value for animal carcinogenicity, *in* Origins of Human Cancer, Book C, Human Risk Assessment, H. H. Hiatt, J. D. Watson, and J. A. Winston, eds., Cold Spring Harbor Laboratory, Cold Spring Harbor, New York, pp. 1431–1450.

McCann, J., E. Choi, E. Yamasaki, and B. N. Ames. 1975. Detection of carcinogens as mutagens in the *Salmonella*/microsome test: Assay of 300 chemicals. Proc. Natl. Acad. Sci. USA 72:5135–5139.

Pienta, R. J., J. A. Poiley, and W. B. Lebherz III. 1977a. Morphological transformation of early passage golden Syrian hamster embryo cells derived from cryopreserved primary cultures as a reliable *in vitro* bioassay for identifying diverse carcinogens. Int. J. Cancer 19:642–655.

Pienta, R. J., J. A. Poiley, and W. B. Lebherz III. 1978. Further evaluation of a hamster embryo cell carcinogenesis bioassay, *in* Cancer Prevention and Detection, Vol. 2. Marcel Dekker, Inc., New York (In press).

Price, P. J., A. E. Freeman, W. T. Lane, and R. J. Huebner. 1971. Morphological transformation of rat embryo cells by the combined action of 3-methylcholanthrene and Rauscher leukemia virus. Nature 230:144–146.

Purchase, I. F. H., E. Longstaff, J. Ashby, J. A. Styles, D. Anderson, P. A. Lefevre, and F. R. Westwood. 1976. Evaluation of six short term tests for detecting organic chemical carcinogens and recommendations for their use. Nature 264:624–627.

Reznikoff, C. A., J. S. Bertram, D. W. Brankow, and C. Heidelberger. 1973. Quantitative and qualitative studies of chemical transformation of clone C3H mouse embryo cells sensitive to postconfluence inhibition of cell division. Cancer Res. 33:3239–3249.

Rhim, J. S., B. Creasy, and R. J. Huebner. 1971. Production of altered cell foci by 3-methylcholanthrene in mouse cells infected with AKR leukemia virus. Proc. Natl. Acad. Sci. USA 68:2212–2216.

Rhim, J. S., and R. J. Huebner. 1973. Transformation of rat embryo cells *in vitro* by chemical carcinogens. Cancer Res. 33:695–700.

Rhim, J. S., D. K. Park, E. K. Weisburger, and J. H. Weisburger. 1974. Evaluation of an *in vitro* assay system for carcinogens based on prior infection of rodent cells with non-transforming RNA tumor virus. J. Natl. Cancer Inst. 52:1167–1173.

Rhim, J. S., W. Vass, H. Y. Cho, and R. J. Huebner. 1971. Malignant transformation induced by 7,12-dimethylbenz[*a*]anthracene in rat embryo cells infected with Rauscher leukemia virus. Int. J. Cancer 7:65–74.

Sanford, K. K. 1974. Biological manifestations of oncogenesis *in vitro:* A critique. J. Natl. Cancer Inst. 53:1481–1485.

Styles, J. A. 1977. A method for detecting carcinogenic organic chemicals using mammalian cells in culture. Br. J. Cancer 36:558–563.

Survey of Compounds Which Have Been Tested for Carcinogenic Activity. 1972–1973. USPHS Publication No. 149 US Public Health Service, Washington, D.C.

Genetics of Carcinogenesis

Carcinogens: Identification and Mechanisms
of Action, edited by A. Clark Griffin and
Charles R. Shaw. Raven Press, New York © 1979.

Aryl Hydrocarbon Hydroxylase in Normal and Cancer Populations

Marilyn S. Arnott,* Toshio Yamauchi,† and Dennis A. Johnston*

*Departments of Biology and Biomathematics, The University of Texas System Cancer Center M. D. Anderson Hospital and Tumor Institute, Houston, Texas 77030; † The University of Texas Medical School at Houston, Houston, Texas 77030

Epidemiological evidence has established an association between cigarette smoking and lung cancer (Hammond et al. 1975, Steinfeld 1971), but the mechanisms involved in the carcinogenic process have not been elucidated. An attractive hypothesis is that components of cigarette smoke, such as polycyclic aromatic hydrocarbons, act on the bronchial epithelium to cause malignant transformation (Huberman and Sachs 1974, Saffiotti et al. 1972).

From the elegant studies of Elizabeth and James Miller has evolved the concept that most chemical carcinogens are not active in the forms in which they are ingested or inhaled. Rather, they must be converted enzymatically into the reactive carcinogenic forms (Miller and Miller 1972, Miller 1970). Figure 1 is a simple representation of the processes of activation and detoxification of chemical carcinogens. The precarcinogen is converted in one step or a series of steps into the proximate carcinogen, which can then be converted to the ultimate carcinogen. It is this form that reacts with cellular macromolecules to begin the process of carcinogenesis. At any point along the activation pathway, the compounds may be converted into noncarcinogenic metabolites and conjugates, which are then excreted. Thus, the amount of the ultimate carcinogen present in the tissues at any time depends not only on exposure to the precarcinogen but also on the balance between activation and detoxification.

Benzo[a]pyrene (BP) is the prototype carcinogenic polycyclic aromatic hydrocarbon whose metabolism has been studied extensively. As shown in Figure 2, the first step in BP metabolism is mediated by the enzyme, aryl hydrocarbon hydroxylase (AHH), one of many mixed function oxygenases (see Jerina and Daly 1974, Sims and Grover 1974, Heidelberger 1975, Nebert et al. 1975, Nebert et al., in press, Nebert and Felton 1976 for reviews). These enzymes are membrane bound, multicomponent electron transfer systems with broad substrate specificity. One of the hallmarks of these enzymes is their inducibility. The enzyme activities, as well as the amounts of the individual components themselves, increase in response to the presence of substrates. Molecular oxygen

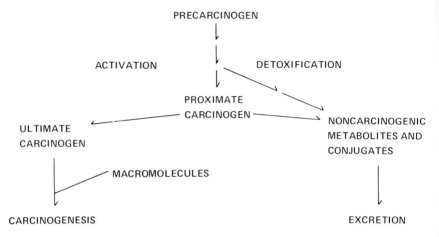

PRECARCINOGEN

ACTIVATION   DETOXIFICATION

PROXIMATE
CARCINOGEN   NONCARCINOGENIC
ULTIMATE   METABOLITES AND
CARCINOGEN   CONJUGATES

MACROMOLECULES

CARCINOGENESIS   EXCRETION

FIG. 1. Relationships among metabolic pathways leading to activation and detoxification of precarcinogens.

and NADPH are required for the various activities, which include ring and N-hydroxylations and N- and O-dealkylations.

The components of the mixed function oxygenases include cytochrome P-450, NADPH-dependent cytochrome P-450 reductase, and phospholipid. The cytochrome derives its name from the wavelength of maximum absorption observed in its carbon monoxide difference spectrum. Several cytochromes exist which differ in their response to specific inducers, in their substrate specificities, and in their spectral characteristics. For example, phenobarbital induces the synthesis of cytochrome P-450, while polycyclic aromatic hydrocarbons, such as BP, 3-methylcholanthrene (MC), and benzanthracene (BA), induce the synthesis of a different cytochrome, with maximum absorption at 448 nm. It is this cytochrome, referred to as cytochrome P-448 or P_1-450, which is a component of AHH.

AHH INDUCIBILITY IN MICE

Genetics

From studies using inbred strains of mice it is apparent that AHH inducibility is genetically controlled (Gielen *et al.* 1972, Thomas *et al.* 1972, Thomas and Hutton 1973, Robinson *et al.* 1974). In crosses between the inducible C57B1/6 (B6) and noninducible DBA/2 (D2) mice, AHH inducibility segregates as an autosomal dominant trait. In crosses between D2 and a different inducible strain, C3H/He (C3), the inducibility is additive. When a particular substrain of the noninducible AKR mice (AKR/N) is crossed with B6, noninducibility segregates as a dominant trait. The genetic control of AHH inducibility in mice obviously must reside in more than a single locus, and the suggestion

BENZO(*a*)PYRENE METABOLISM

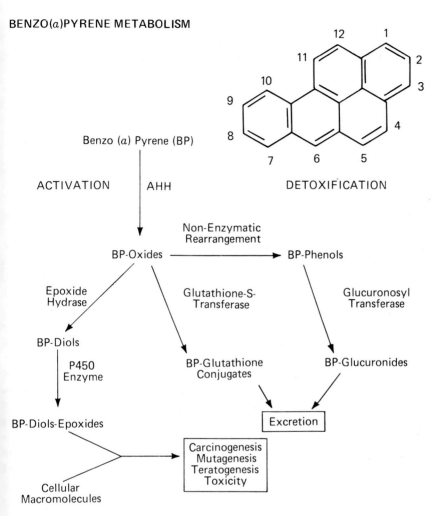

FIG. 2. Metabolism of benzo[*a*]pyrene leading to activation and detoxification.

has been made that at least three alleles at each of two nonlinked loci, plus a structural gene for the cytochrome, must be involved.

Tumor Susceptibility

Despite this complexity, Kouri and co-workers have shown that high AHH inducibility leads to increased susceptibility to tumors caused by hydrocarbons. In a key experiment (Kouri and Nebert 1978), animals were first identified as AHH-inducible or noninducible based on zoxazolamine-induced paralysis time. MC was then instilled intratracheally into B6, D2, and (B6D2)F_1 mice, as well as backcrosses between the F_1 and both parental strains. Lung tumors were found in high frequency in B6, (B6D2)F_1, and (B6D2)F_1 × B6 mice (all AHH inducible). The noninducible D2 animals had a very low tumor incidence. The (B6D2)F_1 × D2 backcross produced both inducible and noninducible animals. The tumor incidence in the inducible offspring was three times that of their noninducible littermates.

AHH IN HUMANS

In 1972, the activity and inducibility of AHH in human cultured leukocytes was reported (Whitlock et al. 1972, Busbee et al. 1972). The method involved the isolation of leukocytes by dextran sedimentation from approximately 20 cc of blood. More recently, Ficoll-Hypaque separation of lymphocytes has been used routinely. In either case, mitogen-stimulated proliferation of lymphocytes is required for induction of appreciable quantities of the enzyme. After two or three days in culture, an inducer of AHH, such as MC or BA, is added to half the cells, while solvent alone is added to the other cells. After an additional 24 hours in culture, the cells are harvested and assayed for their ability to hydroxylate BP. The assay is a modification of the fluorometric assay described by Nebert and Gelboin (1968) which measures the fluorescence of the alkali soluble metabolites of BP. The ratio of activity in induced cultures to activity in noninduced cultures is defined as inducibility.

Using this method, Cantrell, Kellermann, and Shaw reported variation in AHH inducibility in humans (Kellermann et al. 1973a). Population and family studies suggested that the inducibility was under genetic control (Kellermann et al. 1973b,c). The distribution of inducibilities in a population of 353 healthy donors was reported to be trimodal. Kellermann interpreted these results as indicating three distinct subpopulations, based on low, intermediate, or high inducibility, which suggested to him a single locus control of the enzyme.

Since AHH mediates the metabolism of carcinogenic polycyclic aromatic hydrocarbons, including those in cigarette smoke, the AHH activity in lymphocytes from lung cancer patients was of obvious interest. In 1973, Kellermann, Shaw and Kellermann reported that the distribution of AHH inducibilities in lung cancer patients was different from the normal population (1973d). Among 85 normal donors, 45% exhibited low AHH inducibility, 45% intermediate, and 10% high inducibility. A cancer control group, consisting of 46 patients with cancer at sites other than the lung, had a similar distribution of inducibilities. Of the 50 lung cancer patients, however, only 4% were in the low range, 66% intermediate, and 30% high inducibility. The interpretation of these results was that the higher inducibility in cultured lymphocytes from lung cancer patients reflected a higher level of AHH in target cells of the respiratory tract. Persons with higher AHH levels were hypothesized to be at greater risk of developing lung cancer when exposed to cigarette smoke.

In 1973, our understanding of human AHH could be summarized as follows:

1) Variation in AHH inducibility exists in the normal population.
2) The variation in inducibility is under genetic control.
3) The trimodal distribution of inducibilities suggests a single gene control.
4) AHH inducibility is higher in lung cancer patients than in the normal population.

Because of the important implications of these studies, Dr. Toshio Yamauchi, in our laboratory, began measuring human AHH in an attempt to repeat and extend Kellermann's work. For each donor, the age, sex, smoking history, and family history of cancer were recorded, as were the date and time blood was drawn, the lymphocyte yield, several parameters concerning the culture conditions, and the assay results. For the cancer patients, the type and stage of cancer were included, as well as any type of therapy they might have received. In general, only patients who had not undergone chemotherapy or radiotherapy were studied.

During the course of these studies, several changes were incorporated into the culture and assay system, which affected the enzyme levels and inducibilities. This forced us to analyze the populations separately, based on the particular procedures used during that time. Analysis of the large number of variables required a computerized data management system. Since chi-square and Kolmogorov-Smirnov tests of normality showed that the data were not normally distributed, nonparametric statistical methods were used to determine the significance of observed differences. These included the Mann-Whitney test for comparing variables between two groups, and the Kruskal-Wallis one-way analysis of variance for comparing variables in more than two groups. Differences were considered significant when a p value less than 0.05 was obtained. These methods have led to a very conservative interpretation of the data.

The distribution of inducibilities in a normal population is shown in Figure 3. This particular population consists of the normal controls of population II (see below) and is representative of every normal population we have studied. We have never seen any evidence of a trimodal distribution of AHH inducibilities. A unimodal distribution could either reflect the involvement of multiple gene

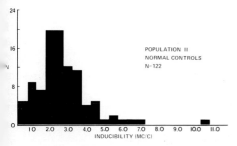

POPULATION II
NORMAL CONTROLS
N=122

INDUCIBILITY (MC/C)

FIG. 3. Distribution of AHH inducibilities in a population of 122 healthy donors over 40 years of age.

loci in the control of AHH inducibility or could simply result from the variability in enzyme measurements. Repeated tests on normal donors indicate that 15% is a conservative estimate of the variation observed in measurements on lymphocytes from a single donor, cultured on different days. Using the frequencies and mean inducibilities of the three groups reported by Kellermann and a 15% variation about each mean, computer simulations of trimodal distributions are indistinguishable from a single log-normal distribution for populations of fewer than 200 individuals. Thus, with the present limitations in the lymphocyte system, it is unlikely that a single locus effect could be observed without testing hundreds of individuals.

Recent support for genetic control of the enzyme system in humans comes from a study of pairs of twins reported by Atlas *et al.* (1976), who observed a high heritability index for AHH inducibility. The number of gene loci involved cannot be determined from these studies. However, recalling the complexity of genetic control of AHH inducibility observed in inbred strains of mice, we feel that the enzyme is probably under polygenic control in the human population.

Among healthy donors, we found no significant differences in AHH inducibility between smokers and nonsmokers or between male and female donors. The family data have not yet been fully analyzed. We did observe, however, that donor age has a significant effect on the observed activity and inducibility of AHH. As we reported in the February 1976 meeting of the National Cancer Institute Carcinogenesis Program in Orlando, Florida, healthy donors over 40 years of age exhibited lower AHH activities and inducibilities than those under 40. The known decline in lymphocyte response to PHA with age (Pisciotta *et al.* 1967, Sample *et al.* 1971, Hagen and Froland 1972, Barnes *et al.* 1975) may contribute to this finding. Since lung cancer patients are primarily among the older age group, the results presented below include only those individuals over the age of 40 years.

In the first population, AHH was measured in cultured leukocytes obtained from dextran sedimentation of whole blood. The results are summarized in

TABLE 1. *Population I*

Diagnosis	N	AHH units/10^6 cells		Inducibility
		C	MC	MC/C
Normal controls	80	.19 ± .01*	.42 ± .03	2.40 ± .10
Cancer controls	78	.21 ± .02	.47 ± .03	2.42 ± .10
Lung cancer	25	.20 ± .02	.56† ± .07	2.70† ± .22

AHH units are defined as fluorescence equivalent to 1 pmole 3-hydroxy benzo*[a]*pyrene per minute.
* Mean ± standard error.
† Significantly different from the normal population (p < .05).

TABLE 2. *Population II*

| Diagnosis | N | AHH units/10^6 cells | | Inducibility |
		C	MC	MC/C
Normal controls	122	.36 ± .03*	.87 ± .05	2.90 ± .13
Cancer controls	100	.31† ± .03	.88 ± .08	3.38 ± .17
Lung cancer	54	.24† ± .03	.81 ± .08	4.06† ± .30
Oropharyngeal cancer	13	.20† ± .03	.69 ± .16	3.90 ± .34

*† See legend for Table 1.

Table 1 for 80 healthy donors, 25 lung cancer patients, and 78 patients with other types of cancer. The noninduced activity was the same for all three groups, but the induced activity for the lung cancer patients was significantly higher than for the normal controls. This resulted in a higher inducibility for the lung cancer patients. The cancer control group was indistinguishable from the normal controls. Although the difference between mean inducibilities for the lung cancer and normal groups is not striking, the nonparametric tests indicated that the distributions of inducibilities in the two groups were significantly different, with the median for the lung cancer group (2.62) being somewhat higher than that of the controls (2.20).

For all subsequent studies, lymphocytes were isolated by centrifugation on Ficoll-Hypaque. The first study done in this manner included 122 normal donors, 100 cancer controls, 54 lung cancer patients, and 13 oropharyngeal cancer patients. As shown in Table 2, the noninduced activity was significantly lower for all the cancer patient groups than for the normal controls. No significant difference was observed in the induced activity between any of the cancer patient groups and the normal population. However, the inducibility for the lung cancer group was significantly higher than for the normal controls. Furthermore, the higher inducibility observed for the oropharyngeal cancer group, compared to the normals, was close to significance (p = 0.056).

After reevaluation of the pH optimum of the lymphocyte enzyme, the pH of the assay was changed from 7.4 to 8.5. This modification resulted in higher activities for all groups in population III.

Using this method, additional samples from oropharyngeal cancer patients were obtained. As shown in Table 3, the inducibility for this group was significantly higher than for the normal controls. AHH inducibilities of lung cancer patients who had undergone chemotherapy or radiotherapy were also examined. The most striking difference between these patients and the normal controls was a marked reduction in the growth of the lymphocytes. Using morphological criteria, the normal controls exhibited 45% blastogenesis (100 × number of lymphoblasts harvested ÷ number of lymphocytes cultured), while the lung cancer patients undergoing therapy exhibited only 23% blastogenesis. This was

TABLE 3. *Population III*

Diagnosis	N	AHH units/10⁶ cells		Inducibility
		C	MC	MC/C
Normal controls	71	.49 ± .05*	1.55 ± .20	3.27 ± .17
Cancer controls	41	.49 ± .06	1.58 ± .22	3.53 ± .29
Lung cancer + therapy	25	.38 ± .06	.72 ± .14	2.12 ± .29
Oropharyngeal cancer	12	.36 ± .06	1.46 ± .24	4.42† ± .36

*† See legend for Table 1.

the only group that showed a significantly decreased capacity for lymphocyte growth. Although the activities and inducibilities were not significantly different from the normal population, they tended to be lower. The myelosuppressive action of virtually all chemotherapeutic and radiotherapeutic methods precludes the use of these patients for any study involving cultured lymphocytes.

The problems of variability have plagued every worker in the human AHH field (Atlas *et al.* 1976, Kouri *et al.*, in press, Gurtoo *et al.* 1977). We have examined the AHH inducibility in a small group of healthy donors, from whom we drew blood on the same day once a week for four weeks. The absolute levels of AHH, and the inducibility, varied for each donor between days. But we found that we could rank these people in order of their inducibilities, and they would maintain that approximate order each week.

With this in mind, we tried a different experimental design to assess AHH inducibility in lung cancer patients. We drew blood from the spouse at the same time we obtained blood from the patient. The spouse served as an approximate age- and environment-matched control. Twenty-four patient-spouse pairs comprise population IV, as shown in Table 4. Because of the design of the experiment, statistical significance was assessed on the basis of paired t-tests. The noninduced enzyme level was significantly lower for the patients than for the spouses. The induced activities were not different, but the inducibility was significantly higher for the patients than for the spouses.

TABLE 4. *Population IV (Lung cancer patient and spouse)*

Subject	N	AHH units/10⁶ cells		Inducibility
		C	MC	MC/C
Patient	24	.06† ± .01*	.40 ± .07	6.39‡ ± .81
Spouse	24	.08 ± .01	.42 ± .07	4.94 ± .68

* Mean ± standard error.
† Significantly different from spouse (p = .011).
‡ Significantly different from spouse (p = .007).

AHH Inducibility versus Absolute Activity

Use of the inducibility, a ratio of two enzyme activities, deserves discussion. The amount of carcinogen metabolized should depend on the absolute amount of enzyme present rather than a ratio of activities. Because the higher inducibility in lung and oropharyngeal cancer patients generally was the result of a lower noninduced activity, rather than a higher induced activity, this is of particular concern. Two possible explanations come to mind.

Several studies have shown that the hepatic enzyme present in male rats induced with hydrocarbons is a different enzyme from that seen in noninduced animals (Wiebel *et al.* 1971, Rasmussen and Yang 1974, Holder *et al.* 1974, Thomas *et al.* 1975). Both enzymes metabolize BP but by different pathways. The noninduced enzyme produces mainly the 4,5-epoxide, while the hydrocarbon-induced enzyme forms relatively more epoxides at the 7,8 and 9,10 positions. Thus the noninduced enzyme may be regarded as a detoxifying enzyme, whereas the induced enzyme metabolizes BP to the proximate carcinogen, the 7,8-diol-9,10-epoxide. The AHH inducibility, then, can be viewed as a ratio of activating to detoxifying enzymes and represents the very crucial balance between activating and detoxifying pathways. If this holds true for the lymphocytes, then whether high AHH inducibility results from a high level of activating enzyme or a low level of detoxifying enzyme is unimportant. In either case, the balance of metabolism has been shifted toward activation of the carcinogen.

It should be noted, however, that studies on rat lung and kidney (Wiebel *et al.* 1971) indicate that the detoxifying enzyme may not be present in extrahepatic tissues. Hence, this interpretation of the significance of AHH inducibility may not be valid for lymphocytes.

Perhaps a more appropriate explanation comes from the many studies on mitogen response of lymphocytes from cancer patients. Using the conventional method of ^{3}H-thymidine incorporation, several workers have reported impairment of mitogen response in lymphocytes from lung cancer patients in particular (Ducos *et al.* 1970, Han and Takita 1972) and from cancer patients in general (Trubowitz *et al.* 1966, Garrioch *et al.* 1970). Other investigators, however, observed no difference in ^{3}H-thymidine incorporation between lymphocytes from recently diagnosed, untreated lung cancer patients and age-matched controls (Barnes *et al.* 1975, Whitcomb and Parker 1977). The latter study by Whitcomb and Parker is particularly relevant to the AHH question. Under culture conditions in which ^{3}H-thymidine incorporation was the same for lung cancer patients and controls, these investigators demonstrated decreased protein synthesis in the cultured lymphocytes from the lung cancer patients. If this holds true in our studies, then the noninduced enzyme level may be serving as a measure of the ability of the lymphocytes to synthesize protein. The higher inducibility in lymphocytes may reflect a higher induced enzyme level in the target tissue. The inducibility in the lymphocytes from cancer patients could then be viewed as a measure of induced activity, corrected for a decreased capacity of the cancer patients' lymphocytes to synthesize protein.

CONCLUSION

Our current view of human AHH can be summarized as follows:

1) Individuals differ in their AHH inducibility.
2) The inducibility difference between people is under genetic control.
3) The unimodal distribution of AHH inducibility in the normal population may be simply a reflection of day-to-day variability in the lymphocyte system but also suggests polygenic control of the enzyme system.
4) Lung and oropharyngeal cancer patients exhibit higher AHH inducibility than the normal population.

Whether the higher AHH inducibility preceded the lung and oropharyngeal cancer or is simply correlated with the presence of the diseases cannot be determined on the basis of these experiments. Such a distinction would require prospective studies. However, the fact that patients with other types of cancer had AHH inducibilities indistinguishable from the normal population indicates that cancer *per se* does not cause high AHH inducibility.

Studies showing a higher incidence of hydrocarbon-induced tumors in AHH-inducible animals suggest that AHH inducibility is a critical factor in susceptibility or resistance to chemically induced tumors. While the human studies reported here are consistent with this concept, the usual cautions in extrapolation from experimental animal systems to man must be observed. Much work remains to be done in developing a more reliable method of assessing AHH inducibility in humans before its role as a determinant of susceptibility to hydrocarbon-induced tumors in man can be established.

ACKNOWLEDGMENTS

The authors sincerely appreciate the generous support of Dr. Charles R. Shaw; the expert technical work of Ms. Betty Bruce, Mr. Richard Branum, Mr. Robert Daimler, and Mr. Timothy Jenkins; the data management provided by Ms. Peggy Wright, Ms. Sheryl Tatar, and Ms. Yvonne Freedman; and the manuscript preparation by Ms. Diane Hicks. This work was supported by Grant GM-15597 from the National Institute of General Medical Sciences, National Cancer Institute Contract NO1 CP 55604, and grants from The Council for Tobacco Research-U.S.A., Inc.

REFERENCES

Atlas, S. A., E. S. Vesell, and D. W. Nebert. 1976. Genetic control of interindividual variations in the inducibility of aryl hydrocarbon hydroxylase in cultured human lymphocytes. Cancer Res. 36:4619–4630.

Barnes, E. W., A. Farmer, W. J. Penhale, W. J. Irvine, P. Roscoe, and N. W. Horne. 1975. Phytohemagglutinin-induced lymphocyte transformation in newly presenting patients with primary carcinoma of the lung. Cancer 36:187–193.

Busbee, D. L., C. R. Shaw, and E. T. Cantrell. 1972. Aryl hydrocarbon hydroxylase induction in human leukocytes. Science 178:315–316.

Ducos, J., J. Migueres, P. Colombies, A. Kessous, and N. Poujoulet. 1970. Lymphocyte response to P.H.A. in patients with lung cancer. Lancet 1:1111–1112.

Garrioch, D. B., R. A. Good, and R. A. Gatti. 1970. Lymphocyte response to P.H.A. in patients with non-lymphoid tumors. Lancet 1:618.

Gielen, J. E., F. M. Goujon, and D. W. Nebert. 1972. Genetic regulation of aryl hydrocarbon hydroxylase induction. II. Simple mendelian expression in mouse tissues *in vivo.* J. Biol. Chem. 247:1125–1137.

Gurtoo, H. L., J. Minowada, B. Paigen, N. B. Parker, and N. T. Hayner. 1977. Factors influencing the measurement and reproducibility of aryl hydrocarbon hydroxylase activity in cultured human lymphocytes. J. Natl. Cancer Inst. 59:787–798.

Hagen, C., and A. Froland. 1972. Lymphocyte transformation and myocardial infarction. Br. Med. J. 1:445.

Hammond, E. C., I. J. Selikoff, and H. Seidman. 1975. Multiple interactions of cigarette smoking. Extrapulmonary cancer, *in* Cancer Epidemiology, Environmental Factors, P. Bucalossi, U. Veronesi, and N. Cascinelli, eds., Vol. 3. Proceedings of the 11th International Cancer Congress, Florence, October 20–26, 1974, Excerpta Medica, Amsterdam, pp. 147–150.

Han, T., and H. Takita. 1972. Immunologic impairment in bronchogenic carcinoma: A study of lymphocyte response to phytohemagglutinin. Cancer 30:616–620.

Heidelberger, C. 1975. Chemical carcinogenesis. Ann. Rev. Biochem. 44:79–121.

Holder, G., H. Yagi, P. Dansette, D. M. Jerina, W. Levin, A. Y. H. Lu, and A. H. Conney. 1974. Effects of inducers and epoxide hydrase on the metabolism of benzo(a)pyrene by liver microsomes and a reconstituted system: Analysis by high pressure liquid chromatography. Proc. Natl. Acad. Sci. USA 71:4356–4360.

Huberman, E., and L. Sachs. 1974. Cell mediated mutagenesis of mammalian cells with chemical carcinogens. Int. J. Cancer 13:326–333.

Jerina, D. M., and J. W. Daly. 1974. Arene oxides: A new aspect of drug metabolism. Science 185:573–582.

Kellermann, G., E. Cantrell, and C. R. Shaw. 1973a. Variation in extent of aryl hydrocarbon hydroxylase induction in cultured human lymphocytes. Cancer Res. 33:1654–1656.

Kellermann, G., M. Luyten-Kellermann, and C. R. Shaw. 1973b. Genetic variation of aryl hydrocarbon hydroxylase in human lymphocytes. Am. J. Hum. Genet. 25:327–331.

Kellermann, G., M. Luyten-Kellermann, and C. R. Shaw. 1973c. Metabolism of polycyclic aromatic hydrocarbons in cultured human leukocytes under genetic control. Humangenetik 20:257–263.

Kellermann, G., C. R. Shaw, and M. Luyten-Kellermann. 1973d. Aryl hydrocarbon hydroxylase inducibility and bronchogenic carcinoma. N. Engl. J. Med. 289:934–937.

Kouri, R. E., R. L. Imblum, and R. A. Prough. 1978. Measurement of aryl hydrocarbon hydroxylase and NADH-dependent cytochrome C reductase activities in mitogen-activated human lymphocytes, *in* Proceedings of the Third International Symposium on the Detection and Prevention of Cancer, H. Nieburgs, ed., Marcel Dekker, New York (In press).

Kouri, R. E., and D. W. Nebert. 1978. Genetic regulation of susceptibility to polycyclic hydrocarbon-induced tumors in the mouse, *in* Cold Spring Harbor Conference on Cell Proliferation, Vol. 4, The Origin of Human Cancer, Cold Spring Harbor Laboratory, Cold Spring Harbor, New York, pp. 811–835.

Miller, E. C., and J. A. Miller. 1972. The presence and significance of bound aminoazo dyes in the livers of rats fed *p*-dimethylaminoazobenzene. Cancer Res. 32:1073–1081.

Miller, J. A. 1970. Carcinogenesis by chemicals: An overview. G. H. A. Clowes Memorial Lecture. Cancer Res. 30:559–576.

Nebert, D. W., and J. S. Felton. 1976. Importance of genetic factors influencing the metabolism of foreign compounds. Fed. Proc. 35:1133–1141.

Nebert, D. W., and H. V. Gelboin. 1968. Substrate-inducible microsomal aryl hydrocarbon hydroxylase in mammalian cell culture. I. Assay and properties of induced enzyme. J. Biol. Chem. 243:6242–6249.

Nebert, D. W., R. E. Kouri, H. Yagi, D. M. Jerina, and A. R. Boobis. 1978. Genetic differences in mouse cytochrome P_1-450-mediated metabolism of benzo[a]pyrene in vitro and carcinogenic index in vivo, *in* Active Intermediates: Formation, Toxicity, and Inactivation, R. Snydor, D. Jollow, and J. R. Gillette, eds., Plenum Press, New York (In press).

Nebert, D. W., J. R. Robinson, A. Niwa, K. Kumaki, and A. P. Poland. 1975. Genetic expression of aryl hydrocarbon hydroxylase activity in the mouse. J. Cell Physiol. 85:393–414.

Pisciotta, A. V., D. W. Westring, C. Deprey, and B. Walsh. 1967. Mitogenic effect of phytohaemagglutinin at different ages. Nature 215:193–194.

Rasmussen, R. E., and I. Y. Wang. 1974. Dependence of specific metabolism of benzo[a]pyrene on the inducer of hydroxylase activity. Cancer Res. 34:2290–2295.

Robinson, J. R., N. Considine, and D. W. Nebert. 1974. Genetic expression of aryl hydrocarbon hydroxylase induction. Evidence for the involvement of other genetic loci. J. Biol. Chem. 249:5851–5859.

Saffiotti, U., R. Montesano, A. R. Sellakumar, F. Cefis, and D. G. Kaufman. 1972. Respiratory tract carcinogenesis in hamsters induced by different numbers of administrations of benz[a]pyrene and ferric oxide. Cancer Res. 32:1073–1081.

Sample, W. F., H. R. Gertner, and P. B. Chretien. 1971. Inhibition of phytohemagglutinin-induced in vitro lymphocyte transformation by serum from patients with carcinoma. J. Natl. Cancer Inst. 46:1291–1297.

Sims, P., and P. L. Grover. 1974. Epoxides in polycyclic aromatic hydrocarbon metabolism and carcinogenesis. Adv. Cancer Res. 20:165–274.

Steinfeld, J. L. 1971. The health consequences of smoking. A report of the surgeon general: 1971. Department of Health, Education and Welfare Publication No. (HSM)71–7513, pp. 239–244.

Thomas, P. E., and J. J. Hutton. 1973. Genetics of aryl hydrocarbon hydroxylase induction in mice: Additive inheritance in crosses between C3H/HeJ and DBA/2J. Biochem. Genet. 8:249–267.

Thomas, P. E., R. E. Kouri, and J. J. Hutton. 1972. The genetics of aryl hydrocarbon hydroxylase induction in mice: A single gene difference between C57BL/6J and DBA/2J. Biochem. Genet. 6:157–168.

Thomas, P. E., A. Y. H. Lu, D. Ryan, S. B. West, J. Kawalek, and W. Levin. 1975. Multiple forms of rat liver cytochrome P-450. Immunochemical evidence with antibody against cytochrome P-448. J. Biol. Chem. 251:1385–1391.

Trubowitz, S., B. Masek, and A. Del Rosario. 1966. Lymphocyte response to phytohemagglutinin in Hodgkin's disease, lymphatic leukemia and lymphosarcoma. Cancer 19:2019–2023.

Whitcomb, M. E., and R. L. Parker. 1977. Abnormal lymphocyte protein synthesis in bronchogenic carcinoma. Cancer 40:3014–3018.

Whitlock, J. P., H. L. Cooper, and H. V. Gelboin. 1972. Aryl hydrocarbon (benzopyrene) hydroxylase is stimulated in human lymphocytes by mitogens and benz[a]anthracene. Science 177:618–619.

Wiebel, F. J., J. C. Leutz, L. Diamond, H. V. Gelboin. 1971. Aryl hydrocarbon (benz[a]pyrene) hydroxylase in microsomes from rat tissues: Differential inhibition and stimulation by benzoflavones and organic solvents. Arch. Biochem. Biophys. 144:78–86.

Carcinogens: Identification and Mechanisms of Action, edited by A. Clark Griffin and Charles R. Shaw. Raven Press, New York © 1979.

Genetic Variation in Metabolism of Chemical Carcinogens Associated with Susceptibility to Tumorigenesis

Daniel W. Nebert, Roy C. Levitt, and Olavi Pelkonen

Developmental Pharmacology Branch, National Institute of Child Health and Human Development, National Institutes of Health, Bethesda, Maryland 20014

An important mechanism of action of environmental carcinogens is related to the genetic control of enzymes that metabolize these substrates to reactive intermediates. In this report we review previous work on the genetic expression of cytochrome P-450-mediated monooxygenase activities, and we examine the degree to which allelic differences at the murine *Ah* locus are correlated with differences in (1) biological activity of polycyclic hydrocarbon carcinogens in the intact animal (i.e., tumorigenesis), (2) DNA binding of reactive metabolites in vivo and in vitro, and (3) mutagenesis of these chemicals in vitro.

THE *Ah* LOCUS

Genetic Expression of AHH and Cytochrome P_1-450 Induction

There are now numerous lines of evidence for at least eight (and probably greater than twelve) different forms of P-450 in mammalian liver (Haugen *et al.* 1975, Thomas *et al.* 1976, Guengerich 1977, Haugen *et al.* 1977). In this report "P-450" in the general sense denotes all forms of CO-binding hemoproteins associated with membrane-bound NADPH-dependent monooxygenase activities. "P_1-450" is defined as that form(s) of cytochrome increased during polycyclic aromatic inducer treatment. It is not yet known whether cytochrome(s) P_1-450 in liver or in any nonhepatic tissue is (are) electrophoretically or catalytically identical to those in any other nonhepatic tissue. There is evidence for at least two forms of microsomal P_1-450 that appear to be closely associated with the induction process by 3-methylcholanthrene (MC) or β-naphthoflavone; in rabbit (Atlas *et al.* 1977) and in rat and mouse liver (Guenthner and Nebert, in press), these two structural gene products are under different temporal control, and we find one form of P_1-450 associated with MC-induced aryl hydrocarbon hydroxylase (AHH) activity and another form (P-448) associated with several other MC-induced monooxygenase activities.

Cyctochrome P_1-450 is highly induced by polycyclic aromatic compounds in the B6 (the inbred C57BL/6 mouse strain) and in other responsive mouse strains, but the induction of this form of cytochrome by polycyclic aromatic compounds is absent in liver and markedly decreased in lung, bowel, kidney, lymph nodes, skin, bone marrow, pigmented epithelium of the eye, brain, mammary gland, uterus, and ovary in the D2 and other nonresponsive mouse strains (reviewed in Thorgeirsson and Nebert 1977, Nebert *et al.* 1978). This "responsiveness" to *a*romatic *h*ydrocarbons was designated (Nebert *et al.* 1972b, Green 1973) the *Ah* locus: The allele *Ah^b* denotes the B6 and *Ah^d* the D2 inbred strain.

Numerous studies (reviewed in Nebert *et al.* 1975) indicate that an important product of the *Ah* (regulatory) locus in mice is a cytosolic receptor (Poland *et al.* 1976) capable of binding to certain polycyclic aromatic inducers (Figure 1). To our knowledge, only foreign chemicals bind with a high degree of specificity. Such a complex in some manner activates structural gene(s), thereby leading to increases in enzymes that metabolize these inducers (and other polycyclic aromatic noninducing compounds). In addition to innocuous products, reactive metabolites may also be generated. These reactive metabolites have been shown to be correlated with genetically determined increases in cancer, mutation, toxicity, birth defects, and detoxication (Thorgeirsson and Nebert 1977, Kouri and

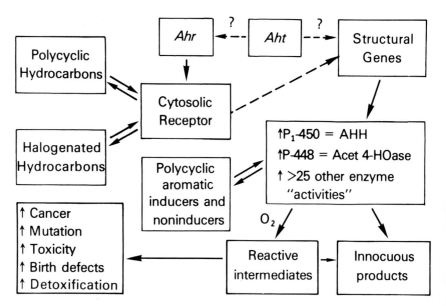

FIG. 1. Simplified scheme demonstrating the relationship of the *Ah* locus in the mouse with cancer, mutagenesis, toxicity, birth defects, and detoxification (modified from Nebert and Jensen, in press). *Ahr,* regulatory, and *Aht,* temporal, gene(s) associated with this genetic system. Acetanilide 4-hydroxylase (Acet 4-HOase) is associated with a form of P-450 which, when reduced and bound with CO, gives a Soret peak at about 448 nm (*i.e.* P-448). (Reproduced from Nebert and Jensen, in press, with permission of CRC Press, Inc.)

Nebert 1977, Nebert *et al.* 1977, Nebert *et al.* 1978), depending on the experimental conditions employed.

The AHH assay is a reliable, simple, and very sensitive assessment of aromatic hydrocarbon responsiveness following treatment of animals with polycyclic hydrocarbon inducers. Using AHH induction as an indicator of phenotype at the *Ah* locus, several laboratories have found that about half, or slightly more than half, of all inbred mouse strains examined are responsive (as are wild mice, randombred mice, and more than 20 inbred strains of rats tested [unpublished data]), and the remaining mouse strains are nonresponsive. There has evolved during the past 60 or 70 years of developing these inbred mouse strains, therefore, a stable mutation whereby certain strains lack (either quantitatively or qualitatively) the gene product of the *Ah* locus, the cytosolic receptor molecule (Poland *et al.* 1976).

Induction of AHH activity and cytochrome P_1-450 by MC is expressed almost exclusively as an autosomal dominant trait among offspring of the appropriate crosses between B6 and D2 (the inbred DBA/2 mouse strain) inbred strains and as an additive trait among offspring of the appropriate crosses between the C3 (the inbred C3H strain) and D2 inbred strains (Thorgeirsson and Nebert 1977). On the other hand, the *lack* of induction of AHH activity and P_1-450 by MC is expressed as an autosomal dominant trait among offspring of the appropriate crosses between C57BL/6N and AKR/N parent strains (Robinson *et al.* 1974). The simplest genetic model to explain most (but still not all) of the data includes a minimum of six alleles and two loci (reviewed in Nebert *et al.* 1975). However, for all intents and purposes, we may regard genetic expression at the *Ah* locus in offspring from the appropriate crosses between B6 and D2 strains and between C3 and D2 strains, respectively, as dominant and additive.

The genetic regulation of an induced enzyme in one tissue need not be the same in other tissues. However, the induction of AHH, and several other monooxygenase activities as well, appears to have similar genetic expression in all tissues examined (reviewed in Thorgeirsson and Nebert 1977). There are difficulties in a very careful genetic analysis of this point because most "control" responsive mice have, in fact, slightly induced AHH activity in many of their tissues which can be lowered by changing the diet. Hence, the slightly higher hepatic and pulmonary AHH activities seen in the responsive "control" B6 and C3 mice (Figure 2) may reflect the enzyme activities slightly induced by environmental factors.

One can also see in Figure 2 that induced AHH in (B6D2)F_1 liver or lung is slightly less than that in B6 liver or lung. The approximately 50:50 bimodal distribution among (B6D2)F_1 × D2 offspring and approximately 25:75 nonresponsive:responsive bimodality among the (B6D2)F_2 generation can be seen clearly in both liver and lung of MC-treated animals. The additive expression of AHH induction is found in the liver (and lung) (data not illustrated) of (C3D2)F_1 × C3 offspring. The approximately 50:50 low:intermediate bimodality among the $(C3D2)F_1 \times D2$ offspring and the approximately $25:50:25$ low:intermediate:high trimodal distribution among the $(C3D2)F_2$ generation that can be seen easily in the liver is not easily demonstrable in the lung because of relatively small differences between these groups and relatively large variation among pulmonary AHH in these MC-treated animals.

Growing evidence over the past 13 years has shown that different forms of P-450 generate different ratios of metabolites from the same substrate. Comparing MC versus phenobarbital as inducers of different forms of P-450 in rat liver,

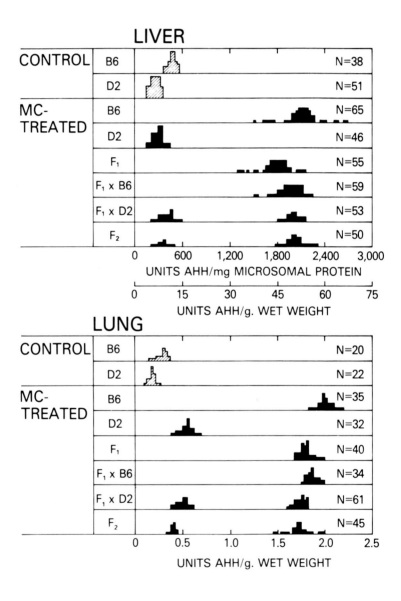

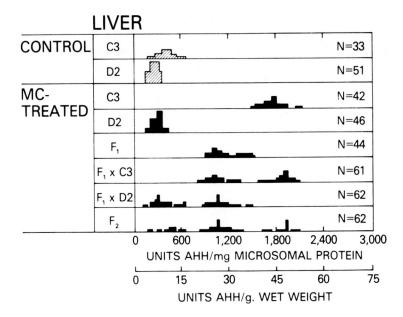

FIG. 2. Genetic variance in hepatic *(top left)* and pulmonary *(bottom left)* AHH activity in control and MC-treated offspring from appropriate crosses between B6- and D2-inbred strains and hepatic AHH activity *(above)* in control and MC-treated offspring from appropriate crosses between C3- and D2-inbred strains (Kouri and Nebert 1977). Histograms for liver samples represent specific AHH activity in control mice and in mice treated intraperitoneally 24 hours previously with MC (100 mg per kg body weight); controls received intraperitoneal corn oil. For lung samples, the mice received MC intratracheally 24 hours beforehand, 500 μg in 20 μl of 0.2% gelatin-0.85% NaCl; controls received the sterile vehicle alone. *One unit* is defined as that amount of enzyme catalyzing per minute at 37°C the formation of the hydroxylated product causing fluorescence equivalent to that of one pmol of 3-hydroxybenzo[*a*]pyrene (Nebert and Gielen 1972). *Specific AHH activity* denotes units per mg of microsomal protein. The mice weighed between 15 and 20 g. The number of mice examined individually is given at the *right* for each group. (Reproduced from Kouri and Nebert 1977, with permission of Cold Spring Harbor Laboratory.)

for example, various groups have shown that oxygenations may occur predominantly in different chemical positions on the molecule for such substrates as biphenyl, testosterone, 2-acetylaminofluorene, bromobenzene, *n*-hexane, and benzo[*a*]pyrene (*cf.* Thorgeirsson and Nebert 1977 for further discussion). Such differences in the metabolite profile of a chemical also suggest that important differences may exist in the nature of the intermediates formed. Differences in the reactivity of these intermediates or products might therefore result in marked dissimilarities in the carcinogenicity or toxicity of a given compound. Recent examples of P-450 differences in the rat in which this hypothesis appears to be true include bromobenzene toxicity (Zampaglione *et al.* 1973) and high blood pressure (Rapp and Dahl 1976). We believe that these same mechanisms are involved in the allelic differences at the *Ah* locus which result in an increased risk of chemical carcinogenesis, mutagenesis, toxicity, and teratogenicity caused by a wide variety of xenobiotics (Thorgeirsson and Nebert 1977). The differences in hepatic and nonhepatic induction of AHH activity (and presumably cytochrome[s] P_1-450) are apparent among B6, (B6D2)F_1, and D2 mice as a function of both time and dose of inducer. A responsive polycyclic hydrocarbon-treated mouse is therefore subject to both quantitative and qualitative increases in the steady-state levels of certain reactive intermediates, because of both an increase in cytochrome(s) P_1-450 content and an increased P_1-450/ P-450 ratio in numerous tissues. The relative content of P_1-450, compared with other forms of P-450, may be especially large (e.g., ratios of $10 : 1$ or $50 : 1$) in tissues such as skin and lung but never reaches even a $1 : 1$ ratio in liver (Kahl *et al.* 1976). This relatively large change in the profile of cytochrome(s) P-450, compared with smaller increments of change in epoxide hydrase (Schmassmann *et al.* 1976), UDP glucuronosyltransferase (Nemoto and Gelboin 1976), and GSH S-transferase (Bend *et al.* 1976) activities with benzo[*a*]pyrene (BP) as substrate, might be a factor in explaining why polycyclic hydrocarbons cause tumors in skin and lung but rarely in liver.

In studies involving the association of the *Ah* locus with cancer, mutation, or toxicity, the routine use of offspring from appropriate crosses between B6 and D2 parent strains (see Figure 2) is ideal because expression of AHH induction by MC most closely approximates a single-gene difference: *Ah*[b] is the dominant allele for responsiveness; *Ah*[d] is the recessive allele, the *Ah*[d]/*Ah*[d] animal being genetically nonresponsive. One therefore can determine if this single allelic difference is advantageous or disadvantageous with respect to risk for cancer or toxicity when all individuals receive the same dose of the same drug. We can thus evaluate the possible importance of steady-state levels of reactive intermediates in the mechanism of chemically induced carcinogenesis, mutagenesis, or toxicity among individuals in the same family or among siblings sharing the same uterus. This genetic probe is a particularly powerful experimental model system in the research areas of pharmacology, toxicology, teratology, and chemical carcinogenesis, because the test compounds studied often cause undesirable side effects (e.g., sedation, diarrhea, malnutrition, hormonal imbalance, etc.) that are hard to distinguish from specific pharmacologic, toxicologic, or carcinogenic effects of the compounds.

The *Ah* Locus and Subcutaneous Tumorigenesis

Fibrosarcomas initiated by subcutaneously administered MC are associated with genetically mediated aromatic hydrocarbon responsiveness among 14 inbred strains of mice (Figure 3). Table 1 demonstrates that the carcinogenesis index for subcutaneous MC in offspring from crosses involving the B6 and D2 inbred parental strains is, in fact, associated with the *Ah*[b] allele: The carcinogenesis index is 43 or greater in all responsive phenotype groups and 11 or less in all nonresponsive phenotype groups.

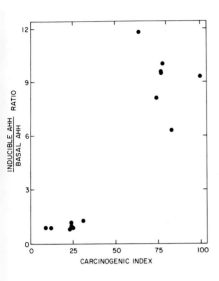

FIG. 3. Relationship between the carcinogenesis index (defined by Iball 1939) for subcutaneous MC and the genetically mediated induction of AHH activity by MC for each of 14 inbred strains; the correlation coefficient *r* is 0.90 (p < 0.001) (Nebert *et al.* 1974). Each *closed circle* represents the average result from a group of 30 inbred mice of a certain strain. The carcinogenesis index was evaluated after a subcutaneous dose of 150 μg of MC had been given to a minimum of 30 weanling mice of each strain. The "inducible AHH/basal AHH ratio" reflects the mean of hepatic AHH activity in MC-treated mice divided by the mean hepatic enzyme activity in control mice (N ≥ 5 for each of the two groups). Whether the MC-inducible AHH activity in the nonhepatic tissues appears to segregate as a single gene with the inducible hepatic AHH activity has not been examined for many of these strains. (Reproduced from Nebert *et al.* 1974, with permission of Marcel-Dekker, Inc.)

With respect to the carcinogenesis index for subcutaneous MC in offspring from crosses involving the C3 and D2 lines, however, unexpected values in Table 1 can be seen. Although the intermediate phenotype has intermediate carcinogenesis index values among $(C3D2)F_1$ individuals and among offspring from the $(C3D2)F_1 \times D2$ backcross (37 and 46, respectively), the values among progeny of the $(C3D2)F_1 \times C3$ backcross and the $(C3D2)F_2$ generation are more susceptible to MC-initiated tumors than can be accounted for by their inducible AHH activity alone (carcinogenesis indices of 60 and 61, respectively). There was also a near doubling (carcinogenesis index of 17) in nonresponsive F_2 individuals. We conclude that there probably exist other genes carried by the C3 mouse that make this strain particularly sensitive to MC tumorigenesis.

Figure 4 illustrates pathways of major importance in the metabolism of BP. Increased K-region oxygenation (at lower left) occurs under conditions of high $P-450/P_1-450$ ratios. Increased oxygenation of the non-K-region (pathway in the center) appears to be very important for covalent binding of metabolites to DNA (reviewed in Nebert *et al.* 1978), and this pathway is favored under conditions of a high $P_1-450/P-450$ ratio in the tissue (Kinoshita *et al.* 1973, Holder *et al.* 1974, 1975, Selkirk *et al.* 1974, 1976). The 7,8-diol-9,10-epoxide of BP is felt to be an ultimate carcinogen. Its extremely short half-life and its inability to be a substrate for UDP glucuronosyltransferase or epoxide-GSH S-transferase apparently account for its marked potential for carcinogenicity and for mutagenicity and toxicity in vitro (reviewed in Nebert *et al.* 1978). From Figure 4, therefore, it would appear likely that differences in BP-initiated subcutaneous fibrosarcomas between B6 and D2 mice would be closely associated with the *Ah* locus.

TABLE 1. *Relationship between aromatic hydrocarbon responsiveness and susceptibility to subcutaneous MC- and BP-initiated tumors among offspring from appropriate crosses involving the B6, C3, and D2 strains of mice* *

Strain or offspring	Expression at *Ah* locus†	Carcinogenesis index for MC	for BP
B6	++	61	
D2	0	11	
B6D2F₁	++	43	
F₁ × B6	++	58	
F₁ × D2	++	54	
	0	8	
F₂	++	63	
	0	6	
C3	++	73	56
D2	0	10	4
C3D2F₁	+	37	19
F₁ × C3	++	74	27
	+	60	24
F₁ × D2	+	46	1
	0	9	1
F₂	++	69	31
	+	61	7
	0	17	2

* Animals received, as weanlings, 150 μg of MC or BP in trioctanoin subcutaneously, and the carcinogenesis index was determined over an eight-month period (Kouri and Nebert 1977). The carcinogenesis index is defined by Iball (1939) as the percent incidence of subcutaneous fibrosarcomas divided by the average latency in days times 100. Further details are described elsewhere (Kouri *et al.* 1974, Kouri 1976).

† The phenotypic expression at the *Ah* locus is ranked as: ++ = fully responsive, 0 = nonresponsive, + = intermediate responsive, as judged by the data illustrated in Figure 2. (Reproduced from Kouri and Nebert 1977, with permission of Cold Spring Harbor Laboratory.)

The carcinogenesis index for subcutaneous BP (far right in Table 1) is disproportionately low among (C3D2)F₁ progeny (value of 19) and among all offspring from both backcrosses and the F₁ × F₁ intercross. The intermediate phenotype of the (C3D2)F₁ × D2 backcross is particularly resistant to BP tumorigenesis, having a carcinogenesis index (value of 1) lower than that for the D2 parent. It seems likely that the D2 strain carries other genes that confer an even higher resistance to BP-induced tumors than would be expected from their AHH content alone. Nonetheless, the *Ah* locus still plays a major role in the susceptibility of these animals to BP tumorigenesis, because both the (C3D2)F₁ × C3 progeny and the (C3D2)F₂ generations demonstrate a close association between tumor susceptibility caused by BP and inducible AHH activity. Thus, although some other genes may also influence susceptibility to BP- and/or MC-initiated tumors,

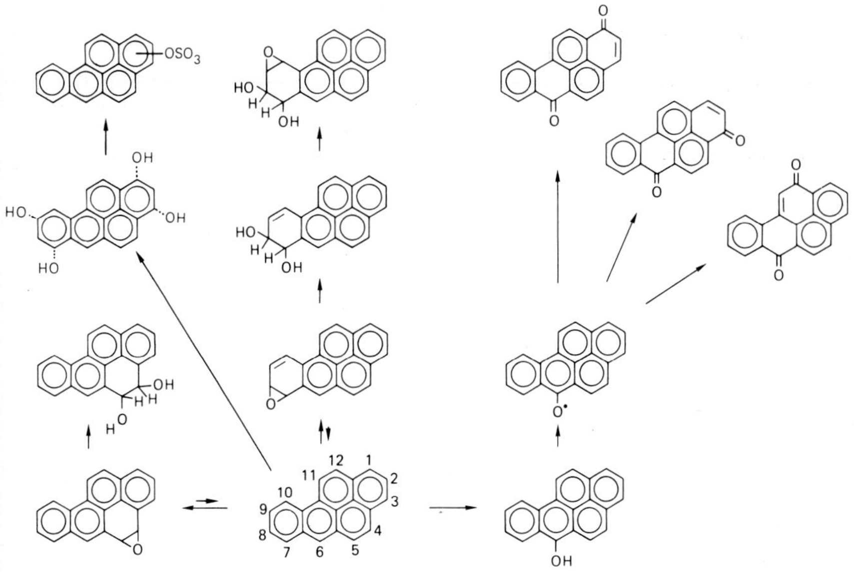

FIG. 4. Chemical structures of known metabolites of BP (*bottom center* with carbon atoms numbered from 1 to 12) (Pelkonen *et al.* 1978b). The in vivo formation of BP phenols in the 1-, 3-, 7-, and 9-positions (Croy *et al.* 1976) and subsequent sulfate conjugation of these phenols (Cohen *et al.* 1977) are shown at *upper left.* The K-region arene oxide *(bottom left)* is formed predominantly by a form(s) of P-450 other than P_1-450 and is subsequently converted to the diol by epoxide hydrase. The 7,8-oxide is formed predominantly by P_1-450; following diol formation via epoxide hydrase, the 7,8-diol-9,10-epoxide is formed predominantly by P_1-450. The 6-phenol can rearrange to the free radical 6-oxybenzo[*a*]pyrene, which subsequently is converted to the three quinones (reviewed in Thorgeirsson and Nebert 1977). (Reproduced from Pelkonen *et al.* 1978b, with permission of Raven Press).

the primary determinant for cancer susceptibility is the allele(s) regulating inducible AHH activity in numerous tissues of the mouse. Among recombinant inbred sublines having C57BL/6N and AKR/N as the progenitor strains, in which the *lack* of induction is expressed as an autosomal dominant trait, susceptibility to MC-initiated tumors remains linked with inducible AHH activity (reviewed in Nebert *et al.* 1978).

The *Ah* Locus and Lung Tumorigenesis

The model system of tumorigenesis initiated by subcutaneous MC or BP suffers from the shortcoming that AHH activity is determined in liver, whereas tumor formation occurs in subcutaneous connective tissue. The lung offers an alternate model system in which pulmonary AHH can be specifically and preferentially induced by intratracheally administered MC (Kouri *et al.* 1974, Kouri 1976). AHH induction in the lung appears to be under similar genetic control as that in the liver (see Figure 2). Mouse lung is known to be susceptible to

MC tumorigenesis; moreover, MC-caused bronchogenic squamous cell carcinomas in mice have been described (Nettesheim and Hammons 1971), and it is well known that carcinomas—not sarcomas—are the most frequently observed type of tumor in man. A statistically significant ($p<0.01$) correlation between lung tumors produced by intratracheal MC and the Ah^b allele has been found (Kouri and Nebert 1977). This correlation is most clearly seen in offspring from the (B6D2)F_1 × D2 backcross, in which the responsive individuals were greater than three times more susceptible to lung cancer than the nonresponsive individuals. Again, some contribution of genes other than the Ah locus seems to be responsible for the increased susceptibility to MC-initiated pulmonary tumors found in the F_1 and F_2 offspring and the progeny from both backcrosses. Most likely, genes controlling DNA repair, susceptibility to oncogenic virus infection, or immunological surveillance (e.g., differences in the H-2 locus) may be important in the overall susceptibility of certain tissues of an individual to chemically induced cancer. Although these other genes may also influence susceptibility to BP- and/or MC-initiated tumors, one primary determinant for cancer susceptibility is the Ah^b allele regulating inducible AHH activity in numerous tissues of the mouse.

The Ah Locus and TCDD as a Cocarcinogen

Hepatic and nonhepatic AHH activity and its associated cytochrome P_1-450 can be stimulated in nonresponsive inbred strains by the potent inducer TCDD (2,3,7,8-tetrachlorodibenzo-p-dioxin) to levels just as high as those in responsive strains; however, the ED_{50} is approximately 15 times higher in nonresponsive strains than in responsive strains (reviewed in Nebert et al. 1978). The carcinogenesis index for subcutaneously administered MC is increased in TCDD-treated nonresponsive D2 mice to about 60% of that of B6 mice in the presence or absence of TCDD (Kouri et al. 1978). We believe the most likely explanation for this effect is that TCDD acts as a cocarcinogen by inducing P_1-450 in the nonresponsive mouse. The newly induced cytochrome is now capable of metabolizing MC to the ultimate carcinogen more readily (Kouri et al. 1978).

In summary, MC and BP are either metabolized to higher steady-state levels of a proximal or ultimate carcinogenic intermediate(s) in the subcutaneous connective tissue or lung of homozygous or heterozygous responsive mice because of increased P_1-450 content, compared with nonresponsive mice, or are predominantly metabolized to a particular proximal or ultimate carcinogen(s) because of a marked change in the P_1-450/P-450 ratio.

DNA BINDING OF CARCINOGENIC METABOLITES

The Ah Locus and BP Metabolites

To understand further the interaction between covalently bound carcinogen and nucleic acid, Baird and Brookes (1973) developed a method for the enzymic degradation of nucleic acid containing bound carcinogens and the fractionatio of the resulting mixture by Sephadex LH20 column chromatography. This method has shown great promise in that distinct peaks eluted from the column can be demonstrated to change in elution profile, depending on the carcinogen incubated with microsomes and cofactors, on whether rat liver microsomes or cells in culture are used (reviewed in Nebert *et al.* 1978), and on the use of microsomal inhibitors in vitro (Boobis *et al.,* in press). The nature of carcinogenic metabolites (from, for example, benzo[*a*]pyrene, 7,12-dimethylbenzo-[*a*]anthracene, and 7-methylbenzo[*a*]anthracene) bound to DNA nucleosides has been studied not only by column chromatography (Baird and Brookes 1973, Sims *et al.* 1974, Boobis and Nebert 1977, Boobis *et al.,* in press, Pelkonen *et al.* 1978a, in press, and 1978b) but also recently by high-pressure liquid chromatography (Jeffrey *et al.* 1976, Moore *et al.* 1977).

Figure 5 illustrates the results obtained by incubating [³H]BP with hepatic microsomes from the control or MC-treated responsive B6 mouse and the control or MC-treated nonresponsive D2 mouse. Instead of five peaks designated A through E by Brookes and co-workers (King *et al.* 1975), nine peaks are reproducibly found in this laboratory. Peaks E and H (which correspond to

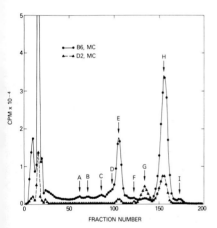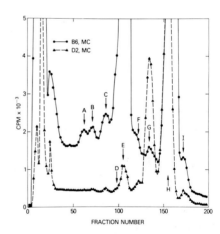

FIG. 5. Sephadex LH20 column chromatograph of an enzyme digest of DNA with [³H]BP metabolites bound during an in vitro incubation with hepatic microsomes from MC-treated B6 or D2 mice (Boobis *et al.,* in press). The treatment of the animals, the preparation of the hepatic microsomes, and the separation of the metabolite-nucleosides after the incubation are previously described (Baird and Brookes 1973, Pelkonen *et al.* 1978c). Deproteinized salmon sperm DNA (20 mg) was incubated with 4 mg of microsomal protein, 25 μmol of MgCl₂, 1 μmol of EDTA, 7 μmol of NADPH, 100 μmol of glucose-6-phosphate, 1.4 units of glucose-6-phosphate dehydrogenase, 1 mmol of potassium phosphate buffer, pH 7.5, and 60 nmol of [³H]BP (1.19 mCi, specific activity 20 Ci/mmol) added in 200 μl of acetone. The 10 ml reaction mixture was incubated at 37°C for 30 minutes. The DNA was reisolated, purified, digested with enzymes, then chromatographed on an 80 cm Sephadex LH20 column, eluted with a 30% to 100% methanol gradient in water at a flow rate of approximately 1 ml per minute. Two hundred fractions of 5.1 ml each were collected. Radioactivity (in cpm) was determined for 1 ml portions of alternate fractions. The ordinate at right is a 10-fold expansion of the ordinate (from the same experiment) at left. (Reproduced from Boobis *et al.,* in press, with permission of Pergamon Press.)

peaks A and D named by Brookes and co-workers [King *et al.* 1975]) were particularly large with microsomes from the responsive B6 mouse. Peaks E, G, and H (which correspond to peaks A, C, and D, respectively, named by Brookes and co-workers [King *et al.*, 1975]) were the largest with microsomes from the nonresponsive MC-treated D2 mouse. Whereas peaks E and H were much larger with the B6 than with the D2 microsomes, peak G was in fact larger with D2 than with B6 microsomes. Peaks A, B, C, D, F, and I were also larger with microsomes from the responsive strain than with microsomes from the nonresponsive strain.

In every incubation with various radioactive polycyclic hydrocarbons and other carcinogens (Pelkonen *et al.* 1978a, in press, and 1978b), there are several (often quite large) peaks eluting between fractions 4 and 40. Part of this material coming off the column early appears to represent metabolites bound to oligonucleotides incompletely hydrolyzed by the DNA digestion procedure. Metabolites already bound to DNA are also possibly oxygenated a second time and bound to a second site on DNA, thereby forming metabolite-dinucleoside complexes that elute from the column in early fractions. The radioactivity eluting early may also represent, in part, metabolites bound to phosphate groups or simply metabolites physically trapped in oligonucleotides (Pelkonen *et al.* 1978c).

Because inbred mouse strains differ at thousands of genetic loci, the definitive experiment is to study responsive *(Ah^b/Ah^d)* and nonresponsive *(Ah^d/Ah^d)* progeny from the B6D2F$_1$ × D2 backcross. In doing this experiment, we found that the result was very similar to that found with the inbred B6 and D2 strains. All peaks, with the exception of peak G, appear to be principally associated with BP metabolism mediated by P$_1$-450 and therefore to be controlled by the *Ah^b* allele (Pelkonen *et al.* 1978b).

With the use of synthetic and biologically produced metabolites (Pelkonen *et al.* 1978c) and on the basis of our studies on the effects of microsomal enzyme inducers and inhibitors (Boobis *et al.*, in press), all peaks are tentatively assigned to one or more metabolites of BP (Figure 6). We suggest that the major reactive intermediate of BP contributing to each peak is as follows: peak A, possibly 4,5-dihydrodiol-7,8-oxide or 4,5-dihydrodiol-9,10-oxide; peaks B, D, F, and I, quinones oxygenated further (or quinone-derived free radicals); peak C, possibly the further metabolism of a dihydrodiol; peak E, both *cis-* and *trans-*7,8-diol-9,10-epoxides; peak G, the 4,5-oxide; and peak H, 9-hydroxybenzo[*a*]pyrene-4,5-oxide (and/or other phenols oxygenated further). Of the nine peaks listed here, it is of interest that eight (all except perhaps peak G) involve more than a single monooxygenation by forms of cytochrome P-450.

BP thus may be metabolized to four different "types" of reactive intermediates capable of binding to DNA: (1) primary arene oxides, (2) diol-epoxides, (3) phenols oxygenated further, and (4) quinones oxygenated further (or quinone-derived free radicals). These last three types of microsomally activated intermediates are therefore the result of two- or three-step enzymic processes in which P-450-mediated monooxygenations occur at least twice.

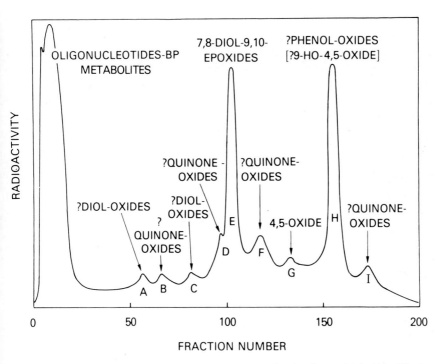

FIG. 6. A typical Sephadex LH20 column chromatograph showing the postulated identification of BP metabolites produced in vitro by mouse liver microsomes that bind to DNA nucleoside(s). The nucleoside(s) contributing to each peak is not known, except for the binding of BP 7,8-diol-9,10-epoxide principally to the 2-amino of guanosine (Weinstein *et al.* 1976).

Attempt to Correlate Differences in the BP Carcinogenesis Index with Differences in DNA Binding

The BP carcinogenesis index for genetically responsive C3 mice is more than five times greater than that for responsive B6 mice and about 15 times greater than that for nonresponsive D2 mice (Table 2). MC-inducible AHH activity and total P-450 content in B6 mice is 30% to 40% greater than that in C3 mice. The MC-inducible AHH activity is about five times greater and the total P-450 content is about two times greater in B6 mice than that in D2 mice. The MC-induced AHH activity and total P-450 content in the responsive $(B6C3)F_1$ and the responsive $(B6D2)F_1$ heterozygotes are similar to values found in the responsive B6 parent, in agreement with data that aromatic hydrocarbon responsiveness is inherited more or less as a single autosomal dominant trait in these genetic crosses. The MC-induced hydroxylase activity and total P-450 content in the $(C3D2)F_1$, on the other hand, are intermediate between both parents, in agreement with previous data that aromatic hydrocarbon responsiveness is inherited additively when C3H/HeJ, C3H/HeN, or C3H/fCum is crossed with DBA/2J, DBA/2N, or DBA/2Cum (reviewed in Kouri and Nebert 1977).

TABLE 2. *BP carcinogenesis index, hepatic AHH, and total cytochrome P-450 content in MC-treated C3, B6, and D2 strains and their F₁ hybrids*

Inbred strain or heterozygote	Number of tumors per number of mice treated	Tumor incidence (%)	Average latency (days)	Carcinogenesis index	Specific AHH activity*	Total P-450 content†
C3	33/42	79	142	56	1620	1020
B6	4/30	13.3	133	10	2260	1330
D2	3/51	5.9	159	3.7	440	690
(B6C3)F₁	21/34	62	130	48	2310	1480
(C3D2)F₁					1040	920
(B6D2)F₁	16/53	30	162	19	2140	1320

* Expressed in units per mg of microsomal protein; six livers were combined (Pelkonen *et al.* 1978a, in press).
† Expressed in pmol per mg of microsomal protein and is principally P-450 in D2 mice and the sum of cytochromes P-450 and P₁-450 in the genetically responsive mice. Six livers were combined for this determination. (Reproduced from Pelkonen *et al.* 1978a, in press, with permission of Waverly Press.)

The carcinogenesis index of 48 for the $(B6C3)F_1$ hybrid is close to the carcinogenesis index of 56 for the C3 parent rather than similar to that of 10 for the B6 parent. The carcinogenesis index of 19 for the $(C3D2)F_1$ is below the expected carcinogenesis index (about 30 would be intermediate for the carcinogenesis index of both parents). These data and a growing body of evidence (reviewed in Kouri 1976, and Kouri and Nebert 1977) indicate that additional genes other than the *Ah* locus may cause a particular inbred strain to be more resistant, or sensitive, to polycyclic hydrocarbon-initiated tumors than expected solely on the basis of AHH inducibility.

Thus, the genetic differences in carcinogenesis index between C3 and D2 (i.e., 56 versus 3.7) or between B6 and D2 (i.e., 10 versus 3.7) might be accounted for by quantitative increases in the generation of BP metabolites that interact with DNA mediated by polycyclic hydrocarbon-induced AHH activity and its associated P_1-450. This correlation breaks down in the comparison between C3 and B6 mice, however. Although the MC-induced AHH activity and total P-450 content are *slightly less* in C3 mice than in B6 mice, the BP carcinogenesis index is at least *five times greater* in C3 than in B6 mice. We therefore wondered if we could find among these three inbred strains any specific chromatographic peaks (representing BP metabolites bound to DNA nucleosides in vitro) that might account for these differences in the biological activity of BP. For example, might there be a single peak that is at least five times greater with C3 than with B6 microsomes and that is three times greater with B6 than with D2 microsomes?

No distinct correlation between the carcinogenesis index and the heights of specific BP metabolite-nucleoside peaks was found (Pelkonen *et al.* 1978a, in press). No peak was more than 60% greater (peak H was 57% greater) in C3 than in B6 mice. The carcinogenesis index in C3 was about three times greater than that in the $(C3D2)F_1$ hybrid, although no peaks were significantly higher in C3 than in the $(C3D2)F_1$; in fact, peak A was more than five times higher in $(C3D2)F_1$ than in C3 mice. The carcinogenesis index of D2 mice was about three times less than that in B6 mice and about 15 times less than that in C3 mice, and the relative quantities of all peaks (except G) were markedly less in D2 mice. Peaks A, B, D, H, and I all demonstrated relative differences among the three inbred strains that were in the same direction as the carcinogenesis index, i.e., greater in C3 than in B6, and both were considerably greater than those in D2 mice (Pelkonen *et al.* 1978a, in press).

In Vitro DNA Binding of BP Metabolites Generated by Skin
and Subcutaneous Tissue

The data shown in Figure 5 represent tests with liver microsomes in vitro, although the tumors (see Table 2) were caused by subcutaneously administered BP. All nine peaks (representing BP metabolite-nucleoside complexes generated with liver microsomes) were also found with skin and subcutaneous tissue microsomes in vitro (Pelkonen *et al.* 1978a, in press). However, there certainly were no peaks in the BP-treated mice that corresponded in any way to the carcinogenesis indices in Table 2, i.e., in which the C3 values are about five times greater than the B6 values.

Why the Lack of Correlation between the BP Carcinogenesis Index and the Binding of BP Metabolites to DNA In Vitro?

We can think of five possible explanations for this apparent lack of correlation. (1) The critical subcellular target for polycyclic hydrocarbon tumorigenesis is not DNA. Indeed, one can just as easily postulate important interactions with nuclear (or cytosolic) proteins or forms of RNA that lead to the initiation of cancer. (2) If there exists an important BP metabolite-nucleoside complex associated with the initiation of tumorigenesis, the complex cannot be detected in the experimental system being used. Most, if not all, of these nine peaks represent more than one BP metabolite binding to DNA (Pelkonen *et al.* 1978c), and some of these peaks may include more than one nucleoside. If the important BP metabolite-nucleoside complex comprises only 1%, or even 10%, of any of these nine peaks, we would not be able to appreciate a fivefold difference between C3 and B6 liver or skin microsomes. (3) Because we are examining isolated microsomes in vitro, we are ignoring any important contribution to the activation of BP or the detoxification of reactive intermediates by UDP glucuronosyltransferase (Nemoto and Gelboin 1976), GSH S-transferase (Bend *et al.* 1976), or β-glucuronidase action on BP phenols (Kinoshita and Gelboin 1978). (4) Perhaps the C3 inbred strain has a greater tendency than B6 to form subcutaneous fibrosarcomas. Tumor susceptibility to BP needs to be examined in other tissues (e.g., skin surface, lung) in these two strains. A carcinogenesis index for MC-initiated subcutaneous fibrosarcomas also should be determined, in order to compare subcutaneous MC with BP. (5) Factors other than metabolic activation and resultant DNA damage, such as DNA repair or immunological competence, may play an important role in one's susceptibility to chemical carcinogenesis. In the present study, the inbred C3 strain seems to be unusually sensitive, or the B6 strain seems to be unusually resistant, to BP-initiated subcutaneous fibrosarcomas.

Comparison of DNA "Repair" in C3 and B6 Skin and Subcutaneous Tissue

We examined DNA repair by observing the rate at which BP metabolites are removed from DNA isolated from the intact mouse skin and subcutaneous tissue (Figure 7). Of the two major peaks observed, the height of peak G decayed more than twice as rapidly as the height of peak E; approximate "half-lives" were 6 and 13 hours, respectively. Such a half-life would be determined by a complex combination of factors such as the persistence and quantity of unmetabolized BP on the skin, the changing rate of P_1-450/P-450 ratio as a function

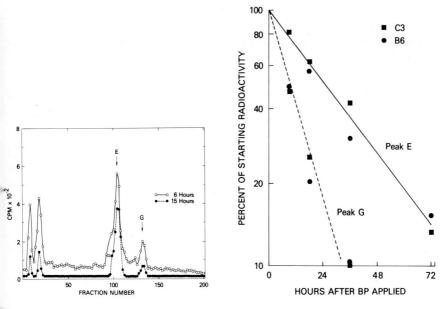

FIG. 7. *Left,* Sephadex LH20 column chromatogram of an enzyme digest of DNA isolated from skin and subcutaneous tissue of B6 mice that had been treated for 6 or 15 hours with [³H]BP topically. *Right,* Rate at which BP 4,5-oxide (peak G) and the BP 7,8-diol-9,10-epoxides (peak E) are removed from the DNA of C3 or B6 skin and subcutaneous tissue in vivo. Each *point* represents a single determination involving the pooled tissues from six mice. A typical experiment, beginning with 24 C3 and 24 B6 mice, is shown. Two other experiments gave similar results. The coefficients of variance for each time point in three experiments ranged between 0.12 and 0.36 (Pelkonen *et al.* 1978a, in press).

of time (i.e., P_1-450 induction), the rate at which DNA repair enzymes remove the various BP metabolites, etc. The total binding of BP equivalents and the radioactivity eluting in the early fractions from the Sephadex LH20 column both decayed with a half-life of about six hours, similar to that of peak G. These data suggest that the BP 7,8-diol-9,10-epoxides (peak E) are removed from DNA with more difficulty than BP or other BP metabolites bound to DNA. Such results are consistent with the possibility (Shinohara and Cerutti 1977) that BP 7,8-diol-9,10-epoxides may bind in the minor groove of the double-stranded DNA helix without causing major conformational distortion. Hence, these lesions might not be recognized and repaired as readily as BP metabolites that bind and distort the DNA helix or as readily as the removal of physically bound parent BP molecules. Perhaps other metabolites such as the 4,5-oxide bound covalently to DNA therefore reside somewhere other than in the minor groove.

Further studies are needed to determine if these differences in the rates of decay of peaks E and G represent biological differences in the efficiency with which DNA repair enzymes remove defective nucleosides or chemical (artifactual) differences associated with the exhaustive degradation scheme (Baird and Brookes 1973, Sims *et al.* 1974, Pelkonen *et al.* 1978c) to produce the nucleoside. We conclude, however, that no significant difference in DNA repair is detectable between C3 and B6 skin and subcutaneous tissue, under the experimental conditions employed here.

We believe that differences in the immune system between C3 and B6 mice may be an important factor in explaining the much greater BP carcinogenesis index in C3 than in B6. For example, the alleles at the major histocompatibility locus, *H-2*, differ between the C3 and B6 strains. C3 has the *H-2^k* allele and B6 has the *H-2^b* allele, and differences in these alleles are associated with the susceptibility to viral-caused tumors and perhaps general immune competence and the occurrence of spontaneous tumors as well (reviewed in Kouri and Nebert 1977). The relationship between these alleles and chemically induced cancers is currently under study in our laboratories (D. W. Nebert and R. E. Kouri, unpublished data) with the use of recombinant inbred and congenic sublines.

DNA Binding of Metabolites of Carcinogens Other Than BP

When MC, 2-acetylaminofluorene, dibenzo[*a,h*]anthracene, dibenzo[*a,c*]anthracene, benzidine, dopamine, benzo[*a*]anthracene, or DMBA is incubated with B6 or D2 liver microsomes, cofactors, and deproteinized salmon sperm DNA, numerous adducts are found (Figure 8). The genetic differences in radioactivity bound per milligram of total DNA (Table 3) are thus exhibited in numerous specific peaks (Figure 8) that are much higher in B6 than in D2 samples. These increased peaks in B6 presumably represent P_1-450-catalyzed metabolites bound to DNA.

It should be noted that the B6/D2 increased ratio for dibenzo[*a,c*]anthracene (i.e., 3.8 in Table 3) cannot be seen as an important genetic difference when specific metabolite-nucleoside peaks are sought (see Figure 8). Definitive experiments with MC-treated *Ah^b/Ah^d* and *Ah^d/Ah^d* individuals from the B6D2F$_1$ × D2 backcross have been performed with BP in vitro (Pelkonen *et al.* 1978b) and with MC in vitro (unpublished data) but not on the other seven compounds on which DNA binding studies are listed in Table 3. In the case of BP and of MC, all peaks shown to be greater in B6 samples than in D2 samples were found to be associated with the *Ah^b* allele (i.e., increased P_1-450 content).

Several recent studies suggest the identity of some of the peaks seen in Figure 8 with mouse liver microsomes. The two largest peaks for MC that are different between the B6 and D2 samples (see Figure 1) are believed to represent the 9,10-diol-7,8-epoxide and the 1-phenol-9,10-diol-7,8-epoxide of MC (King *et al.* 1977). The largest peak difference for benzo[*a*]anthracene and for DMBA between B6 and D2 samples probably represents the 3,4-diol-7,8-epoxide of these polycyclic hydrocarbons (Malaveille *et al.* 1975, Moschel *et al.* 1977, Wood *et al.* 1977). There are no studies, as far as we know, on the identification of

Compound	Concentration in assay for metabolites binding to DNA* (µM)	Total amount presumed to be covalently bound to DNA (pmol/mg DNA)†		Estimated percent of total added compound that is bound covalently	Ratio (B6/D2)	Concentration at which genetic differences in mutagenesis were maximal (µg/plate)	Bacterial tester strain in which genetic differences in mutagenesis were maximal	Revertants per plate	
BP	6	B6	12	0.30	5.4	1.0	TA98	B6	540
		D2	2.2	0.055				D2	150
MC	6	B6	10.7	0.27	3.0	100	TA1538	B6	180
		D2	3.6	0.089				D2	40
Benzo[a]anthracene	60	B6	108	0.27	6.6	10	TA100	B6	830
		D2	16.5	0.042				D2	540
Dibenzo[a,h]anthracene	6	B6	6.7	0.17	13	10	TA100	B6	1240
		D2	0.52	0.014				D2	310
Dibenzo[a,c]anthracene	6	B6	21	0.47	3.8	10	TA100	B6	1250
		D2	5.6	0.18				D2	410
DMBA	6	B6	23	0.57	2.7	10	TA100	B6	820
		D2	8.6	0.22				D2	580
2-acetylamino-fluorene	60	B6	35	0.088	2.5	10	TA1538	B6	4100
		D2	14	0.036				D2	980
Dopamine	6	B6	3.6	0.090	2.0				
		D2	1.8	0.045					
Benzidine	60	B6	23	0.057	1.0				
		D2	23	0.058					
6-aminochrysene						10	TA1538	B6	11,900
								D2	850
α-naphthylamine						100	TA100	B6	750
								D2	500
β-naphthylamine						100	TA100	B6	650
								D2	320

* For technical and practical reasons (such as expense of some of the compounds and relatively low specific radioactivity of ^{14}C-labeled compounds), the test compounds were used at varying concentrations in the in vitro assay (Pelkonen et al. 1978a, in press, 1978b). Experiments with BP concentrations of 0.6, 6.0, and 60 µM, however, showed little difference in the relative heights of all nine peaks (unpublished data). The results in this Table are based on two different experiments, except with dopamine and the steroids in which only one experiment was performed. Because two separate experiments never differed more than 20–30%, however, we believe these results are accurate.

† Values representing "noncovalent" binding (radioactivity bound to DNA in the presence of heat-denatured microsomes) were subtracted from values obtained with active microsome.

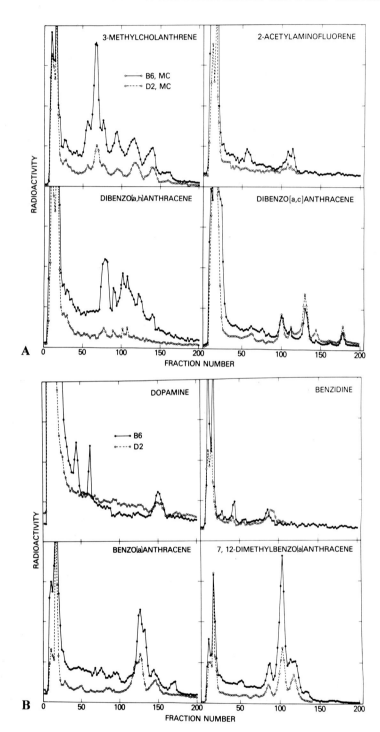

specific metabolites of any of the other chemicals by Sephadex LH20 column chromatography shown in Figure 8.

The strain difference in the binding of reactive intermediates of dopamine to DNA (Figure 8) is interesting because dopamine is an endogenous substrate rather than a xenobiotic, but much further work will be needed before any conclusions can be made concerning the correlation of dopamine metabolite-nucleoside complexes with P_1-450 and, therefore, the Ah^b allele. Sephadex LH20 column chromatography is most likely not the best method for separating such a polar compound as dopamine and its metabolite-nucleoside complexes.

2-Acetylaminofluorene binds covalently to proteins much more avidly than to DNA (Miller and Miller 1974). At least three distinct 2-acetylaminofluorene metabolite-nucleoside peaks in B6 but relatively little in D2 (Figure 8), however, were found. Although the total benzidine radioactivity covalently bound to gross DNA (Table 3) exhibited no genetic difference, at least one distinct benzidine metabolite-nucleoside peak (Figure 8) was found in B6 and not in D2. Further success of such studies with 2-acetylaminofluorene and benzidine might be achieved with compounds having higher specific radioactivity than those available to us at the time of this study.

MUTAGENICITY OF CARCINOGENIC METABOLITES

A sensitive and simple bacterial test for the detection of chemical carcinogens has been developed (Ames et al. 1975). About 300 carcinogens and noncarcinogens of widely varying chemical structures have been tested, and there exists a high correlation between carcinogenicity and mutagenicity: about 90% (157 of 175 compounds) of carcinogens were mutagenic, and few chemicals believed to be "noncarcinogens" showed any degree of mutagenicity (Ames et al. 1975, McCann et al. 1975, McCann and Ames 1976).

The *Ah* Locus and Mutagenesis In Vitro

Can genetic differences in P_1-450 content be detected as differences in this in vitro mutagenicity test? We previously have shown that the Ah^b allele is highly correlated with the activation of MC, 2-acetylaminofluorene, and 6-amino-chrysene to mutagens in vitro (reviewed in Thorgeirsson and Nebert 1977) and with the activation of BP in vitro (Levitt et al. 1977, and in press). Figure 9 illustrates that MC in vitro, in the presence of the S-9 fraction from MC-treated B6 mice (i.e., increased P_1-450 content), is more mutagenic (per molecule of CO-binding cytochrome) than that from phenobarbital-treated or control B6

IG. 8. Sephadex LH20 column chromatograms of enzyme digests of DNA with various metabolites bound during an in vitro incubation with hepatic microsomes from MC-treated B6 or D2 mice. *Top,* MC, 2-acetylaminofluorene, dibenzo[*a,h*]anthracene, dibenzo[*a,c*]anthracene. *Bottom,* dopamine, benzidine, benzo[*a*]anthracene, DMBA.

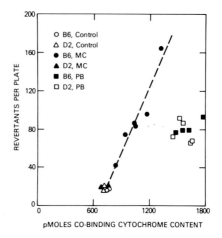

FIG. 9. Relationship between total CO-binding hemoprotein content and MC as a mutagen in vitro (Felton and Nebert 1975). S-9 liver fractions from control (0), MC-treated (●), or phenobarbital-treated (PB) (■) B6 mice, and control (△), MC-treated (▲), or phenobarbital-treated (□) D2 mice were used. B6 mice were sacrificed 6, 9, 12, 18, 20, and 48 hours after MC treatment in vivo. Control mice treated with either corn oil or 0.85% NaCl solution gave similar results. Each closed circle or triangle (●,▲) represents the liver combined from two MC-treated mice. Each closed or open square (■,□) denotes an individual phenobarbital-treated mouse. The dashed line drawn between the closed triangles and circles (▲,●) was calculated with the Monro-matic computer program for least-squares analysis. The CO-binding cytochrome content is expressed in picomoles per milligram of microsomal protein. In this study 100 μg of MC per plate was added in vitro. (Reproduced from Felton and Nebert 1975, with permission of American Society of Biological Chemists, Inc.)

or D2 mice or MC-treated D2 mice. With regard to cytochrome P_1-450 content and either 6-aminochrysene or 2-acetylaminofluorene mutagenesis in vitro, we found (Felton and Nebert 1975) this same relationship. We thus conclude that P_1-450 is more effective than other forms of P-450 in the metabolic conversion of MC to an intermediate that is mutagenic. Similar relationships probably hold true for 2-acetylaminofluorene, 6-aminochrysene, and BP.

Genetic differences in mutagenicity with the bacterial test system catalyzed by liver S-9 from MC-treated B6 and D2 mice with ten nonradioactive substrates are also shown in Table 3. The mutagenicity displayed distinct strain differences with BP, MC, benzo[*a*]anthracene, dibenzo[*a,h*]anthracene, dibenzo[*a,c*]anthracene, 2-acetylaminofluorene, 6-aminochrysene, and β-naphthylamine. The "background" revertant rates/plate are approximately 30, 35, and 250 for TA1538, TA98, and TA100, respectively, but somewhat variable between experiments; therefore, it is difficult to describe "fold increases" in B6 samples compared with D2 samples. DMBA and α-naphthylamine, however, showed only very small differences between B6 and D2.

Figure 10 shows typical experiments in which revertants per plate were studied as a function of mutagen concentration. The *concentration* of each compound and the bacterial tester *strain* in which genetic differences in mutagenicity were

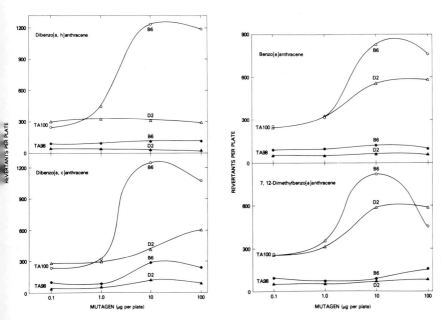

FIG. 10. *Left,* Dibenzo[*a,h*]anthracene and dibenzo[*a,c*]anthracene and *right,* benzo[*a*]anthracene and DMBA mutagenesis in vitro as a function of concentration of the mutagens. The liver S-9 fractions were from MC-treated B6 or D2 mice, and protein concentrations were 2.4 mg/plate. Results with both bacterial tester strains TA100 and TA98 are shown.

maximal under these test conditions are listed in Table 3. The striking genetic differences for dibenzo[*a,h*]anthracene and dibenzo[*a,c*]anthracene mutagenesis can be compared with the less striking genetic differences for benzo[*a*]anthracene and β-naphthylamine and with the least striking genetic differences for DMBA and α-naphthylamine.

Dramatic genetic differences in DNA binding of metabolites (see Figure 8) and in mutagenicity in vitro (Figure 10) are found for dibenzo[*a,h*]anthracene. For dibenzo[*a,c*]anthracene, however, genetic differences in the specific metabolite-nucleoside peaks (Figure 8) are not found, although there exist genetic differences in mutagenesis for both stereoisomers (Figure 10). With liver microsomes from Aroclor 1254-treated rats, dibenzo[*a,c*]anthracene mutagenesis is more than 15 times greater than dibenzo[*a,h*]anthracene mutagenesis (McCann *et al* 1975). However, dibenzo[*a,h*]anthracene/dibenzo[*a,c*]anthracene ratios for metabolism of these two isomers have been reported as approximately 14 for mouse embryo cultures (Brookes *et al.* 1974) and 1.9 for CD-1 mouse epidermis (Slaga *et al.,* 1976). Studies in the mouse indicate that both dibenzo[*a,h*]anthracene and dibenzo[*a,c*]anthracene are potent carcinogens (Arcos and Argus 1974). There are, therefore, distinct discrepancies for these two isomers between the mutagenesis data and results with tumorigenesis, metabolism, or DNA bind-

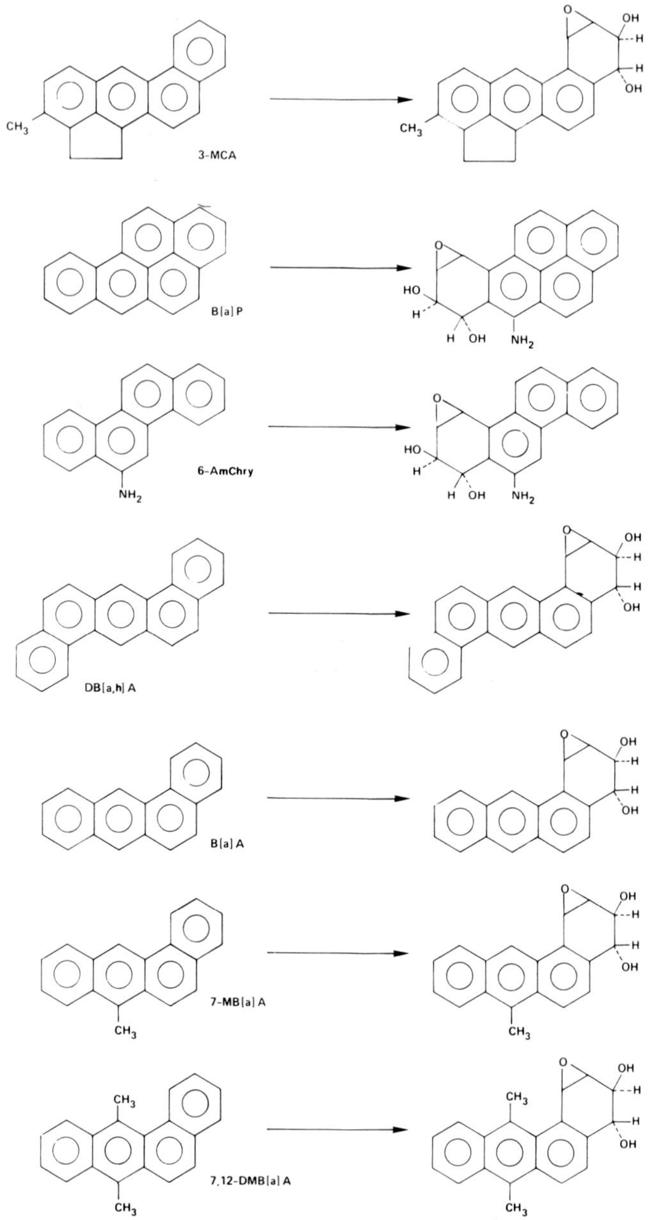

FIG. 11. Postulated reactive intermediates catalyzed predominantly by cytochrome P_1-450, the "bay region" theory holds true for a large number of polycyclic hydrocarbons (Pelkonen et al. 1978b). From top to bottom, structures of substrates shown are MC, BP, 6-aminochrysene, dibenzo[a,h]anthracene, BA, 7-methylbenzo[a]anthracene, and DMBA. (Reproduced from Pelkonen et al. 1978b, with permission of Raven Press.)

ing in vitro. A better understanding of these discrepancies will require further studies.

HYPOTHESIS THAT OXYGENATION OF POLYCYCLIC HYDROCARBONS BY P₁-450 OCCURS PREDOMINANTLY IN THE "BAY REGION"

It is very tempting to speculate that the enzyme active-site(s) of cytochrome(s) P_1-450 preferentially attacks the benzylic ring at the bond farther from the "bay region." Following hydration by the closely coupled (Oesch and Daly 1972) epoxide hydrase, the *trans*-dihydrodiol is formed. The benzylic ring now contains only a nonaromatic bond adjacent to the bay region, and P_1-450 preferentially oxygenates the *trans*-dihydrodiol to the diol-epoxide (Pelkonen *et al.* 1978b, Boobis *et al.*, in press). Figure 11 shows such postulated diol-epoxides for seven polycyclic aromatic compounds of interest to this review. All these different chemicals have been shown to be at least weakly carcinogenic in one or another experimental model system (Malaveille *et al.* 1975, McCann *et al.* 1975, Kapitulnik *et al.* 1977, Wood *et al.* 1977, and reviewed by Thorgeirsson and Nebert 1977). During the next few years it will be interesting to find out if P_1-450 catalyzes (predominantly) each of these carcinogens to the diol-epoxide of the benzylic ring adjacent to the bay region, providing a common molecular basis for the initiation of polycyclic aromatic hydrocarbon-induced tumorigenesis—a hypothesis recently advanced by Jerina and Daly (1976). Among the compounds examined in the present report, DMBA exhibited about the least genetic difference in mutagenicity with any of the bacterial strains (Table 3 and Felton and Nebert 1975), whereas genetic differences in the binding of metabolites to DNA were quite prominent (see Figure 8). It is of interest that no correlations were found between DMBA tumorigenesis and the *Ah* locus in an earlier study (Nebert *et al.* 1972a). Moreover, because there is evidence for differences at the human *Ah* locus (reviewed in Kouri and Nebert 1977 and Atlas and Nebert 1978), elucidation of P_1-450-catalyzed metabolites of numerous environmental carcinogenic pollutants becomes extremely important.

SUMMARY

The *Ah* locus regulates the inducibility by MC and numerous other polycyclic aromatic compounds of at least 20 monooxygenase "activities" and associated cytochrome(s) P_1-450, including AHH activity. Regulation of responsiveness in mice probably involves several alleles at more than one locus, but differences between B6 (responsive, Ah^b) and D2 (nonresponsive, Ah^d) can be almost completely explained by the difference at the *Ah* locus. Heterozygotes *(Ahᵇ/Ahᵈ)* are responsive. Responsiveness occurs not only in the liver but also in numerous nonhepatic tissues such as lung, kidney, bowel, skin, lymph nodes, bone marrow, retinal pigmented epithelium of the eye, brain, mammary gland, uterus, and ovary. A major product of the regulatory *Ah* gene is a cytosolic receptor protein, which has a high affinity (apparent $K_d \cong 1$ nM) for potent polycyclic aromatic inducers and which appears to be defective (i.e., has diminished affinity) in nonresponsive mice.

Important differences among individual mice, with regard to chemical carcinogenesis, mutagenesis, teratogenesis, and several forms of drug toxicity, all have been attributed to allelic differences at the *Ah* locus. Genetic differences, associated with the *Ah* locus and therefore metabolism catalyzed predominantly by cytochromes P_1-450, have been demonstrated in vitro for mutagenesis of numerous chemical carcinogens in the *Salmonella*/liver system and for the binding of BP, MC, benzo[*a*]anthracene, DMBA, dibenzo[*a,h*]anthracene, 2-acetylaminofluorene, benzidine, and dopamine metabolites to DNA. Whereas genetic differences show, in general, an excellent correlation between mutagenicity and binding of metabolites to DNA in vitro, there are exceptions when one attempts to extrapolate these in vitro tests to the intact animal (i.e., genetic differences in tumorigenesis). Knowing that differences at the *Ah* locus are also present in the human, we suggest that these findings may have important implications to environmentally caused cancers in man.

ACKNOWLEDGMENTS

We acknowledge valuable discussions about various aspects of this work with Dr. Richard E. Kouri and Dr. Allan B. Okey. We appreciate the expert secretarial assistance of Ms. Ingrid E. Jordan.

REFERENCES

Ames, B. N., J. McCann, and E. Yamasaki. 1975. Methods for detecting carcinogens and mutagens with the *Salmonella*/mammalian-microsome mutagenicity test. Mutat. Res. 31:347–364.

Arcos, J. C., and M. F. Argus. 1974. Chemical Induction of Cancer. Vol. IIA. Academic Press New York, p. 19.

Atlas, S. A., A. R. Boobis, J. S. Felton, S. S. Thorgeirsson, and D. W. Nebert. 1977. Ontogenetic expression of polycyclic aromatic compound inducible monooxygenase activities and forms of cytochrome P-450 in rabbit. Evidence for temporal control and organ specificity of two genetic regulatory systems. J. Biol. Chem. 252:4712–4721.

Atlas, S. A., and D. W. Nebert. 1978. Pharmacogenetics: A possible pragmatic perspective in neoplasm predictability. Semin. Oncol. 5:89–106.

Baird, W. M., and P. Brookes. 1973. Isolation of the hydrocarbon-deoxyribonucleoside products from the DNA of mouse embryo cells treated in culture with 7-methylbenz[a]anthracene-³H Cancer Res. 33:2378–2385.

Bend, J. R., Z. Ben-Zvi, J. Van Anda, P. M. Dansette, and D. M. Jerina. 1976. Hepatic and extrahepatic glutathione S-transferase activity toward several arene oxides and epoxides in the rat, in Polynuclear Aromatic Hydrocarbons: Chemistry, Metabolism and Carcinogenesis, R. I. Freudenthal and W. W. Jones, eds., Raven Press, New York, pp. 63–75.

Boobis, A. R., and D. W. Nebert. 1977. Genetic differences in the metabolism of carcinogen and in the binding of benzo[a]pyrene metabolites to DNA, in Advances in Enzyme Regulation G. Weber, ed. Vol. 15. Pergamon Press, New York and Oxford, pp. 339–362.

Boobis, A. R., D. W. Nebert, and O. Pelkonen. 1978. The effects of microsomal enzyme inducer *in vivo* and inhibitors *in vitro* on the covalent binding of benzo[a]pyrene metabolites to DNA catalyzed by liver microsomes from genetically responsive and nonresponsive mice. Biochem Pharmacol. (In press).

Brookes, P., W. M. Baird, and A. Dipple. 1974. Interaction of the carcinogen 7-methylbenz(a)anthracene with DNA of mammalian cells, *in* Chemical Carcinogenesis, P. O. P. Ts'o and J. A. Di Paolo, eds., Marcel-Dekker, Inc., New York, pp. 149–157.

Cohen, G. M., B. P. Moore, and J. W. Bridges. 1977. Organic solvent soluble sulphate ester conjugates of monohydroxybenzo(a)pyrenes. Biochem. Pharmacol. 26:551–553.

Croy, R. G., J. K. Selkirk, R. G. Harvey, J. F. Engel, and H. V. Gelboin. 1976. Separation of ten benzo[a]pyrene phenols by recycle high pressure liquid chromatography and identification of four phenols as metabolites. Biochem. Pharmacol. 25:227–230.

Felton, J. S., and D. W. Nebert. 1975. Mutagenesis of certain activated carcinogens *in vitro* associated with genetically mediated increases in monooxygenase activity and cytochrome P_1-450. J. Biol. Chem. 250:6769–6778.

Green, M. C. 1973. Guideline for genetically determined biochemical variants in the house mouse, *Mus musculus.* Biochem. Genet. 9:369–374.

Guengerich, F. P. 1977. Separation and purification of multiple forms of microsomal cytochrome P-450. Activities of different forms of cytochrome P-450 towards several compounds of environmental interest. J. Biol. Chem. 252:3970–3979.

Guenthner, T. M., and D. W. Nebert. 1978. Evidence in rat and mouse liver for temporal control of two polycyclic aromatic-inducible forms of cytochrome P-450. Eur. J. Biochem. (In press).

Haugen, D. A., L. G. Armes, K. T. Yasunobu, and M. J. Coon. 1977. Amino-terminal sequence of phenobarbital-inducible cytochrome P-450 from rabbit liver microsomes: Similarity to hydrophobic amino-terminal segments of preproteins. Biochem. Biophys. Res. Commun. 77:967–973.

Haugen, D. A., T. A. van der Hoeven, and M. J. Coon. 1975. Purified liver microsomal cytochrome P-450. Separation and characterization of multiple forms. J. Biol. Chem. 250:3567–3570.

Holder, G., H. Yagi, P. Dansette, D. M. Jerina, W. Levin, A. Y. H. Lu, and A. H. Conney. 1974. Effects of inducers and epoxide hydrase on the metabolism of benzo[a]pyrene by liver microsomes and a reconditioned system: Analysis by high pressure liquid chromatography. Proc. Natl. Acad. Sci. USA, 71:4356–4360.

Holder, G. M., H. Yagi, D. M. Jerina, W. Levin, A. Y. H. Lu, and A. H. Conney. 1975. Metabolism of benzo[a]pyrene. Effect of substrate concentration and 3-methylcholanthrene pretreatment on hepatic metabolism by microsomes from rats and mice. Arch. Biochem. Biophys. 170:557–566.

Iball, J. 1939. The relative potency of carcinogenic compounds. Am. J. Cancer 35:188–190.

Jeffrey, A. M., S.H. Blobstein, B. Weinstein, and R. G. Harvey. 1976. High-pressure liquid chromatography of carcinogen-nucleoside conjugates: Separation of 7,12-dimethylbenzanthracene derivatives. Anal. Biochem. 73:378–385.

Jerina, D. M., and J. W. Daly. 1976. Oxidation at carbon, *in* Drug Metabolism—From Microbe to Man, D. W. Parke and R. L. Smith, eds. Taylor and Francis Ltd., London, pp. 13–32.

Kahl, G. F., R. Kahl, K. Kumaki and D. W. Nebert. 1976. Association of the *Ah* locus with specific changes in metyrapone and ethylisocyanide binding to mouse liver microsomes. J. Biol. Chem. 251:5397–5407.

Kapitulnik, J., W. Levin, A. H. Conney, H. Yagi, and D. M. Jerina. 1977. Benzo[a]pyrene 7,8-dihydrodiol is more carcinogenic than benzo[a]pyrene in newborn mice. Nature 266:378–380.

King, H. W. S., M. R. Osborne, and P. Brookes. 1977. The metabolism and DNA binding of 3-methylcholanthrene. Int. J. Cancer 20:564–571.

King, H. W. S., M. H. Thompson, and P. Brookes. 1975. The benzo[a]pyrene deoxyribonucleoside products isolated from DNA after metabolism of benzo[a]pyrene by rat liver microsomes in the presence of DNA. Cancer Res. 34:1263–1269.

King, H. W. S., M. H. Thompson, and P. Brookes. 1976. The role of 9-hydroxybenzo[a]pyrene in the microsome mediated binding of benzo[a]pyrene to DNA. Int. J. Cancer 18:339–344.

Kinoshita, N., and H. V. Gelboin. 1978. β-glucuronidase catalyzed hydrolysis of benzo[a]pyrene-3-glucuronide and binding to DNA. Science 199:307–309.

Kinoshita, N., B. Shears, and H. V. Gelboin. 1973. K-region and non-K-region metabolism of benzo[a]pyrene by rat liver microsomes. Cancer Res. 33:1937–1944.

Kouri, R. E. 1976. Relationship between levels of aryl hydrocarbon hydroxylase activity and susceptibility to 3-methylcholanthrene and benzo[a]pyrene-induced cancers in inbred strains of mice, *in* Polynuclear Aromatic Hydrocarbons: Chemistry, Metabolism and Carcinogenesis, R. I. Freudenthal and P. W. Jones, eds. Raven Press, New York, pp. 139–151.

Kouri, R. E., and D. W. Nebert. 1977. Genetic regulation of susceptibility to polycyclic hydrocarbon-induced tumors in the mouse, *in* Origins of Human Cancer, H. H. Hiatt, J. D. Watson, and

J. A. Winsten, eds., Vol. 4. Cold Spring Harbor Laboratory, Cold Spring Harbor, New York, pp. 811–835.

Kouri, R. E., H. Ratrie, and C. E. Whitmire. 1974. Genetic control of susceptibility to 3-methycholanthrene-induced subcutaneous sarcomas. Int. J. Cancer 13:714–720.

Kouri, R. E., T. H. Rude, R. Joglekar, P. M. Dansette, D. M. Jerina, S. A. Atlas, I. S. Owens, and D. W. Nebert. 1978. 2,3,7,8-tetrachlorodibenzo-*p*-dioxin: Cocarcinogen which enhances 3-methylcholanthrene-initiated subcutaneous tumors in mice genetically "nonresponsive" at *Ah* locus. Cancer Res. 38:2777–2783.

Levitt, R. C., C. Legraverend, D. W. Nebert, and O. Pelkonen. 1977. Effects of harman and norharman on the mutagenicity and binding to DNA of benzo[a]pyrene metabolites *in vitro* and on aryl hydrocarbon hydroxylase induction in cell culture. Biochem. Biophys. Res. Commun. 79:1167–1175.

Levitt, R. C., O. Pelkonen, A. B. Okey, and D. W. Nebert. 1978. Genetic differences in metabolism of polycyclic aromatic carcinogens and aromatic amines by mouse liver microsomes. Detection by DNA binding of metabolites and by mutagenicity in histidine-dependent *Salmonella typhimurium in vitro*. J. Natl. Cancer Inst. (In press).

Malaveille, C., H. Bartsch, P. L. Grover, and P. Sims. 1975. Mutagenicity of non-K-region diols and diol-epoxides of benz[a]anthracene and benzo[a]pyrene in *S. typhimurium* TA 100. Biochem. Biophys. Res. Commun. 66:693–700.

McCann, J., and B. N. Ames. 1976. Detection of carcinogens as mutagens in the *Salmonella/*microsome test: Assay of 300 chemicals: Discussion. Proc. Natl. Acad. Sci. USA 73:950–954.

McCann, J., E. Choi, E. Yamasaki, and B. N. Ames. 1975. Detection of carcinogens as mutagens in the *Salmonella/*microsome test: Assay of 300 chemicals. Proc. Natl. Acad. Sci. USA 72:5135–5139.

Miller, E. C., and J. A. Miller, 1974. Biochemical mechanisms of chemical carcinogenesis, *in* Molecular Biology of Cancer, H. Busch, ed., Academic Press, New York, pp. 377–402.

Moore, P. D., M. Koreeda, P. G. Wislocki, W. Levin, A. H. Conney, H. Yagi, and D. M. Jerina. 1977. *In vitro* reactions of the diastereomeric 9,10-epoxides of (+) and (−)-trans-7,8-dihydroxy-7,8-dihydrobenzo[a]pyrene with polyguanylic acid and evidence for formation of an enantiomer of each diastereomeric 9,10-epoxide from benzo[a]pyrene in mouse skin, *in* Drug Metabolism Concepts (American Chemical Society Symposium Series, Number 44), D. M. Jerina, ed., American Chemical Society, pp. 127–154.

Moschel, R. C., W. M. Baird, and A. Dipple. 1977. Metabolic activation of the carcinogen 7,12-dimethylbenz[a]anthracene for DNA binding. Biochem. Biophys. Res. Commun. 76:1092–1098.

Nebert, D. W., S. A. Atlas, T. M. Guenthner, and R. E. Kouri. 1978. The *Ah* locus: Genetic regulation of the enzymes which metabolize polycyclic hydrocarbons and the risk for cancer, *in* Polycyclic Hydrocarbons and Cancer: Chemistry, Molecular Biology and Environment, P. O. P. Ts'o and H. V. Gelboin, eds., Academic Press, New York, pp. 345–390.

Nebert, D. W., W. F. Benedict, J. E. Gielen, F. Oesch, and J. W. Daly. 1972a. Aryl hydrocarbon hydroxylase, epoxide hydrase, and 7,12-dimethylbenz[a]anthracene-produced skin tumorigenesis in the mouse. Mol. Pharmacol. 8:374–379.

Nebert, D. W., W. F. Benedict, and R. E. Kouri. 1974. Aromatic hydrocarbon-produced tumorigenesis and the genetic differences in aryl hydrocarbon hydroxylase induction, *in* Chemical Carcinogenesis, P. O. P. Ts'o and J. A. Di Paolo, eds., Marcel-Dekker, Inc., New York, pp. 271–288.

Nebert, D. W., and J. E. Gielen. 1972. Genetic regulation of aryl hydrocarbon hydroxylase induction in the mouse. Fed. Proc. 31:1315–1325.

Nebert, D. W., J. E. Gielen, and F. M. Goujon. 1972b. Genetic expression of aryl hydrocarbon hydroxylase induction. III. Changes in the binding of *n*-octylamine to cytochrome P-450. Mol. Pharmacol. 8:651–666.

Nebert, D. W., and N. M. Jensen. 1978. The *Ah* locus: Genetic regulation of the metabolism of carcinogens, drugs, and other environmental chemicals by cytochrome P-450-mediated monooxygenases, *in* Critical Reviews in Biochemistry. CRC Press, Inc., Cleveland (In press).

Nebert, D. W., R. C. Levitt, N. M. Jensen, G. H. Lambert, and J. S. Felton. 1977. Birth defects and aplastic anemia: Differences in polycyclic hydrocarbon toxicity associated with the *Ah* locus. Arch. Toxicol. 39:109–132.

Nebert, D. W., J. R. Robinson, A. Niwa, K. Kumaki, and A. P. Poland. 1975. Genetic expression of aryl hydrocarbon hydroxylase activity in the mouse. J. Cell. Physiol. 85:393–414.

Nemoto, N., and H. V. Gelboin. 1976. Enzymatic conjugation of benzo[a]pyrene oxides, phenols and dihydrodiols with UDP-glucuronic acid. Biochem. Pharmacol. 25:1221–1226.

Nettesheim, P., and A. S. Hammons. 1971. Induction of squamous cell carcinoma in the respiratory tract of mice. J. Natl. Cancer Inst. 47:697–701.

Oesch, F., and J. Daly. 1972. Conversion of naphthalene to *trans*-naphthalene dihydrodiol: Evidence for the presence of coupled aryl monooxygenase-epoxide hydrase system in hepatic microsomes. Biochem. Biophys. Res. Commun. 46:1713–1720.

Pelkonen, O., A. R. Boobis, R. C. Levitt, R. E. Kouri, and D. W. Nebert. 1978a. Genetic differences in the metabolic activation of benzo[a]pyrene in mice. Attempts to correlate tumorigenesis with binding of reactive intermediates to DNA and with mutagenesis *in vitro*. J. Natl. Cancer Inst. (In press).

Pelkonen, O., A. R. Boobis, and D. W. Nebert. 1978b. Genetic differences in the binding of reactive carcinogenic metabolites to DNA, *in* Carcinogenesis, Polynuclear Aromatic Hydrocarbons, P. W. Jones and R. I. Freudenthal, eds., Vol. 3. Raven Press, New York, pp. 383–400.

Pelkonen, O., A. R. Boobis, H. Yagi, D. Jerina, and D. W. Nebert. 1978c. The tentative identification of benzo[a]pyrene metabolite-nucleoside complexes produced *in vitro* by mouse liver microsomes. Mol. Pharmacol. 14:306–322.

Poland, A. P., E. Glover, and A. S. Kende. 1976. Stereospecific, high affinity binding of 2,3,7,8-tetrachlorodibenzo-*p*-dioxin by hepatic cytosol. Evidence that the binding species is the receptor for the induction of aryl hydrocarbon hydroxylase. J. Biol. Chem. 251:4936–4946.

Rapp, J. R., and L. K. Dahl. 1976. Mutant forms of cytochrome P-450 controlling both 18- and 11β-steroid hydroxylation in the rat. Biochemistry 15:1235–1242.

Robinson, J. R., N. Considine, and D. W. Nebert. 1974. Genetic expression of aryl hydrocarbon hydroxylase induction. Evidence for the involvement of other genetic loci. J. Biol. Chem. 249:5851–5859.

Schmassmann, H. U., H. R. Glatt, and F. Oesch. 1976. A rapid assay for epoxide hydratase activity with benzo[a]pyrene 4,5-(K-region-)oxide as substrate. Anal. Biochem. 74:94–106.

Selkirk, J. K., R. G. Croy, and H. V. Gelboin. 1974. Benzo[a]pyrene metabolites: Efficient and rapid separation by high pressure liquid chromatography. Science 183:169–171.

Selkirk, J. K., R. G. Croy, F. J. Wiebel, and H. V. Gelboin. 1976. Differences in benzo[a]pyrene metabolism between rodent liver microsomes and embryonic cells. Cancer Res. 36:4476–4479.

Shinohara, K., and P. A. Cerutti. 1977. Excision repair of benzo[a]pyrene-deoxyguanosine adducts in baby hamster kidney 21/C13 cells and in secondary mouse embryo fibroblasts C57BL/6J. Proc. Natl. Acad. Sci. USA 74:979–983.

Sims, P., P. L. Grover, A. Swaisland, K. Pal, and A. Hewer. 1974. Metabolic activation of benzo[a]pyrene proceeds by a diol-epoxide. Nature 252:326–328.

Slaga, T. J., D. L. Berry, M. R. Juchau, S. Thompson, S. G. Buty, and A. Viaje. 1976. Effects of benzoflavones and trichloropropene oxide on polynuclear aromatic hydrocarbon metabolism and initiation of skin tumors, *in* Polynuclear Aromatic Hydrocarbons: Chemistry, Metabolism and Carcinogenesis, R. I. Freudenthal and P. W. Jones, eds., Raven Press, New York, pp. 127–138.

Slaga, T. J., W. M. Bracken, A. Viaje, W. Levin, H. Yagi, D. M. Jerina, and A. H. Conney. 1977. Comparison of the tumor-initiating activities of benzo[a]pyrene arene oxides and diol-epoxides. Cancer Res. 37:4130–4133.

Thomas, P. E., A. Y. H. Lu, D. Ryan, S. B. West, J. Kawalek, and W. Levin. 1976. Immunochemical evidence for six forms of rat liver cytochrome P450 obtained using antibodies against purified rat liver cytochromes P450 and P448. Mol. Pharmacol. 12:746–758.

Thorgeirsson, S. S., and D. W. Nebert. 1977. The *Ah* locus and the metabolism of chemical carcinogens and other foreign compounds. Adv. Cancer Res. 25:149–193.

Weinstein, I. B., A. M. Jeffrey, K. W. Jennette, S. H. Blobstein, R. G. Harvey, C. Harris, H. Autrup, H. Kasai, and K. Nakanishi. 1976. Benzo[a]pyrene diol epoxides as intermediates in nucleic acid binding *in vitro* and *in vivo*. Science 193:592–595.

Wood, A. W., R. L. Chang, W. Levin, R. E. Lehr, M. Schaefer-Ridder, J. M. Karle, D. M. Jerina, and A. H. Conney. 1977. Mutagenicity and cytotoxicity of benz[a]anthracene diol epoxides and tetrahydro-epoxides: Exceptional activity of the bay region 1,2-epoxides. Proc. Natl. Acad. Sci. USA 74:2746–2750.

Zampaglione, N., D. J. Jollow, J. R. Mitchell, B. Stripp, M. Hamrick, and J. R. Gillette. 1973. Role of detoxifying enzymes in bromobenzene-induced liver necrosis. J. Pharmacol. Exp. Ther. 187:218–227.

Carcinogens: Identification and Mechanisms
of Action, edited by A. Clark Griffin and
Charles R. Shaw. Raven Press, New York © 1979.

Perspectives and Future Developments in Research on Environmental Carcinogenesis

John Higginson

International Agency for Research on Cancer, Lyon, France

The potential role of environmental factors in cancer has been discussed extensively elsewhere (Doll 1967, Higginson 1969, Doll 1977, Higginson and Muir 1977). Accordingly, I propose to limit this paper first to a review of the magnitude of the problem of environmental carcinogenesis and second to a discussion of those factors—both scientific and nonscientific—that have prevented society from developing effective control, since such considerations will have increasing influence on future research priorities.

It is often forgotten that the term "environment" embraces exposure not only to such common habits as smoking but also widespread exposures of a general nature, in addition to the limited risks of the workplace. Further, although its importance has long been recognized (Wynder *et al.* 1959, Higginson and Oettlé 1960), the role of "life-style" has become again of renewed interest to oncologists (Phillips 1975, Wynder and Gori 1977). The term life-style can be defined as the complex interplay of all factors, whether as initiators, promoters or inhibitors, that modify an individual's reaction to the environment and may even include physical exercise, which modifies calorie intake and utilization.

THE ETIOLOGY OF HUMAN CANCER

More is known about the cause of human cancer than is generally realized, although the implications for control are frequently misunderstood (Higginson and Muir 1977, Doll 1977, Wynder and Gori 1977). For 80 to 90 percent of cancers, the role of the environmental background is already well established or can be supported by strong circumstantial evidence, even when the stimuli have not yet been fully defined.

Known Etiological Factors

Cultural Factors

The recognition of the overwhelming role of the cultural environment has been the most important development in our knowledge of cancer etiology in the last 30 years. In addition to lung cancer, cigarette smoking has been implicated in cancers of the mouth, larynx, pharynx, gastric cardia, esophagus, bladder, and possibly pancreas. In several sites, alcoholic beverages play a synergistic role and are directly related to cancers of the mouth, larynx, pharynx, esophagus, and liver (Higginson and Muir 1977, Doll 1977). In India, approximately 30 percent of all cancers are related to betel chewing. The great importance of voluntary exposure to sunlight as a causal factor is frequently forgotten due to the effectiveness of treatment for skin cancer.

Cancers Related to the Workplace

The recognition of such cancers has formed the basis of modern environmental carcinogenesis (Doll 1975). Industrial cancers are important in terms of point source exposures of individual workers to carcinogens, which may also escape to involve larger population groups. However, available epidemiological data would indicate that the proportion of all cancers in males due to "point source" industrial pollution is probably between one and five percent, depending on the country (Doll 1977, Higginson and Muir 1977, Wynder and Gori 1977). Although relatively small, this could imply as many as 15,000 cancers in males per year in the United States.

More recently, it has been recognized that there are some cancers which are "job-associated," being influenced by the social milieu related to the job rather than to direct carcinogen exposure. In a recent report on occupational mortality from the United Kingdom (Her Majesty's Stationery Office 1978), a number of occupations showed an increase in cancer mortality at certain sites that cannot easily be ascribed to direct industrial exposures. Examples include gastric cancer in coal miners and textile workers, cancer of the large intestine in farmers and executives, cancers of the esophagus and lung in the food, drink, tobacco, and transport industries workers, as well as in the armed forces (Table 1).

When the cancer frequency in each occupation was standardized according to social class, which in the United Kingdom is an index to some extent of "life-style," the differences between occupations were often considerably reduced (Table 2). This would suggest that factors other than occupation per se were involved. This view is further supported by the fact that women classified by their husbands' occupation also tended to show the same unusual disease patterns, apart from accidents (Table 3). While some job-associated cancers are of course due to use of alcoholic beverages or cigarettes (Table 4), as in Danish brewery workers (International Agency for Research on Cancer 1977), others are more difficult to understand.

Thus, although many direct occupational hazards have now been identified, e.g., beta-naphthylamine, their nature may often require complex analysis of the total as well as the limited environment. Further, past exposures to a potential risk often cannot be measured, and many workplace studies are complicated

TABLE 1. *Standardized mortality (SM) by occupation and cancer site in males aged 15–64**

Occupation	All sites	Esophagus	Stomach	Large intestine	Lung	Lymphomas
Farmers, foresters, fishermen	92	113	97	120	84	112
Miners, quarrymen	120	83	171	111	116	123
Gas, coke, and chemical workers	118	120	150	108	123	97
Woodworkers	107	127	108	84	113	99
Clothing workers	97	91	82	135	104	106
Transport workers	120	128	124	103	128	109
Sales workers	89	90	69	105	85	107
Administrators and managers	74	75	65	99	60	102
Armed forces	161	289	114	146	148	109

* After Office of Population Censuses and Surveys 1978

by the synergistic effect of smoking, e.g., in asbestos workers (Hammond and Selikoff 1973).

Drug-Related Cancers

The association of cancer with use of certain drugs is well recognized. However, the increasing use of drugs over prolonged periods by healthy individuals has expanded the problem of surveying for toxic effects, as most available registries for reporting side effects are inadequate for diseases with long induction periods.

TABLE 2. *Mortality from cancer in males aged 15–64 (SM) standardized for social class (All neoplasms*)*

Occupation	Nonstandardized†	Standardized‡
Farmers, foresters, fishermen	92	92
Miners, quarrymen	120	105
Gas, coke, and chemical workers	118	102
Woodworkers	107	95
Clothing workers	97	86
Transport workers	120	106
Sales workers	89	104
Administrators and managers	74	94
Armed forces	161	—

* After Office of Population Censuses and Surveys 1978
† The nonstandardized compares mortality with total population.
‡ The standardized compares mortality with people in the same social group and therefore is a more accurate indication of the effects of occupation.

TABLE 3. *Differences between married men and women in mortality (SM)*
according to occupation, 15–64 years: significance at p < 0.01*

Occupation	All Neoplasms Men	All Neoplasms Woment	Circulatory Diseases Men	Circulatory Diseases Woment	Accidents Men	Accidents Woment
Farmers, foresters, fishermen	89	105	78	110	124	100
Miners, quarrymen	118	133	131	190	176	105
Gas, coke, and chemical workers	—	—	112	144	—	—
Transport workers	—	—	108	124	129	84
Sales workers	90	102	96	80	—	—
Professional	73	95	85	66	76	100

* After Office of Population Censuses and Surveys 1978
† Married women classified according to husband's occupation

It should be remembered that there is often a tendency to consider the role of drugs only in terms of ill effects and to forget both the intended and possible auxiliary beneficial effects. Thus, hormonal contraceptives probably reduce benign or preneoplastic disease of the breast (Cole 1977), suggesting new approaches to cancer control (chemoprevention).

The Study of Etiological Factors in Cancers of Presumed Environmental Origin

While it would appear that most of the obvious, major causal carcinogenic factors—cultural or occupational—have been identified, the evidence for an environmental role in tumors at many sites, e.g., gastrointestinal and genitourinary systems, breast, etc., remains predominantly circumstantial, being based

TABLE 4. *Relationship between smoking habits and lung cancer for men aged*
15–64 in selected occupations*

	Ratio of current smoking habit to meant	Lung SM
Coal miners underground	131	114
Coal miners above ground	160	118
Rubber workers	129	114
Bus drivers	128	125
Managers	77	60
Farmers	65	57
Ministers, MPs, senior government officials	31	37
Doctors	33	32
University teachers	52	15

* After Office of Population Censuses and Surveys 1978
† This is the ratio of the number of smokers in the group to the numbers expected in the general population

TABLE 5. *Incidence of primary liver cancer in selected areas of Europe 1968–1972**

Country or city	World standardized rates (per 100,000)	
	Male	Female
Geneva	9.4	1.4
Warsaw	8.5	5.8
Zaragoza	7.8	6.2
Hamburg	3.6	1.8
German Democratic Republic	3.2	1.4
Sweden	2.9	1.4
Birmingham, England	1.0	0.5

* Data based on Waterhouse *et al.* 1976.

on geographical and temporal variations and on migrant studies. The investigation of these cancers is difficult, as it requires a more sophisticated multidisciplinary approach to provide testable hypotheses, as illustrated in the case of tumors of the liver and the role of diet and life-style.

Primary Cancer of the Liver

The relatively high frequency of liver cancer in North America and Europe due to alcoholic beverages (Table 5) is well known. The evidence for the etiology, however, is as much based on histopathological as epidemiological data (Higginson 1977). In contrast, increasing evidence in Africa and Asia suggests the possible role of a mycotoxin, e.g., aflatoxin, produced by fungal contamination of foodstuffs (Linsell and Peers 1977).

The possible promoting role of viral hepatitis put forward in the 1940s (Bergeret 1947) was largely neglected because it did not fit prevailing fashions or available animal models, despite the pathological supporting data and the evidence against malnutrition (Higginson 1963, 1977). Recently, new evidence for the association between hepatitis B virus and primary liver cancer has become available (Table 6), and the cofactor theory is now seriously considered (Larouzé

TABLE 6. *Association between hepatitis B virus (HBV) infection and primary liver cancer (PLC)*

Country	No. of patients		Active HBV infection*		RR
	PLC	Control	PLC (%)	Control (%)	
Zambia†	19	40	68.4	12.5	15.2
Uganda†	47	50	72.3	8.0	30.1
USA†	27	200	40.7	1.0	68.1

* Positive for HBsAg (with or without anti-HBs) or for anti-HBc (without anti-HBs)
† Data based on Tabor *et al.* 1977

et al. 1977, Blumberg 1977, Nayak *et al.* 1977). Thus, lines for research and control have been identified, including evaluation of aflatoxin exposure and possible use of hepatitis vaccines. It is important, however, to note that real progress only became possible due to the development of the technology to measure and identify mycotoxins and hepatitis viruses in a less traditionally conditioned scientific climate.

Dietary and Life-Style Factors

Whereas the existence of direct carcinogens as dietary contaminants is a straightforward idea, the role of dietary nutrient patterns per se has been virtually ignored in man.

In a study carried out from 1953 to 1955 on cancer in the South African Bantu, including the role of diet and life-style (Higginson and Oettlé 1960), it was reported that many cancers could not be explained by current theory, and it was emphasized that the dietary patterns appeared, if anything, to reduce the risk for those cancers of major importance in Western populations. The authors concluded that "to find the cause of these differences, we need to compare the manner of life of these populations (that is Bantu and Western Europeans). Such a comparison is made difficult by the lack of possible hypotheses regarding the causes of many of these neoplasms and, where one does not know what aspects to compare, the task of adequately describing the manner of life of the group studied here becomes impossibly great." Today, I have little to add to these remarks except that there has been a marked change in accepting the possible role of life-styles. Further, we are now in a position for the first time to study such hypotheses on a more objective basis, although surprisingly few new theories on the effects of life-style have been put forward. However, the important studies on Mormons and Seventh-Day Adventists by Wynder *et al.* (1959), Enstrom (1975), and Phillips (1975) have had a major influence in expanding this approach, as have Burkitt's views on the role of fiber in intestinal cancer (Burkitt *et al.* 1972). However, "absence of fiber" in the diet cannot be described as "a direct carcinogen" but only as "a carcinogenic risk factor" (Lancet 1977a).

Cancers of the stomach and large intestine illustrate some of the other difficulties in studying such factors, including possible noncarcinogenic precursors. For example, gastric cancer has been ascribed to excessive nitrate ingestion, with resultant in vivo formation of nitrosamines (Lancet 1977b). Yet in contrast, there is general agreement that persons who eat dairy products, fresh fruit, and raw vegetables have a lower risk of gastric cancer, even though these foods may be a major source of nitrites. Moreover, in many countries, gastric cancer has decreased despite increased use of fertilizers. Thus, for each hypothetical causal agent, whether nitrates, malnutrition, fat or meat intake, etc., it is nearly always possible to find contrary data from elsewhere, indicating the necessity for more definitive investigation. These complexities are well illustrated by the difficulties

TABLE 7. *Clinical and latent prostate cancer rates**

Area	Mortality (per 10^5 per year)	Incidence	Prevalence %† (latent cancer)
Singapore	—	3.6	13.2
Hong Kong	2.2	—	15.8
Uganda	—	4.4	19.5
Israel	7.9	14.3	22.0
Jamaica	13.9	20.7	29.8
Federal Republic of Germany	13.9	21.1	28.4
Sweden	18.4	38.8	31.6

* Data based on Breslow 1977
† Prevalence rates (%) of positive cancer directly standardized to pooled age distribution

encountered in identifying the causal factors in esophageal cancer in Central Asia and Iran (Kmet *et al.,* in press). Finally, a vast number of potential carcinogens and promoters may occur under natural cooking conditions (Sugimura *et al.* 1977).

The role of promoting factors possibly related to life-style may also explain the observation that between different countries the prevalence of latent carcinoma of the prostate is only partly paralleled by differences in the prevalence of invasive carcinoma (Table 7) (Tulinius 1977).

The indirect effects of diet are difficult to examine in animal models, which tend to be more suited to studies with high dose levels of carcinogens or extreme dietary modifications than for the study of those subtle life-style modifications that may be important in man. Such investigations in human populations, termed "metabolic epidemiology," include studies of individual and population susceptibilities to the action of carcinogens in terms other than the measure of simple exposures to carcinogens. Research in this field may, in due course, present the possibility of "chemoprevention," as, for example, the addition of ascorbic acid to the diet to prevent in vivo nitrosamine formation.

Hereditary and Racial Factors

Hereditary and racial factors in cancer etiology have been extensively discussed (Fraumeni 1975). Apart from skin cancers, susceptibility to which is influenced by skin pigmentation, nasopharyngeal carcinoma, and possibly adenocarcinoma of the lung in Cantonese females, cancers clearly related to these factors are limited to a few relatively rare congenital conditions. Individual susceptibility may also be modified by exogenous stimuli, such as enzyme inducers (Conney *et al.* 1977). Where such susceptibility differences are expressed in biochemical changes, mutagenic tests may prove useful for their investigation in human tissues, fluids, or excreta.

Congenital abnormalities have been suggested as a crude index of exposure to exogenous toxic agents, but most studies show the frequency of such abnormalities to be very similar over a wide variety of environments. It has been estimated that approximately one third of congenital malformations are associated with chromosomal abnormalities occurring in children born to women over 35 years of age (Yunis and Chandler 1977), and the frequency of cancers associated with such abnormalities, e.g., Down's syndrome, could be reduced if older women did not bear children. Such an approach to control, however, is unlikely to receive widespread support.

Cancers of Unknown Origin

There is little evidence that environmental factors are involved in most cancers of the lymph glands, hemopoietic system, soft tissues and bone, and childhood tumors, with certain exceptions, e.g., radiation-induced leukemia. Furthermore, in contrast to the incidence of epithelial tumors in adults, the incidence of such tumors (except, for example, Burkitt's lymphoma) tends to be similar over a wide variety of environments. It is for this group of tumors that viruses are considered probable etiological agents (de Thé *et al.* 1975).

IMPLICATIONS FOR CANCER CONTROL

I have presented this rather lengthy summary of data on cancer causation, putting emphasis on life-style, because I am concerned that available observations are often misinterpreted by the public and scientists alike, with detrimental effects not only on preventive strategy but also on research priorities.

In his textbook written in 1947, Willis discussed the etiology of several cancers, stating, for example, that breast cancer was due to "unnatural reproductive habits," but he appeared reasonably certain about the cause of only ten percent of tumors (Willis 1947). His discussion on lung cancer was limited, in the main, to industrial hazards, and he wrote that the role of tobacco in lung cancer in man would be almost impossible to prove, and in any case the evidence would never convince smokers. He denied the existence of mesothelioma. Today, proposals based on sound scientific observations are available which, if practiced, could prevent up to 50 percent of cancers in males in certain societies. However, it is now clearly recognized that this level of prevention is not achievable for a variety of scientific and nonscientific reasons. Furthermore, there are certain methods, apart from elimination of exposures, that could ensure effective cancer control but that are simply *not* acceptable to most societies—even if today one third of U. S. females have agreed to a hysterectomy (Table 8).

Experience has shown that individuals are very resistant to changes in cultural habits. The pleasures of smoking, chewing, and drinking are often more important to those whose life tends to be boring and frustrating, whether they are industrial employees or Asian peasants. For such people, the immediate pleasures outweigh the theoretical risk of cancer to a greater extent than for the more

TABLE 8. *Cancer prevention—effective but impractical*

Procedures	Gain*	Sex
No smoking	40%	Male
No drinking	5–10%	Male
Prostatectomy (60 yrs)	20–30%	Male
Nipplectomy (< 14 yrs)	30%	Female
Subtotal hysterectomy	10%	Female
Total hysterectomy (< 35 yrs)	30%	Female
Personnel engineering	2%	Both sexes
Arab dress	20–30%	Both sexes
Celibacy	10–40%	Both sexes

* Gain = proportion of all cancers likely to be affected by procedure

fortunate members of society whose life is easier and more pleasant. Furthermore, the puritan or elitist view usually assumes that these habits are voluntary and susceptible to individual control. The addictive effect of smoking is thus often ignored, although alcoholism is increasingly regarded as a disease. In contrast, there is little difficulty in getting society to accept control of iatrogenic, industrial, and other imposed hazards where the individual is not personally involved. Unfortunately, however, the *overall* impact of control of such factors in terms of reduction of cancer rates will be very limited.

Factors Inhibiting Cancer Control

Despite the increase in knowledge of potential control methods, at no time have cancer research workers been under greater attack for lack of success. The fact that many cancers can now be attributed definitively, or partly, to environmental causes has been considered by the public to imply that all cancers are preventable *now,* through simple regulatory action. Such an attitude indicates a lack of understanding of the problems involved, which include:

1) Unwillingess to accept that cigarette smoking is the major causal factor so far identified in human cancer;
2) Belief in a predominant role in cancer causation of industrial pollution—whether point source or ambient—an exposure assumed to be controllable with resultant ignoring of other environmental factors;
3) Failure to understand the complex biology of cancer in man, and the technical difficulties of analyzing and defining the role of "life-style," in its widest sense;
4) Failure to distinguish between the identification and control of existing hazards, and identification and control of future hazards—and the relative weight to be given to evaluating the implications of experimental studies in each situation. This is compounded by a failure to appreciate the present technological and biological limitations to rational quantitative extrapolation from the results of animal experiments to man;

5) Failure to understand that exposure standards only protect against future and not past exposures;

6) Insufficient understanding of the different types of statistical risks, e.g., relative, absolute, etc., so that "real" and "potential" hazards are not separated. Thus, there may be no appreciation of the different options involved in controlling a hazard;

7) A failure to understand that "safety" is a statistical concept and not a biological absolute (Lowrance 1976);

8) A failure to accept that regulatory decisions are based on many considerations, not only on the scientific data (Bates, in press);

9) The widespread opinion that "everything is dangerous," which has led to neglect of control of obvious hazards;

10) Unwarranted hope in the development of a "miracle" cure or preventive vaccine in the immediate future, which has diminished support for prevention.

Certain of the above problems merit further discussion.

Presentation of Risks

In presenting data to the public, the concept of "life-time risk" is probably the most useful, as it is relatively easy to express and understand (Pochin 1974). Further, additive risks can be described according to occupational hazard, etc. For example, nonsmokers in the United Kingdom have a 30 percent chance of dying by 65 years of age, compared with smokers, who have a 40 percent risk. The one-third increase in death risk is due to their tenfold increased risk of lung cancer. Although the "relative risk" for angiosarcoma in workers exposed to high levels of vinyl chloride may be exceedingly high (400-fold), the "additive risk" of 0.3 percent by 65 years of age (i.e., 30.3 percent chance of dying by that age) is modest as compared to that due to smoking. On the other hand, the combined effects of smoking and asbestos lead to a massive "additive increase" in risk (possibly more than 50-fold) over nonsmoking asbestos workers (Hammond and Selikoff 1973), although the "relative risk" is actually less than that with vinyl chloride (Higginson 1976). It is possible to combine a number of different risks to give an approximation of the hazards of an occupation in relation to the general population not only for cancer but also for other diseases, and such real risks are of great value in determining cost-benefits.

The word "safe" is a statistical concept and does not mean absence of risk. A "safe" exposure could be described as the probability of either a "real" or "potential" risk that society accepts as being of a "reasonable" order, the magnitude varying with the type of risk and other considerations. Proof of safety can only be presented as probable figures for a "real risk," and a subjective estimate based on expert opinion of a "potential" risk. The terminology difficulties of safety are illustrated in a recent editorial in Lancet (1977c) comparing two reports. The first report stated that there was *no convincing* evidence of increased risk through true ambient exposure to asbestos—in air, water, drugs, etc.—although the possibility of such a risk could not be denied categorically. The editorial then described the second report as being "more pessimistic," since it stated *"it is not possible* to assess whether there is a level of exposure in humans below which an increased risk of cancer would not occur." Thus, although both reports utilized the same evidence to make essentially identical judgments, the latter are regarded as being quantitatively different. It is not surprising that the public is confused and often considers all potential risks as equal, and equivalent to real risks.

These comments of course do not imply that preventable risks should not be controlled because they are small. There is no justification for ignoring a minor hazard because a greater evil exists (Ashford 1976), but conversely, there is no justification for overemphasizing a minor risk to the detriment of control of a major hazard. Unfortunately, the emotive problems associated especially with industrial hazards, however small, make dispassionate discussion in the real world difficult, where political or other considerations are involved.

Nonetheless, an oversimplistic approach to defining risks is dangerous, as it prevents reasoned discussion of the options open to society in evaluating cost-benefits. This is true of all types of situations, including the risks associated with drugs. Certain drugs, e.g., sodium penicillin G and isoniazide, are carcinogens to certain animal species and therefore present potential risks, but they have not been shown to be carcinogenic to man at normal dose levels. Yet today it is possible that the risk of using isoniazide would be considered unreasonable, for attitudes to risks may be highly subjective. Those doctors who have personally witnessed the revolution caused by antibiotics are much less likely to be impressed by the extent of the problem of drug usage than a young toxicologist.

Comparison of Direct Carcinogen Exposure at Low-Dose Versus Life-Style

The identification and control of point source exposures to identified human or animal carcinogens is becoming a relatively clear-cut problem, but the difficulties associated with ambient exposures are more complex. The widespread impression that industrial and environmental pollution due to the summation of multiple carcinogens in minute doses is responsible for much of our present cancer patterns represents a return to the concept of Livingstone that cancer is a "disease of civilization."

Without excluding the importance of examining and controlling, where necessary, ambient exposures, it is desirable to examine the available epidemiological data on the role of such exposures within the overall picture of cancer etiology. There is no clear-cut correlation between the overall incidence of cancer in most European countries and the degree of industrialization, e.g., industrial Birmingham, United Kingdom, versus Geneva, Switzerland (Table 9). Further-

TABLE 9. *Standardized morbidity rates per 100,000 per year for lung and other cancers**

Area		Lung Male	All cancers (Excluding skin and lung) Male	Female
U.S.:	White	55	222	248
Alameda County, Calif.	Black	70	259	207
Utah		29	184	190
Israel:	Jews	29	189	221
	Non-Jews	27	103	74
Singapore:	Chinese	56	197	135
	Indian	10	119	171
Norway:	Urban	33	195	193
	Rural	14	159	166
U.K.:	Ayrshire	65	173	156
	Birmingham	77	163	171
Geneva:		60	217	207
New Zealand:	Maori	67	169	212
	Non-Maori	48	173	182

* Data based on Waterhouse *et al.* 1976

more, apart from the increase in cigarette-related cancer, the overall patterns
of cancer observed today in most industrial and nonindustrial states are very
similar to those at the turn of the century. Thus, the environmental agents
involved have been present for many years. Stomach or large intestinal cancer
cannot simply and uncritically be ascribed to food additives. The relative importance of smoking in lung cancer and the minor role of ambient air pollution,
except as a synergistic factor, illustrate the problem of confounding variables
in seeking to analyze the role of ambient pollutants. While certain cancers,
e.g., breast, colon, and corpus uteri, are relatively rare in some developing countries, others, such as tumors of the liver, prostate, and cervix, may be more
common in Africa than in some European countries (Tables 10 and 11). There

TABLE 10. *Incidence of malignant neoplasms in males per 100,000 per year (standardized)**

Site	Geneva 1970–1972	Bulawayo (Rhodesia, African) 1968–1972
Liver	9.4	64.6
Prostate	29.9	32.3
Skin	24.9	9.8
Colon	18.9	7.0
Stomach	18.1	12.4
All sites	303.0	355.8

* Data based on Waterhouse *et al.* 1976

TABLE 11. *Incidence of malignant neoplasms in females per 100,000 per year (standardized)**

Site	Geneva 1970–1972	Bulawayo (Rhodesia, African) 1968–1972
Breast	70.6	13.8
Corpus uteri	16.3	10.2
Cervix uteri	16.1	28.4
Skin	14.7	0.9
Colon	13.5	5.8
Ovary	10.9	8.1
Liver	1.4	25.4
All sites	229.7	148.3

* Data based on Waterhouse *et al.* 1976

is no consistent pattern, and each site must be considered as a separate etiological entity. Instead of accepting these observations with some relief as scientific facts that imply no immediate environmental, universal catastophe, many would prefer to regard such a conclusion as smug and lacking in responsibility, since it contradicts certain political, societal, and quasi-scientific dogmas.

The above comments do not mean that we should not control ambient pollution of the environment or that some types of ambient pollution may not be dangerous. They do mean that many cancers cannot easily be explained on such a basis, not even where urban-rural differences exist (Blot *et al.* 1977). It is necessary to investigate the total life-style of such societies in addition to cultural smoking and drinking habits, as described by Lyon *et al.* (1976, 1977) and Weisburger *et al.* (1977), and also earlier occupational exposures. Furthermore, the potential role of chemical inhibitors in the environment needs further investigation (Wattenberg 1977).

The Difficulties of Extrapolation from Animal and In Vitro Systems

The scientific difficulties of generalizing from animals to man are well recognized. Failure by the public to appreciate the implications has been responsible for much of the confrontation that surrounds regulatory control of environmental hazards, as is the failure to distinguish between past and future hazards. In relation to future putative hazards, animal studies would appear a reasonable and effective method of preventing the introduction of potentially hazardous new compounds into the environment without good cause, and, in this context, the value of the Delaney Clause is generally accepted. Problems do, however, arise relative to the evaluation for man of compounds that are carcinogenic in an animal species and that have been present in the environment for many years, where many interests are involved, where human exposures are widespread, and where the only epidemiological data available are inadequate.

Due to animal/human differences in ingestion, absorption, metabolism, and variations between species, the concept of a "weak" or "strong" carcinogen, as extrapolated from animal experience to man, has little validity, although there are an increasing number of parameters that may provide guidance. Thus, it is probable that animal carcinogens which are strongly electrophilic are carcinogenic in several species, are metabolized similarly in man and animals, and, where human exposures are high and prolonged, should perhaps receive priority as being more likely to be dangerous than those which do not show some of these characteristics, although there are exceptions.

Thus, it must be emphasized to the public that extensive basic research is still required into the mechanism of action of carcinogens. The organization of appropriate epidemiological surveys should be established where human exposures have occurred in the past to provide more concrete data on which methods for rational extrapolation may be developed in the future. This in no way implies that such exposures should not be controlled immediately, but where they have occurred, whether through inadvertent carelessness or ignorance, the maximum scientific information should be obtained for future benefits to man.

THE CONCEPT OF NONEFFECT EXPOSURES

Our views on noneffect exposures to carcinogens are governed by the view that noncarcinogenic dose levels to a carcinogen do not exist, and, further, they cannot be calculated from animal studies. In this context the experience of radiobiologists may be instuctive. Although all levels of ionizing radiation are regarded as carrying a potential hazard, standards of permitted exposures were established based on existing knowledge, and these have been regularly up-dated with new developments. It is possible that a similar approach would facilitate rational legislation for carcinogens.

There are many epidemiological and statistical problems in proving the existence of a noneffect level in man. These include the inadequacy of the available epidemiological material, which is often limited to small groups of exposed individuals. Nonetheless, a number of case-history and correlation studies suggest that there are situations in which no significant additive risk has been documented in man after exposures to known animal carcinogens, e.g., saccharin, DDT, isoniazide, and sodium penicillin G. Since the results of experimental studies have been very influential in developing cancer control strategies, the existence of data supporting noncarcinogenic exposure levels should not be ignored. The majority of hyperplastic nodules produced in the liver by carcinogens are reversible (Quinn and Higginson 1965, Farber 1976, Pitot 1977), and although subject to statistical limitations, the doses given would not appear always to produce tumors within the lifetime of the animals. I cannot accept the view that since one cannot distinguish between reversible and irreversible nodules, they should all be called "neoplastic," presumably on the grounds that it is better to be 98 percent wrong and two percent right than 98 percent right and two percent wrong, a somewhat dubious scientific base to the objective reporting of tests on potential animal carcinogens. Studies on the bladder (Jacobs *et al.* 1977) also suggest reversibility after carcinogen exposure. A noneffect level is also implicit in most two-stage experiments in that initiation, although irreversible, does not result in tumors without the interaction of other stimuli. In contrast, studies in mutational in vitro systems have not produced supportive evidence for a noneffect dose (H. Bartsch, personal communication).

Examining the statistical problems, Cornfield (1977), in a recent elegant study of noneffect dose levels, concluded that even if "this analysis establishes that carcinogenesis is an irreversible, one-hit phenomenon between the ultimate carcinogen and DNA . . . the existence of a noneffect or threshold level for the carcinogenic compound administered is not precluded." Clearly, this represents a research field to which both experimentalists and epidemiologists should give the highest priority, to clarify the issues.

Decision Making

Space does not permit a detailed discussion of the decision-making process and the role of conflicting interests that have been widely discussed elsewhere (New Scientist 1977a, McGinty and Atherley 1977, International Commission on Radiobiological Protection 1977, Weisburger *et al.* 1977, Manos 1977, Thomas 1977, Federation Proceedings 1977, Martin 1978). The role of the regulator and scientist in decision making has never been better expressed than by Ashby (1976) who wrote: "For many political decisions (not only decisions about the environment) there has to be an ingredient of hard data: scientific, technological, economic, statistical. But before the decision can be made, another ingredient has to be added. I called it 'hunch' but a more respectable name for it is 'political judgement.' This can be shallow, as it is when it is mere vote-catching; but it can be profound, and sometimes it tips the balance even against the weight of cognitive evidence." Regulation is growing and will continue to do so, possibly without a comparable increase in effectiveness; our job is to control the quality of regulation and to advise on pragmatic action, recognizing that for the moment we may be unable often to give definitive answers. This should make us sympathize with the invidious position of the regulator who is required to decide between many different options, which are frequently highly emotive.

THE ETHICAL RESPONSIBILITY OF THE SCIENTIST IN RELATION TO ENVIRONMENTAL CARCINOGENESIS

Outside medicine there is no code that contains any explicit criteria regarding the conduct of scientists in applying or evaluating scientific knowledge in practical life. Unfortunately, such judgments take place in circumstances more compatible with the advocatory confrontation of law courts where the brilliance of a lawyer's arguments is more important than the objective merits of his case. Experience in legal medicine has confirmed the inadequacy of such an approach.

André Cournand (1977) has ascribed the following characteristics to the scientist, notably: objectivity, tolerance, doubt of certitude, recognition of error, unselfish engagement, and communal spirit.

Objectivity

If we wish to guard our reputation as experts and guides for the public well-being, objectivity must never be forgotten. The vested interests of industrialists, trade unionists, and politicians are well publicized; however, the possibility that a scientist under the stresses of modern academic life, including the quest for research support, may overemphasize the importance of his research or a new test or chemical carcinogen and thus unconsciously exaggerate a danger, should not be completely forgotten. Furthermore, a scientist may get locked into a certain conceptual approach that may affect his objective evaluation of data conflicting with his own research. He may instinctively tend to favor what he believes *should* happen as distinct from what *does* happen.

This is well illustrated by the "Great Cancer Scare of 1975" when an apparently large increase in cancer mortality in the U.S. was described unhesitantly by many scientists as the leading edge of the wave of cancer resulting from the petrochemical pollution of our environment, a view widely publicized in the press and which, not unnaturally, led to great public concern and anxiety. When the artefactual nature of the increase was demonstrated, retractions were notable by their absence (Chiazze *et al.* 1976). Such uncritical evaluation of data can only be highly detrimental to our image as experts and may have the additional danger of diverting public attention from real and more pressing hazards.

The situation regarding asbestos is also instructive. All commercial types of asbestos may be responsible for the induction of mesothelioma, but some are less dangerous than others (Harington and Allison 1977). Yet crocidolite has only been restricted in a few countries, and between 1960 and 1973, the exports from South Africa doubled. Further, the synergism between cigarettes and asbestos enormously increases the risk of lung cancer (Hammond and Selikoff 1973), but, in contrast to coal miners or workers in some breweries, cigarette smoking has not been forbidden among asbestos workers. In reviewing this history, one has the impression that the failure to take action on crocidolite and amosite has been partly motivated by a wish to prove that exposures to all forms of asbestos are equally dangerous, and thus the benefits of reduced smoking and of eliminating exposures to the more dangerous types of asbestos have not been implemented. Some people still believe that to forbid smoking in the workplace does not reduce smoking exposures, contrary to the evidence in coal miners, for example (Table 12). For this failure, environmental scientists must take some responsibility. However, lack of definite data on comparative hazards has

TABLE 12. *Male smoking habits by occupation (mean)* *

| Occupation | Cigarette consumption by current smokers | | |
	Weekday	Weekend	Weekly
Coal miners,			
Underground	14.8	20.7	115.7
Above ground	21.6	22.7	153.6
Managers	16.6	17.2	119.6
Armed Forces	17.8	19.7	128.6

* After Office of Population Censuses and Surveys 1978

been compounded by the failure in the past of employers to accept that a problem existed and, therefore, to ensure generation of the epidemiological data necessary to evaluate critically the risks from the different types of asbestos.

Tolerance and Doubt of Certitude

In making pronouncements on the potential role of certain factors in human cancer, scientists frequently lack the certitude on which to base definitive proposals. Therefore, control proposals have both subjective and objective components. This incertitude should render us humble and not dogmatic in a highly complex field and guard us from offering simple solutions.

Recognition of Error

Jurists and legislators will continue to demand certainty, but the interests of the public will not be served by unjustified simplification of complex problems, no matter how well intentioned. This is well illustrated by the banning of DDT, often regarded as a triumph by environmentalists. In Pakistan, one third of sprayers applying malathion developed symptoms of poisoning, following the switch from DDT (Baker *et al.* 1978). A recent report from India indicated that following the discontinuation of DDT use in the malaria program, there had been a resurgence of kala-azar with 100,000 cases and 4,000 deaths in 1976. Control of this disease was a side benefit of the DDT program, and a decision to reintroduce the pesticide has now been made (New Scientist 1977b). To blame this decision only on politicians or public health officials is to beg the question, since their attitude was largely conditioned by the oversimplification in the scientific community, which has not always recognized that there are other causes of morbidity and other benefits required by society that are outside scientists' field of competence (Black and Pole 1975).

Although DDT had been widely distributed for over 30 years, with marked variations in the levels of exposure between communities, there has been no evidence ever that local cancer patterns in any way reflect such variations in exposure, and, as Doll concluded at the XIth International Cancer Congress,

Florence, 1974: "If DDT is a carcinogen to man, it is certainly an exceedingly weak one" (R. Doll, personal communication). Yet instead of regarding such an observation as a reason for caution, many people have rather emphasized the potential dangers, with the result, however unintentional, that the Indian farmer was exposed to a real hazard. Tolerance clearly requires that we listen to the opinion of others. Certainly, where decisions are subjective, there is no justification for casting aspersions on the integrity of colleagues when their value judgments on the available data are different from our own. Nor is the danger of cancer the only reason for controlling the environment.

Communal Spirit

The quality and effectiveness of environmental control will largely depend on an educated legislature and public whose attitudes are largely governed by the media (Abelson 1976) and are thus dependent on the ability of the latter to provide objective reports. If the view in the National News Council (Carter 1977) represents policy, the outlook is indeed poor: "What is essential in a documentary is that its conclusions be based on verifiable information—that is on documentation—and not that it be fully objective. A major function of journalism is responsible interpretation." How can one regard responsible journalism as ignoring a balanced judgment of *all* the verifiable information?

For the scientist, it should be a rule that reports on health hazards be submitted to peer review in a scientific journal rather than presentation in the public press, as was done in the New Orleans drinking water controversy (DeRouen and Diem 1975). It was publication in scientific journals that exposed the flimsy supportive data for the carcinogenic effects ascribed to fluoridization of water (Doll and Kinlen 1977).

The scientist must accept his limitations, remain objective, and as far as health science is concerned, in its widest sense, follow the dictates of the Hippocratic Oath. I believe it is completely irresponsible for scientists and regulators to alarm people merely to satisfy scientific curiosity or a legal requirement, e.g., by informing them of a past and possibly harmless exposure, where no benefit to the individual can be offered. Such an attitude attacks the base of medical practice—to always consider the maximum good of the individual patient and avoid causing unnecessary anxiety.

In conclusion, there are a number of problems both in understanding carcinogenic mechanisms and also in relation to improved environmental and epidemiological techniques that bear on the common problem of environmental carcinogenesis. In the application of these data there will be also a number of societal questions that will require answers. In Table 13, both the scientific and nonscientific questions are summarized that, in my opinion, are of greatest immediate importance.

Having drawn attention to many of the failures of the scientific community,

TABLE 13. *The $64,000 questions in carcinogenesis*

1) Are there noneffect exposure levels in man?
2) Can biological responses for man be extrapolated from nonhuman systems in terms of exposures?
3) Can "life-style" be defined?
4) Can individual susceptibility be defined?
5) Can a potential risk be measured?
6) Can a real risk be measured?
7) How should a negative result be evaluated?
8) Who is an expert?
9) Who makes value judgments?

I prefer to end more positively and suggest that as a community we should cease to be defensive about what we have already done in identifying causes of cancer. I have already emphasized the great progress made in the last 30 years, not only in the field of epidemiology but also in the field of chemical carcinogenesis since Boyland (1947, 1950) first suggested the role of metabolites as ultimate carcinogens. It is time we indicated to society and its leaders their responsibilities and re-affirm our position as experts, which includes the presentation of hazards and risks objectively.

When we draw attention to major risks such as smoking, we should reject accusations that we are condoning minor risks. There is no excuse for selling cigarettes to minors when the sale of alcohol is forbidden; there is no excuse for continuing the use of crocidolite when other forms of asbestos are less hazardous, and there is no excuse for not developing the epidemiological studies that, for pragmatic purposes, we must use for evaluating existing hazards: This includes not only those relevant to direct chemical carcinogens but all those problems which fall under the heading of "life-style" and which will need further development in expressing individual susceptibility in biochemical and immunological terms. To retain the confidence of the public we must ensure that our role as experts remains intact and that our communication with the public is such that it facilitates an understanding of the complex issues involved. This cannot be done in a spirit of confrontation and, if we do not take steps to ensure that our profession maintains its scientific integrity, it may well be that we shall find that governments and others will undertake the task at our expense. Finally, we must be prepared to accept that it will be many years before full cancer prevention will be possible, if ever. I would agree with Weiner and Newberne (1977) who stated that "our ability to better predict human safety from animal toxicologic studies will not come from irrationally expanding the variety and magnitude of 'routine' tests but by selectively augmenting an appropriate spectrum of empirical toxicologic studies consistent with the nature of each specific problem." If society wishes a balanced plan of cancer control and prevention, it should be prepared to support the basic research that such an effort will require, rather than ask "What is its value?"

To quote de Tocqueville: "They (the Americans) had a lively faith in the perfectibility of man. They judged that the diffusion of knowledge must necessarily be advantageous and the consequence of ignorance fatal."

REFERENCES

Abelson, P. H. 1976. Communicating with the publics. Science 194:565.

Ashby, The Rt. Hon. Lord. 1976. Protection of the environment: The human dimension (Jephcott Lecture). Proc. R. Soc. Med. 69:721–730.

Ashford, N. A. 1976. Crisis in the Workplace: Occupational Disease and Injury (A Report to the Ford Foundation). MIT Press, Cambridge, Mass.

Baker, E. L., M. Warren, M. Zack, R. D. Dobbin, J. W. Miles, S. Miller, L. Alderman, and W. R. Teeters. 1978. Epidemic malathion poisoning in Pakistan malaria workers. Lancet I:31–34.

Bates, R. 1978. Regulation of carcinogenic food additives and drugs in the U.S., *in* Carcinogenic Risks-Strategies for Intervention. W. Davis and C. Rosenfeld, eds., IARC Scientific Publication No. 25, International Agency for Research on Cancer, Lyon, France (In press).

Bergeret, C., and F. Roulet. 1947. Au sujet des ictères graves de la cirrhose et du cancer primitif chez le noir d'Afrique. Acta Trop. 4:210–240.

Black, D. A., and J. D. Pole. 1975. Priorities in biomedical research (indices of burden). Br. J. Prev. Soc. Med. 29:222–227.

Blot, W. J., L. A. Brinton, J. F. Fraumeni, and B. J. Stone. 1977. Cancer mortality in U.S. counties with petroleum industries. Science 198:51–53.

Blumberg, B. S. 1977. Australia antigen and the biology of hepatitis B. Science 197:17–25.

Boyland, E., and F. Weigert. 1947. Metabolism of carcinogenic compounds. Br. Med. Bull. 4:354–359.

Boyland, E. 1950. The biological significance of metabolism of polycyclic hydrocarbons, *in* Biological Oxidation of Aromatic Rings. R. T. Williams, ed., Biochemical Society Symposia No. 5, Cambridge University Press, London, England, pp. 40–54.

Breslow, N., C. W. Chan, G. Dhom, R. A. B. Drury, L. M. Franks, B. Gellei, Y. S. Lee, S. Lundberg, B. Sparke, N. H. Sternby, and H. Tulinius. 1977. Latent carcinoma of prostate at autopsy in seven areas. Int. J. Cancer 20:680–688.

Burkitt, D. P., A. R. P. Walker, and N. S. Painter. 1972. Effect of dietary fibre on stools and transit-times and its role in the causation of disease. Lancet II:1408–1411.

Carter, L. J. 1977. A mixed verdict on NBC nuclear waste documentary. Science 198:1232–1233.

Chiazze, L., D. T. Silverman, and D. L. Levin. 1976. The cancer mortality scare—problems of estimation using monthly data. JAMA 236:2310–2312.

Cole, P. 1977. Oral contraceptives and breast neoplasia. Cancer 39:1906–1908.

Conney, A. H., E. J. Pantuck, K.-C. Hsiao, R. Kuntzman, A. P. Alvares, and A. Kappas. 1977. Regulation of drug metabolism in man by environmental chemicals and diet. Fed. Proc. 36:1647–1652.

Cornfield, J. 1977. Carcinogenic risk assessment. Science 198:693–699.

Cournand, A. 1977. The code of the scientist and its relationship to ethics. Science 198:699–705.

de Thé, G., M. A. Epstein, and H. zur Hausen, eds. 1975. Oncogenesis and Herpesviruses II (Parts 1 and 2). IARC Scientific Publication No. 11, International Agency for Research on Cancer, Lyon, France.

DeRouen, T. A., and J. E. Diem. 1975. The New Orleans drinking water controversy—a statistical perspective. Am. J. Public Health 65:1060–1062.

Doll, R. 1967. Prevention of cancer—pointers for epidemiology. The Rock Carling Fellowship 1967—Nuffield Provincial Hospitals Trust 1967. Whitefriars Press Ltd., London, England.

Doll, R. 1975. Pott and the prospects for prevention. (7th Walter Hubert Lecture). Br. J. Cancer 32:263–272.

Doll, R. 1977. Strategy for detection of cancer hazards to man. Nature 265:589–596.

Doll, R., and L. Kinlen. 1977. Fluoridation of water and cancer mortality in the USA. Lancet I:1300–1302.

Enstrom, E. J. 1975. Cancer mortality among Mormons. Cancer 36:825–841.

Farber, E. 1976. On the pathogenesis of experimental hepatocellular carcinoma, *in* Hepatocellular Carcinoma, K. Okuda and R. L. Peters, eds., John Wiley and Sons, New York, pp. 1–24.

Federation Proceedings. 1977. Conducting scientific analyses. Fed. Proc. 36:2534–2543.

Fraumeni, J. F., ed. 1975. Persons at High Risk of Cancer: An Approach to Cancer Etiology and Control. Academic Press, New York.

Hammond, E. C., and I. J. Selikoff. 1973. Relation of cigarette smoking to risk of death of asbestos-associated disease among insulation workers in the United States, *in* Biological Effects of Asbestos, P. Bogovski, J. C. Gilson, V. Timbrell, and J. C. Wagner, eds., IARC Scientific Publication No. 8, International Agency for Research on Cancer, Lyon, France, pp. 312–317.

Harington, J. S., and A. C. Allison. 1977. Tissue and cellular reactions to particles, fibers, and aerosols retained after inhalation, *in* Handbook of Physiology-Reactions to Environmental Agents. Williams and Wilkins, Baltimore, pp. 263–383.

Higginson, J. 1963. The geographical pathology of primary liver cancer. Cancer Res. 23:1624–1633.

Higginson, J. 1969. Present trends in cancer epidemiology, *in* Proceedings of the Eighth Canadian Cancer Conference, Honey Harbour, Ontario, 1968. J. F. Morgan, ed., Pergamon Press, Canada, pp. 40–75.

Higginson, J. 1976. A hazardous society? Individual versus community responsibility in cancer prevention. (Third Annual Matthew B. Rosenhaus Lecture). Am. J. Public Health 66:359–366.

Higginson, J. 1977. The role of the pathologist in environmental medicine and public health (review article). Am. J. Pathol. 86:460–484.

Higginson, J., and C. S. Muir. 1977. Détermination de l'importance des facteurs environnementaux dans le cancer humain: role de l'épidémiologie. Bull. Cancer 64:365–384.

Higginson, J., and A. G. Oettlé. 1960. Cancer incidence in the Bantu and "Cape Colored" races of South Africa: Report of a cancer survey in the Transvaal (1953–1955). J. Natl. Cancer Inst. 24:589–671.

International Agency for Research on Cancer Annual Report. 1977. International Agency for Research on Cancer, Lyon, France.

International Commission on Radiological Protection (ICRP). 1977. Problems involved in developing an index of harm. Ann. ICRP 1:(4).

Jacobs, A. R., M. Arai, S. M. Cohen, and G. H. Friedell. 1977. A long-term study of reversible and progressive urinary bladder cancer lesions in rats fed N-(4-(5-nitro-2-furyl)-2-thiazolyl)formamide. Cancer Res. 37:2817–2821.

Kmet, J., D. MacLaren, and F. Siassi. 1978. Epidemiology of oesophageal cancer with special reference to nutritional studies among the Turkomen of Iran. Advances in Human Nutrition (In press).

Lancet. 1977a. Dietary fibre. II:337–338.

Lancet. 1977b. Nitrate and human cancer. II:281–282.

Lancet. 1977c. Asbestos. II:1211–1212.

Larouzé, B., B. S. Blumberg, W. T. London, E. D. Lustbader, M. Sankalé, and M. Payet. 1977. Forecasting the development of primary hepatocellular carcinoma by the use of risk factors: Studies in West Africa. J. Natl. Cancer Inst. 58:1557–1561.

Linsell, C. A., and F. S. Peers. 1977. Aflatoxin and liver cancer. Trans. R. Soc. Trop. Med. Hyg. 71:471–473.

Lowrance, W. W. 1976. Of Acceptable Risk (Science and the Determination of Safety). William Kaufman Inc., Los Altos, California.

Lyon, J. L., J. W. Gardner, M. R. Klauber, and C. R. Smart. 1977. Low cancer incidence and mortality in Utah. Cancer 39:2608–2618.

Lyon, J. L., M. R. Klauber, J. W. Gardner, and C. R. Smart. 1976. Cancer incidence in Mormons and non-Mormons in Utah, 1966–1970. N. Engl. J. Med. 294:129–133.

Manos, J. 1977. Going on the defensive. Nature 267:194–195.

Martin, J. A. 1978. The "Science Court"—It should be tried. Chemical and Engineering News, 30 January 1978, p. 5.

McGinty, L., and G. Atherley. 1977. Acceptability versus democracy. New Scientist 74:323–325.

Nayak, N. C., A. Dhar, R. Sachdeva, A. Mittal, H. N. Seth, D. Sudarsanam, B. Reddy, U. L. Wagholikar, and C. R. R. M. Reddy. 1977. Association of human hepatocellular carcinoma and cirrhosis with hepatitis B virus surface and core antigens in the liver. Int. J. Cancer 20:643–654.

New Scientist. 1977a. The health hazard of coal power. 74:693.

New Scientist. 1977b. DDT's Indian comeback. 76:73.

Office of Population Censuses and Surveys. 1978. Occupational Mortality: England and Wales 1970–1972 (decennial supplement). Her Majesty's Stationery Office, London, England.

Phillips, R. L. 1975. Role of life-style and dietary habits in risk of cancer among Seventh-Day Adventists. Cancer Res. 35:3513–3533.

Pitot, H. C. 1977. The stability of events in the natural history of neoplasia. Am. J. Pathol. 89:703–716.

Pochin, E. E. 1974. Occupational and other fatality rates. Community Health 6:2–13.

Quinn, P. S., and J. Higginson. 1965. Reversible and irreversible changes in experimental cirrhosis. Am. J. Pathol. 47:353–369.

Sugimura, T., M. Nagao, T. Kawachi, M. Honda, T. Yahagi, Y. Seino, S. Sato, N. Matsukura, T. Matsushima, A. Shirai, M. Sawamura, and H. Matsumoto. 1977. Mutagen-carcinogens in food, with special reference to highly mutagenic pyrolytic products in broiled foods, *in* Origins of Human Cancer (Book C). Human Risk Assessment. H. H. Hiatt, J. D. Watson and J. A. Winsten, eds., Vol. 4. Cold Spring Harbor Laboratory, Cold Spring Harbor, New York, pp. 1561–1577.

Tabor, E., R. J. Gerety, C. L. Vogel, A. C. Bayley, P. P. Anthony, C. H. Chan, and L. F. Barker. 1977. Hepatitis B virus infection and primary hepatocellular carcinoma. J. Natl. Cancer Inst. 58:1197–1200.

Thomas, L. 1977. Notes of a biology-watcher (The hazards of science). N. Engl. J. Med. 296:324–328.

Waterhouse, J. A. H., P. Correa, C. S. Muir, and J. Powell, eds. 1976. Cancer Incidence in Five Continents. Volume III. IARC Scientific Publication No. 15. International Agency for Research on Cancer, Lyon, France.

Wattenberg, L. W. 1977. Inhibition of chemical carcinogenesis (Guest editorial). J. Natl. Cancer Inst. 60:11–18.

Weiner, M., and J. W. Newberne. 1977. Drug metabolites in the toxicologic evaluation of drug safety (Editorial). Toxicol. Appl. Pharmacol. 41:231–233.

Weisburger, J. H., L. A. Cohen, and E. L. Wynder. 1977. On the etiology and metabolic epidemiology of the main human cancers, *in* Origins of Human Cancer (Book A). Incidence of Cancer in Humans. H. H. Hiatt, J. D. Watson and J. A. Winsten, eds. Vol. 4. Cold Spring Harbor Laboratory, Cold Spring Harbor, New York, pp. 567–602.

Willis, R. A. 1947. Pathology of Tumours. Butterworth and Co. Ltd., London, England.

Wynder, E. L., F. R. Lemon, and I. J. Bross. 1959. Cancer and coronary artery disease among Seventh-Day Adventists. Cancer 12:1016–1028.

Wynder, E. L., and G. B. Gori. 1977. Contribution of the environment to cancer incidence: An epidemiologic exercise (Guest editorial). J. Natl. Cancer Inst. 58:825–832.

Yunis, J. Y., and M. E. Chandler. 1977. The chromosomes of man—Clinical and biologic significance (A review). Am. J. Pathol. 88:466–496.

Mechanisms of Carcinogenesis

Carcinogens: Identification and Mechanisms of Action, edited by A. Clark Griffin and Charles R. Shaw. Raven Press, New York © 1979.

Species and Tissue Variations in the Metabolic Activation of Aromatic Amines

Charles C. Irving

Veterans Administration Hospital and Department of Urology, University of Tennessee Center for the Health Sciences, Memphis, Tennessee 38104

It has been well over 100 years since aromatic amines were first discovered and introduced into industry (reviewed by Scott 1962). These compounds have been widely used in the chemical, textile, dyeing, rubber, pigment, and paper industries. Several aromatic amines, including 2-naphthylamine, 4-aminobiphenyl, and benzidine, are known to be carcinogenic for the human urinary bladder (IARC 1972, 1974). Others are highly suspect. Indeed, 9 of the 14 carcinogens for which Federal Standards have been promulgated by the Department of Labor are aromatic amines or amides or compounds that can be converted to aromatic amines (Federal Register 1973). The most active compound in this series is 2-acetylaminofluorene (AAF). AAF was patented for use as an insecticide, but its carcinogenicity was discovered before it was ever used as such (Wilson *et al.* 1941). In the late 1940's, an intensive effort to learn the biochemical mechanisms involved in the induction of cancer by this class of compounds was undertaken by a small group of investigators in several different laboratories: those of Drs. Elizabeth and James Miller at the University of Wisconsin, Drs. Elizabeth and John Weisburger at the National Cancer Institute, Dr. Helmut Gutmann at the University of Minnesota, and Drs. Eric Boyland and David Clayson in the United Kingdom. The American groups worked primarily with AAF, and the English groups concentrated mainly on 4-aminobiphenyl and 2-naphthylamine.

STRUCTURE-ACTIVITY RELATIONSHIPS

Aromatic amines have certain properties that confer strong carcinogenic activity and other properties that make them inactive. This subject has been covered in an excellent review by Arcos and Argus (1974). In general, monocyclic aromatic amines are inactive or at best very weak carcinogens. Aniline and its N-acetyl derivative (acetanilide) are noncarcinogenic (IARC 1974). Methyl substitution on the ring, such as in *o*-toluidine and 2,4,6-trimethylaniline, yields compounds with weak carcinogenic activity. Phenacetin is carcinogenic in the rat (Johansson and Angervall 1976), and chronic abuse of phenacetin or phenacetin-containing analgesics is associated with carcinoma of the renal pelvis and urinary bladder in man (Johansson *et al.* 1974, Rathert *et al.* 1975). The most active aromatic amine carcinogens are those that have two or three aromatic rings. These include benzidine, 2-naphthylamine, 4-aminobiphenyl, 2-aminofluorene, 2-aminophenanthrene, and 2-aminoanthracene. Compounds in which two benzenic nuclei are separated by an azo or ethylenic double bond, such as 4-aminostilbene and 4-aminoazobenzene, are also included. In each of these aromatic amines, the position of the amino substituent is critical for carcinogenic activity. The highest level of carcinogenic activity is obtained with di- and tricyclic aromatic amines when the amino substituent is located at the terminal carbon atom of the longest conjugated chain (Arcos and Argus 1974).

Even among the active di- and tricyclic aromatic amines, there are strong differences in species and tissue susceptibilities to cancer induction. These differences in species and tissue susceptibility appear to be accounted for by differences in the metabolism of the aromatic amines and in the reactivity of certain metabolites. The metabolism of aromatic amines is complex because of the large number of possible reactions these compounds can undergo (for reviews see Miller and Miller 1969, Irving 1970, Weisburger and Weisburger 1973, Kriek 1974). In general, it doesn't matter whether the free aromatic amine or its N-acetyl derivative is administered. Most species, with the exception of the dog, establish an equilibrium between the amine and the N-acetyl compound which favors acetylation. Most of the urinary metabolites of aromatic amines are N-acetylated. The major urinary metabolites are ring hydroxylated phenolic compounds, which are excreted primarily as sulfate or glucuronide conjugates. The relative amounts of these two types of conjugates depend on the species.

N-HYDROXYLATION

N-hydroxylation of carcinogenic aromatic amines and their N-acetyl derivatives, catalyzed by cytochrome P450-dependent monooxygenases, is the initial step in the activation of this class of carcinogens and is an absolute requirement for their carcinogenicity. Evidence for this was first obtained with AAF (Cramer *et al.* 1960), and the studies were later extended to include other aromatic amines (or their N-acetyl derivatives) (Miller and Miller 1969). However, it appears that the N-oxidation of N-methyl-4-aminoazobenzene, a more active derivative of 4-aminoazobenzene, is catalyzed by a mixed-function oxidase that does not require cytochrome P450 (Kadlubar *et al.* 1976b). The N-hydroxylation of AAF occurs in the livers of all mammals examined to date (Weisburger and Weisburger 1973), including the guinea pig (Gutmann and Bell 1977), a species earlier found to have no detectable activity (Irving 1964, Lotlikar *et al.* 1967).

Several drugs containing an arylamine or N-acetylarylamine group are N-hydroxylated also, and it seems likely that N-hydroxylation of such drug plays an important role in the toxicity of these compounds in humans. Thes drugs include 4,4'-diaminodiphenylsulfone (Dapsone) (Cucinell *et al.* 1972, Uehleke and Tabarelli 1973), phenacetin (Hinson and Mitchell 1976), and acetaminophen (paracetamol) (Calder *et al.* 1978, Nelson *et al.* 1978). Many other drugs containing nitrogen, such as pentobarbital (Tang *et al.* 1977) are N-hydroxylated or N-oxidized (Gorrod 1978).

It is now realized that N-hydroxylation is not a sufficient condition for the carcinogenicity of aromatic amines or their N-acetyl derivatives and that additional metabolism is required for activation of these N-hydroxy metabolites.

CONJUGATION REACTIONS

Conjugation reactions play an important role in the metabolic activation of N-arylhydroxylamines and N-acetyl-N-arylhydroxylamines, such as has been demonstrated for the induction of liver cancer in rats with AAF and N-hydroxy-AAF (DeBaun *et al.* 1970a,b). Attention was first directed to the reactivity of this type of conjugate by the discovery that synthetic esters, such as the benzoic and acetic acid esters of N-hydroxy-N-methylaminoazobenzene and N-hydroxy-AAF, were very reactive with proteins and nucleic acids in vitro (Lotlikar *et al.* 1966, Kriek *et al.* 1967). Following the discovery of the reactivity of these synthetic esters, a great deal of attention was focused on a search for similar metabolically formed esters or conjugates of the N-hydroxy metabolites of aromatic amines and amides.

Sulfate Conjugates

A number of N-acetyl-N-arylhydroxylamines have now been shown to be metabolized to their sulfuric acid esters (O-sulfonates or N-sulfates). This reaction is catalyzed by one or more sulfotransferases present in the soluble fraction of rat liver and requires adenosine-3'-phospho-5'-phosphosulfate (PAPS) (Figure 1). Formation of this type of conjugate was first demonstrated for N-hydroxy-AAF, and this reaction results in the formation of the highly reactive AAF-N-sulfate (DeBaun *et al.* 1970a). The enzyme, referred to as N-hydroxy-AAF sulfotransferase, has been purified 2,000-fold from livers of male Sprague-Dawley rats (Wu and Straub 1976). The final enzyme preparation was homogeneous on analytical disc gel electrophoresis. The purified enzyme also had appreciable

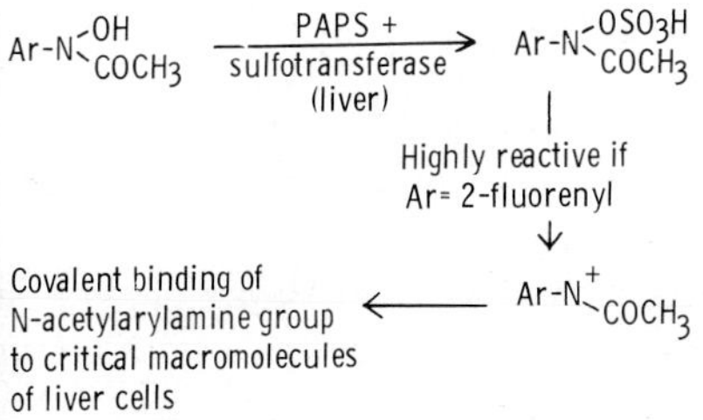

$$Ar-N\!\!<^{OH}_{COCH_3} \xrightarrow[\substack{\text{sulfotransferase}\\ \text{(liver)}}]{\text{PAPS +}} Ar-N\!\!<^{OSO_3H}_{COCH_3}$$

$$\Big|$$

Highly reactive if
Ar= 2-fluorenyl

$$\downarrow$$

Covalent binding of
N-acetylarylamine group $\longleftarrow$ $Ar-N\!\!<^{+}_{COCH_3}$
to critical macromolecules
of liver cells

FIG. 1. Formation of sulfate conjugates of N-acetyl-N-arylhydroxylamines. (Ar = aryl group)

activity towards p-nitrophenol, but it had almost no detectable activity towards various steroids, serotonin, and L-tyrosine methyl ester. Although these findings are consistent with earlier conclusions that N-hydroxy-AAF sulfotransferase and phenol sulfotransferase were possibly identical (DeBaun *et al.* 1970a), there are differences in the purified enzymes, which led Wu and Straub (1976) to conclude that the two sulfotransferases may not be identical.

Only small amounts of the N-hydroxy-AAF sulfotransferase are present in livers of female Sprague-Dawley rats (DeBaun *et al.* 1970a, Jackson and Irving 1972, Wu and Straub 1976). However, the presence of considerable N-hydroxy-AAF sulfotransferase activity in livers of female Fischer and female Wistar rats has been demonstrated (Irving 1975). In these experiments, the level of hepatic N-hydroxy-AAF sulfotransferase correlated well with the LD_{50} of an acute i.p. injection of N-hydroxy-AAF in both sexes of several strains of rats. N-hydroxy-AAF sulfotransferase activity was not detected in livers of the mouse, hamster, or guinea pig (DeBaun *et al.* 1970a), and enzyme activity is absent in all extrahepatic tissues examined (DeBaun *et al.* 1970a, Irving *et al.* 1971), including tissues quite susceptible to induction of cancer with N-hydroxy-AAF (Irving *et al.* 1971).

Hepatic N-hydroxy-AAF sulfotransferase activity has been assayed by measuring the PAPS-dependent production of o-methylmercapto-AAF (a mixture of the 1- and 3-isomers) from N-hydroxy-AAF in the presence of excess methionine added to trap the reactive AAF-N-sulfate (DeBaun *et al.* 1970a). The initial product, o-(methion-S-yl)AAF, is decomposed by heat to yield the o-methylmercapto-AAF. Using the methionine-trapping assay, N-hydroxy-4-acetylaminobiphenyl, N-hydroxy-4-acetylaminostilbene, and N-hydroxy-4-acetylaminoazobenzene were also shown to serve as substrates for the hepatic N-hydroxy-AAF sulfotransferase. Activity with N-hydroxy-2-acetylaminophenanthrene (N-hydroxy-AAP) as a substrate was very low, and activity with N-hydroxy-1-acetylaminonaphthalene (N-hydroxy-1-AAN) or N-hydroxy-2-acetylaminonaphthalene (N-hydroxy-2-AAN) was not detectable. It is obvious that the methionine-trapping assay cannot be used to demonstrate the enzymatic formation of weakly reactive or nonreactive O-sulfonate conjugates of N-acetyl-N-arylhydroxylamines. One alternative method for assaying sulfotransferase activity is to measure the PAPS-dependent conversion of carbon-14 or tritium-labeled substrates to water-soluble metabolites. This method is illustrated by the data in Table 1 in which N-hydroxy-[G-³H]AAP was used as a substrate for rat liver sulfotransferase. The relative sulfotransferase activity with several other substrates (1-hydroxy-AAF, estradiol, and dehydroepiandrosterone) are also shown in Table 1. Formation of the O-sulfonate conjugate of N-hydroxy-AAP was not detected in the methionine-trapping assay at 30 minutes incubation (Table 2).

Another method for the indirect measurement of the rate of enzymatic formation of O-sulfonate conjugates of these N-hydroxy metabolites in rat liver was recently published (Mulder *et al.* 1977). In this assay, 3′,5′-adenosine diphos-

TABLE 1. *Sulfotransferase activities in male rat liver*

Substrate*	Sulfotransferase activity† (nmoles conjugated/hr/mg protein)
N-hydroxy-[G-³H]AAP	30.9 ± 0.5
1-hydroxy-[1-¹⁴C]AAF	17.5 ± 1.1
Estradiol-17-β-6,7-³H	13.1 ± 0.6
Dehydroepiandrosterone-7-³H	1.5 ± 0.4

* The labeled N-hydroxy-AAP (Irving 1977) and 1-hydroxy-AAF (Irving and Williard 1962) were synthesized in the author's laboratory, and the labeled estradiol and dehydroepiandrosterone were obtained from New England Nuclear Corp.
† Reaction mixtures contained in a final volume of 1 ml: 100 μmoles Tris-HCl buffer, pH 7.4; 5 μmoles $MgCl_2$; 0.6 μmole PAPS; 0.4 μmole substrate; and 105,000 × g supernatant (1 mg protein) prepared from livers of male Sprague-Dawley rats. After 60 minutes at 37°C, the mixtures were extracted five times with 3 ml of toluene, and an aliquot of the remaining aqueous phase was counted. PAPS was omitted from control mixtures, and sulfotransferase activity was calculated from the PAPS-dependent formation of water-soluble metabolites. Values given represent mean ± S.E. for three to four rats.

phate and p-nitrophenyl sulfate were used as a PAPS-generating system. The release of p-nitrophenol, which was measured spectrophotometrically, was used to estimate sulfotransferase activity. N-hydroxy-AAF, N-hydroxyphenacetin, N-hydroxyacetanilide, N-hydroxy-p-chloroacetanilide, and N-hydroxy-2-AAN served as substrates for the sulfotransferase. It is also interesting to note that sulfotransferase activity for N-hydroxy-2-AAN was picked up in this assay but was not detectable in rat liver with the methionine-trapping assay (DeBaun *et al.* 1970a).

The lack of activity of N-hydroxy-1-AAN and N-hydroxy-2-AAN and the extremely low activity of N-hydroxy-AAP in the methionine-trapping assay probably indicates that the O-sulfonate conjugates of these N-hydroxy compounds are not very reactive with methionine. Since one might argue that these particular conjugates quickly rearrange to nonreactive phenolic O-sulfonates (see Irving 1970), this question can only be resolved by synthesis of the O-sul-

TABLE 2. *Comparison of the reaction of methionine with enzymatically generated O-sulfonate conjugates of N-hydroxy-AAF and N-hydroxy-AAP*

Substrate	o-Methylmercapto derivative formed* (nmoles/30 min./mg protein)
N-Hydroxy-AAF	72.2
N-Hydroxy-AAP	0

* The assay was carried out using 105,000 × g supernatant prepared from livers of male Sprague-Dawley rats as previously described (DeBaun *et al.* 1970a, Irving *et al.* 1971). The values given were corrected for controls in which PAPS was omitted from the reaction mixture.

fonate conjugates of these N-hydroxy compounds and by study of their stability in aqueous solution.

The O-sulfonate conjugate of N-hydroxy-AAF (AAF-N-sulfate) is very reactive with proteins and with nucleic acids (Miller and Miller 1969, DeBaun *et al.* 1970a,b) and is a strong mutagen (Maher *et al.* 1970). Current evidence shows that the hepatotoxicity and the hepatocarcinogenicity of N-hydroxy-AAF are markedly dependent on the levels of N-hydroxy-AAF sulfotransferase activity in liver (DeBaun *et al.* 1970a,b, Irving 1975, Jackson and Irving 1972, Weisburger *et al.* 1972). N-hydroxy arylamine sulfotransferase also appears to be involved in the activation of N-hydroxy-N-methyl-4-aminoazobenzene (Kadlubar *et al.* 1976a). O-sulfonate conjugates may be responsible for the biological activity of other N-hydroxy compounds. For example, it has recently been demonstrated that the enzymatically formed O-sulfonate conjugate of N-hydroxyphenacetin binds covalently to proteins (Mulder *et al.* 1977). Since phenacetin is known to be N-hydroxylated by liver microsomes (Hinson and Mitchell 1976), it is possible that these coupled reactions (N-hydroxylation and sulfate conjugation) might play some role in causing the toxic effects of high doses of phenacetin in vivo. O-sulfonate conjugates do not appear to be involved in the further activation of N-hydroxy metabolites of aromatic amines and amides in nonhepatic tissues of the rat (DeBaun *et al.* 1970a, Irving *et al.* 1971), and so we must look for other mechanisms of activation of N-hydroxylated aromatic amines and amides in other tissues.

Glucuronide Conjugates

O-Glucuronide Conjugates of N-Acetyl-N-Arylhydroxylamines

The O-glucuronide of N-hydroxy-AAF (N-GlO-AAF) is the most reactive compound of this type, but this glucuronide has a much lower rate of reaction with nucleic acids or proteins than does N-acetoxy-AAF or AAF-N-sulfate (Irving 1970, 1971). However, the reactivity of these glucuronides is enhanced markedly at slightly alkaline pH. The enhanced reactivity appears to be due to the generation of the O-glucuronide of the N-arylhydroxylamine under slightly alkaline conditions. The reaction products are characterized by loss of the acetyl group of the reacting glucuronide. The aryl group has a strong effect on the rate of reaction of this type of glucuronide with nucleophiles (Irving 1977). A comparison of the rates of reaction of N-GlO-AAF with the glucuronides of N-hydroxy-4-acetylaminostilbene (N-GlO-AAS), N-hydroxy-4-acetylaminobiphenyl (N-GlO-AABP), and N-hydroxy-2-acetylaminophenanthrene (N-GlO-AAP) with tRNA, rRNA, DNA, polyA, polyG, polyU, and polyC has been made (Table 3). The relative order of reactivity of these glucuronides with nucleic acids was N-GlO-AAF > N-GlO-AAS > N-GlO-AABP > N-GlO-AAP. N-GlO-AAP showed only marginal or negligible reactivity. N-GlO-AAF showed greater reactivity with polyG than with polyA, but the reverse was

TABLE 3. *Effect of the aryl group on the reactivity of glucuronide conjugates of various N-acetyl-N-arylhydroxylamines with nucleic acids and homopolynucleotides**

Ar-N-COCH$_3$	Covalent binding to polynucleotide						
|	(mmoles aryl group/mole polynucleotide P)						
O-glucuronide							
Ar- group =	tRNA	rRNA	DNA	polyA	polyG	polyU	polyC
2-fluorenyl	14.9	11.6	8.8	3.0	18.7	1.0	0.2
4-stilbenyl	2.6	2.8	0.9	34.2	4.1	0.8	0.6
4-biphenylyl	0.3	0.2	0.1	0.5	0.2	nd†	nd
2-phenanthryl	nd	0.1	0.1	nd	0.1	nd	nd

* The incubation mixtures contained in a final volume of 0.5 ml: polynucleotide P, 1 μmole; glucuronide conjugate, 1 μmole; dextran sulfate, 50 μg; NaCl, 0.5 mmole; Tris-HCl buffer, pH 7.7 (at 38°C), 0.02 mmole. After incubation at 38°C for 24 hours, the nucleic acids and homopolynucleotides were precipitated by addition of 3 volumes of cold ethanol and purified as described previously (Irving 1977).
† nd = not detectable (less than 0.1)

true for N-GlO-AAS; both of these glucuronides had much lower reactions with polyU and polyC. Except for the low reaction of N-GlO-AABP with polyA, there was no detectable reaction of this glucuronide or of N-GlO-AAP with the homopolynucleotides. The relative rates of the reactions of this series of glucuronides with nucleic acids parallel the hepatocarcinogenicity of their N-hydroxy compounds. The O-glucuronides are major excretory forms of the parent N-acetyl-N-arylhydroxylamines. For example, as much as 30% of a single oral dose of AAF was excreted in 24 hours in the urine of rabbits as the glucuronide of N-hydroxy-AAF (Irving 1962). It is interesting to note that the epithelial lining of the urinary tract of the rabbit is one tissue of this species known to be susceptible to carcinogenesis by AAF or N-hydroxy-AAF (Irving *et al.* 1967). Since the rabbit excretes a fairly alkaline urine (average pH 8.5, but frequently running as high as pH 8.9–9.0), it is tempting to speculate that the increased reactivity of the glucuronide of N-hydroxy-AAF at pH 8.5–9.0 plays an important role in the susceptibility of the epithelium of the urinary tract of the rabbit to AAF. A mechanism by which this might occur is shown in Figure 2.

The glucuronide of N-hydroxy-AAF, when administered by s.c. injection, also induces a low incidence of tumors at the site of injection and in mammary gland, liver, and ear duct sebaceous gland (Irving and Wiseman 1971).

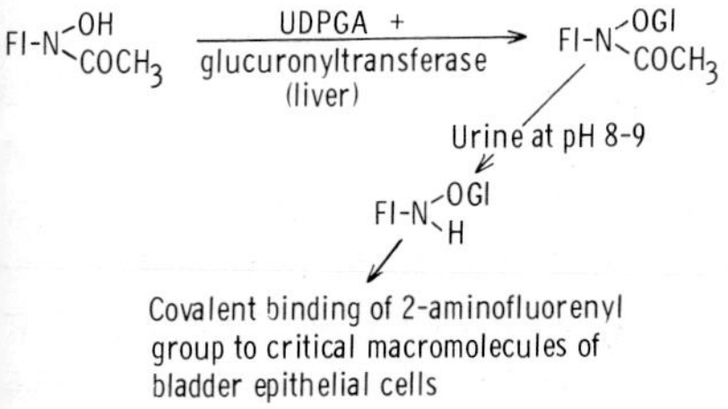

FIG. 2. Possible metabolic pathway involved in the induction of bladder cancer in the rabbit by N-hydroxy-AAF. (Fl = 2-fluorenyl; Gl = glucuronyl)

Little information is available on the reactivity of O-glucuronides of other N-acetyl-N-arylhydroxylamines. In a recent report it was found that the O-glucuronide of N-hydroxyphenacetin, formed in an in vitro system, lead to covalent binding to protein in the system, and it was suggested that covalent binding might play some role in the toxicity of high doses of phenacetin, especially in the kidney and bladder (Mulder *et al.* 1977).

O-Glucuronide Conjugates of N-Arylhydroxylamines

Two O-glucuronides of N-arylhydroxylamines have been reported in the literature. The O-glucuronide of N-2-fluorenylhydroxylamine (N-GlO-AF) was prepared by the deacetylation of the O-glucuronide of N-hydroxy-AAF (Irving and Russell 1970). Synthesis of the O-glucuronide of N-4-biphenylylhydroxylamine by a similar method has been claimed, but the authors have not reported any data on the characterization of the compound by analytical or spectroscopic methods (Radomski *et al.* 1977). N-GlO-AF is unstable in aqueous solution and reacts at neutral pH with nucleic acids, with methionine, and with tryptophan. The glucuronide reacts with guanosine-5'-monophosphate to give 8-(N-2-fluorenylamino)-guanosine 5'-monophosphate but does not react with the 5'-monophosphates of uridine, cytidine, or adenosine. When assayed using the *Bacillus subtilis* transformation system, the mutagenic activity of N-GlO-AF equaled or surpassed that reported for N-acetoxy-AAF and AAF-N-sulfate (Maher and Reuter 1973). It was proposed that N-GlO-AF might be formed as a metabolite of N-hydroxy-AAF via the O-glucuronide of N-hydroxy-AAF and might account for the observed binding of N-hydroxy-AAF to rat liver DNA in vivo (Irving 1970, 1971). Cardona and King (1976) recently showed that the O-glucuronide of N-hydroxy-AAF could be activated by deacetylation in guinea pig liver to give N-GlO-AF. The deacetylation of the glucuronide of N-hydroxy-AAF could be involved in the activation of this compound in extrahepatic tissues, including the bladder (see previous section and Figure 2).

N-Glucuronide Conjugates of N-Arylhydroxylamines

Kadlubar *et al.* (1977) reported that several N-arylhydroxylamines can be converted to their N-glucuronides by microsomes prepared from livers of dogs, rats, and humans. These N-glucuronides were relatively stable and nonreactive at neutral pH. At pH 5, however, the N-glucuronides of N-1-naphthylhydroxylamine, N-2-naphthylhydroxylamine, and N-4-biphenylylhydroxylamine were rapidly hydrolyzed to the corresponding free arylhydroxylamines that were then converted to reactive derivatives capable of covalent binding to nucleic acids (Figure 3). This mechanism is quite distinct from the mechanism of reaction of the O-glucuronide of N-2-fluorenylhydroxylamine (see Figure 2), which is highly reactive per se at neutral pH and for which reactivity does not proceed

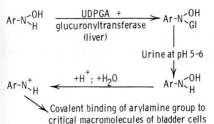

FIG. 3. Possible metabolic pathway involved in the induction of bladder cancer in the dog and man by the arylhydroxylamine metabolites derived from arylamines. (Ar = aryl group; Gl = glucuronyl)

through the intermediate formation of the free N-2-fluorenylhydroxylamine (Irving and Russell 1970).

There is evidence that this type of N-glucuronide is formed in vivo in the dog (Radomski *et al.* 1977), but its formation in vivo in other species has not yet been demonstrated. The N-glucuronide of N-4-biphenylylhydroxylamine was isolated from urine of dogs given 4-aminobiphenyl, and the conjugate was reported to be mutagenic at pH 5.5 or 6.8 in strains TA1538 and TA98 of *Salmonella typhimurium* (Radomski *et al.* 1977). It has been proposed that N-glucuronides of this type serve as stable transport forms for carcinogenic aromatic amines. Kadlubar *et al.* (1977) suggested that hydrolysis of these N-glucuronides and conversion of the resulting free arylhydroxylamines to reactive electrophilic arylnitrenium ions occurs in the normally acidic urine of dogs and humans and that these reactions may be critical for the induction of bladder cancer with aromatic amines in these species.

OTHER REACTIONS

Acetylation and Deacetylation

Acetylation of Arylamines

Some years ago it was postulated that N-arylhydroxylamines were somehow involved in the induction of cancer of the urinary bladder, whereas in liver, the N-acetyl-N-arylhydroxylamine was required for carcinogenesis (Poirier *et al.* 1963). This postulate was based on the observation that the dog, unlike other species (see Lower and Bryan 1973), was not able to acetylate aromatic amines but was quite susceptible to the induction of bladder cancer by these compounds. This idea was strengthened by further studies carried out in a dog by Radomski and Brill (1970, 1971).

The role that acetylation of aromatic amines may play in the determination of species and tissue susceptibility has recently become clearer with the studies of Lower and Bryan (1976), Radomski *et al.* (1977), and Kadlubar *et al.* (1977). The type of urinary metabolite that appears to be involved in the induction of bladder cancer in the dog by aromatic amines is the N-glucuronide of the N-arylhydroxylamine (see previous section on N-glucuronides). Using 2-amino-

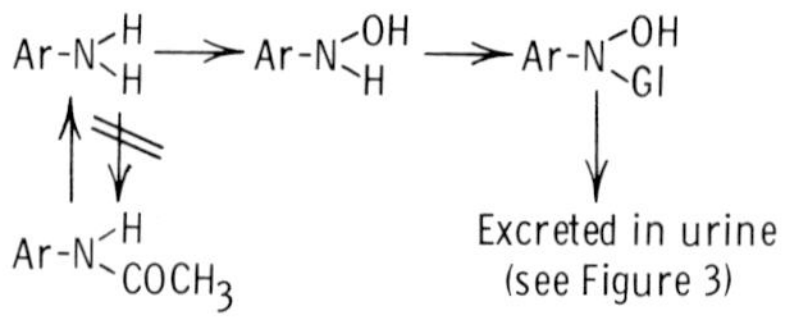

$$Ar\text{-}N{<}^H_H \longrightarrow Ar\text{-}N{<}^{OH}_H \longrightarrow Ar\text{-}N{<}^{OH}_{Gl}$$

$$Ar\text{-}N{<}^H_{COCH_3}$$

Excreted in urine
(see Figure 3)

FIG. 4. Possible role of lack of N-acetylation (dog) or slow rate of N-acetylation (man) of arylamines in the induction of bladder cancer. Metabolism of the arylamine is shifted toward formation of the N-glucuronide of the aryl-hydroxylamine. (Ar = aryl group; Gl = glucuronyl)

fluorene (AF) as an example, tissue specificity would be conferred in this case by (1) the inability of the dog to acetylate AF, (2) N-hydroxylation of AF, followed by the formation of the N-glucuronide conjugate which is stable at neutral pH, (3) excretion of the N-glucuronide in the urine, and (4) the hydrolysis of the N-glucuronide to N-2-fluorenylhydroxylamine and its conversion to the reactive arylnitrenium ion in the acidic urine of dogs.

This sequence of events may also be involved in the induction of bladder cancer in man by aromatic amines. Carcinogenic aromatic amines are N-acety-lated at variable rates by human hepatic enzymes. The known genetic regulation and polymorphic distribution of this hepatic enzyme system in humans and the known enhanced susceptibility of patients with the genetically distinct "slow acetylator" phenotype to various aromatic amine toxicities has suggested a possi-ble correlation between acetylator phenotype and urinary bladder cancer induc-tion (Lower 1978). Acetylator phenotyping of bladder cancer patients having received exposures to known carcinogenic aromatic amines is being carried out by Lower (1978). Lower's studies in the human combined with the findings of Kadlubar et al. (1977) would suggest that the conditions most favorable for the induction of bladder cancer in humans exposed to aromatic amines would be for an individual to be a slow acetylator and to excrete an acidic urine (Figure 4). The complexity of the factors involved in determining species and tissue specificity for the induction of cancer by aromatic amines can be illustrated by comparing the postulated sequence of events for induction of bladder cancer in the rabbit, dog, and man with that for the induction of liver cancer in rats as shown in Figure 5.

Now, let us consider some mechanisms that might be involved in the activation of aromatic amines in other susceptible tissues.

Deacetylation of N-Acetyl-N-Arylhydroxylamines

N-hydroxy-AAF is readily deacetylated (Figure 5, reaction 11) by enzymes present in the microsomal fractions of livers from rats, rabbits, hamsters, and guinea pigs to yield N-hydroxy-2-aminofluorene (N-hydroxy-AF) (Irving 1966, unpublished observations). The rates of deacetylation found (μmoles per hour per mg of protein) were rat 0.05, rabbit 0.21, hamster 1.58, and guinea pig 3.48. Some of these results were confirmed by Jarvinen et al. (1971), who also reported N-hydroxy-AAF deacetylase activity in brain and kidney of guinea

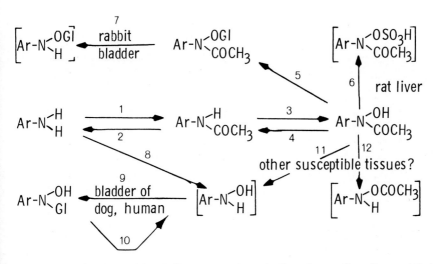

FIG. 5. Summary of multiple metabolic pathways for activation of aromatic amines and their N-acetyl derivatives in susceptible tissues of several species. (Ar = aryl group; GI = glucuronyl)

pigs. Other N-acetyl-N-arylhydroxylamines are also deacetylated (Booth and Boyland 1964).

Durston and Ames (1974) have shown that N-hydroxy-AF and 2-nitrosofluor-ene, an oxidation product of N-hydroxy-AF, are strong mutagens in *S. typhimurium* TA1538. More recently, Stout *et al.* (1976) showed that a mutagen was produced from N-hydroxy-AAF by an enzyme from the soluble fraction of rat liver, and they identified the mutagenic agent as N-hydroxy-AF. Since earlier studies with the guinea pig led to the conclusion that there was no N-hydroxy-AAF deacetylase activity in liver soluble fraction (Irving 1966), these studies have been repeated using a more sensitive procedure for determination of deacetylase activity. With the more sensitive procedure, a considerable fraction (22%) of the total homogenate deacetylase activity in the rat was found to be present in the soluble fraction (Table 4), while only 3% of the deacetylase

TABLE 4. *Deacetylation of N-hydroxy-AAF by fractions of rat and guinea pig liver homogenates*

Liver cell fraction	Rat		Guinea pig	
	Activity*	%	Activity	%
Whole homogenate	3.10	100	154.0	100
Nuclei	0.30	9	8.8	5
Mitochondria	0.16	5	5.2	3
Microsomes	2.19	64	146.0	89
Soluble fraction	0.76	22	4.8	3

* Deacetylation of N-hydroxy-AAF was determined by the radiochemical procedure described earlier (Irving 1966), and enzyme activity is expressed as μmoles of N-hydroxy-AAF deacety-lated per hour by the fraction obtained from 1 g of liver.

TABLE 5. Deacetylation of N-hydroxy-AAF by rat tissues

Tissue	Deacetylase activity* (μmoles/hr/gm)	
	male	female
Zymbal's gland	6.04 ± 0.28	7.27 ± 0.30
Liver	2.41 ± 0.17	3.21 ± 0.10
Adrenal	0.57 ± 0.02	—
Kidney	0.49 ± 0.05	—
Brain	0.31 ± 0.02	—
Small intestine	0.27 ± 0.02	—
Lung	0.21 ± 0.02	—
Spleen	0.18 ± 0.01	—
Testes	0.13 ± 0.01	—
Muscle	0.12 ± 0.02	—
Mammary gland		
whole gland	0.04 ± 0.002	0.05 ± 0.003
parenchymal tissue	0.08 ± 0.002	0.10 ± 0.009

* Deacetylase activity was determined in whole homogenates as described in Table 4.

activity was found in the soluble fraction from guinea pig liver. Recentrifugation of the soluble fraction for two hours at 105,000 x g did not change the results shown in Table 4 for the soluble fraction. Because of the much higher deacetylase activity in guinea pig liver, the absolute N-hydroxy-AAF deacetylase activity in the soluble fraction from guinea pig liver was much greater than that found in the soluble fraction from rat liver (Table 4). These data demonstrate quite clearly that there is no relationship between the ability of the liver to activate N-hydroxy-AAF in vivo and the capability of liver cell fractions to form mutagenic products in vitro.

Although there is certainly no relationship between deacetylation of N-hydroxy-AAF in the liver and susceptibility of various species to liver cancer induction with N-hydroxy-AAF, this reaction might be important as a mechanism of activation of N-acetyl-N-arylhydroxylamines in extrahepatic tissues. The ability of a number of tissues of the rat to deacetylate N-hydroxy-AAF has been examined (Table 5). It is interesting to note that the highest deacetylase activity was found in the sebaceous gland of the ear duct (Zymbal's gland), a tissue of the rat that is highly susceptible to carcinogenesis by AAF, N-hydroxy-AAF, and a number of other aromatic amines or amides. On the other hand, deacetylase activity was barely detectable in the mammary gland of female rats, a tissue that is also highly susceptible to cancer induction with these compounds.

Mammary gland tissue from 50 to 60-day-old Sprague-Dawley rats was used for the experiments reported in Table 5. Deacetylase activity in parenchymal cells isolated from whole mammary glands of female Sprague-Dawley rats (Irving *et al.* 1971) was also very low.

N-Acyltransferase

Another enzymatic reaction that may be of importance involves transfer of the N-acetyl group from an N-acetyl-N-arylhydroxylamine to the oxygen (N-O acyltransferase) to form the O-acetyl derivative of the N-arylhydroxylamine (see Figure 5, reaction 12). Rat liver N-O acyltransferase can also utilize other N-acylated derivatives of N-2-fluorenylhydroxylamine as substrates (King *et al.* 1978). N-O acyltransferase as a mechanism of activation of N-hydroxy metabolites of aromatic amides was first reported by Bartsch *et al.* (1972, 1973), and the reaction has been studied extensively by King (King 1974, King and Olive 1975, King *et al.* 1976). The O-acyl derivatives of N-arylhydroxylamines are too reactive to be isolated, but their formation can be detected by trapping them with various nucleophiles, such as N-acetyl-methionine and guanosine or tRNA. The enzyme is found in the 105,000 x g supernatant of cell homogenates and has been purified 1,000-fold from livers of Sprague-Dawley rats (Alleban and King 1977, Weeks *et al.* 1978). N-O acyltransferase activity is present in other tissues, such as stomach, small intestine, colon, and kidney. Enzyme activity is also present in mammary gland from pregnant rats, but it has not been studied in the immature mammary gland of female rats, which is the susceptible gland. Bartsch *et al.* (1973) were not able to detect enzyme activity in the ear duct sebaceous gland (Zymbal's gland) under a variety of conditions using the N-acetylmethionine trapping assay. However, King (personal communication) has been able to detect acyltransferase activity in this tissue using tRNA to trap the reactive electrophile generated from N-hydroxy-AAF.

The enzymatic formation of the O-acetyl derivatives of N-2-fluorenylhydroxylamine and N-4-biphenylylhydroxylamine from N-hydroxy-AAF and N-hydroxy-4-acetylaminobiphenyl, respectively, may account for a significant amount of the covalent binding of these carcinogens to DNA in vivo, since it has been observed that most of the residues bound in vivo are the aminoaryl moieties (acetyl group lost) (Irving 1970, Irving and Veazey 1971, Irving *et al.* 1972). The relationship between acyltransferase-induced nucleic acid adduct formation and mutagenic potential of N-hydroxy-AAF in an *S. typhimurium* (TA1538) system has been studied (Weeks *et al.* 1978). These authors found that *S. typhimurium* did not detect the reactive electrophile generated from N-hydroxy-AAF by the partially purified acyltransferase (presumably N-acetoxy-AF) and speculated that the mutagen produced in the system might be N-hydroxy-AF. Weeks *et al.* (1978) also showed that there was not a good correlation between the ability of AF derivatives to bind covalently to nucleic acids and their mutagenic potential in the *S. typhimurium* system, raising the possibility that mutagenic events detected in *S. typhimurium* with aromatic amines and mammalian activation systems do not measure the production of the reactive electrophiles thought to be involved in the induction of cancer by aromatic amines. McGregor (1975) also found a much closer correlation between the ability of AAF and N-hydroxy-AAF to induce liver cancer and its covalent binding to nucleic acids than between hepatocarcinogenicity and liver-mediated mutagenicity in *S. typhimurium* TA1538.

SUMMARY

Today we are confronted with a variety of chemicals that have been shown to produce cancer in man or which serve as excellent models for the study of mechanisms of carcinogenesis in experimental animals. It has taken over 30 years for us to reach our present state of knowledge of the metabolism and mechanisms of metabolic activation of one such class of carcinogens, the aromatic amines. Yet we do not fully understand the biochemical mechanisms involved in the activation of this class of compounds. Several important findings and general concepts have emerged, however. (1) The aromatic amines and their N-acetyl derivatives are activated in vivo by multiple pathways. Differences in these metabolic pathways largely account for the differences in tissue and species susceptibilities to cancer induction. It is likely that multiple pathways for the activation of other classes of carcinogens, e.g., the polycyclic aromatic hydrocarbons and the dialkylnitrosamines, also exist. (2) At least with AAF and its metabolites, there does not appear to be a relationship between the ability of the liver to activate metabolites in vivo and the capability of liver cell fractions to form mutagenic products in vitro. (3) The term metabolic activation should not be equated with carcinogenicity. Although metabolic activation represents an essential facet of the initiation of cancer by most chemicals, it is by no means a sufficient condition for the induction of cancer by these compounds. The rodent liver, for example, has a tremendous capacity to activate a large number of chemicals, but only a few of these will actually induce liver cancer in the normal adult rodent. Additional factors involved in the carcinogenic process have been reviewed by Miller and Miller (1977) and by Solt et al. (1977).

ACKNOWLEDGMENTS

The generous support of my work by the U. S. Veterans Administration is gratefully acknowledged. This work has also been supported in part by the National Cancer Institute Research Grant CA-05490.

REFERENCES

Allaben, W. T., and C. M. King. 1977. Purification and characterization of arylhydroxamic acid acyltransferase. (Abstract) Fed. Proc. 36:349.
Arcos, J. C., and M. F. Argus. 1974. Chemical Induction of Cancer. Structural Bases and Biological Mechanisms, Vol. IIB. Academic Press, New York.
Bartsch, H., M. Dworkin, J. A. Miller, and E. C. Miller. 1972. Electrophilic N-acetoxyaminoarenes derived from carcinogenic N-hydroxy-N-acetylaminoarenes by enzymatic deacetylation and trans-acetylation in liver. Biochim. Biophys. Acta 286:272–298.
Bartsch, H., C. Dworkin, E. C. Miller, and J. A. Miller. 1973. Formation of electrophilic

N-acetoxyarylamines in cytosols from rat mammary gland and other tissues by transacetylation from the carcinogen N-hydroxy-4-acetyl-aminobiphenyl. Biochim. Biophys. Acta 304:42–55.

Booth, J., and E. Boyland. 1964. The biochemistry of aromatic amines. 10. Enzymic N-hydroxylation of arylamines and conversion of arylhydroxylamines into o-aminophenols. Biochem. J. 91:362–369.

Calder, I. C., K. Healey, A. C. Yong, C. A. Crowe, K. N. Ham, and J. D. Tange. 1978. N-hydroxyparacetamol: Its role in the metabolism of paracetamol, *in* Biological Oxidation of Nitrogen, J. W. Gorrod, ed., Elsevier, Amsterdam, pp. 309–318.

Cardona, R. A., and C. M. King. 1976. Activation of the O-glucuronide of the carcinogen N-hydroxy-N-2-fluorenylacetamide by enzymatic deacetylation in vitro: Formation of fluorenylamine-tRNA adducts. Biochem. Pharmacol. 25:1051–1056.

Cramer, J. W., J. A. Miller, and E. C. Miller. 1960. N-hydroxylation: A new metabolic reaction observed in the rat with the carcinogen 2-acetylaminofluorene. J. Biol. Chem. 235:885–888.

Cucinell, S. A., Z. H. Israeli, and P. G. Dayton. 1972. Microsomal N-oxidation of Dapsone as a cause of methemoglobin formation in human red cells. Am. J. Trop. Med. Hyg. 21:322–331.

DeBaun, J. R., E. C. Miller, and J. A. Miller. 1970a. N-hydroxy-2-acetylaminofluorene sulfotransferase: Its probable role in carcinogenesis and in protein(methion-S-yl)-binding in rat liver. Cancer Res. 30:577–595.

DeBaun, J. R., J. Y. R. Smith, E. C. Miller, and J. A. Miller. 1970b. Reactivity in vivo of the carcinogen N-hydroxy-2-acetylaminofluorene: Increase by sulfate ion. Science 167:184–186.

Durston, W. E., and B. N. Ames. 1974. A simple method for the detection of mutagens in urine: Studies with the carcinogen 2-acetylaminofluorene. Proc. Natl. Acad. Sci. USA 71:737–741.

Federal Register. 1973. Vol. 38, No. 144.

Gorrod, J. W., ed. 1978. Biological Oxidation of Nitrogen. Elsevier, Amsterdam.

Gutmann, H. R., and P. Bell. 1977. N-hydroxylation of arylamides by the rat and guinea pig. Evidence for substrate specificity and participation of cytochrome P_1-450. Biochim. Biophys. Acta 498:229–243.

Hinson, J. A., and J. R. Mitchell. 1976. N-hydroxylation of phenacetin by hamster liver microsomes. Drug Metab. Disposition 4:430–435.

IARC. 1972. Monographs on the Evaluation of Carcinogenic Risk of Chemicals to Man. Vol. 1. International Agency for Research on Cancer, Lyon.

IARC. 1974. Monographs on the Evaluation of Carcinogenic Risk of Chemicals to Man. Vol. 4. International Agency for Research on Cancer, Lyon.

Irving, C. C. 1962. N-hydroxylation of 2-acetylaminofluorene in the rabbit. Cancer Res. 22:867–873.

Irving, C. C. 1964. Enzymatic N-hydroxylation of the carcinogen 2-acetylaminofluorene and the metabolism of N-hydroxy-2-acetylaminofluorene-9-C^{14} in vitro. J. Biol. Chem. 239:1589–1596.

Irving, C. C. 1966. Enzymatic deacetylation of N-hydroxy-2-acetylaminofluorene by liver microsomes. Cancer Res. 26:1390–1396.

Irving, C. C. 1970. Conjugates of N-hydroxy compounds, *in* Metabolic Conjugation and Metabolic Hydrolysis, W. H. Fishman, ed., Academic Press, New York, pp. 53–119.

Irving, C. C. 1971. Metabolic activation of N-hydroxy compounds by conjugation. Xenobiotica 1:387–398.

Irving, C. C. 1975. Comparative toxicity of N-hydroxy-2-acetylaminofluorene in several strains of rats. Cancer Res. 35:2959–2961.

Irving, C. C. 1977. Influence of the aryl group on the reaction of glucuronides of N-arylacethydroxamic acids with polynucleotides. Cancer Res. 37:524–528.

Irving, C. C., D. H. Janss, and L. T. Russell. 1971. Lack of N-hydroxy-2-acetylaminofluorene sulfotransferase activity in the mammary gland and Zymbal's gland of the rat. Cancer Res. 31:1468–1472.

Irving, C. C., and L. T. Russell. 1970. Synthesis of the O-glucuronide of N-2-fluorenylhydroxylamine. Reaction with nucleic acids and with guanosine-5′-monophosphate. Biochemistry 9:2471–2476.

Irving, C. C., L. T. Russell, and E. Kriek. 1972. Biosynthesis and reactivity of the glucuronide of N-hydroxy-4-acetylaminobiphenyl. Chem.-Biol. Interact. 5:37–46.

Irving, C. C., and R. A. Veazey. 1971. Differences in the binding of 2-acetylaminofluorene and its N-hydroxy metabolite to liver nucleic acids of male and female rats. Cancer Res. 31:19–22.

Irving, C. C., and R. F. Williard. 1962. Synthesis of N-(1-hydroxy-2-fluorenyl-l-C^{14})acetamide with a high specific activity. J. Org. Chem. 27:2260–2261.

Irving, C. C., and R. Wiseman, Jr. 1971. Studies on the carcinogenicity of the glucuronides of

N-hydroxy-2-acetylaminofluorene and N-2-fluorenylhydroxylamine in the rat. Cancer Res. 31:1645–1648.

Irving, C. C., R. Wiseman, Jr., and J. M. Young. 1967. Carcinogenicity of 2-acetylaminofluorene in the rabbit. Cancer Res. 27:838–848.

Jackson, C. D., and C. C. Irving. 1972. Sex differences in cell proliferation and N-hydroxy-2-acetylaminofluorene sulfotransferase levels in rat liver during 2-acetylaminofluorene administration. Cancer Res. 32:1590–1594.

Jarvinen, M., R. S. S. Santti, and V. K. Hopsu-Havu. 1971. Partial purification and characterization of two enzymes from guinea pig liver microsomes that hydrolyze carcinogenic amides 2-acetylaminofluorene and N-hydroxy-2-acetylaminofluorene. Biochem. Pharmacol. 20:2971–2982.

Johansson, S., and L. Angervall. 1976. Urothelial hyperplasia of the renal papillae in female Sprague-Dawley rats induced by long term feeding of phenacetin. Acta Pathol. Microbiol. Scand. 84:353–354.

Johansson, S., L. Angervall, U. Bengtsson, and L. Wahlquist. 1974. Uroepithelial tumors of the renal pelvis associated with phenacetin-containing analgesics. Cancer 33:743–753.

Kadlubar, F. F., J. A. Miller, and E. C. Miller. 1976a. Hepatic metabolism of N-hydroxy-N-methyl-4-aminobenzene and other N-hydroxy arylamines to reactive sulfuric acid esters. Cancer Res. 36:2350–2359.

Kadlubar, F. F., J. A. Miller, and E. C. Miller. 1976b. Microsomal N-oxidation of the hepatocarcinogen N-methyl-4-aminoazobenzene and the reactivity of N-hydroxy-N-methyl-4-aminoazobenzene. Cancer Res. 36:1196–1206.

Kadlubar, F. F., J. A. Miller, and E. C. Miller. 1977. Hepatic microsomal N-glucuronidation and nucleic acid binding of N-hydroxy arylamines in relation to urinary bladder carcinogenesis. Cancer Res. 37:805–814.

King, C. M. 1974. Mechanism of reaction, tissue distribution, and inhibition of arylhydroxamic acid acyltransferase. Cancer Res. 34:1503–1515.

King, C. M., W. T. Allaben, E. J. Lazear, S. C. Louie, and C. E. Weeks. 1978. Influence of the acyl group on aryl-hydroxamic acid N-O acyltransferase-catalyzed mutagenicity and metabolic activation of N-acyl-N-2-fluorenylhydroxylamines, *in* Biological Oxidation of Nitrogen, J. W. Gorrod, ed., Elsevier, Amsterdam, pp. 335–340.

King, C. M., and C. W. Olive. 1975. Comparative effects of strain, species, and sex on the acyltransferase-catalyzed activations of N-hydroxy-N-2-fluorenylacetamide. Cancer Res. 35:906–912.

King, C. M., N. R. Traub, R. A. Cardona, and R. B. Howard. 1976. Comparative adduct formation of 4-aminobiphenyl and 2-aminofluorene derivatives with macromolecules of isolated liver parenchymal cells. Cancer Res. 36:2374–2381.

Kriek, E. 1974. Carcinogenesis by aromatic amines. Biochim. Biophys. Acta 355:177–203.

Kriek, E., J. A. Miller, U. Juhl, and E. C. Miller. 1967. 8-(N-2-fluorenylacetamido)guanosine, an arylamidation reaction product of guanosine and the carcinogen N-acetoxy-N-2-fluorenylacetamide in neutral solution. Biochemistry 6:177–182.

Lotlikar, P. D., M. Enomoto, J. A. Miller, and E. C. Miller. 1967. Species variations in the N- and ring-hydroxylation of 2-acetylaminofluorene and effects of 3-methylcholanthrene pretreatment. Proc. Soc. Exp. Biol. Med. 125:341–346.

Lotlikar, P. D., J. D. Scribner, J. A. Miller, and E. C. Miller. 1966. Reaction of esters of aromatic N-hydroxy amines and amides with methionine in vitro: A model for in vivo binding of amine carcinogens to protein. Life Sci. 5:1263–1269.

Lower, G. M., Jr. 1978. Metabolic factors involved in bladder carcinogenesis. (Abstract) National Bladder Cancer Project Investigators' Workshop, Sarasota, Florida, p. 14.

Lower, G. M., Jr., and G. T. Bryan. 1973. Enzymatic N-acetylation of carcinogenic aromatic amines by liver cytosol of species displaying different organ susceptibility. Biochem. Pharmacol. 22:1581–1588.

Lower, G. M., Jr., and G. T. Bryan. 1976. Enzymatic deacetylation of carcinogenic arylacetamides by tissue microsomes of the dog and other species. J. Toxicol. Environ. Health 1:421–432.

Maher, V. M., J. A. Miller, E. C. Miller, and W. C. Summers. 1970. Mutations and loss of transforming activity of *Bacillus subtilis* DNA after reaction with esters of carcinogenic N-hydroxy aromatic amides. Cancer Res. 30:1473–1480.

Maher, V. M., and M. A. Reuter. 1973. Mutations and loss of transforming activity caused by the O-glucuronide conjugate of the carcinogen N-hydroxy-2-aminofluorene. Mutation Res. 21:63–71.

McGregor, D. 1975. The relationship of 2-acetamidofluorene mutagenicity in plate tests with its in vivo liver cell component distribution and its carcinogenic potential. Mutation Res. 30:305–316.

Miller, J. A., and E. C. Miller. 1969. The metabolic activation of carcinogenic aromatic amines and amides. Prog. Exp. Tumor Res. 11:273–301.

Miller, J. A., and E. C. Miller. 1977. Ultimate chemical carcinogens as reactive mutagenic electrophiles, *in* Origins of Human Cancer, Vol. B. H. H. Hiatt, J. D. Watson, and J. A. Winsten, eds., Cold Spring Harbor Laboratory, Cold Spring Harbor, New York, pp. 605–627.

Mulder, G. J., J. A. Hinson, and J. R. Gillette. 1977. Generation of reactive metabolites of N-hydroxyphenacetin by glucuronidation and sulfation. Biochem. Pharmacol. 26:189–196.

Nelson, S. D., R. J. McMurtry, and J. R. Mitchell. 1978. N-oxidation and O-dealkylation pathways underlying acetaminophen and phenacetin hepatotoxicity, *in* Biological Oxidation of Nitrogen, J. W. Gorrod, ed., Elsevier, Amsterdam, pp. 319–323.

Poirier, L. A., J. A. Miller, and E. C. Miller. 1963. The N- and ring-hydroxylation of 2-acetylaminofluorene and the failure to detect N-acetylation of 2-aminofluorene in the dog. Cancer Res. 23:790–800.

Radomski, J. L., and E. Brill. 1970. Bladder cancer induction by aromatic amines: Role of N-hydroxy metabolites. Science 167:992–993.

Radomski, J. L., and E. Brill. 1971. The role of N-oxidation products of aromatic amines in the induction of bladder cancer in the dog. Arch. Toxicol. 28:159–175.

Radomski, J. L., W. L. Hearn, T. Radomski, H. Moreno, and W. E. Scott. 1977. Isolation of the glucuronic acid conjugate of N-hydroxy-4-aminobiphenyl from dog urine and its mutagenic activity. Cancer Res. 37:1757–1762.

Rathert, P., H. Melchior, and W. Lutyeyer. 1975. Phenacetin: A carcinogen for the urinary tract? J. Urol. 113:653–657.

Scott, T. S. 1962. Carcinogenic and Chronic Toxic Hazards of Aromatic Amines. Elsevier Publishing Co., New York.

Solt, D. B., A. Medline, and E. Farber. 1977. Rapid emergence of carcinogen-induced hyperplastic lesions in a new model for the sequential analysis of liver carcinogenesis. Am. J. Pathol. 88:595–618.

Stout, D. L., J. N. Baptist, T. S. Matney, and C. R. Shaw. 1976. N-hydroxy-2-aminofluorene: The principal mutagen produced from N-hydroxy-2-acetylaminofluorene by a mammalian supernatant enzyme preparation. Cancer Letters 1:269–274.

Tang, B. K., T. Inaba, and W. Kalow. 1977. N-hydroxylation of pentobarbital in man. Drug Metab. Dispos. 5:71–74.

Uehleke, H., and S. Tabarelli. 1973. N-hydroxylation of 4,4'-diaminodiphenylsulfone (Dapsone) by liver microsomes and in dogs and humans. Arch. Pharmacol. 278:55–68.

Weeks, C. E., W. T. Allaben, S. C. Louie, E. J. Lazear, and C. M. King. 1978. Role of arylhydroxamic acid acyltransferase in the mutagenicity of N-hydroxy-N-2-fluorenylacetamide in *Salmonella typhimurium.* Cancer Res. 38:613–618.

Weisburger, J. H., and E. K. Weisburger. 1973. Biochemical formation and pharmacological, toxicological, and pathological properties of hydroxylamines and hydroxamic acids. Pharmacol. Rev. 25:1–66.

Weisburger, J. H., R. S. Yamamoto, G. M. Williams, P. H. Grantham, T. Matsushima, and E. K. Weisburger. 1972. On the sulfate ester of N-hydroxy-N-2-fluorenylacetamide as a key ultimate hepatocarcinogen in the rat. Cancer Res. 32:491–500.

Wilson, R. H., F. DeEds, and A. J. Cox, Jr. 1941. The toxicity and carcinogenic activity of 2-acetylaminofluorene. Cancer Res. 1:595–608.

Wu, S-C. G., and K. D. Straub. 1976. Purification and characterization of N-hydroxy-2-acetylaminofluorene sulfotransferase from rat liver. J. Biol. Chem. 251:6529–6536.

Carcinogens: Identification and Mechanisms
of Action, edited by A. Clark Griffin and
Charles R. Shaw. Raven Press, New York © 1979.

Carcinogen-Induced Damage to DNA

Bernard Strauss, Manuel Altamirano, Kallol Bose, Robert Sklar,
and Kouichi Tatsumi

Department of Microbiology, The University of Chicago, Chicago, Illinois 60637

An initial step in the long chain of events leading to cancer is set off by the combination of an activated molecule, the ultimate carcinogen, with the DNA of a single cell. The evidence that DNA is, in fact, the target molecule is based in part on the increased tumor susceptibility of individuals with metabolic disease affecting DNA repair, such as xeroderma pigmentosum (Miller 1977, Kraemer 1977). These conditions are discussed in detail by Dr. Paterson elsewhere in this volume (1979, see pages 251 to 276).

The target cell may respond to the combination with carcinogen in at least three ways (Strauss 1977): (1) An enzymatic sequence may remove (excise) the region of DNA containing the adduct and replace the damaged region with a normal sequence of nucleotides, thereby restoring the genetic material to its original state. (2) Cellular systems may recognize the DNA as altered and produce breaks in the phosphodiester chain, thereby initiating the processes leading to cell death. The accumulation of unrepaired DNA breaks leads to chromatid aberrations after DNA synthesis (Figure 1); the consequence of the replication of cells with chromatid breaks is cell death due to an "imbalance" in the genetic material. Active cellular participation is required to bring about cell death. Nondividing cells with breaks in their DNA may remain viable, and it is only after cell division that these breaks are converted to lethal damage. The result of replication is illustrated in the response of a human lymphoblastoid line to treatment with methyl methanesulfonate (MMS) (Figure 2). At some critical concentration, the population size first increases and then growth ceases and the culture decays. Adherent human epithelial carcinoma (HEp.2) cells can form microcolonies after treatment with MMS, and these microcolonies consist of swollen cells, unable to divide but still able to metabolize (Myers and Strauss 1971). MMS, monofunctional alkylating agents in general, and ionizing radiation produce numerous breaks in DNA (Karran *et al.* 1977, and below), and it is reasonable to suppose that this reaction pattern is responsible for their efficient cytotoxic behavior and that the induction of irreparable DNA breaks is the basis for much efficient chemotherapeutic action. (3) A third possible response is lack of response: the cell may behave as though it has failed to recognize that changes have occurred. Methylation of guanine to form 7-methyl

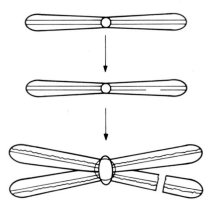

FIG. 1. Interpretation of the probable relationship between DNA synthesis using DNA containing single-strand interruptions as a template and the production of chromatid interruptions.

guanine residues has such a result, since bacteria alkylated with MMS reproduce their DNA even though it contains numerous 7-methyl guanine residues (Prakash and Strauss 1970, Lawley and Orr 1970). The spontaneous production of apurinic or apyrimidinic sites (AP sites) by the loss of alkylated bases does result in activation of the excision response, but as far as we know 7-methyl guanine adducts per se have no effect. Normal methylations, particularly of the amino groups of adenine, may have regulatory effects (Holliday and Pugh 1975), but such changes are certainly not seen as "damage."

Cells may also ignore changes that are recognized as damage, by a mechanism in which the DNA replicating machinery "senses" that an altered template is present but nonetheless replicates past the lesion. How this occurs is still a mystery, as will be discussed below. One possibility is that the damage is ignored because the synthetic machinery is allowed to make "mistakes" in the course of replication, and it is these mistakes that lead to mutation and constitute

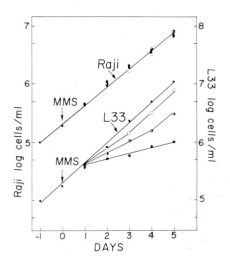

FIG. 2. Effect of treatment of two lymphoid cell lines with MMS. Cultures were maintained in a rapidly growing state by daily dilution. At day "0," they were treated with 0, 0.1, 0.2, or 0.3 mM MMS for one hour. The cultures were centrifuged and the medium replaced. Cultures were counted daily and the population size adjusted to 4.0×10^5/ml. The fractional increase was used to calculate an apparent cell concentration assuming no dilution, and this is shown in the Figure. Filled circles, control; open boxes, 0.1 mM; half-filled circles, 0.2 mM; closed boxes, 0.3 mM MMS. Left-hand scale, Raji; right-hand scale, L33.

the initial steps in carcinogenesis. However, although most carcinogens are mutagens (McCann and Ames 1976), it is not necessary to suppose that mutation is the primary carcinogenic process even though DNA is the critical reactant. For example, a recent hypothesis by Holliday (personal communication) supposes that excision repair, occurring before enzymatic methylation of a newly synthesized daughter strand, might remove controlling elements from the parental strand and therefore result in uncontrolled growth that would be propagated from cell generation to generation. The importance of the hypothesis is not only that it may be correct but also that it demonstrates how an epigenetic change in the DNA could have an effect on cellular regulation that would persist from generation to generation.

We have been concerned with some of these features of cellular response and would like to discuss the following in greater detail: (1) some characteristics of the different excision repair mechanisms; (2) evidence that lesions present in the DNA can be bypassed by the DNA synthetic machinery; and (3) some possible mechanisms for the bypass. Before proceeding, it is necessary to point out that the consequence of reaction of DNA with carcinogen depends critically on the exact adduct formed. Single carcinogens can react at a number of sites within the DNA. Methyl nitronitrosoguanidine (MNNG), for example, may produce up to 15 different reaction products with DNA (Singer 1976). Although some adducts are produced in very small yield, even a minor reaction product may be present in sufficient amount to have important biological consequences, since a single reaction product within a genome may be effective if carcinogenesis is even quasimutational. One would like to be able to analyze what happens to individual lesions, since the analysis of the complete action of compounds is too complex. However, producing DNA with only one type of lesion is still beyond our capabilities. We consider the compounds acetoxy acetylaminofluorene (AAAF) and MMS as relatively simple, since they produce single major adducts in DNA, and, therefore, these substances are used to indicate major repair pathways. By contrast, compounds such as MNNG or treatment with ionizing radiation must be considered as extremely complex because of the wide range of lesions induced (Strauss *et al.* 1975, Cerutti, in press).

EXCISION REPAIR PATHWAYS

It is possible to divide the different excision repair mechanisms into three main pathways: nucleotide excision, base excision, and apurinic-apyrimidinic (AP) repair (Figure 3). Nucleotide excision is the paradigm of the three, since it is the major pathway for the repair of ultraviolet (UV)-induced pyrimidine dimers and was discovered first (Setlow and Carrier 1964, Boyce and Howard-Flanders 1964). In nucleotide excision there is an endonucleolytic incision at or near the site of the lesion, an exonucleolytic removal of an oligonucleotide stretch, the replacement of the removed stretch by a "patch," and a closing of the remaining single-strand interruption by a ligase reaction. The "patch

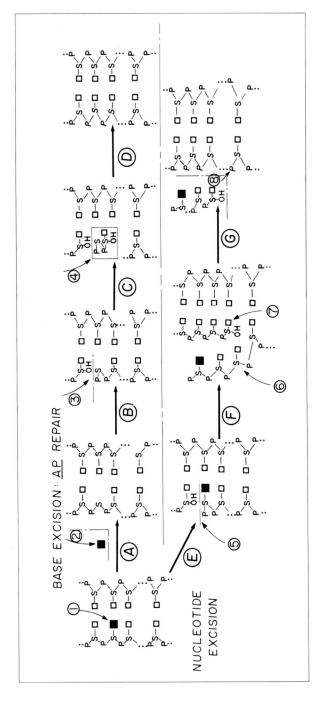

FIG. 3. Pathways of DNA excision repair. A, removal of damaged base (spontaneous in AP repair, DNA N-glycosylase catalyzed in base excision); B, AP endonuclease; C, 5'-3' exonuclease; D, polymerase; E, incising endonuclease; F, strand displacement and polymerase catalyzed chain elongation; G, exonuclease, polymerase + ligase action. 1, Damaged base; 2, free base as product of reaction A; 3, free 3' OH as product of apurinic endonuclease; 4, removal of dinucleotides by 5'-3' exonuclease; 5, endonucleolytic cleavage liberating a free 3' OH; 6, strand displacement as a result of polymerase action; 7, newly synthesized "patch"; 8, exonuclease action liberating damaged base as part of an oligonucleotide.

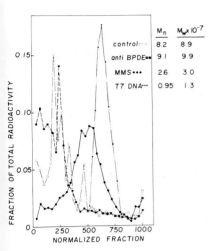

FIG. 4. Lack of detectable anti-BPDE-induced breaks in DNA. Raji lymphoma cells were prelabeled by 48 hours incubation in medium with ^{14}C-thymidine (0.05 μCi/ml), followed by 16 hours incubation in non-labeled medium. Cell suspensions (2 ml, 8 × 10[5]/ml) were then incubated with MMS (600 μg/ml) or anti-BPDE (5 μg/ml). The suspensions were incubated 45 minutes at 37°C, harvested, washed, and suspended in SSC, and 100 μl were lysed on top of an alkaline sucrose gradient. A marker T7 DNA preparation was centrifuged at the same time. Treatment at 0.1 μg/ml anti-BPDE gave the same result as the higher concentration.

size" in simple nucleotide excision in mammalian cells is variously estimated as between 30 (Edenberg and Hanawalt 1972) and 100 (Regan and Setlow 1974) nucleotides, depending on the methodology. (The details of the repair mechanisms seem to differ in bacteria, in which simple excision repair occurs with patches of about 30 and complex excision repair with longer patches of over 1,000 nucleotides [Cooper and Hanawalt 1972].)

Although an endonucleolytic step is critical, single-strand breaks in the DNA are relatively rare and difficult to detect (Karran *et al.* 1977), and it has been suggested (Ahmed and Setlow 1977) that a complete repair complex for the sequence is involved. For example, treatment of the human lymphoma line Raji with anti-benzpyrene diolepoxide (anti-BPDE) at two concentrations, one reducing survival to 60% and the other sufficient to kill all the cells and completely inhibit DNA synthesis, did not result in breaks in the parental DNA strand as detected by alkaline sucrose gradient centrifugation after 45 minutes of incubation (Figure 4). (A more recent quantitative determination indicates that about 0.1 of the number of MMS-induced breaks are observed after anti-BPDE treatment at doses of 440 μg/ml of MMS and 5 μg/ml of anti-BPDE, which result in the same number of adducts in the DNA of treated Raji cells.)

An alternative method for the detection of single-strand breaks involves the lysis of cells on top of neutral sucrose gradients containing Sl nuclease in the top layer: single-strand breaks are converted to double-strand breaks easily detected by centrifugation. Cells treated with AAAF or with bromomethylbenz*[a]*anthracene (BMBA) do not show breaks (Karran *et al.* 1977). These experiments involved relatively short incubation times of about one hour. However, the activated compounds used react rapidly with cells, and breaks, if abundant, would have been expected to be present as with other compounds (see below). Repair induced by the polycyclic aromatic hydrocarbons (PAH) is likely to proceed mainly by the nucleotide excision pathway (Heflich *et al.* 1977). There-fore, the lack of detectable breaks in parental DNA implies that the initial endonuclease step is limiting. DNA strand interruptions *have* been detected in nucleotide excision, but such detection requires methodologies such as alkaline elution (Fornace *et al.* 1976) that can scan large molecular weight fragments for single interruptions and are therefore very sensitive.

AP repair results when an unstable adduct such as 3-methyl adenine or 7-methyl guanine is produced and then spontaneously depurinates to leave an AP site. Apurinic endonuclease recognizes such sites (Ljungquist 1977); an exonuclease removes the AP site and an adjacent nucleotide, a small patch is inserted by polymerase, and ligation occurs. The patch size in AP repair is only two to three nucleotides long in vivo (Painter and Young 1972, Regan and Setlow 1974). Many free DNA strand interruptions are readily detected in AP repair by the Sl nuclease method described above, by shearing DNA with interruptions creating single-stranded regions that make the DNA adhere to benzoylated napthoylated DEAE cellulose (BND cellulose) (Karran *et al.* 1977), or by any methodology that detects single-strand breaks. A simple expla-nation for the characteristics of AP repair is that in contrast to nucleotide excision, there is an excess of endonucleolytic activity, but the exonuclease activ-ity is both distributive and limiting. This hypothesis accounts for the accumula-tion of DNA with breaks and for the small patch size, since one might expect a limiting, distributive exonuclease to be displaced by polymerase.

We have constructed an in vitro model of AP repair with these properties. In this system, T7 DNA containing about 10 MMS- and heat-induced AP sites per strand is incubated with an endonuclease-exonuclease preparation from the human lymphoma line Daudi, a Daudi DNA polymerase α, and, after a period of incubation, a ligase derived from phage T4 (Bose *et al.* 1978). This system repairs T7 DNA as seen by the loss of alkaline-labile sites (Figure 5). The data indicate that repair activity is limited by the activity of the exonuclease preparation, and this exonuclease activity is increased in the presence of DNA polymerase α (Figure 6), even though the polymerase alone has no nuclease activity. A similar phenomenon has been observed with the *Escherichia coli* polymerase I (Setlow and Kornberg 1972). Proteolytic treatment of this enzyme separates a $5'-3'$ exonuclease without polymerase activity from a DNA polymer-ase without $5'-3'$ exonuclease activity. Setlow and Kornberg (1972) showed that the mixture of the separate fragments and the addition of nucleoside tri-phosphates increased exonuclease activity. In our case, activity is enhanced even in the absence of added nucleoside triphosphate. We calculate that when ligase is added after 30 minutes, the patch size is about two nucleotides, and, as would be expected, the first major reaction product of exonucleolytic reaction in vitro is a dinucleotide (Bose *et al.* 1978).

Base excision differs from AP repair in requiring a DNA N-glycosylase to remove the altered base (Lindahl 1976). Glycosylases have been reported that act on uracil in DNA and on 3-methyl adenine (Lindahl *et al.* 1978, Laval 1977). So far, there has been no confirmed report of a DNA N-glycosylase

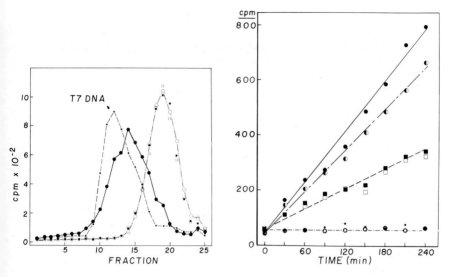

FIG. 5, left. Repair of alkali-labile sites in T7 DNA. T7 DNA (5.7 μg, 5600 ³H cpm/μg), alkylated and depurinated to give 10 apurinic sites per strand, was incubated with 8 μg of DNA polymerase or 1.9 μg of nuclease, or both, and with unlabeled nucleoside triphosphates for 30 minutes at 37°C. Ligase (10 units) and ATP (final concentration 100 μM) were added where indicated. The reaction mixture was then incubated an additional 30 minutes at 30°C, after which 200 μl of 0.2 M NaOH/0.1 M NaCl/20 mM EDTA/1% sucrose was added to stop the reaction. The mixtures were incubated for 15 minutes at room temperature, and then 100 μl was layered on top of a preformed 5–20% linear sucrose gradient containing 0.3 M NaOH/0.5 M NaCl/10 mM EDTA. The gradients were centrifuged at 44,800 rpm for 2.5 hours at 5°C. Samples were collected from the bottom of the tube on filter paper discs (Whatmann 3MM), dried, washed with 5% trichloroacetic acid, 95% ethanol, and acetone, and dried; radioactivity was then determined. •, untreated T7 DNA; ●, MMS-treated DNA plus nuclease plus polymerase plus ligase (complete system); ○, complete system minus polymerase; □, complete system minus polymerase and minus ligase; ■, complete system minus ligase. The curve for the complete system (polymerase plus ligase) but without nuclease is not shown, but these results superimpose on the results for the complete system minus polymerase or minus ligase. (Reprinted from Bose *et al.* 1978.)

FIG. 6, right. Exonuclease assay using ³H-labeled T5 DNA. Effect of DNA polymerase and nucleotide triphosphates on exonuclease activity. Exonuclease with (□) and without (■) nucleotide triphosphate removed 7.6 × 10¹¹ nucleotides per μg protein per 30 minutes. Exonuclease with DNA polymerase (◐) removed 1.4 × 10¹² nucleotides per μg protein per 30 minutes. Exonuclease with DNA polymerase and nucleotide triphosphate (●) removed 1.8 × 10¹² nucleotides per μg protein per 30 minutes. (•) no enzyme. (○) DNA polymerase only.

using 6-methoxyguanine as a substrate, but the biological data (see below) make the existence of such an enzyme very likely. The biological properties of base excision repair are largely unknown; there are no data showing the patch size, and it is not clear whether an accumulation of breaks is to be expected. However, insofar as the uracil N-glycosylase is responsible for a proportion of Okazaki fragments (Tye *et al.* 1977), it would appear that base excision may also produce free breaks, which, however, are quickly repaired. DNA synthesis occasionally misincorporates uracil into the DNA. The uracil N-glycosylase recognizes this misincorporation and removes the uracil, creating an AP site that is then attacked by the endonuclease. Formation of these fragments in newly synthesized DNA accounts for a portion of the Okazaki pieces observed (Tye *et al.* 1978). Although all types of excision repair involve breaks in the DNA, there is evidence that nucleotide excision and AP repair are independent metabolic pathways. Cells deficient in nucleotide excision may be perfectly capable of carrying out AP repair. For example, xeroderma pigmentosum lymphoblastoid cells (Andrews *et al.* 1974), relatively deficient in their ability to repair UV- or AAAF-induced damage, are able to perform MMS- or MNNG-induced repair at initial rates equivalent to or greater than those of control lymphoma cells without repair defects (Figure 7). Nucleotide excision is reported to be low in adult rodent cells, but rodent cells are perfectly capable of performing AP repair (Table 1). A number of in vitro studies demonstrate that the initial endonucleolytic incision is different in UV and in AP repair; AP endonucleases are not UV endonucleases (Ljungquist 1977). There is some evidence that the steps subsequent to the endonucleolytic cut are also different, as would be expected for different pathways. The difference in patch size reported for nucleotide excision and AP repair makes it unlikely that a single process starting from a common intermediate is involved. Furthermore, although it is not known what the physiologically important exonucleases may be, the activity involved in the in vitro repair of AP sites liberates primarily dinucleotides and can produce an in vitro patch size of about two (Bose *et al.* 1978), whereas the exonuclease isolated from human placenta by Doniger and Grossman (1976), and suggested by them to have the properties required of a nucleotide excision repair exonuclease, excises fragments of an average size of four and processes for stretches of about 30–40. It is therefore at least possible to find enzymes with the different properties required for two separate and independent metabolic pathways.

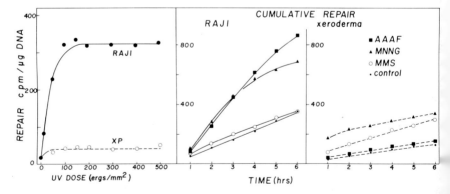

FIG. 7. Repair activity of Raji lymphoma and XPA-3 xeroderma lymphoblastoid lines. Repair was measured as described by Scudiero *et al.* (1975, 1976). Concentrations of carcinogen that reduced DNA synthesis to 10% of control were added as follows: AAAF: Raji 20 μg; XP-3 10 μg; MMS: Raji 90 μg, XP-3 150 μg; MNNG: Raji 5 μg, XP-3 10 μg.

TABLE 1. *Repair activity of three cell lines*

Compound	% Residual DNA synthesis	Repair: cpm/μg DNA* Line		
		Raji (human)	XP-3 (human)	L5178Y (mouse)
AAAF	100	17	12	29
	37	81 (5)†	17 (5)	51 (2)
	10	245 (20)	35 (10)	66 (10)
BMBA	100	20	12	13
	37	37 (0.1)	17 (0.04)	16 (0.75)
	10	123 (3)	13 (3)	23 (4)
MMS	100	17	12	32
	37	42 (70)	70 (90)	102 (100)
	10	80 (100)	100 (200)	102 (200)
MNNG	100	17	12	32
	37	41 (2.5)	156 (5)	84 (4)
	10	70 (5)	196 (10)	175 (10)

* Repair was measured by the BND cellulose technique (Scudiero *et al.* 1975) as cpm ^{3}HdT incorporated per μg of DNA in the 1 M NaCl eluate. Rapidly growing cells were preincubated for 30 minutes with 10 mM hydroxyurea, then incubated in medium for 60 minutes with 10 mM hydroxyurea, ^{3}HdT (10 μCi/ml, 13 Ci/mole), and carcinogen. Treatment with carcinogen was to a level giving about 37% and 10% residual DNA synthesis. The nontreated controls are indicated as 100% residual synthesis. Rates of DNA synthesis were estimated from the amounts of ^{3}HdT incorporated by cultures incubated in the absence of hydroxyurea.
† Values in parentheses indicate the actual amount of compound added in μg/ml.

Xeroderma pigmentosum has long been thought of as a disease in which nucleotide excision is deficient (Cleaver and Bootsma 1975), and at one time was thought to be a simple metabolic defect in which the lesion was a deficiency in the UV-incision enzyme. Recent studies by Goth-Goldstein (1977) indicate that fibroblasts of a complementation group A xeroderma patient are also deficient in their ability to excise 06 alkyl guanine residues. We have confirmed this result with cells of a lymphoblastoid line derived from a complementation group C patient. These cells do not remove 06 methyl guanine residues when compared to excision-competent Raji lymphoma cells after treatment with doses of MNNG (0.5 μg/ml) that are only slightly inhibitory (Table 2). However, they remain competent in the rapid removal of 3-methyl adenine.

Since it is not yet clear whether 06 methyl guanine groups are removed by nucleotide or base excision, we also decided to determine whether *uvr* A and *uvr* B *E. coli* mutants were able to remove such groups. We treated suspensions of *E. coli* K12 and the closely related *uvr* A, *uvr* B, and *uvr* AB mutants (Howard-Flanders *et al.* 1966) with 5.0 μg/ml of MNNG for 60 minutes and then incubated for an additional hour. The cells were then lysed, the DNA isolated and hydrolyzed, and the hydrolysis products separated by Sephadex G 10 chromatography. *Uvr* bacterial mutants do excise 06 methyl guanine residues (Table 2), and in bacteria, therefore, this excision is not due to the UV

TABLE 2. Removal of 0–6 methyl guanine from DNA after treatment of cells with MNNG

Strain	Time incubated	7-Methyl guanine			3-Methyl adenine				0–6 Methyl guanine			
		cpm	cpm/µg G	corrected cpm/µg G	cpm	cpm/µg G	corrected cpm/µg G	3 MeA / 7 MeG	cpm	cpm/µg G	corrected cpm/µg G	0–6 MeG / 7 MeG
Raji	0	1628	12.8		226	1.78		13.9	61	0.64		3.7
	36 hrs	892	3.3	4.1	14	0.06	0.075	1.6	7	0.03	0.04	0.8
XPA-3	0	1978	12.2		184	1.13		9.3	174	1.07		8.8
	36 hrs	1490	4.6	7.3	11	0.03	0.05	0.7	162	0.5	0.8	11.0
Escherichia coli												
K12	0	2224	4.8		37	0.1		1.7	220	0.5		9.9
	1 hr	3739	3.5		5	0.005		0.1	0	—		—
uvr A	0	2536	4.9		45	0.1		1.8	265	0.5		10.5
	1 hr	1812	2		9	0.01		0.5	26	0.03		1.4
uvr B	0	4771	5.3		221	0.2		4.6	267	0.3		5.6
	1 hr	4259	2.9		16	0.01		0.4	9	0.006		0.2
uvr AB	0	989	1.6		78	0.13		7.9	29	0.05		2.9
	1 hr	2462	1.7		26	0.02		1.1	2	—		—

* Rapidly growing cultures were concentrated by centrifugation, resuspended, and treated with ^{14}C-MNNG (New England Nuclear, 14.3 mCi/mM) in a total volume of 40 ml. Lymphoid cell lines were treated at 0.5 µg/ml; bacteria were incubated with 5 µg/ml MNNG. After 15 minutes incubation, cultures were harvested and either resuspended in medium for incubation or harvested. After incubation the cells were lysed with 0.2% sodium dodecyl sulfate. The lysates were digested for one hour at 37°C with 50 µg/ml of pancreatic ribonuclease and then for one hour with 1.5 mg/ml of heat-treated Pronase. The solution was then extracted three times with phenol. DNA was hydrolyzed with 0.1 N HCl for 20 minutes at 70°C and chromatographed along with authentic markers on a column of Sephadex G10 (8.0 × 1.5 cm) and eluted with ammonium formate (0.005 M, pH 6.8). The fractions were collected, pooled, evaporated, and counted in an Aquasol scintillation cocktail for periods long enough to ensure statistical significance. The cpm/µg G after incubation were corrected for growth on the basis of actual cell counts.

endonuclease. It is clearly a long jump from *uvr* bacterial strains to xeroderma lymphoblasts, but these results do make it unlikely that a mammalian UV endonuclease participates in the excision of 06 alkyl guanine. Xeroderma cells therefore are deficient in two separate metabolic reactions. In addition, there is evidence that UV- and AAAF-induced damage in mammalian cells is attacked by different endonucleases (Ahmed and Setlow 1977, Amacher *et al.* 1977) and that xeroderma cells are deficient in both. The xeroderma cell is therefore deficient in three separate metabolic steps but behaves normally with respect to AP repair and also in the base-excision of 3-methyl adenine. Not only does this illustrate the independence of AP and nucleotide excision, but it also suggests that the xeroderma mutations which occur in five or more complementation groups (Kraemer 1977) are unlikely to be explicable on a simple gene-enzyme basis.

BYPASS REPAIR

Replication does not wait for the excision of adducts, and cell systems relatively or absolutely deficient in excision ability are able to replicate even though adducts are present. It is generally supposed that special mechanisms, variously called postreplication repair or replication repair to indicate their connection with DNA synthesis, are involved. We are particularly interested in the mode of action of benzpyrene as a carcinogen. In order to demonstrate that cells can replicate DNA containing benzpyrene adducts, we reacted excision-competent Raji and excision-defective xeroderma lymphoblastoid cells with ^{3}H-labeled anti-BPDE. The cells were then incubated in medium containing bromodeoxyuridine (BrdUrd) for 36 to 40 hours. The dose of anti-BPDE was low enough (0.05 μg/ml) to permit replication. Raji cells are not inactivated, and xeroderma cells give about 60% survival at this dose. The DNA was isolated and centrifuged through a CsCl gradient. The hybrid DNA (from replicated samples) was isolated, dialyzed, and centrifuged again through alkaline CsCl (Figure 8). All of the radioactivity was found at the hybrid density after the first centrifugation through neutral CsCl, indicating that the nonexcised label was in replicated DNA. After alkaline CsCl centrifugation, almost all of the remaining radioactivity was recovered in the parental strand. This means that whatever the mechanism of replication, a major recombination step is not involved. We also calculated the specific activity of the DNA before and after replication (Table 3). It can be seen that replication occurs with almost no change in specific activity in xeroderma cells. Even the excision-competent Raji cells retain about one third of the residues after 36 hours. Either there is some particular BPDE-induced lesion that is not subject to excision, or the excision process is unable to recognize certain lesions in particular locations, possibly in replicated DNA.

These results are in agreement with those of Dipple and Roberts (1977), who estimated from excision data that at nonlethal doses of BMBA about 50% of carcinogen-induced adduct remained in cells that had replicated their DNA.

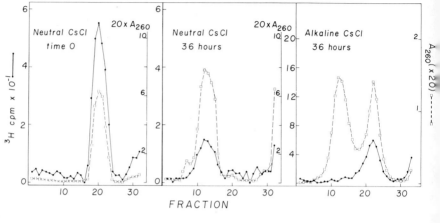

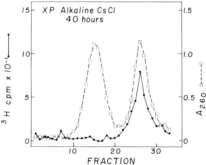

FIG. 8. A (top), CsCl gradients of DNA from BPDE-treated Raji cells. Solid lines, radioactivity; dashed lines, absorbancy. Cultures were incubated 30 minutes with 0.05 μg/ml of BPDE (222 mCi/mmol). The cells were washed and suspended in medium containing 33 μM of BrdUrd and 1 μM FdUrd. Fractions from the neutral CsCl gradient were dialyzed and sedimented in alkaline CsCl. Radioactivity is given as cpm/50 μl for neutral gradients and cpm/ml for alkaline gradients. B (bottom), Alkaline gradient from XPA-3 cells treated and incubated as described above.

It is possible to devise models to account for the appearance of PAH residues in replicated DNA without bypass by supposing that DNA is synthesized with nicks or gaps opposite each adduct, but such schemes predict extensive chromosome fragmentation in subsequent divisions, which is not compatible with the 100% viability retained at the doses we use.

The dose of BPDE at which these experiments were done (0.05 μg/ml) is very low, and at higher doses both inhibition of DNA synthesis and inactivation of cloning ability occur. The question might well be: "What kills cells after BPDE reaction?" rather than "How does replication occur?" At the doses we used, there were about 1.5 adducts per 10^8 daltons of DNA (see Table 3). This is equivalent to about 45,000 per cellular equivalent of DNA or 1 in 3 μm of DNA. Since this corresponds to about one per replicon, e^{-1} or 37% of the replicons had no adducts, 37% had one adduct, and only 26% had two or more per replicon. All of the DNA seemed to be replicated (Figure 8) and we conclude, therefore, that even a large number of adducts can be replicated if sparsely distributed.

A simple explanation is that at low doses some critical adduct is not formed or there is some peculiar distribution of adducts so that none is formed at low concentrations at some critical location. A second "explanation" of this

TABLE 3. *Specific activity of DNA from anti-BPDE-treated cells*

Cell	Time after treatment	Binding: BP/10^8 daltons DNA*
Raji	0	2.5
	36 hrs	0.82
XPA-3	0	1.5
	40 hrs	1.4

* Binding of benzpyrene residues was determined from the radioactivity and absorbancy of the DNA in the peak fraction of an alkaline CsCl gradient using the value 26 absorbancy units at 260 μm = 1 mg to calculate the denatured DNA concentration.

replication is that no explanation is needed, that is, that benzpyrene (BP) adducts are not recognized as damage by the replication machinery. However, the observed toxicity of anti-BPDE and its enhanced toxicity for xeroderma cells (Heflich *et al.* 1977) indicates that unexcised BP lesions in DNA can be effective inhibitors and that some special reaction sequence must account for the ability of cells to ignore lesions remaining in the DNA. By definition, "bypass" occurs only when there is DNA synthesis, and therefore the process is called replication or postreplication repair, depending on the mechanism proposed. Replication repair can be visualized by alkaline sucrose gradients of lysates of cells treated with carcinogen and incubated with radioactive thymidine. The newly synthesized DNA appears in smaller pieces than observed in controls and then elongates; the elongation is inhibited by hydroxyurea as is normal replication (Lehmann 1972a). Supposing there to be a special process distinct from replication is particularly attractive because of the relatively well-understood postreplication repair mechanism observed in *E. coli*. This repair proceeds via a "recombination" mechanism in which DNA synthesis is blocked on the damaged template strand but proceeds past the point of a lesion on both strands, leaving a single-strand "gap" in one of the daughter double helices. The gap is then filled in by insertion (recombination) of a section of parental DNA into the newly synthesized strand (Figure 9). When lesions occur at intervals along both strands, the transfer of a section of parental DNA containing lesions to a daughter strand can occur and has been observed in bacteria (Ganesan 1974). Therefore, the report that UV-induced lesions were detectable in daughter strands in a mammalian cell system (Meneghini and Hanawalt 1976) implied the existence of a recombination mechanism in these cells. However, recent studies make it possible to account

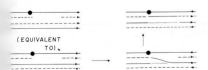

FIG. 9. Model of recombination repair via strand displacement. ——————, parental DNA; - - - - ......, daughter DNA; ●, block to replication.

for these results by supposing the addition of isotope to preexisting DNA chains containing pyrimidine dimers (Lehman and Kirk-Bell 1978), and therefore it appears that the amount of recombination repair in mammalian cells is very low. Our results (Figure 8) also imply that strand exchange does not play a major role in the bypass reactions.

At least two hypotheses can account for the bypass of lesions. The first hypothesis suggests that as in the bacteria, a nonreplicated gap results on one strand as a result of the progress of replication and that this gap is later "filled in" by some process, possibly by the induction of a system that alters the proofreading function of the replicating system so that an error in replication due to the misreading of a carcinogen-altered base is not recognized as a mistake (Caillet-Fauquet et al. 1977). The idea of an inducible system is interesting and important and is applicable to any of the bypass mechanisms that have been suggested. Evidence for such an inducible mechanism is accumulating (cf. Bockstahler et al. 1976, Sarasin and Hanawalt 1978), but its existence in mammalian cells has yet to be firmly established.

A second hypothesis supposes that DNA synthesis along both strands halts near the point of the lesion and that the actual bypass is the result of reactions at the DNA growing point. We recently suggested a particular model of how this might occur (Higgins et al. 1976) based on the processes of DNA strand displacement and branch migration (Thompson et al. 1976). Displacement of DNA strands at growing points can lead to the restoration of the original helical structure associating two parental strands. The process also results in movement of the growing point fork or branch, and hence in branch migration and strand displacement (Figure 10). If branch migration proceeded far enough to displace both daughter strands, association between the two complementary, newly synthesized strands could occur, and if synthesis had been blocked on one strand and had proceeded for some distance past the point of the lesion along the other, these daughter strands would be of unequal length. Higgins et al. (1976) suggested that one strand could then serve as a template for elongation of the other. Reversal of the branch migration process would then result in a daughter molecule containing lesions but not gaps. If replication occurs in the presence of the density analogue BrdUrd, the model predicts that bifilarly substituted molecules should be found within the first generation as a result of the shearing of DNA at growing points (Figure 11). Such DNA_{HH} (DNA with both strands substituted with "heavy" analogue) is readily observed (Higgins et al. 1976). Also observed is a fraction of DNA of intermediate density (DNA_{int}) that originates from DNA growing points (Kato and Strauss 1974) and contains both parental and daughter DNA connected by single-strand regions.

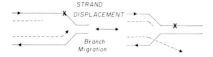

FIG. 10. Branch migration and strand displacement.

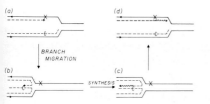

FIG. 11. Model of replication repair by branch migration.

The proportion of DNA$_{HH}$ observed compared to the total radioactivity incorporated was very high, amounting at times to 25% (see below), and this implied that branch migration had occurred at every DNA growing point. We wondered, therefore, whether the branch migration process might not occur in vitro as a consequence of isolating growing points with single-stranded regions. Results show that most DNA$_{HH}$ does originate during or after cell lysis. This in vitro formation was demonstrated by a cross-linking experiment in which human lymphoma cells were treated with mutagen, incubated, and then treated with trioxsalen and near-UV light immediately before lysis. This treatment cross-links DNA at intervals of about 200 nucleotides (Hanson et al. 1976) and effectively blocks branch migration (Tatsumi and Strauss 1978). In contrast to the cells not cross-linked by this procedure, no DNA$_{HH}$ was observed in the trioxsalen-treated cells (Figure 12). Cross-linking with trioxsalen and near-UV light did not affect the yield of DNA$_{HH}$ when carried out after cell lysis. We interpret this result to mean that cross-linking in vivo prevented branch migration and that disruption of the chromosome by detergent is responsible for the formation of such fragments. The limits of detection are 1–2% of the incorporated label,

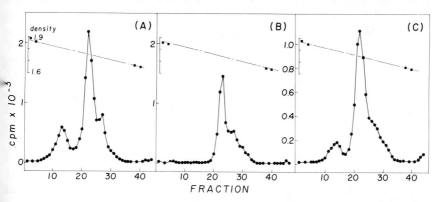

IG. 12. Effect of trioxsalen and near-UV light on DNA$_{HH}$. XPA-3 cells were treated with AAAF 36.8 μM) for 30 minutes and incubated with ^{3}HdT in the presence of BrdUrd and FdUrd. ollowing the labeling, the cells were suspended in phosphate buffered saline with hydroxyurea nd treated with trioxsalen (5 μg/ml) and near-UV light (2 mW/cm^2) for 20 minutes. Phenol-xtracted DNA was sheared three times through a 22-gauge needle and centrifuged through CsCl gradient (Tatsumi and Strauss 1978). A, Without cross-linking; B, cross-linking in vivo; , cross-linking in vitro after SDS, RNase, and Pronase treatment.

and the experiments therefore set an upper limit on the amount of DNA_{HH} that could result from in vivo reactions. The origin of DNA_{HH} from DNA_{int} was shown by subjecting isolated DNA_{int} preparations to extensive shear (Figure 13). DNA_{HH} was produced, indicating its origin from near the growing point.

It is much easier to separate DNA_{HH} from the nearest DNA density species (hybrid DNA) than it is to separate hybrid DNA from DNA_{int}. In addition, the alternative method we use for isolating DNA growing points by BND cellulose chromatography (Scudiero and Strauss 1974) depends on the presence of single-stranded regions and therefore does not distinguish between growing points and single-stranded regions due to gaps within replicons (Iyer and Rupp 1971). We therefore decided to measure DNA_{HH} as an indication of the proportion of newly synthesized DNA located near growing points, since even though DNA_{HH} is formed in vitro, it can only be formed from fragments associated with growing points. An indication of the usefulness of this probe is seen in the following experiment: A lymphoblastoid line of xeroderma pigmentosum (XPA-3) was treated with 10 mM caffeine to inhibit DNA synthesis to about 50% of the control. Both the absolute and relative amount of DNA_{HH} increased in the caffeine-treated cells even when the time of incubation was adjusted so that approximately the same amount of radioactivity was incorporated into DNA (Table 4). Over 25% of the radioactivity was detected as DNA_{HH} in the caffeine-treated samples. At least two models account for these observations (Figure 14). Either strand displacement results in long stretches of DNA_{HH} in the presence of caffeine (Figure 14A) or inhibition by caffeine slows down the rate of chain elongation but does not inhibit the start of new replicons so that there is an increase in the number of growing points (Figure 14B). The number average molecular weight of DNA_{HH} in neutral sucrose gradients was 2.7 ×

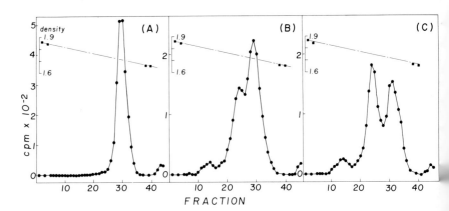

FIG. 13. DNA_{HH} originates from DNA_{int}. DNA_{int} was isolated by rebanding of density 1.69 1.73 g/cm³ material from neutral CsCl gradients similar to those shown in Figure 12A. After dialysis, DNA_{int} was further sheared by 10 passages through a 26-gauge needle or treated with *N. crassa* endonuclease. A, No treatment; B, sheared; C, treated with endonuclease.

TABLE 4. *Effect of caffeine on yield of DNA$_{HH}$ and on the size of nascent DNA in alkaline sucrose gradients**

Concentration of caffeine (mM)	Labeling time (min)	Overall incorporation of ^{3}HdT (cpm/μg of total DNA)	Incorporation into HH region (cpm/μg of total DNA)	Relative yield of DNA$_{HH}$ (%)	Mol. weight of nascent DNA† ($\times 10^{-7}$ daltons)
0	10	690	102	14.8	11.2
	20	1479	115	7.8	13.1
10	20	833	198	25.7	1.97
	40	1255	254	24.9	5.83

* DNA$_{HH}$ was prepared by 10 passages through a 26-gauge needle and treatment with *Neurospora crassa* endonuclease followed by CsCl gradient centrifugation, as described by Tatsumi and Strauss (1978).

† XPA-3 cells were preincubated with caffeine for 30 minutes before labeling with ^{3}HdT (66 Ci/mmol; 30 μCi/ml) in the presence of BrdUrd (3.3 $\times$ 10^{-5} M) and FdUrd (10^{-6} M). Weight-average molecular weights were calculated from sedimentation profiles of DNA in alkaline sucrose gradients.

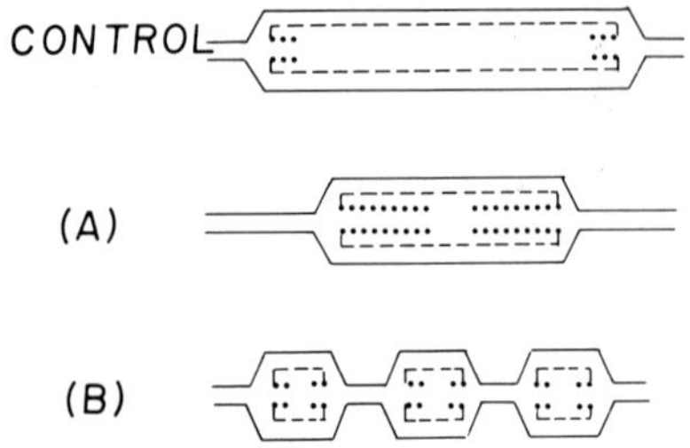

FIG. 14. Models for the accumulation of DNA_{HH} in caffeine-treated cells.

10^6 for caffeine-treated cultures and 5.3×10^6 for controls, but since DNA_{HH} is produced as a result of extensive shear, this result alone is not conclusive. However, we also found that the molecular weight of the newly synthesized strands as determined in an alkaline sucrose gradient was much lower in the presence of caffeine (Table 4), implying that model B (Figure 14), which indicates an accumulation of growing forks, is more likely. This agrees with a suggestion of Lehmann (1972b) that DNA is synthesized in smaller units in the presence of caffeine.

We then tested the effect of treatment of cells with AAAF or with BPDE on both the yield of DNA_{HH} and on the size of the newly synthesized DNA in alkaline sucrose gradients (Table 5). Incubation of excision-defective XPA-3 cells with concentrations of AAAF or BPDE sufficient to inhibit DNA synthesis to the 50% level resulted in an increased yield of DNA_{HH}. The yield was inversely related to the size of the daughter DNA produced; the smaller the size of the nascent DNA, the higher the proportion of label in DNA_{HH}. The lower molecular weight of DNA synthesized after treatment with AAAF or BPDE can be accounted for by supposing either that DNA synthesis proceeds past lesions, leaving single-stranded "gaps" in the DNA, or that the newly synthesized DNA occurs in shortened replicating units resulting from a temporary block to synthesis (Figure 15).

The finding of an increased yield of DNA_{HH} accompanying the shortened

TABLE 5. *Effect of anti-benzpyrene diolepoxide (BPDE) and acetoxy acetyl aminofluorene (AAAF) on the yield of DNA_{HH} and on the size of nascent DNA in alkaline sucrose gradients*

Treatment	Dose (M)	Rate of DNA synthesis (% of control)	Labeling time (min)	Relative yield of DNA_{HH} (%)	Molecular weight of nascent DNA ($\times 10^7$ daltons)
Control XPA-3	—	100	20	5.6	12.7
BPDE	0.5	51.5	40	9.2	7.4
AAAF	7.0	53.5	40	15.8	4.3

* Drug was added to rapidly growing cultures for 30 minutes before the addition of ^3Hd (66 Ci/mmol; 20 μCi/ml), BrdUrd (3.3×10^{-5} M), and FdUrd (10^{-6} M). Samples were handled and calculations done as described in the legend to Table 4.

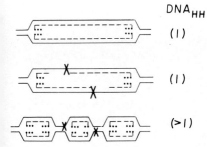

FIG. 15. Models for replication repair. Top, nondamaged DNA; middle, gap formation; bottom, bypass at growing points.

pieces of newly synthesized DNA is most easily accounted for by supposing that a block does occur when a growing point encounters a lesion and that DNA synthesis in these XPA-3 cells is held up near the site of lesions. This conclusion depends on the supposition that DNA_{HH} does not form from DNA containing internal, single-strand gaps. It is possible to construct models in which DNA_{HH} does originate from such internal gaps, but these models require single-strand breaks in a parental strand for each branch migration event (Lavin 1978). The two models (branch migration and internal gap formation) are indistinguishable under such conditions. DNA_{HH} molecules can be generated by true recombination mechanisms such as must be involved in sister chromatid exchange (Moore and Holliday 1976), but such DNA_{HH} fragments are not chased into hybrid DNA on further incubation. In our experiments, both DNA_{int} and DNA_{HH} fractions are chased into hybrid DNA on continued incubation; therefore, our data are best accounted for by the notion that bypass reactions occur at the DNA growing point. We think that the inhibition of postreplication repair by caffeine may also result from the accumulation of unfinished replicons rather than by an inhibition of internal gap filling. In fact, the notion of a separate postreplication repair process is probably unnecessary, since the events that occur when synthesis encounters a strand containing a lesion are part of the general process of DNA replication. An understanding of the phenomena of DNA replication in mammalian cells is therefore a fundamental prerequisite to an understanding of carcinogenesis and mutagenesis.

SUMMARY

Human cells respond to carcinogen-induced damage in their DNA in at least two ways. The first response, excision repair, proceeds by at least three variations, depending on the nature of the damage. Nucleotide excision results in relatively large repair patches but few free DNA breaks, since the endonuclease step is limiting. Apurinic repair is characterized by the appearance of numerous breaks in the DNA and by short repair patches. The pathways behave as though they function independently. Lymphoid cells derived from a xeroderma pigmentosum complementation group C patient are deficient in their ability to perform nucleotide excision and also to excise 6 methoxyguanine adducts, but they are apurinic-repair competent. Since the UV endonuclease is not involved in excision of 6 methoxyguanine residues, the defect in xeroderma is multiple.

Organisms may bypass damage in their DNA. Lymphoblastoid cells, including those derived from xeroderma pigmentosum treated with ^{3}H-anti-BPDE, can replicate their DNA at low doses of carcinogen. Unexcised ^{3}H is found in the light or parental strand of the resulting hybrid DNA when replication occurs in medium with BrdUrd. We think that this observation indicates a bypass reaction occurring by a mechanism involving branch migration at DNA growing points. We have observed branch migration in DNA preparations, but the evidence is that most occurs in BrdUrd-containing DNA during cell lysis. The measurement of the bifilarly substituted DNA resulting from branch migration is a convenient method of estimating the proportion of new synthesis remaining in the vicinity of the DNA growing point. Treatment with carcinogens or caffeine results in accumulation of DNA growing points accompanied by the synthesis of shortened pieces of daughter DNA.

ACKNOWLEDGMENTS

The experimental work reported from this laboratory was supported by grants from the National Institutes of Health (GM 07816–19 and CA–14599) and Department of Energy (EY76 S–02–2040). We appreciate the aid of the National Cancer Institute, Carcinogenesis Research Program, in supplying radioactive benzpyrene diolepoxide. Kouichi Tatsumi is a fellow of the Leukemia Society of America.

REFERENCES

Ahmed, F., and R. Setlow. 1977. Different rate-limiting steps in excision repair of ultraviolet- and N-acetoxy-2 acetylaminofluorene-damaged DNA in normal human fibroblasts. Proc. Natl. Acad. Sci. USA 74:1548–1552.
Amacher, D., J. Elliott, and M. Lieberman. 1977. Differences in removal of acetylaminofluorene and pyrimidine dimers from the DNA of cultured mammalian cells. Proc. Natl. Acad. Sci. USA 74:1553–1557.
Andrews, A., J. Robbins, K. Kraemer, and D. Buell. 1974. *Xeroderma pigmentosum* long term lymphoid lines with increased ultraviolet sensitivity. J. Natl. Cancer Inst. 53:691–693.
Bockstahler, L., C. D. Lytle, J. Stafford, and K. Haynes. 1976. Ultraviolet enhanced reactivation of a human virus: Effect of delayed infection. Mutat. Res. 35:189–198.
Bose, K., P. Karran, and B. Strauss. 1978. Repair of depurinated DNA *in vitro* by enzymes purified from human lymphoblasts. Proc. Natl. Acad. Sci. USA 75:794–798.
Boyce, R., and P. Howard-Flanders. 1964. Release of ultraviolet light-induced thymine dimers from DNA in *E. coli* K-12. Proc. Natl. Acad. Sci. USA 51:293–300.
Caillet-Fauquet, P., M. Defais, and M. Radman. 1977. Molecular mechanisms of induced mutagenesis. Replication *in vivo* of bacteriophage ΦX174 single-stranded, ultraviolet light-irradiated DNA in intact and irradiated host cells. J. Mol. Biol. 117:95–110.
Cerutti, P. 1978. Repairable damage in DNA, *in* DNA Repair Mechanisms, P. Hanawalt, E. Friedberg, and C. Fox, eds. Academic Press, New York. (In press).
Cleaver, J., and D. Bootsma. 1975. Xeroderma pigmentosum: biochemical and genetic characteristics. Ann. Rev. Genet. 9:19–38.

Cooper, P., and P. Hanawalt. 1972. Heterogeneity of patch size in repair replicated DNA in *Escherichia coli.* J. Mol. Biol. 67:1–10.

Dipple, A., and J. Roberts. 1977. Excision of 7-bromomethyl benz *(a)* anthracene adducts in replicating mammalian cells. Biochemistry 16:1499–1503.

Doniger, J., and L. Grossman. 1976. Human correxonuclease. Purification and properties of a DNA repair exonuclease from placenta. J. Biol. Chem. 251:4579–4587.

Edenberg, H., and P. Hanawalt. 1972. Size of repair patches in the DNA of ultraviolet-irradiated HeLa cells. Biochim. Biophys. Acta 272:361–372.

Fornace, A., K. Kohn, and H. Kann. 1976. DNA single-strand breaks during repair of UV damage in human fibroblasts and abnormalities of repair in xeroderma pigmentosum. Proc. Natl. Acad. Sci. USA 73:39–43.

Ganesan, A. 1974. Persistence of pyrimidine dimers during postreplication repair in ultraviolet light irradiated *Escherichia coli* K12. J. Mol. Biol. 87:103–119.

Goth-Goldstein, R. 1977. Repair of DNA damaged by alkylating carcinogens is defective in xeroderma pigmentosum-derived fibroblasts. Nature 267:81–82.

Hanson, C., C. Chen, and J. Hearst. 1976. Cross-linking of DNA *in situ* as a probe for chromatin structure. Science 193:62–64.

Heflich, R., D. Dorney, V. Maher, and J. McCormick. 1977. Reactive derivatives of benzo(a)pyrene and 7,12-dimethylbenz(a)anthracene cause S_1 nuclease sensitive sites in DNA and "UV-like" repair. Biochem. Biophys. Res. Commun. 77:634–641.

Higgins, N. P., K. Kato, and B. Strauss. 1976. A model for replication repair in mammalian cells. J. Mol. Biol. 101:417–425.

Holliday, R., and J. Pugh. 1975. DNA modification mechanisms and gene activity during development. Science 187:226–232.

Howard-Flanders, P., R. Boyce, and L. Theriot. 1966. Three loci in *Escherichia coli* K-12 that control the excision of pyrimidine dimers and certain other mutagen products from DNA. Genetics 53:1119–1136.

Iyer, V., and W. Rupp. 1971. Usefulness of benzoylated naphthoylated DEAE cellulose to distinguish and fractionate double stranded DNA bearing different extents of single stranded regions. Biochim. Biophys. Acta 228:117–126.

Karran, P., N. P. Higgins, and B. Strauss. 1977. Intermediates in excision repair by human cells: Use of Sl nuclease and BND cellulose to reveal single strand breaks. Biochemistry 16:4483–4490.

Kato, K., and B. Strauss. 1974. Accumulation of an intermediate in DNA synthesis by HEp.2 cells treated with methyl methanesulfonate. Proc. Natl. Acad. Sci. USA 71:1969–1973.

Kraemer, K. 1977. Progressive degenerative diseases associated with defective DNA repair: Xeroderma pigmentosum and ataxia telangiectasia, *in* DNA Repair Processes, W. Nichols and D. Murphy, eds., Symposia Specialists, Miami, pp. 37–71.

Laval, J. 1977. Two enzymes are required for strand incision in repair of alkylated DNA. Nature 269:829–832.

Lavin, M. 1978. A model for postreplication repair of UV damage in mammalian cells. J. Supramol. Struct. (Suppl.) 2:83.

Lawley, P., and D. Orr. 1970. Specific excision of methylation products from DNA of *Escherichia coli* treated with N-methyl-N′-nitro-N-nitrosoguanidine. Chem. Biol. Interac. 2:154–157.

Lehmann, A. 1972a. Postreplication repair of DNA in ultraviolet-irradiated mammalian cells. J. Mol. Biol. 66:319–337.

Lehmann, A. 1972b. Effect of caffeine on DNA synthesis in mammalian cells. Biophys. J. 12:1316–1325.

Lehmann, A., and S. Kirk-Bell. 1978. Pyrimidine dimer sites associated with the daughter DNA strands in UV-irradiated human fibroblasts. Photochem. Photobiol. 27:297–308.

Lindahl, T. 1976. New class of enzymes acting on damaged DNA. Nature 259:64–66.

Lindahl, T., P. Karran, and S. Riazuddin. 1978. DNA glycosylases of *Escherichia coli.* J. Supramol. Struct. (Suppl.) 2:12.

Ljungquist, S. 1977. A new endonuclease from *Escherichia coli* acting at apurinic sites in DNA. J. Biol. Chem. 252:2808–2814.

McCann, J., and B. Ames. 1976. Detection of carcinogens as mutagens in the *Salmonella/*microsome test: Assay of 300 chemicals: Discussion. Proc. Natl. Acad. Sci. USA 73:950–954.

Meneghini, R., and P. Hanawalt. 1976. T4-endonuclease V-sensitive sites in DNA from ultraviolet-irradiated human cells. Biochim. Biophys. Acta 425:428–437.

Miller, R. 1977. Cancer and congenital malformations: Another view, *in* The Genetics of Human Cancer, J. Mulvihill, ed., Raven Press, New York, pp. 77–79.

Moore, P., and R. Holliday. 1976. Evidence for the formation of hybrid DNA during mitotic recombination in Chinese hamster cells. Cell 8:573–579.

Myers, T., and B. Strauss. 1971. Effect of methyl methanesulfonate on synchronized cultures of HEp.2 cells. Nature New Biol. 230:143–144.

Painter, R., and B. Young. 1972. Repair replication in mammalian cells after X-irradiation. Mutat. Res. 14:225–235.

Paterson, M. C. 1979. Environmental carcinogenesis and imperfect repair of damaged DNA in *Homo sapiens:* Causal relation revealed by rare hereditary disorders, *in* Carcinogens: Identification and Mechanisms of Action (The University of Texas System Cancer Center 31st Annual Symposium on Fundamental Cancer Research, 1978), A. C. Griffin and C. R. Shaw, eds., Raven Press, New York, pp. 251–276.

Prakash, L., and B. Strauss. 1970. Repair of alkylation damage: Stability of methyl groups in *Bacillus subtilis* treated with methyl methanesulfonate. J. Bacteriol. 102:760–766.

Regan, J., and R. Setlow. 1974. Two forms of repair in the DNA of human cells damaged by chemical carcinogens and mutagens. Cancer Res. 34:3318–3325.

Sarasin, A., and P. Hanawalt. 1978. Carcinogens enhance survival of UV-irradiated simian virus 40 in treated monkey kidney cells: Induction of a recovery pathway? Proc. Natl. Acad. Sci. USA 75:346–350.

Scudiero, D., and B. Strauss. 1974. Accumulation of single-stranded regions in DNA and the block to replication in a human cell line alkylated with methyl methane sulfonate. J. Mol. Biol. 83:17–32.

Scudiero, D., E. Henderson, A. Norin, and B. Strauss. 1975. The measurement of chemically induced DNA repair synthesis in human cells by BND-cellulose chromatography. Mutat. Res. 29:473–488.

Scudiero, D., A. Norin, P. Karran, and B. Strauss. 1976. DNA excision-repair deficiency of human peripheral blood lymphocytes treated with chemical carcinogens. Cancer Res. 36:1397–1403.

Setlow, R., and W. Carrier. 1964. The disappearance of thymine dimers from DNA: An error-correcting mechanism. Proc. Natl. Acad. Sci. USA 51:226–231.

Setlow, P., and A. Kornberg. 1972. Deoxyribonucleic acid polymerase: Two distinct enzymes in one polypeptide. II. A proteolytic fragment containing the $5'$-$3'$ exonuclease function. Restoration of intact enzyme functions from the two proteolytic fragments. J. Biol. Chem. 247:232–240.

Singer, B. 1976. All oxygens in nucleic acids react with carcinogenic ethylating agents. Nature 264:333–339.

Strauss, B. 1977. Molecular biology of the response of cells to radiation and to radiomimetic chemicals. Cancer 40:471–480.

Strauss, B., D. Scudiero, and E. Henderson. 1975. The nature of the alkylation lesion in mammalian cells, *in* Molecular Mechanisms for Repair of DNA, Part A, P. Hanawalt and B. Setlow, eds., Plenum Press, New York, pp. 13–24.

Tatsumi, K., and B. Strauss. 1978. Production of DNA bifilarly substituted with bromodeoxyuridine in the first round of synthesis: Branch migration during isolation of cellular DNA. Nucleic Acids Res. 5:331–347.

Thompson, B., M. Camien, and R. Warner. 1976. Kinetics of branch migration in double-stranded DNA. Proc. Natl. Acad. Sci. USA 73:2299–2303.

Tye, B., J. Chien, I. Lehman, B. Duncan, and H. Warner. 1978. Uracil incorporation: A source of pulse-labeled DNA fragments in the replication of the *Escherichia coli* chromosome. Proc. Natl. Acad. Sci. USA 75:233–237.

Tye, B., P. Nyman, I. Lehman, S. Hochhauser, and B. Weiss. 1977. Transient accumulation of Okazaki fragments as a result of uracil incorporation into nascent DNA. Proc. Natl. Acad. Sci. USA 74:154–157.

Carcinogens: Identification and Mechanisms
of Action, edited by A. Clark Griffin and
Charles R. Shaw. Raven Press, New York © 1979.

Environmental Carcinogenesis and Imperfect Repair of Damaged DNA in *Homo sapiens:* Causal Relation Revealed by Rare Hereditary Disorders

M. C. Paterson

*Biology and Health Physics Division, Atomic Energy of Canada Limited,
Chalk River, Ontario KOJ 1JO, Canada*

One of the most significant advances in cancer research during the last two decades has been the realization that most human malignancies have their causes in the environment (see Higginson 1979, pages 187 to 208, this volume, Doll 1977). In recent years much effort has been expended in the identification of physical and chemical carcinogens in the environment, and standards have been introduced to minimize exposures in the workplace in particular (see Shubik 1979, pages 39 to 49, this volume, Brusick 1979, pages 95 to 107, this volume, and Bridges 1976). The concept of a carcinogen-free biosphere seems unattainable in practice, however, even if a list of all environmental hazards were readily at hand. From experience with cigarette smoking and lung cancer, it appears unlikely that society would appreciably alter its life-style even when confronted with an association between a known "cultural" carcinogen and increased risk of malignancy (e.g., dietary factor and colon neoplasm). In many cases we are therefore left with the difficult task of conducting risk-benefit assessments to assist society in evaluating the dangers and benefits of any given agent. Quantitative risk estimates are currently obtained by extrapolation from limited experiences with animals and humans at relatively high levels of exposure. The more relevant exposure-effect data at very low levels (where practical thresholds may exist) are simply not, nor are they likely to become, available. The consensus among researchers is that refinement in these estimates will require clarification of the basic mechanisms by which normal cells give rise to tumors. Moreover, a fuller understanding of the fundamental processes involved may be expected to point out improved strategies for preventive and curative measures.

Other contributions in this volume indicate that steady progress is being made in elucidating the chain(s) of events leading to the inception of the cancerous state. This article bears on a particular aspect of the problem, namely, the role of carcinogen-induced damage to DNA and its inefficient enzymatic repair in the initiation of neoplastic transformation. Evidence that such damage to

251

the genetic material can be an etiologic factor stems largely from the discovery that in certain rare genetic disorders, affected individuals are predisposed to cancer and their cells in culture exhibit hallmarks of deficient repair of DNA damage. This association is well documented for the prototype disease, xeroderma pigmentosum (XP), and to a lesser extent for two others, ataxia telangiectasia (AT) and Fanconi's anemia (FA). My primary intention here is to review the current state of knowledge concerning these three diseases, with emphasis on the most recent data, and to discuss the implications of these findings to general theories of environmental carcinogenesis.

BASIC DNA REPAIR MECHANISMS IN HUMAN CELLS

The following brief description of popular models of the three basic repair mechanisms operative in cultured human cells—excision repair, postreplication repair, and photoenzymatic repair—is provided as background to the main topic, namely, repair characteristics of XP, AT, and FA cells. These three mechanisms are in fact ubiquitous throughout the animal and plant kingdoms (Cleaver 1974). (A current comprehensive treatise on the subject of DNA repair mechanisms is that of Hanawalt *et al.,* in press.)

Excision Repair

As is implicit in the name, in the excision-repair process, remedial action is accomplished by the release of a defective single-strand region followed by replacement with undamaged nucleotides, utilizing the complementary intact strand for base-pairing instructions. Two different modes are known: (1) nucleotide excision repair (Grossman, in press) and (2) base excision repair (Friedberg *et al.,* in press). In the former, a damaged base residue is excised, presumably within an oligonucleotide, by two sequential single-strand nicks, the first by a specific damage-recognizing endonuclease and the second by an exonuclease; a DNA polymerase then inserts correct nucleotides into the gap, and finally the site is sealed by a polynucleotide ligase. In the latter mode, a modified base, such as uracil (deaminated cytosine) or 3-methyladenine, is released as a free base by a DNA glycosylase (formerly called N-glycosidase). The site containing the remaining denuded sugar moiety (apurinic/apyrimidinic site) is then replaced in the same fashion as described above for nucleotide excision repair; that is, the combined action of an apurinic/apyrimidinic endonuclease and exonuclease cuts out the damage, and the site is restored to a normal configuration by repair synthesis and strand ligation. It is not clear why different excision strategies are effected by different lesions. Generally, lesions expected to cause major alterations in base pairing and base stacking, such as cyclobutyl pyrimidine dimers induced by ultraviolet (UV) radiation and adducts produced by reactive metabolites of 2-acetylaminofluorene (AAF), are supposedly removed as part of oligonucleotides, whereas those lesions causing only minor helix distortion such as uracil and 3-methyladenine, are released as free bases prior to incision of the DNA backbone. This preliminary step may ensure that the damage site, once incised, is committed to excision/resynthesis before ligation and not to abortive rounds of incision/ligation without site restoration.

A virtue of the excision-repair mechanism is its extreme versatility; it can act on a seemingly limitless range of alterations in the heterocyclic bases including mono- and difunctional base defects, bulky adducts, intercalation damage, and DNA-protein cross-links. This capacity derives from a battery of lesion-attacking DNA glycosylases and endonucleases. In addition, single-strand breaks produced directly in the sugar-phosphate backbones by ionizing radiation, for example, are believed to be rejoined by exonucleolytic degradation, repair synthesis, and ligation. Enzymes possessing the properties deemed necessary for mediating steps in the two modes of excision repair have been detected in human cell extracts. These include uracil DNA glycosylase (Kuhnlein *et al.* 1978a), apurinic/apyrimidinic and UV (pyrimidine dimer-recognizing) endonucleases (Linsley *et al.* 1977, Moses and Beaudet 1978, Kuhnlein *et al.* 1978b, Mortelmans *et al.* 1976), exonucleases (Cook and Friedberg 1978), DNA β-polymerase (Bertazzoni *et al.* 1976), and polynucleotide ligase (Söderhäll and Lindahl 1976). While many of these human enzymes have been purified to varying extents, efforts to isolate the putative UV endonuclease have been futile, presumably foiled at least in part by the freezing-lability of the enzyme (or a related activity) (Duncan *et al.* 1975).

A large number of physical and chemical carcinogens are capable of inflicting damage on DNA, and the number of reaction products is even larger because each agent generally produces a broad spectrum of alterations (Cerutti, in press). The vast majority of these chemically distinct lesions seems to be handled by the two modes of excision repair. The size of the "repair patches" inserted at sites of excised damage can vary greatly, depending on the lesion and, to a certain extent, the repair mode utilized; patches arising from base excision repair are expected to be much shorter (possibly one to several nucleotides in length) than those resulting from nucleotide excision repair (known, in some cases, to contain as many as 100 nucleotides or more [Cleaver 1974]). As a general rule, bulky lesions (e.g., pyrimidine dimers) give rise to much longer patches than do those causing only minor distortions in the double helix (e.g., alkylation products of methyl methanesulfonate [MMS]). Regan and Setlow (1974) have classified chemical carcinogens on the basis of patch size induced and the kinetics of the repair process: Those, such as MMS, giving rise to short patches (several nucleotides) during a brief period (<60 minutes) mimic ionizing radiation and are referred to as "ionizing-like"; those, such as N-acetoxy-AAF, that induce long patches (~100 nucleotides) over an extended period (~20 hours) mimic UV radiation and are thus "UV-like"; and those, such as 4-nitroquinoline-1-oxide (4NQO), that elicit both responses are "ionizing- and UV-like."

Postreplication Repair

DNA synthesized in mammalian cells shortly after UV irradiation is initially smaller than that made in unirradiated cells. Upon subsequent incubation the nascent DNA is converted to parental size molecules. Postreplication repair (also termed replicative or bypass repair) is the name given to this poorly understood conversion process (Lehmann 1974). Two basic models have been proposed: (1) Upon encountering UV photoproducts, such as dimers, the replication apparatus skips past and reinitiates beyond, leaving large gaps that are eventually closed by de novo synthesis (Lehmann 1974); (2) the replication machinery pauses momentarily when reaching lesions and in some fashion eventually circumvents the lesions (Edenberg 1976). Both models may in fact exist, depending upon experimental conditions and cell type (Lehmann, in press). Regardless of the strategy, albeit by discontinuous (model 1) or continuous (model 2) synthesis, it is necessary to allow for the insertion of the correct nucleotide sequence opposite a lesion-containing site. The information could be obtained by recombinational exchanges between sister or homologous chromatids. Detection of dimers induced in parental DNA at later times in daughter DNA would argue for the occurrence of recombination events; however, the evidence for dimer exchanges is controversial (Lehmann, in press). (Since man is diploid, recombination exchanges between homologous genetic material need not be confined to G_2 phase but could conceivably occur at any time in the cell cycle; in fact, there is some evidence for prereplicative recombination repair in fungi [Gentner 1977].) An alternative proposal for which there is limited experimental evidence permits information retrieval by continuous de novo synthesis (Higgins et al. 1976); that is, upon reaching a lesion, DNA synthesis proceeds in the strand not containing the lesion but is impeded in the other strand by the presence of the lesion. This newly synthesized single strand could then be displaced and serve as a template for continuation of synthesis in the second strand, thereby circumventing the lesion,\using a native template. For some obscure reason, cells start to synthesize DNA pieces of normal size at later times after UV treatment (see Lehmann, in press). While the manner in which damaged cells replicate their DNA is currently highly controversial, it is nevertheless crucial to gain greater insight into the steps involved, because postreplication repair, unlike excision repair, appears to have an error-prone component (Roberts 1978).

Photoenzymatic Repair

Conceptually at least, this is the simplest of the three mechanisms. Pyrimidine dimers are the sole lesions acted upon by this mechanism. In this process, dimers are monomerized in situ by a photolyase in a two-step reaction: The photoreactivating enzyme binds to a dimer-containing site, and then, upon absorption of photon energy in the wavelength range 300–600 nm by the enzyme-DNA complex, the photoproduct is converted back to two normal monomers

(Sutherland, in press). Such photolyases have been detected in human lymphocytes and cultured cells (Sutherland 1974, Sutherland *et al.* 1975). Light-dependent disappearance of pyrimidine dimers from DNA has also been observed in UV-damaged human fibroblasts (Sutherland *et al.* 1975); this can be ascribed to photoenzymatic repair. The light-induced dimer loss is only seen under strict culture conditions (Sutherland and Oliver 1976; Mortelmans *et al.* 1977), thereby possibly explaining why, despite extensive efforts, evidence for this photorepair mechanism has gone undetected for so long (Cook 1970).

The requirement for visible light as a cofactor in dimer monomerization by the photolyase enables the investigator to employ photoenzymatic repair selectively. This property has been exploited as an analytical tool to implicate dimers as the photoproducts responsible for many of the effects of UV radiation; dimers can, for example, decrease survival of UV-damaged herpes simplex virus (assayed on human cells) and inhibit de novo DNA synthesis in irradiated human fibroblasts (Sutherland 1977).

The discovery of photoenzymatic repair in human cells sets us the task of determining the role of this process in ameliorating the deleterious effects of solar ultraviolet radiation in vivo. Since skin neoplasms attributed to actinic damage are the most prevalent human cancers, advances in this line of research would seem particularly relevant to the study of environmental carcinogenesis.

Novel Repair Mechanisms

There is some evidence that the battery of repair mechanisms in mammalian systems is not limited to the three mechanisms discussed here. Extracts of human origin have been reported to contain an activity of an enzyme that is capable of simply inserting a normal base at an apurinic/apyrimidinic site (Linn *et al.*, in press). Repair might then be achieved by the concerted actions of a DNA glycosylase and an "insertase" without cutting the DNA backbone. An activity has also been detected in extracts of rat liver tissue which can apparently remove the methyl group in the O^6 position of guanine (Pegg 1977, Pegg and Hui, in press); in this case, there would be no need to excise the modified base. O^6-alkylguanine products are regarded as the critical lesions formed by many alkylating agents, and it will be of importance to assay for the presence of a "demethylase" in tissue of human origin.

EFFECT OF CHROMATIN STRUCTURE ON INDUCTION AND REPAIR OF DNA DAMAGE

The study of DNA repair in mammals has been greatly influenced over the years by models derived from more sophisticated experimentation in bacteria, especially *Escherichia coli*. It is now quite evident, however, that these prokaryotic models do have certain limitations when applied to eukaryotes. In particular, there is a growing awareness of the need to take into account the complex structural organization of mammalian chromatin. Mammalian DNA is now believed to be structurally organized into nucleosomes consisting of core DNA (~140 base pairs wrapped around four pairs of histones) and linker DNA (up to 50 base pairs [Kornberg 1977]). Consideration of chromatin structure would appear to be necessary not only when studying the intragenomic distribution of carcinogen-induced damage but also when monitoring the remedial actions of repair processes. Reaction products formed by chemical carcinogens are generally not distributed randomly throughout the genome but are usually found in higher yield in micrococcal nuclease-accessible regions of the DNA (Moses *et al.* 1976, Ramanathan *et al.* 1976, Jahn and Litman 1977, Metzger *et al.* 1977). These findings presumably reflect the relative ease of accessibility of chemical carcinogens to targets in linker DNA compared to core DNA. Recent data also suggest that chromatin structure influences the rate of excision repair. For example, methylated products arising from dimethylnitrosamine treatment disappear more slowly from nuclease-inaccessible than from nuclease-accessible fractions of DNA in rat liver cells in vivo (Ramanathan *et al.* 1976). Furthermore, analysis of the distribution of repair patches in UV-damaged human fibroblasts at various times after UV exposure indicates that photoproducts are preferentially excised from linker DNA (Cleaver 1977a). This is consistent with earlier studies in which dimers were shown to disappear from DNA at two different rates (Paterson *et al.* 1973), those associated with nuclear proteins being removed at the slower rate (Wilkins and Hart 1974). These results raise the possibility that cofactors may be required in order for a putative UV endonuclease to gain access to its substrate in DNA associated with nuclear proteins. Whether a single repair process acts on all dimers regardless of their intragenomic location or different repair processes preferentially remove dimers from core DNA than from linker DNA is an open question.

Within the same eukaryotic species, DNA repair capacity can vary greatly from one cell type to another. This is presumably due to changes in the pattern of gene expression during development. The rate of de novo DNA synthesis typically decreases with increasing cellular differentiation, and this change is usually accompanied by a reduction in the ability to carry out various modes of DNA repair. Terminally differentiated cells, such as myotubes and neurons, are less capable of repairing damage induced by various physical and chemical carcinogens (e.g., UV and ionizing radiations, MMS, AAF, and 4NQO) than are their proliferating progenitor cells (Hahn *et al.* 1971, Stockdale 1971, Chan *et al.* 1976, McCombe *et al.* 1976, Karran *et al.* 1977). The capacity to excise pyrimidine dimers is closely linked with developmental state in the mouse (Peleg *et al.* 1976). Early passage cells cultured from 13- to 15-day embryos are excision proficient, whereas similar passage cells from 17- to 19-day embryos are not nor are cells from adult animals. The excision competence of the cells from 13- to 15-day embryos decreases with passage number, and this closely parallels a reduction in growth rate. In two highly differentiated model systems, mouse neuroblastoma cells (McCombe *et al.* 1976) and human peripheral blood lymphocytes (Scudiero *et al.* 1976) (but not in a third—neural retinal cells of embryonic chick origin [Karran *et al.* 1977]), artificially induced stimulation of de novo DNA synthesis is accompanied by increased repair capacity. A relatively low repair competence has been causally implicated in tissue-specific tumorigenesis in fetal rats: Ethylnitrosourea (ENU) selectively induces tumors in neural tissue, and this correlates with the persistence of O^6-ethylguanine (one of the alkylation products caused by ENU) in brain, compared to liver, DNA (Goth and Rajewsky 1974). These data, taken together, indicate that the genes coding for mammalian repair enzymes may be turned on and off at different stages in development, and understanding the control of their expression represents one of the most exciting challenges to researchers in the field.

HUMAN DISEASES LINKED WITH DNA REPAIR DEFECTS

XP, AT, and FA—the three diseases for which an association between high cancer risk and defective DNA repair is best established—are multisystem, degenerative disorders that are inherited as simple autosomal recessive traits (Kraemer 1977, Setlow 1978). All three afflictions are rare; XP and FA occur at a frequency of ~2 per million, whereas AT is about 10-fold more common, i.e., ~25 per million. Both XP and FA patients often result from consanguinous matings (Mulvihill 1975, Gmyrek and Syllm-Rapoport 1964); however, there is no indication that the incidence of inbreeding is any higher in AT families than in the society-at-large. A high incidence of XP has been reported among Arabs in North America (Miller 1977), while AT is unusually high among Moroccan Jews in Israel (Levin and Perlov 1971).

Xeroderma pigmentosum

The clinical features of this disease are outlined in Table 1 (for details, consult Robbins *et al.* 1974, Kraemer 1977). The major target organ is the skin, and the most notable abnormality is hypersensitivity to solar radiation as chiefly reflected by pigmentation changes, elevated erythema, and multiple neoplasms. Basal and squamous cell carcinomas are the most prevalent types, although malignant melanomas are also seen. Tumor incidence increases with age, and by puberty as many as 100 or more cancers per patient are common. Death usually occurs by the fourth decade due to metastatic carcinoma and wasting (Pathak and Epstein 1971). Various ocular changes, including photophobia, develop in parallel with the skin lesions. Clinicians distinguish two forms of the disease: (1) classical XP, displaying skin (and ocular) complications only, and (2) neurological XP, in which a wide range of central nervous system (CNS) deficiencies accompany the skin lesions (Robbins *et al.* 1974, Kraemer 1977). The vast majority of the neurological XP patients develop only a few of the CNS abnormalities listed in Table 1; however, in the extreme case, de Sanctis-Cacchione syndrome, most and often all seven changes are present. The two clinical forms are approximately equal in prevalence and appear to be geneti-

TABLE 1. *Clinical hallmarks of xeroderma pigmentosum*

Cutaneous Abnormalities (sun-exposed areas)
  Dryness and scaling, hypo- and hyperpigmentation, erythema, keratoses, excessive freckling
  Multiple cancers (basal and squamous cell carcinomas, melanomas)
Ocular Abnormalities
  Photophobia, pigment and telangiectatic changes (lids)
  Cancers (as above, plus epitheliomas)
Neurological Abnormalities (variable*)
  Microcephaly, mental retardation, ataxia, areflexia, dwarfism, sexual dysfunction, choreoathetosis
Etiology
  Autosomal recessive trait, Prevalence—1–4 per 10^6
  Blood relatives—elevated risk of skin cancer

---

* Two clinical forms: classical, neurological.
From Robbins *et al.* 1974, Kraemer 1977.

cally distinct. The disease has been successfully diagnosed prenatally by observing an abnormal response of cultured amniotic cells to UV irradiation (Ramsay *et al.* 1974). Early detection is critical to proper prophylatic care, as XP patients, if placed on a well-planned photoprotection regimen from birth, can enjoy reasonably long and productive lives (Lynch *et al.* 1977).

Colony survival after a given UV fluence is lower in XP cells than in normal cells. The degree of hypersensitivity varies greatly from one XP strain to another, ranging from slightly above normal to 30-fold (Table 2). XP strains display cross-sensitivity to certain chemical carcinogens, including reactive forms of polycyclic hydrocarbons (e.g., "K-region" epoxides of benzo[a]pyrene) and aromatic amides (e.g., 4NQO) but respond normally to ionizing radiation, monofunctional alkylating agents (e.g., N-methyl-N′-nitro-N-nitrosoguanidine [MNNG]), and the DNA–cross-linking agent, mitomycin C (MMC) (Maher *et*

TABLE 2. *Sensitivities of XP, AT and FA fibroblasts*

Cell type	Complementation group	Carcinogen	Ratio of 10% survival treatments
XP	A	UV	6,18
	C	UV	4–7
	D	UV	12
	Variant	UV	1–1.4
AT	A	X-, γ-rays	3.2
	B	X-, γ-rays	3.1
	Variant	X-, γ-rays	3.2
FA	?	MMC	5
	?	MMC	15

Data from Cleaver 1977b, Paterson, in press.

al. 1975, Maher and McCormick 1976, Arlett 1977, Fujiwara et al. 1977, Setlow 1978). Cells from affected individuals also have a reduced capacity to reactivate UV-inactivated phage, assayed on the basis of either plaque-forming ability (Day 1974) or production of viral structural antigens (Rainbow 1978).

On the basis of knowledge gained from studies on microbial systems (see Grossman et al. 1975), the abnormal UV response of XP cells in these two measures of cell function (colony-forming ability and host-cell reactivation) suggests that the molecular defect in XP cells lies in the repair of UV-induced DNA damage. There are now extensive biochemical and biophysical data on the DNA repair properties of UV-treated XP strains in support of this notion (Cleaver and Bootsma 1975, Kraemer 1977, Setlow 1978). All strains are defective in one or more of the three basic repair mechanisms operating on UV photoproducts (Table 3). Cells established from all neurological XP patients and from most classical XP patients are deficient, to varying extents, in excision repair. This conclusion is supported by data on several molecular endpoints: removal of dimers (Cleaver 1974, Cleaver and Bootsma 1975), disappearance of UV endonuclease-sensitive sites (Paterson et al. 1973), and repair-synthesis level as monitored directly by unscheduled DNA synthesis (UDS) or repair replication (Cleaver 1974), or indirectly by photolysis of incorporated bromo deoxyuridine (BrdUrd) (Regan et al. 1971). Comparative clinical and biochemical analyses of patients whose cells are deficient in excision repair have revealed that the degree of deficiency in excision repair in vitro correlates directly with the severity of the clinical complications of the disease (Bootsma 1977). There are several exceptions to this correlation; these may reflect variable environmental factors that can affect the clinical picture, e.g., amount of solar radiation received by a patient.

The XP strains that are deficient in excision repair have been subdivided

TABLE 3. *DNA repair properties of different genetic forms of XP*

Group	Clinical features Cutaneous	Clinical features Neurological	Excision repair (% of normal)	Postreplication repair	Photolyase (% of normal)
A*	+	+	<2	Partly def.	36
B	+	?	3–7	Partly def.	0
C	+	−	10–20	Partly def.	16
D	+	+	25–50	Partly def.	8
E	+	−	>60	Proficient	49
F	+	−	10	?	?
G	+	?	?	?	?
Variant	+	−	100	Markedly def.	<20

+, present; −, absent; ?, unknown.
* De Sanctis-Cacchione syndrome.
   Data from Robbins et al. 1974, Lehmann et al. 1975, Sutherland et al. 1975, Sutherland 1977, Takebe 1978, Bootsma, in press.

on the basis of a complementation analysis, using the technique of somatic cell hybridization (Kraemer *et al.* 1975). Two strains are assigned to different complementation groups if, upon cell fusion, both nuclei of binuclear hybrid cells exhibit near-normal levels of UV-induced UDS; alternatively, if the UDS levels remain reduced in the hybrids, the two strains are allocated to the same group. To date, seven complementation groups have been identified (see Table 3) (Kraemer *et al.* 1975, Takebe 1978, Bootsma, in press), and there is no reason to conclude that the list is complete—that is, mutations in no less than seven different loci affecting dimer excision can give rise to the XP phenotype. In binuclear hybrids from two strains of different complementation groups, execution of repair replication, removal of UV endonuclease-sensitive sites, and host-cell reactivation are also normal in all combinations tested (deWeerd-Kastelein *et al.* 1973, Paterson *et al.* 1974, Day *et al.* 1975).

Despite the multiplicity of complementation groups, all excision repair-deficient XP strains appear to be blocked at the incision step. Not only are fewer single-strand nicks observed in these XP cells than in normal cells during post-UV incubation (Fornace *et al.* 1976, Cleaver 1974) but the introduction of dimer-specific T4 endonuclease V into such UV-damaged XP cells restores repair replication to normal and enhances colony-forming ability (Tanaka *et al.* 1977). The simplest explanation for the basic molecular defects in these XP strains— alterations in different subunits comprising the putative human UV endonuclease—does not seem likely for groups A, C, and D, at least, because cell extracts from representative strains of each of these groups excise dimers from UV-treated "naked" DNA with normal kinetics (Table 4) (Mortelmans *et al.* 1976). However, group A-cell extracts are defective in removing dimers from UV-damaged chromatin, despite the presence of normal levels of exonuclease activity. Thus, the mutated loci in group A cells may possibly code for a cofactor, such as a DNA-unwinding protein, involved in the repair of chromatin.

Other data suggest that certain XP loci may regulate genes controlling the expression of multiple repair enzymes or related proteins that affect different repair pathways. Strains falling into groups A-D are partially deficient in postreplication repair, while a group A strain does not recover normal rates of de novo DNA synthesis several hours after UV exposure (Rudé and Friedberg 1977); moreover, strains belonging to groups A-E have reduced levels of photolyase (see Table 3), and those in groups A and D do not possess normal levels of apurinic/apyrimidinic endonuclease activity (Kuhnlein *et al.* 1976,1978b). (None of these studies has been performed as yet on strains in groups F and G.) The repair properties of rodent cells, as discussed earlier, are consistent with the notion that mammalian DNA repair processes are under complex genetic control. Others have argued that repair enzymes might possibly form part of a coordinated complex and that defects in XP loci may lead to instability of the complex; this has been invoked to explain the existence of different rate-limiting steps for the removal of dimers and N-acetoxy-AAF adducts in human cells (Ahmed and Setlow 1977). It is also possible that artificial cell fusion,

TABLE 4. *Excision of dimers by crude extracts of human cells*

Cell type	UV-damaged substrate	
	Purified DNA	Chromatin
Normal	+	+
XP A	+	−
XP C	+	?
XP D	+	+
XP Variant	+	−

+, proficient; −, deficient; ?, unknown.
Data from Friedberg *et al.* 1977.

employing inactivated Sendai virus, may modify gene expression to the extent that complementation in vitro does not reflect the number of different genotypes giving rise to the XP phenotypes (Cleaver 1977b). An explanation of the primary biochemical defect(s) in XP is crucial to a fuller understanding of the relation between imperfect DNA repair and the biological consequences of exposure to carcinogens.

The so-called XP variants constitute a minority of the strains from persons having the classical form of XP. Such XP strains are proficient in excision repair but are deficient in postreplication repair after UV treatment (see Table 3) (Lehmann *et al.* 1975). These variants, like the excision-repair deficient strains, possess reduced levels of photolyase activity; the residual levels vary greatly from strain to strain (Table 3) (Sutherland 1977). It would thus appear that the variant strains are also impaired in photoenzymatic repair. Nonetheless, their post-UV colony-forming ability is only slightly below normal. However, in many variants, caffeine greatly potentiates cell killing by UV light. Although complementation analysis has not been conducted on these strains as yet, different degrees of caffeine potentiation of UV-induced killing suggest genetic heterogeneity in the variant group (Fujiwara 1978).

The mutation frequency induced by UV is well above normal in the XP variant strains, not only when expressed per unit UV fluence but also per survivor (Maher *et al.* 1976). In contrast, the XP strains deficient in excision repair are only hypermutable when the mutation frequency is given as a function of UV fluence, and not survival (Maher and McCormick 1976). These observations provide good biological evidence that postreplication repair is relatively error prone, whereas excision repair is error free, at least in response to UV damage.

A capacity to repair damaged DNA seems to be particularly critical for the maintenance of a functional nervous system. Andrews and co-workers (1976) have found, for a number of XP patients, an inverse correlation between the post-UV colony-forming ability of a strain and the severity of the neurological complications in the donor. Neurons in the CNS cease to divide after two years of age (Robbins *et al.* 1974); hence, efficient DNA repair processes are

TABLE 5. Cytogenetic features of XP, AT, and FA cells

Cell type	Chromosome aberrations		SCE's*	
	Spontaneous	Induced	Spontaneous	Induced
XP	N	+	N	+/Nt
AT	+	+	N	N
FA	+	+	N	−

* Sister chromatid exchanges.
† Varies from one complementation group to another.
Data from Cleaver 1977b, Paterson, in press.

apparently required to prevent accelerated loss of neurons (due to death), as observed in XP patients with neurological abnormalities. As noted elsewhere, XP variant strains (proficient in excision repair) are derived exclusively from classical XP patients (free of CNS deficits), indicating that the excision-repair process is especially important to nonregenerating tissues, including those of the nervous system.

The cytogenetic picture in XP is summarized in Table 5. The yields of chromosome aberrations and sister chromatid exchanges (SCE's) in untreated XP cells do not differ significantly from those in normal cells (German 1972, Wolff et al. 1975). Consequently, the repair defects in XP cells do not appear to influence the spontaneous occurrence of either type of cytogenetic event. XP strains display more chromosome breakage than normal cells upon treatment with UV light or "UV-like" carcinogens but not "ionizing-like" carcinogens (Bartram et al. 1976, Sasaki 1973, Wolff et al. 1977). All three types of carcinogens induce above normal frequencies of SCE's in most, but not all, XP strains deficient in excision repair; in contrast, UV exposure results in normal levels of SCE's in XP variants (Wolff et al. 1977, deWeerd-Kastelein et al. 1977). Such data, coupled with the observation that chromosome aberrations but not SCE's can be prevented by photoreactivation, led Wolff (1978) to hypothesize that chromosome aberrations arise from inefficient repair of major lesions (e.g., pyrimidine dimers), whereas SCE's reflect the persistence in damaged DNA of unidentified minor lesions.

Transformation by SV40 virus occurs at a normal rate in XP strains, both when untreated and when UV-treated prior to viral infection (Parrington et al. 1971, Key and Todaro 1974).

Ataxia telangiectasia

As can be seen in Table 6, this progressive multifaceted disorder features the simultaneous occurrence of neurological, oculocutaneous, and immunological complications (for clinical details, see Sedgwick and Boder 1972, Kraemer 1977). Diagnosis is typically made in early childhood from the joint appearance of

TABLE 6. *Clinical hallmarks of ataxia telangiectasia*

Neurological Abnormalities
   Progressive cerebellar ataxia
   Atrophy of cerebellar cortex (purkinje and granular cells)
   Other (ocular dyspraxia, hyporeflexia, choreoathetosis)
Oculocutaneous Abnormalities
   Progressive telangiectases
     Bulbar conjunctiva, exposed and friction areas of skin
   Progeric changes of hair and skin in adults
Immunological Abnormalities (variable)
   Repeated sinopulmonary infections
   Absent or hypoplastic thymus
   Impaired cell-mediated and humoral systems
   Lymphoproliferative cancers (lymphomas, lymphatic leukemias)
Other Abnormalities
   Unusual sensitivity to radiotherapy
   Hepatic dysfunction (elevated α-fetoprotein)
   Short stature, gonadal dysgenesis (variable)
Etiology
   Autosomal recessive trait, prevalence—25 per 10^6, universal
   Mild clinical signs in heterozygous carriers (sporadic)

From Sedgwick and Boder 1972, Kraemer 1977.

cerebellar ataxia and telangiectases of the bulbar conjunctivae and skin. Persons with the syndrome are prone to repeated bouts of respiratory infection in association with immune deficiencies, involving the humoral and/or cell-mediated systems. The immunodeficiencies are attributable to an absent or rudimentary thymus. It is estimated that afflicted patients stand a 10% chance of developing cancers at an early age, 85% of which are lymphomas and lymphatic leukemias. This cancer risk is over 100 times greater than that of an age-matched control population. Patients seldom live beyond early adulthood, typically succumbing to various respiratory ailments and/or lymphoproliferative neoplasms. A consistent in vitro feature of the disease is an elevated level of α-fetoprotein. The recent discovery that AT patients react adversely (sometimes fatally) to standard radiotherapy (e.g., see Cunliffe *et al.* 1975) has stimulated laboratory studies into the radioresponses of AT cells in vitro.

There are scattered reports that an AT gene can also have some clinical effect in the heterozygous state. Some AT heterozygotes exhibit certain characteristics of the disorder; these include defective immunity (e.g., autoimmunity) (Friedman *et al.* 1977), oculocutaneous telangiectases (Sedgwick and Boder 1972), and propensity to cancer (Swift *et al.* 1976). The last complication is of some public health concern, as it can be estimated that ~1% of the general population is heterozygous for AT.

Increased sensitivity to inactivation by ionizing radiation is characteristic of diploid fibroblasts from affected patients. Furthermore, the extent of hypersensitivity is far less variable than that for UV-induced killing of XP cells. X- and γ-ray survival data have been obtained for no less than 11 strains to date, and all 11 strains are ~3.2 times more sensitive to inactivation by acute exposure to these two types of low LET (linear energy transfer) radiation than are normal cells (see Table 2) (Taylor *et al.* 1975, Paterson, in press, our unpublished data) AT strains are also more sensitive to high LET radiation; in this case the differ- ence in sensitivity is only ~1.4 for neutrons (Myers *et al.,* in press), indicating that the genetic defect in AT strains is less crucial to the repair of damage inflicted by high than low LET radiation. AT strains are also more sensitive to MNNG and actinomycin D (Scudiero 1978, Hoar and Sargent 1976), and some, but not all, are more sensitive to MMC and possibly MMS (Hoar and Sargent 1976, but see Arlett 1977). However, UV irradiation, both near and far, and N-hydroxy-AAF inactivate AT cells at the same rate as normal cells (Arlett 1977). It will be recalled that this pattern of response is the converse of that described earlier for XP strains.

In striking contrast to the hypermutability of XP cells by UV exposure, AT cells are *hypomutable* by X-rays (Arlett 1978). This reduced mutation frequency in AT compared to normal cells may mean that a larger fraction of the X- ray-induced mutations are lethal in an AT genotype than in a normal genotype. Alternatively, AT cells may possibly be deficient in an error-prone repair pathway (Arlett 1978).

As was observed for XP cells, SV40 virus transforms AT cells normally; hence, neither the XP nor AT genotype affects the recombination mechanism promoting the insertion of the viral DNA into the human host genome.

Various hallmarks of DNA repair have been measured in AT strains following exposure to ionizing radiation and certain radiomimetic chemicals. Whereas all AT strains tested to date rejoin both single- and double-strand breaks as efficiently as normal strains (Vincent *et al.* 1975, Taylor *et al.* 1975, Lehmann and Stevens 1977), the majority of strains (7 of 12 tested) have depressed levels of repair replication in response to anoxic irradiation (Paterson *et al.* 1977). (Unlike the case of strand breaks, the yield of base defects is not increased by the presence of oxygen during irradiation; consequently, the ratio of base defects to single-strand breaks is higher under anoxic conditions [Paterson, in press].) The pattern of repair replication for AT strains treated with MNNG mimics that for X-ray exposure (5 of the above 12 tested; 3 deficient and 2 proficient in γ-ray-induced repair replication) (Scudiero 1978).

Consistent with the γ-ray data, three of the AT strains deficient in repair replication are partially defective in removing those γ-induced base defects that are detected as γ-induced sites sensitive to endonuclease activity in a crude extract from *Micrococcus luteus* (Paterson *et al.* 1976, 1977). Preliminary data utilizing endonuclease S_1 from *Aspergillus oryzae* as the lesion probe suggest that AT strains deficient in repair replication are imparied in acting upon bulky γ-radioproducts, possibly DNA-protein cross-links (Paterson, in press).

The chemical nature of the unrepaired lesions in AT cells is unknown. They are probably not thymine glycols because cell homogenates of all AT strains (both repair replication-deficient and -proficient) remove these base defects from irradiated chromatin with normal kinetics (Remsen and Cerutti 1977). The situation in intact cells may be different, however; for example, sonicates of XP variants are deficient in the excision of dimers from UV-damaged chromatin, and yet whole cells are proficient (Mortelmans *et al.* 1977, Lehmann *et al.* 1975).

Conventional cell fusion studies have assigned three AT strains deficient in γ-induced repair replication to two complementation groups: AT1BE (CRL 1312) and AT3BI to group A, and AT2BE (CRL 1343) to group B (Paterson *et al.* 1977). The discovery of biochemical complementation and the existence of AT strains proficient in repair replication (referred to as AT variants by analogy to XP variants) reinforce the clinical evidence cited earlier for genetic heterogeneity in the disease.

Fibroblasts cultured from AT donors seem to possess normal capacities to cope with UV- and MMS-induced damage. AT strains remove UV endonuclease-sensitive sites as rapidly as normal strains, are proficient in postreplication repair after UV treatment, and exhibit a normal repair-replication response to UV irradiation and MMS (Paterson *et al.* 1976, Lehmann *et al.* 1977, Scudiero, in press).

There are biological and biochemical indications that many, but perhaps not all, cells heterozygous for AT are moderately sensitive to ionizing radiation. This is true for both transformed lymphoblastoid cell lines (Lavin *et al.* 1978) and diploid fibroblasts (Paterson *et al.* 1978). Blood relatives of AT patients are also predisposed to malignancy (Swift *et al.* 1976). Since AT heterozygous carriers may comprise ~1% of the general population, it would seem that a significant fraction of the public who are known to be cancer prone may also be moderately sensitive to certain environmental agents, including ionizing radiation and presumably some radiomimetic chemicals. Development of a laboratory test to detect AT heterozygotes, in combination with identification of particularly hazardous agents in our biosphere, would be of obvious practical importance.

AT cells, both lymphocytes and dermal fibroblasts, tend to present chromosome aberrations of all types at frequencies in excess of normal (see Table 5) (German 1972, Harnden 1974, McCaw *et al.* 1975). The most characteristic spontaneous change involves the highly specific translocation of the long arm of chromosome 14 with band 14q12 as the preferred breakpoint. In the case of one AT patient with chronic lymphocytic leukemia, a lymphocyte clone with this translocation appears to have been the progenitor of the leukemic cells (McCaw *et al.* 1975). The molecular defect(s) giving rise to an AT phenotype does not appear to be of any significance to the production of SCE's, since these cytogenetic changes occur at normal rates in AT lymphocytes, both spontaneously (Changanti *et al.* 1974) and following treatment with either X-rays or any one of three chemicals: MMC, ethyl methanesulfonate (EMS), and Adriamycin (Galloway 1977).

AT cells display an unusual pattern of chromosome aberrations in the mitosis following irradiation in either G_0/early G_1 or G_2 phase (Taylor *et al.* 1976).

The simplest interpretation of the data is that any AT strain, irrespective of whether it is deficient in repair replication or not, is defective in the repair of both single-strand and double-strand lesions. Such considerations have led Lehmann (1977) to hypothesize that the lesions responsible for enhanced lethality in AT cells are unrejoined single- or double-strand breaks rather than unexcised base damage. These "critical" breaks would constitute a minute fraction of the total yield and would go undetected by present biophysical methodology. While AT may be classified as the ionizing radiation analogue of XP, we are far from understanding the disease at the molecular level.

Fanconi's anemia

The predominant clinical features of this complex syndrome (also termed Fanconi's pancytopenia) are hematological disturbances (involving all elements of the bone marrow), diverse anatomic malformations, cutaneous lesions and growth retardation (both intrauterinal and postnatal) (see Table 7 for summary and Gmyrek and Syllm-Rapoport [1964] or German [1972] for review of the clinical picture). A postnatal increase of fetal-type hemoglobin is common; this abnormality is useful for early diagnosis. Like XP and AT, this disorder is chronic and progressive; affected individuals typically die in childhood from excessive bleeding or overwhelming infection, two manifestations of bone marrow failure. Those who survive to adulthood are prone to (a) acute leukemia, particularly myelomonocytic, (b) squamous cell carcinoma of mucocutaneous junctions surrounding the oral and anal cavities, and (c) hepatic adenoma (see Mulvihill 1975). Predisposition to the hepatic neoplasm is attributed to prolonged exposure to androgenic steroids as therapy for bone marrow failure. The spectrum of

TABLE 7. *Clinical hallmarks of Fanconi's anemia*

Hematological Abnormalities
  Progressive hypoplastic pancytopenia
  Frequent infection, hemorrhage
  Elevated fetal hemoglobin
Anatomic Abnormalities
  Renal, cardiac, ocular, and aural anomalies
  Skeletal malformations (hypoplastic radius and thumb)
Cutaneous Abnormalities
  Hyperpigmentation (melanin overproduction)
  Café-au-lait spots
Other Abnormalities
  Cancers (acute myelomonocytic leukemia, squamous cell carcinoma, hepatic adenoma)
  Short stature, microcephaly, mental retardation
Etiology
  Autosomal recessive trait, Prevalence—3 per 10^6
  Blood relatives—Elevated risk of cancer

From Gmyrek and Syllm-Rapoport 1964, German 1972, Hecht and McCaw 1977.

anatomic anomalies varies greatly from patient to patient as does age of onset of bone marrow disturbances; variability in these two clinical abnormalities provides evidence for genetic heterogeneity in the disease.

FA fibroblasts are abnormally sensitive to different physical and chemical carcinogens than are XP or AT fibroblasts. FA cells are hypersensitive to bifunctional alkylating agents (e.g., MMC, nitrogen mustard) or to psoralen-plus-black light but are at most only slightly more sensitive than normal cells to far UV or γ-radiation, 4NQO, or MMS (Sasaki *et al.* 1977, Fujiwara *et al.* 1977). A complementation analysis has not as yet been carried out on FA strains; however, their broad range of sensitivity to MMC (5- to 15-fold above normal, see Table 2) supports the suggestion from the clinical picture that the syndrome has a heterogeneous genetic basis.

The modal karyotype is typically normal in FA (this also holds true for XP and AT) (German 1972). Nonetheless, cells from afflicted donors display an abnormal cytogenetic behavior (see Table 5). Both blood lymphocytes and dermal fibroblasts are characterized by a high spontaneous frequency of chromosome aberrations; chromatid-type breaks and gaps predominate, although rearrangements leading to dicentric chromosomes and interchanges between nonhomologous chromosomes resulting in asymmetric quadriradials are also common (see German 1972). The incidence of chromatid-type alterations in particular is markedly elevated in FA lymphocytes by MMC (Sasaki and Tonomura 1973) or X-ray exposure (Higurashi and Conen 1973). Diepoxybutane (DEB), another bifunctional alkylating agent, also increases the yield of chromosome anomalies at concentrations that produce no increase in normal cells (Auerbach and Wolman 1976). On the other hand, the spontaneous frequency of SCE's is normal in FA fibroblasts (Kato and Stich 1976), and the induction of SCE's by MMC is actually *reduced* in FA lymphocytes compared to normal lymphocytes (Latt *et al.* 1975).

A possible biochemical explanation for the cellular and cytogenetic abnormalities in FA cells is provided by the molecular studies of Fujiwara and collaborators (1977). The agents to which FA cells are hypersensitive are known to induce, among other alterations, interstrand DNA cross-links; FA strains are defective, to varying extents, in initiating the repair of such lesions, i.e., they are impaired in unhooking one arm of the cross-link. Elucidation of the mechanism by which such a class of defects might lead to an increased yield of chromosome aberrations and a reduced frequency of SCE's in response to MMC should provide insight into the genesis of chromosome anomalies. DNA repair defects have been reported in FA strains after exposure to high UV fluences (retarded rate of dimer excision in one strain, attributed to malfunctional exonuclease) (Poon *et al.* 1974) and after γ-irradiation (reduced ability, in two of four strains, of cell nuclear preparations to excise thymine glycols from exogenous DNA) (Remsen and Cerutti 1976). Consistent with these findings, FA cells show a reduced capacity to produce viral structural antigens after infection with UV- or γ-irradiated adenovirus (Rainbow and Howes 1977a).

FA cells are hypomutable by an agent to which they exhibit sensitivity, namely MMC (Finkelberg *et al.* 1977); in this respect they behave like AT, but not XP cells. FA cells also generate a reduced incidence of spontaneous and EMS-induced mutants relative to normal cells. In contrast to fibroblasts from the other two disorders, FA fibroblasts are transformed at an elevated rate by SV40 virus (Todaro *et al.* 1966), implying that FA cells may possibly be hypersensitive to the elusive human oncogenic virus.

Close relatives of FA patients are at increased risk (~threefold) of malignancy (Swift 1971); this may reflect cancer proneness in heterozygous carriers. FA heterozygotes can be readily distinguished from FA homozygotes and normal individuals on the basis of the relative yields of chromosome damage induced by DEB (Auerbach and Wolman 1978). Aside from its utility in prenatal diagnosis (Auerbach *et al.* 1978), this cytogenetic assay should prove to be important because it is believed that ~0.3% of the population is heterozygous for the disease.

OTHER POSSIBLE REPAIR-DEFICIENT DISORDERS

At present, only in XP, AT, and FA are defects in the repair of damaged DNA a characteristic property of cultured cells. However, there are other clinically similar syndromes in which repair defects are suspected: Bloom's syndrome, Cockayne's syndrome, Rothmund-Thomson syndrome, Werner's syndrome, basal cell nevus syndrome, D-deletion-type retinoblastoma, and progeria (see Cleaver 1977b, Hecht and McCaw 1977, German, in press). The mode of inheritance of the first four is autosomal recessive, whereas the next two are transmitted in an autosomal dominant fashion; the genetic etiology of progeria has not been established, due to its extreme rarity. In five of the seven listed here (Cockayne's syndrome and progeria are the exceptions), affected individuals show an increased propensity for developing one or more types of cancer, the most common being cutaneous carcinomas. Progeroid patients could possibly be at high risk of cancer, but the rarity of the disorder may preclude uncovering this trait. Cockayne's and Werner's syndromes and progeria share many clinical features in common, including premature aging and severe growth retardation. Skin pigmentation changes, immune deficiency, and neurological disturbances are other abnormalities variously present in the seven disorders.

Clinical manifestations of sensitivity to solar radiation are common to the first five, and fibroblasts from patients with either Bloom's or Cockayne's syndrome are hypersensitive to killing by UV irradiation (Giannelli *et al.* 1977, Schmickel *et al.* 1977). In contrast, cells established from individuals with either of the last two syndromes show hallmarks of moderate sensitivity to ionizing radiation; retinoblastoma fibroblasts are sensitive to inactivation by X-irradiation (Weichselbaum *et al.* 1977), and progeroid fibroblasts have a reduced capacity to reactivate γ-irradiated adenovirus (Rainbow and Howes 1977b). Progeroid cells senesce prematurely in culture and, under certain conditions, are defective in rejoining single-strand breaks induced in DNA by X-rays (see Cleaver 1977b, Setlow 1978).

Bloom's syndrome is of particular significance because it is the prototype of the so-called "chromosome breakage syndromes," which share as common clinical features chromosome instability and cancer proneness; the other members are AT, FA, and XP (German 1972). In both lymphocytes and fibroblasts from persons with Bloom's syndrome, the incidence of chromosome aberrations (notably symmetric exchanges leading to quadriradials) and SCE's is much above normal. The only known defect in cultured cells is a reduced rate of DNA chain elongation (Hand and German 1975). However, this impairment does not alter synthesis past pyrimidine dimers in template DNA, i.e., postreplication repair is normal (Giannelli *et al.* 1977).

Of the remaining six disorders, chromosome instability is only seen in the basal cell nevus syndrome (Hecht and McCaw 1977). Nevertheless, the tendency to undergo chromosomal change may be "conditional" in the other five, that is, normally latent and requiring (as in the case of UV light for XP) exposure to certain DNA-damaging agents for expression (German, in press).

RELEVANCY OF REPAIR DEFICIENCIES TO ENVIRONMENTAL CARCINOGENESIS

What have the studies associating defective DNA repair with cancer proneness in these human disorders taught us about the underlying mechanism of neoplastic transformation? At present, XP is the only disease for which a relation between the laboratory and clinical observations is obvious. This syndrome provides a dramatic example of the interplay of environmental and host factors in cancer induction. The hypermutability of cultured XP cells by UV-irradiation is encouraging to proponents of the somatic mutation theory of cancer; accumulation of UV lesions, due to incomplete or faulty repair, could give rise to mutations in critical regions of the genome, and in turn these genetic alterations may predispose a skin cell to malignant conversion. However, the disease may prove to be a special case, rather than the rule. The hypomutability of AT and FA cells by carcinogens eliciting abnormal repair responses does not lend ready support to the mutation theory. Instead, aberrant tissue differentiation during early embryonic development has been invoked to explain many clinical features of AT, including the immunological, hepatic, and gonadal disturbances (e.g., see McFarlin *et al.* 1972). Assuming that defective DNA repair is also manifest in vivo, at least two possibilities may be considered: A repair deficiency is the primary cause, leading to developmental malformations. Alternatively, a repair defect may be a concurrent feature of the initiation of the disease, possibly resulting from misdirected gene repression events. Repair studies in differentiated systems may yield information on the genetic control of DNA repair functions and other functions differentially expressed during embryogenesis.

CONCLUDING REMARKS AND PROSPECTUS

The studies on the human disorders discussed here have yielded considerable insight into the importance of DNA repair processes in man. That unrepaired damage to DNA can lead to malignancy in normal individuals is a reasonable prediction. Elucidation of the precise biochemical defect(s) and explanation of the apparent genetic heterogeneity in these diseases are of high priority. Persons heterozygous for certain genes associated with DNA repair (i.e., FA, XP, and AT genes) may be at increased risk to certain environmental agents. The evaluation of this possibility and its contribution to the overall cancer burden would seem germane to the study of environmental carcinogenesis.

ACKNOWLEDGMENTS

I thank Dr. P. J. Smith for helpful discussions, and Drs. N. E. Gentner, D. K. Myers and P. J. Smith for critical commentary on the manuscript.

REFERENCES

Ahmed, F. E., and R. B. Setlow. 1977. Different rate-limiting steps in excision repair of ultraviolet- and N-acetoxy-2-acetylaminofluorene-damaged DNA in normal human fibroblasts. Proc. Natl. Acad. Sci. USA 74:1548–1552.

Andrews, A. D., S. F. Barrett, and J. H. Robbins. 1976. Relation of DNA repair processes to pathological ageing of the nervous system in xeroderma pigmentosum. Lancet 1:1318–1320.

Arlett, C. F. 1977. Lethal response to DNA damaging agents in a variety of human fibroblast cell strains. Mutat. Res. 46:106.

Arlett, C. F. 1978. Cell killing and mutagenesis in repair defective cultured human cells. J. Supramol. Struct. (Suppl.) 2:40.

Auerbach, A. D., D. Warburton, and R. S. K. Chaganti. 1978. Prenatal detection of the Fanconi's anemia gene by cytogenetic methods. J. Supramol. Struct. (Suppl.) 2:84.

Auerbach, A. D., and S. R. Wolman. 1976. Susceptibility of Fanconi's anemia fibroblasts to chromosome damage by carcinogens. Nature 261:494–496.

Auerbach, A. D., and S. R. Wolman. 1978. Carcinogen-induced chromosome breakage in Fanconi's anemia heterozygous cells. Nature 271:69–71.

Bartram, C. R., T. Koske-Westphal, and E. Passarge. 1976. Chromatid exchanges in ataxia telangiectasia, Bloom syndrome, Werner syndrome, and xeroderma pigmentosum. Ann. Human Genet. 40:79–86.

Bertazzoni, U., M. Stefanini, G. Pedrali-Noy, E. Giulotto, F. Nuzzo, A. Falaschi, and S. Spadari 1976. Variations of DNA polymerases-α and -β during prolonged stimulation of human lymphocytes. Proc. Natl. Acad. Sci. USA 73:785–789.

Bootsma, D. 1977. Defective DNA repair and cancer, *in* Research in Photobiology, A. Castellani ed., Plenum Press, New York, pp. 455–468.

Bootsma, D. 1978. Xeroderma pigmentosum, *in* DNA Repair Mechanisms, P. C. Hanawalt, E. C. Friedberg, and C. F. Fox, eds., Academic Press, New York (In press).

Bridges, B. A. 1976. Short term screening tests for carcinogens. Nature 261:195–200.

Brusick, D. 1979. Bacterial mutagenesis and its role in the identification of potential animal carcinogens, *in* Carcinogens: Identification and Mechanisms of Action (The University of Texas System Cancer Center 31st Annual Symposium on Fundamental Cancer Research, 1978), A. C. Griffin and C. R. Shaw, eds., Raven Press, New York, pp. 95–107.

Cerutti, P. A. 1978. Repairable damage in DNA, *in* DNA Repair Mechanisms, P. C. Hanawalt, E. C. Friedberg, and C. F. Fox, eds., Academic Press, New York (In press).

Chan, A. C., S. K. C. Ng, and I. G. Walker. 1976. Reduced DNA repair during differentiation of a myogenic cell line. J. Cell Biol. 70:685–691.

Chaganti, R. S. K., S. Schonberg, and J. German. 1974. A manyfold increase in sister chromatid exchanges in Bloom's syndrome lymphocytes. Proc. Natl. Acad. Sci. USA 71:4508–4512.

Cleaver, J. E. 1974. Repair processes for photochemical damage in mammalian cells. Adv. Radiat. Biol. 4:1–75.

Cleaver, J. E. 1977a. Nucleosome structure controls rates of excision repair in DNA of human cells. Nature 270:451–453.

Cleaver, J. E. 1977b. DNA repair processes and their impairment in some human diseases, *in* Progress in Genetic Toxicology, D. Scott, B. A. Bridges, and F. H. Sobels, eds., Elsevier/North-Holland Press, Amsterdam, pp. 29–42.

Cleaver, J. E., and D. Bootsma. 1975. Xeroderma pigmentosum: Biochemical and genetic characteristics. Annu. Rev. Genet. 9:19–38.

Cook, J. S. 1970. Photoreactivation in animal cells, *in* Photophysiology, A. C. Giese, ed. Vol 5. Academic Press, New York, pp. 191–233.

Cook, K. H., and E. C. Friedberg. 1978. Partial purification, isolation and characterization of three nuclease activities from human KB cells which can excise thymine-containing pyrimidine dimers. J. Supramol. Struct. (Suppl.) 2:10.

Cunliffe, P. N., J. R. Mann, A. H. Cameron, K. D. Roberts, and H. W. C. Ward. 1975. Radiosensitivity in ataxia-telangiectasia. Br. J. Radiol. 48:374–376.

Day, R. S., III. 1974. Studies on repair of adenovirus 2 by human fibroblasts using normal, xeroderma pigmentosum, and xeroderma pigmentosum heterozygous strains. Cancer Res. 34:1965–1970.

Day, R. S., III, K. H. Kraemer, and J. H. Robbins. 1975. Complementing xeroderma pigmentosum fibroblasts restore biological activity to UV-damaged DNA. Mutat. Res. 28:251–255.

de Weerd-Kastelein, E. A., W. J. Kleijer, M. L. Sluyter, and W. Keijzer. 1973. Repair replication in heterokaryons derived from different repair-deficient xeroderma pigmentosum strains. Mutat. Res. 19:237–243.

de Weerd-Kastelein, E. A., W. Keijzer, G. Rainaldi, and D. Bootsma. 1977. Induction of sister chromatid exchanges in xeroderma pigmentosum cells after exposure to ultraviolet light. Mutat. Res. 45:253–261.

Doll, R. 1977. Strategy for detection of cancer hazards to man. Nature 265:589–596.

Duncan, J., H. Slor, K. Cook, and E. C. Friedberg. 1975. Thymine dimer excision by extracts of human cells, *in* Molecular Mechanisms for Repair of DNA, P. C. Hanawalt and R. B. Setlow, eds., Plenum Press, New York, pp. 643–649.

Edenberg, H. J. 1976. Inhibition of DNA replication by ultraviolet light. Biophys. J. 16:849–860.

Finkelberg, R., M. Buchwald, and L. Siminovitch. 1977. Decreased mutagenesis in cells from patients with Fanconi's anemia. Am. Soc. Human Genet. Annu. Meeting (Abstract) 54A.

Fornace, A. J., Jr., K. W. Kohn, and H. E. Kann, Jr. 1976. DNA single-strand breaks during repair of UV damage in human fibroblasts and abnormalities of repair in xeroderma pigmentosum. Proc. Natl. Acad. Sci. USA 73:39–43.

Friedberg, E. C., C. Anderson, T. Bonura, R. Cone, and R. Simmons. 1978. Base excision repair, *in* DNA Repair Mechanisms, P. C. Hanawalt, E. C. Friedberg, and C. F. Fox, eds., Academic Press, New York (In press).

Friedberg, E. C., K. H. Cook, K. Mortelmans, and J. Rudé. 1977. Studies on the enzymology of excision repair in extracts of mammalian cells, *in* Research in Photobiology, A. Castellani, ed., Plenum Press, New York, pp. 299–306.

Friedman, J. M., P. J. Fialkow, S. D. Davis, H. D. Ochs, and R. J. Wedgwood. 1977. Autoimmunity in the relatives of patients with immunodeficiency diseases. Clin. Exp. Immunol. 28:375–388.

Fujiwara, Y. 1978. Postreplication DNA repair (PRR) in UV-irradiated xeroderma pigmentosum (XP) and XP variant cells. J. Supramol. Struct. (Suppl.) 2:17.

Fujiwara, Y., M. Tatsumi, and M. S. Sasaki. 1977. Cross-link repair in human cells and its possible defect in Fanconi's anemia cells. J. Mol. Biol. 113:635–649.

Galloway, S. M. 1977. Ataxia telangiectasia: the effects of chemical mutagens and X-rays on sister chromatid exchanges in blood lymphocytes. Mutat. Res. 45:343–349.

Gentner, N. E. 1977. Evidence for a second "prereplicative G2" repair mechanism, specific for γ-induced damage, in wild-type *Schizosaccharomyces pombe*. Molec. Gen. Genet. 154:129–133.

German, J. 1972. Genes which increase chromosomal instability in somatic cells and predispose to cancer. Prog. Med. Genet. 8:61–101.

German, J. 1978. DNA repair defects and human disease, *in* DNA Repair Mechanisms, P. C. Hanawalt, E. C. Friedberg, and C. F. Fox, eds., Academic Press, New York (In press).

Giannelli, F., P. F. Benson, S. A. Pawsey, and P. E. Polani. 1977. Ultraviolet light sensitivity and delayed DNA-chain maturation in Bloom's syndrome fibroblasts. Nature 265:466–469.

Gmyrek, D., and I. Syllm-Rapoport. 1964. Fanconi anemia (FA): Analysis of 129 described cases. Z. Kinderheilk. 91:297–337.

Goth, R., and M. F. Rajewsky. 1974. Persistence of O6-ethylguanine in rat-brain DNA: Correlation with nervous system-specific carcinogenesis by ethylnitrosourea. Proc. Natl. Acad. Sci. USA 71:639–643.

Grossman, L. 1978. Nucleotide excision repair, *in* DNA Repair Mechanisms, P. C. Hanawalt, E. C. Friedberg, and C. F. Fox, eds., Academic Press, New York (In press).

Grossman, L., A. Braun, R. Feldberg, and I. Mahler. 1975. Enzymatic repair of DNA. Annu Rev. Biochem. 44:19–43.

Hahn, G. M., D. King, and S. J. Yang. 1971. Quantitative changes in unscheduled DNA synthesis in rat muscle cells after differentiation. Nature New Biol. 230:242–244.

Hanawalt, P. C., E. C. Friedberg, and C. F. Fox. 1978. DNA Repair Mechanisms. Academic Press, New York (In press).

Hand, R., and J. German. 1975. A retarded rate of DNA chain growth in Bloom's syndrome Proc. Natl. Acad. Sci. USA 72:758–762.

Harnden, D. G. 1974. Ataxia telangiectasia syndrome: Cytogenetic and cancer aspects, i. Chromosomes and Cancer, J. German, ed., John Wiley and Sons, New York, pp. 619–636.

Hecht, F., and B. K. McCaw. 1977. Chromosome instability syndromes, *in* Genetics of Human Cancer, J. J. Mulvihill, R. W. Miller, and J. F. Fraumeni, Jr., eds., Raven Press, New York pp. 105–123.

Higgins, N. P., K. Kato, and B. Strauss. 1976. A model for replication repair in mammalian cells. J. Mol. Biol. 101:417–425.

Higginson, J. 1979. Perspectives and future developments in research in environmental carcinogen esis, *in* Carcinogens: Identification and Mechanisms of Action (The University of Texas System Cancer Center 31st Annual Symposium on Fundamental Cancer Research, 1978), A. C. Griffi and C. R. Shaw, eds., Raven Press, New York, pp. 187–208.

Higurashi, M., and P. E. Conen. 1973. *In vitro* chromosomal radiosensitivity in "chromosoma breakage syndromes." Cancer 32:380–383.

Hoar, D. I., and P. Sargent. 1976. Chemical mutagen hypersensitivity in ataxia telangiectasia Nature 261:590–592.

Jahn, C. L., and G. W. Litman. 1977. Distribution of covalently bound benzo(a)pyrene in chromatir Biochem. Biophys. Res. Commun. 76:534–540.

Karran, P., A. Moscona, and B. Strauss. 1977. Developmental decline in DNA repair in neura retina cells of chick embryos: Persistent deficiency of repair competence in a cell line derive from late embryos. J. Cell Biol. 74:274–286.

Kato, H., and H. F. Stich. 1976. Sister chromatid exchanges in ageing and repair-deficient huma fibroblasts. Nature 260:447–448.

Key, D. J., and G. J. Todaro. 1974. Xeroderma pigmentosum cell susceptibility to SV40 viru transformation: Lack of effect of low dosage ultraviolet radiation in enhancing viral-induce transformation. J. Invest. Dermatol. 62:7–10.

Kornberg, R. D. 1977. Structure of chromatin. Annu. Rev. Biochem. 46:931–954.

Kraemer, K. H. 1977. Progressive degenerative diseases associated with defective DNA repai Xeroderma pigmentosum and ataxia telangiectasia, *in* Cellular Senescence and Somatic Cell Gene ics: DNA Repair Processes, W. W. Nichols and D. G. Murphy, eds., Symposia Specialist: Miami, pp. 37–71.

Kraemer, K. H., E. A. deWeerd-Kastelein, J. H. Robbins, W. Keijzer, S. F. Barrett, R. A. Peting and D. Bootsma. 1975. Five complementation groups in xeroderma pigmentosum. Mutat. Re 33:327–340.

Kuhnlein, U., B. Lee, and S. Linn. 1978a. Human uracil DNA N-glycosidase: Studies in norm. and repair defective cultured fibroblasts. Nucleic Acids Res. 5:117–125.

Kuhnlein, U., B. Lee, E. E. Penhoet, and S. Linn. 1978b. Xeroderma pigmentosum fibroblasts the D group lack an apurinic DNA endonuclease species with a low apparent K_m. Nucle Acids Res. 5:951–960.

Kuhnlein, U., E. E. Penhoet, and S. Linn. 1976. An altered apurinic DNA endonuclease activity in group A and group D xeroderma pigmentosum fibroblasts. Proc. Natl. Acad. Sci. USA 73:1169–1173.

Latt, S. A., G. Stetten, L. A. Juergens, G. R. Buchanan, and P. S. Gerald. 1975. Induction by alkylating agents of sister chromatid exchanges and chromatid breaks in Fanconi's anemia. Proc. Natl. Acad. Sci. USA 72:4066–4070.

Lavin, M. F., P. C. Chen, and C. Kidsen. 1978. Ataxia telangiectasia: Characterization of heterozygotes. J. Supramol. Struct. (Suppl.) 2:75.

Lehmann, A. R. 1974. Postreplication repair of DNA in mammalian cells. Life Sci. 15:2005–2016.

Lehmann, A. R. 1977. Ataxia telangiectasia and the lethal lesion produced by ionizing radiation, *in* Cellular Senescence and Somatic Cell Genetics: DNA Repair Processes, W. W. Nichols and D. G. Murphy, eds., Symposia Specialists, Miami, pp. 167–175.

Lehmann, A. R. 1978. DNA replication in normal and defective human cells after UV-irradiation, *in* DNA Repair Mechanisms, P. C. Hanawalt, E. C. Friedberg, and C. F. Fox, eds., Academic Press, New York (In press).

Lehmann, A. R., S. Kirk-Bell, C. F. Arlett, S. A. Harcourt, E. A. deWeerd-Kastelein, W. Keijzer, and P. Hall-Smith. 1977. Repair of ultraviolet light damage in a variety of human fibroblast cell strains. Cancer Res. 37:904–910.

Lehmann, A. R., S. Kirk-Bell, C. F. Arlett, M. C. Paterson, P. H. M. Lohman, E. A. deWeerd-Kastelein, and D. Bootsma. 1975. Xeroderma pigmentosum cells with normal levels of excision repair have a defect in DNA synthesis after UV-irradiation. Proc. Natl. Acad. Sci. USA 72:219–223.

Lehmann, A. R., and S. Stevens. 1977. The production and repair of double strand breaks in cells from normal humans and from patients with ataxia telangiectasia. Biochim. Biophys. Acta 474:49–60.

Levin, S., and S. Perlov. 1971. Ataxia-telangiectasia in Israel with observations on its relationship to malignant disease. Isr. J. Med. Sci. 12:1535–1541.

Linn, S., W. S. Linsley, U. Kuhnlein, E. E. Penhoet, and W. A. Deutsch. 1978. Enzymes for the repair of apurinic/apyrimidinic sites in human cells, *in* DNA Repair Mechanisms, P. C. Hanawalt, E. C. Friedberg, and C. F. Fox, eds., Academic Press, New York (In press).

Linsley, J. S., E. E. Penhoet, and S. Linn. 1977. Human endonuclease specific for apurinic/apyrimidinic sites in DNA: Partial purification and characterization of multiple forms from placenta. J. Biol. Chem. 252:1235–1242.

Lynch, H. T., J. Lynch, and P. Lynch. 1977. Management and control of familial cancer, *in* Genetics of Human Cancer, J. J. Mulvihill, R. W. Miller, and J. F. Fraumeni, Jr., eds., Raven Press, New York, pp. 235–256.

Maher, V. M., and J. J. McCormick. 1976. Effect of DNA repair on the cytotoxicity and mutagenicity of UV irradiation and of chemical carcinogens in normal and xeroderma pigmentosum cells, *in* Biology of Radiation Carcinogenesis, J. M. Yuhas, R. W. Tennant, and J. D. Regan, eds., Raven Press, New York, pp. 129–145.

Maher, V. M., L. M. Ouellette, R. D. Curren, and J. J. McCormick. 1976. Frequency of ultraviolet light-induced mutations is higher in xeroderma pigmentosum variant cells than in normal human cells. Nature 261:593–595.

Maher, V. M., L. M. Ouellette, M. Mittlestat, and J. J. McCormick. 1975. Synergistic effect of caffeine on the cytotoxicity of ultraviolet irradiation and of hydrocarbon epoxides in strains of xeroderma pigmentosum. Nature 258:760–763.

McCaw, B. K., F. Hecht, D. G. Harnden, and R. L. Teplitz. 1975. Somatic rearrangement of chromosome 14 in human lymphocytes. Proc. Natl. Acad. Sci. USA 72:2071–2075.

McCombe, P., M. Lavin, and C. Kidson. 1976. Control of DNA repair linked to neuroblastoma differentiation. Int. J. Radiat. Biol. 29:523–531.

McFarlin, D. E., W. Strober, and T. A. Waldmann. 1972. Ataxia-telangiectasia. Medicine 51:281–314.

Metzger, G., F. X. Wilhelm, and M. L. Wilhelm. 1977. Non-random binding of a chemical carcinogen to the DNA in chromatin. Biochem. Biophys. Res. Commun. 75:703–710.

Miller, R. W. 1977. Ethnic differences in cancer occurrence: Genetic and environmental influences with particular reference to neuroblastoma, *in* Genetics of Human Cancer, J. J. Mulvihill, R. W. Miller, and J. F. Fraumeni, Jr., eds., Raven Press, New York, pp. 1–14.

Mortelmans, K., J. E. Cleaver, E. C. Friedberg, M. C. Paterson, B. P. Smith, and G. H. Thomas. 1977. Photoreactivation of thymine dimers in UV-irradiated human cells: Unique dependence on culture conditions. Mutat. Res. 44:433–446.

Mortelmans, K., E. C. Friedberg, H. Slor, G. Thomas, and J. E. Cleaver. 1976. Defective thymine dimer excision by cell-free extracts of xeroderma pigmentosum cells. Proc. Natl. Acad. Sci. USA 73:2757–2761.

Moses, H. L., R. A. Webster, G. D. Martin, and T. C. Spelsberg. 1976. Binding of polycyclic aromatic hydrocarbons to transcriptionally active nuclear subfractions of AKR mouse embryo cells. Cancer Res. 36:2905–2910.

Moses, R. E., and A. L. Beaudet. 1978. Apurinic DNA endonuclease activities in repair-deficient human cell lines. Nucleic Acids Res. 5:463–473.

Mulvihill, J. J. 1975. Congenital and genetic diseases, *in* Persons at High Risk of Cancer, J. F. Fraumeni, Jr., ed., Academic Press, New York, pp. 3–37.

Myers, D. K., M. C. Paterson, N. E. Gentner, P. Unrau, and F. K. Zimmermann. 1978. DNA repair and the assessment of the biological hazards of ionizing radiation, *in* IAEA Proceedings of International Symposium on Late Biological Effects of Ionizing Radiation, March 13–17, 1978, Vienna (In press).

Parrington, J. M., J. D. A. Delhanty, and H. P. Baden. 1971. Unscheduled DNA synthesis, UV-induced chromosome aberrations and SV_{40} transformation in cultured cells from xeroderma pigmentosum. Ann. Human Genet. 35:149–160.

Paterson, M. C. 1978. Ataxia telangiectasia: A model inherited disease linking deficient DNA repair with radiosensitivity and cancer proneness, *in* DNA Repair Mechanisms, P. C. Hanawalt, E. C. Friedberg, and C. F. Fox, eds., Academic Press, New York (In press).

Paterson, M. C., P. H. M. Lohman, and M. L. Sluyter. 1973. Use of a UV endonuclease from *Micrococcus luteus* to monitor the progress of DNA repair in UV-irradiated human cells. Mutat. Res. 19:245–256.

Paterson, M. C., P. H. M. Lohman, A. Westerveld, and M. L. Sluyter. 1974. DNA repair monitored by an enzymatic assay in multinucleate xeroderma pigmentosum cells after fusion. Nature 248:50–52.

Paterson, M. C., B. P. Smith, P. A. Knight, and A. K. Anderson. 1977. Ataxia telangiectasia: An inherited human disease involving radiosensitivity, malignancy and defective DNA repair, *in* Research in Photobiology, A. Castellani, ed., Plenum Press, New York, pp. 207–218.

Paterson, M. C., B. P. Smith, P. H. M. Lohman, A. K. Anderson, and L. Fishman. 1976. Defective excision repair of γ-ray-damaged DNA in human (ataxia telangiectasia) fibroblasts. Nature 260:444–447.

Paterson, M. C., B. P. Smith, P. J. Smith, and A. K. Anderson. 1978. Radioresponse of fibroblasts from ataxia telangiectasia heterozygotes. Radiat. Res. (Abstract) 74:83–84.

Pathak, M. A., and J. H. Epstein. 1971. Normal and abnormal reactions of man to light, *in* Dermatology in General Medicine, T. B. Fitzgerald, K. A. Arndt, W. H. Clark, Jr., A. Z. Eisen, E. J. VanScott, and J. H. Vaughn, eds., McGraw-Hill, New York, pp. 977–1036.

Pegg, A. E. 1977. Alkylation of rat liver DNA by dimethylnitrosamine: Effect of dosage on O^6 methylguanine levels. J. Natl. Cancer Inst. 58:681–687.

Pegg, A. E., and G. Hui. 1978. Formation and subsequent removal of O^6-methylguanine from deoxyribonucleic acid in rat liver and kidney after small doses of dimethylnitrosamine. Biochem. J. 173:739–748.

Peleg, L., E. Raz, and R. Ben-Ishai. 1976. Changing capacity for DNA excision repair in mouse embryonic cells *in vitro*. Exp. Cell Res. 104:301–307.

Poon, P. K., R. L. O'Brien, and J. W. Parker. 1974. Defective DNA repair in Fanconi's anaemia. Nature 250:223–225.

Rainbow, A. J. 1978. Production of viral structural antigens by irradiated adenovirus as an assay for DNA repair in human fibroblasts. J. Supramol. Struct. (Suppl.) 2:35.

Rainbow, A. J., and M. Howes. 1977a. Defective repair of ultraviolet- and gamma-ray-damaged DNA in Fanconi's anaemia. Int. J. Radiat. Biol. 31:191–195.

Rainbow, A. J., and M. Howes. 1977b. Decreased repair of gamma ray damaged DNA in progeria. Biochem. Biophys. Res. Commun. 74:714–719.

Ramanathan, R., S. Rajalakshmi, D. S. R. Sarma, and E. Farber. 1976. Nonrandom nature of *in vivo* methylation by dimethylnitrosamine and the subsequent removal of methylated products from rat liver chromatin DNA. Cancer Res. 36:2073–2079.

Ramsay, C. A., T. M. Coltart, S. Blunt, S. A. Pawsey, and F. Giannelli. 1974. Prenatal diagnosis of xeroderma pigmentosum: Report of the first successful case. Lancet 2:1109–1112.

Regan, J. D., and R. B. Setlow. 1974. Two forms of repair in the DNA of human cells damaged by chemical carcinogens and mutagens. Cancer Res. 34:3318–3325.

Regan, J. D., R. B. Setlow, and R. D. Ley. 1971. Normal and defective repair of damaged DNA in human cells: A sensitive assay utilizing the photolysis of bromodeoxyuridine. Proc. Natl. Acad. Sci. USA 68:708–712.

Remsen, J. F., and P. A. Cerutti. 1976. Deficiency of gamma-ray excision repair in skin fibroblasts from patients with Fanconi's anemia. Proc. Natl. Acad. Sci. USA 73:2419–2423.

Remsen, J. F., and P. A. Cerutti. 1977. Excision of gamma-ray induced thymine lesions by preparations from ataxia telangiectasia fibroblasts. Mutat. Res. 43:139–146.

Robbins, J. H., K. H. Kraemer, M. A. Lutzner, B. W. Festoff, and H. G. Coon. 1974. Xeroderma pigmentosum: An inherited disease with sun sensitivity, multiple cutaneous neoplasms, and abnormal DNA repair. Ann. Intern. Med. 80:221–248.

Roberts, J. J. 1978. The repair of DNA modified by cytotoxic, mutagenic, and carcinogenic chemicals. Adv. Radiat. Biol. 7:211–436.

Rudé, J. M., and E. C. Friedberg. 1977. Semi-conservative deoxyribonucleic acid synthesis in unirradiated and ultraviolet-irradiated xeroderma pigmentosum and normal human skin fibroblasts. Mutat. Res. 42:433–442.

Sasaki, M. S. 1973. DNA repair capacity and susceptibility to chromosome breakage in xeroderma pigmentosum cells. Mutat. Res. 20:291–293.

Sasaki, M. S., K. Toda, and A. Ozawa. 1977. Role of DNA repair in the susceptibility to chromosome breakage and cell killing in cultured human fibroblasts, *in* Biochemistry of Cutaneous Epidermal Differentiation, M. Seiji and I. A. Bernstein, eds., University of Tokyo Press, Tokyo, pp. 167–180.

Sasaki, M. S., and A. Tonomura. 1973. A high susceptibility of Fanconi's anemia to chromosome breakage by DNA cross-linking agents. Cancer Res. 33:1829-1836.

Schmickel, R. D., E. H. Y. Chu, J. E. Trosko, and C. C. Chang. 1977. Cockayne syndrome: Cellular sensitivity to ultraviolet light. Pediatrics 60:135-139.

Scudiero, D. A. 1978. Repair deficiency in N-methyl-N′-nitro-N-nitrosoguanidine treated ataxia telangiectasia (AT) fibroblasts. J. Supramol. Struct. (Suppl.) 2:83.

Scudiero, D., A. Norin, P. Karran, and B. Strauss. 1976. DNA excision-repair deficiency of human peripheral blood lymphocytes treated with chemical carcinogens. Cancer Res. 36:1397–1403.

Sedgwick, R. P., and E. Boder, 1972. Ataxia-telangiectasia, *in* Handbook of Clinical Neurology, P. J. Vinken and G. W. Bruyn, eds. Vol. 14. North-Holland Publishing Co., Amsterdam, pp. 267–339.

Setlow, R. B. 1978. Repair deficient human disorders and cancer. Nature 271:713–717.

Shubik, P. 1979. Identification of environmental carcinogens: Animal test models, *in* Carcinogens: Identification and Mechanisms of Action (The University of Texas System Cancer Center 31st Annual Symposium on Fundamental Cancer Research, 1978), A. C. Griffin and C. R. Shaw, eds., Raven Press, New York, pp. 39–49.

Söderhäll, S., and T. Lindahl. 1976. DNA ligases of eukaryotes. FEBS Lett. 67:1–8.

Stockdale, F. E. 1971. DNA synthesis in differentiating skeletal muscle cells: Initiation by ultraviolet light. Science 171:1145–1147.

Sutherland, B. M. 1974. Photoreactivating enzyme from human leukocytes. Nature 248:109–112.

Sutherland, B. M. 1977. Human photoreactivating enzymes, *in* Research in Photobiology, A. Castellani, ed., Plenum Press, New York, pp. 307–315.

Sutherland, B. M. 1978. Enzymatic photoreactivation of DNA, *in* DNA Repair Mechanisms, P. C. Hanawalt, E. C. Friedberg, and C. F. Fox, eds., Academic Press, New York (In press).

Sutherland, B. M., and R. Oliver. 1976. Culture conditions affect photoreactivating enzyme levels in human fibroblasts. Biochim. Biophys. Acta 442:358–367.

Sutherland, B. M., M. Rice, and E. K. Wagner. 1975. Xeroderma pigmentosum cells contain low levels of photoreactivating enzyme. Proc. Natl. Acad. Sci. USA 72:103–107.

Swift, M. 1971. Fanconi's anaemia in the genetics of neoplasia. Nature 230:370–373.

Swift, M., L. Sholman, M. Perry, and C. Chase. 1976. Malignant neoplasms in the families of patients with ataxia-telangiectasia. Cancer Res. 36:209–215.

Takebe, H. 1978. Relationship between DNA repair defects and skin cancers in xeroderma pigmentosum. J. Supramol. Struct. (Suppl.) 2:30.

Tanaka, K., H. Hayakawa, M. Sekiguchi, and Y. Okada. 1977. Specific action of T4 endonuclease V on damaged DNA in xeroderma pigmentosum cells *in vivo.* Proc. Natl. Acad. Sci. USA 74:2958–2962.

Taylor, A. M. R., D. G. Harnden, C. F. Arlett, S. A. Harcourt, A. R. Lehmann, S. Stevens, and B. A. Bridges. 1975. Ataxia telangiectasia: A human mutation with abnormal radiation sensitivity. Nature 258:427–429.

Taylor, A. M. R., J. A. Metcalfe, J. M. Oxford, and D. G. Harnden. 1976. Is chromatid-type damage in ataxia telangiectasia after irradiation at G$_0$ a consequence of defective repair? Nature 260:441–443.

Todaro, G. J., H. Green, and M. R. Swift. 1966. Susceptibility of human diploid fibroblast strains to transformation by SV40 virus. Science 153:1252–1254.

Vincent, R. A., Jr., R. B. Sheridan, III, and P. C. Huang. 1975. DNA strand breakage repair in ataxia telangiectasia fibroblast-like cells. Mutat. Res. 33:357–366.

Weichselbaum, R. R., J. Nove, and J. B. Little. 1977. Skin fibroblasts from a D-deletion type retinoblastoma patient are abnormally X-ray sensitive. Nature 266:726–727.

Wilkins, R. J., and R. W. Hart. 1974. Preferential DNA repair in human cells. Nature 247:35–36.

Wolff, S. 1978. Relation between DNA repair, chromosome aberrations, and sister chromatid exchanges, *in* DNA Repair Mechanisms, P. C. Hanawalt, E. C. Friedberg, and C. F. Fox, eds. Academic Press, New York (In press).

Wolff, S., J. Bodycote, G. H. Thomas, and J. E. Cleaver. 1975. Sister chromatid exchange in xeroderma pigmentosum cells that are defective in DNA excision repair or post-replication repair. Genetics 81:349–355.

Wolff, S., B. Rodin, and J. E. Cleaver. 1977. Sister chromatid exchanges induced by mutagenic carcinogens in normal and xeroderma pigmentosum cells. Nature 265:347–349.

Carcinogens: Identification and Mechanisms of Action, edited by A. Clark Griffin and Charles R. Shaw. Raven Press, New York © 1979.

Sarc and Leuk Oncogene-Transforming Proteins as Antigenic Determinants of Cause and Prevention of Cancer in Mice and Rats

Robert J. Huebner and Donald C. Fish

Laboratory of RNA Tumor Viruses, National Cancer Institute, Bethesda, Maryland 20014; and Frederick Cancer Research Center, Frederick, Maryland 21701

Numerous reports describing the molecular, oncogenic, and antigenic properties of sarcoma and leukemia viruses as inducers of cancer suggested that oncogene expressions provided the specific determinants (transforming proteins) not only for transformation and tumor induction but also determinants that would be useful in prevention of cancer within species (Huebner and Todaro 1969, Todaro and Huebner 1972). This deduction was derived from definitive molecular and immunological findings that have been correlated with the successful prevention of cancer described in this report. Acting on the concepts derived from the viral oncogene theory, we and our associates embarked on a series of studies aimed at immunoprevention of chemically induced cancer in mice and rats, the animal species most often used for investigations of carcinogenesis and for identifying environmental carcinogens.

PREVENTION OF SPONTANEOUS AND CHEMICALLY INDUCED CANCER

In early studies with Carrie Whitmire of Microbiological Associates, formalin-inactivated radiation leukemia virus (RadLV), furnished by Lieberman and Kaplan, provided significant, active immunoprotection against 3-methylcholanthrene (3MC)-induced subcutaneous sarcomas in C57BL/6 mice (Whitmire and Huebner 1972). In the same experiment, a "wild"-type leukemia virus isolated from C57BL/6 mice processed as a killed vaccine also provided comparable protection. When, in subsequent experiments, we failed to protect against 3MC sarcomas with similar "inactivated" vaccines, we found that the viruses had not been completely inactivated and that small amounts of live RadLV had replicated and thus had produced sufficient immunity to account for the protection observed.

Acting on this lead, Whitmire used RadLV at $10^{1.0}$ to $10^{1.5}$ infectious doses as a live vaccine given to C57BL/6 mice during the early newborn period 8

TABLE 1. *Use of infectious RadLV and Graffi virus given to newborn C57BL/6Cum mice in protection against chemically (3MC) induced subcutaneous sarcomas*

Experiment	Viral dosage	3MC dosage (µg)	(Interval)	Sarcomas/ total (%)	p value	Mean latency (months)	Total period of observation (months)
1	RadLV $10^{1.5}$	150	(10 weeks)	4/18 (22)*		>4	8
	PBS controls	150		16/20 (80)	<.001	<4	
2	RadLV $10^{1.1}$	25	(8 days)	9/31 (29)		>5	8
	PBS controls	25		19/30 (63)	<.007	4½	8
3	RadLV $10^{1.1}$	100	(8 days)	12/27 (44)		5	8
	PBS controls	100		20/21 (95)	<<.001	4½	
4	Graffi (LV)† ($\approx10^{1.9}$)	100	(30 days)	15/25 (60)		<5	8
	HBSS controls	100		15/28 (54)‡	NS	5	

Abbreviations: PBS, phosphate buffered saline; HBSS, Hanks' balanced salt solution.

* Three leukemias of RadLV type also observed; RadLV is the endogenous ecotropic virus of C57BL/6 mice.

† Graffi virus is immunologically distinct from RadLV.

‡ Four leukemias also occurred, three at five months of age. (These data are summarized from Whitmire 1973, Whitmire and Salerno 1973.)

to 30 days prior to 3MC inoculations. The live RadLV vaccines provided highly significant protection against 3MC tumors in each of three experiments, while a heterotypic virus vaccine, a live Graffi virus used as a control, failed to protect (Whitmire 1973, Whitmire and Salerno 1973) (Table 1). The successful protection experiments in large part were based on earlier observations that RadLV of low infectivity, when injected into young C57BL/6 mice, produced both neutralizing and complement-fixing antibodies to RadLV (R. J. Huebner, unpublished observation, Igel *et al.* 1969).

The suggestion that immunity to RadLV could be utilized to provide protection against chemically induced cancer was confirmed when banded viral concentrates of RadLV cultured in large quantities were used to immunize goats, which yielded high titers of passive antibodies giving equivalent neutralizing responses as high as 1:3,200 to both the ecotropic and xenotropic viruses in the XC and focus-forming tests and thus establishing the RadLV-immunizing virus as a recombinant expressing leuk oncogene specified tumor antigens. When given to mice, the goat antisera processed as IgG not only prevented the oncogenic effects of the RadLV recombinant itself but also the oncogenic capability of other related viruses, such as AKR, GLV and MSV(GLV). In contemporary experiments, the use of passive IgG immunity to clearly establish recombinant viruses provided highly significant protection against 3MC-induced sarcomas when given prior to, during, and following administration of 3MC (Huebner, in press) and as described below.

PREVENTION OF SARCOMAS INDUCED BY 3MC IN VIRUS-FREE C3H/f MICE

Passive immunity to RadLV and GLV, demonstrated to have the properties of a recombinant type C oncornavirus (Hartley *et al.* 1977, Staal *et al.* 1977), was produced in goats by periodic immunizations with banded high titer RadLV virus preparations. The methods and materials used have been published elsewhere (Huebner *et al.* 1976a, b, c).

Four separate experiments (Tables 2–4) were performed in weanling C3H/f mice with individual IgG preparations previously tested in XC and focus-forming assays for antibody responses to ecotropic (AKR) and xenotropic (AT124) viruses. Some preparations (processed as IgG) revealed equivalent neutralizing responses to both viruses and furnished the specifications of a recombinant, while the responses of other IgG preparations did not show equivalent titers to both viruses and thus did not meet specifications for a recombinant virus. Also, mixtures of IgG preparations having equivalent high titers to both viruses did not qualify as recombinants, failed to protect against 3MC tumors, and were abandoned. In each of the experiments, neutralization titers versus both ecotropic and xenotropic viruses, days of administration, total dosage of the IgG given, tumor incidences, and the significance of protection are shown directly on each table.

TABLE 2. *Prevention of 3-methylcholanthrene (3MC) tumors in weanling C3H MTV⁻ mice by passive immunization with antiviral IgG*

Experiment	Goat IgG used	Days of administration	Total volume administered (ml)	Neutralization titer versus		150 μg 3MC administered on day	Tumor incidence day 122	% Tumors	p value
				AKR	AT124				
1	RadLV*	0, 3, 6	0.6	3,200	3,200	3	14/27	52	0.006
	Control	—	—	—	—	3	25/29	86	
2	RadLV	0, 3, 6, 9, 12	1.0	3,200	3,200	12	11/30	37	0.002
	Control	—	—	—	—	12	29/39	74	

* Radiation leukemia virus (RadLV of Lieberman and Kaplan), a recombinant virus, was used to produce antibodies in goats, which were then processed as IgG. The RadLV hyperimmune IgG antibodies were demonstrated in the XC test to provide specific immunity directed against the AKR (ecotropic) and AT124 (xenotropic) recombinant viruses (Hartley *et al.* 1977). The RadLV immunity apparently specifies immunity to the transforming proteins of the "leukemia" and "sarcoma" oncogenes.

TABLE 3. *Prevention of 3-methylcholanthrene (3MC) tumors in weanling C3H MTV⁻ mice by passive immunization with antiviral IgG*

Goat IgG used	Days of administration	Total volume administered (ml)	Neutralization titer versus		150 µg 3MC administered on day	Tumor incidence day 150	% Tumors	Tumor incidence day 250	% Tumors	p value
			AKR	AT124						
RadLV*	0, 2, 4, 6, 8, 10	1.2	1,600	800	4	6/20	30	7/20	35	0.003
GLV†	0, 2, 4, 6, 8, 10	1.2	800	200	4	11/22	50	13/22	59	NS
C57L‡	0, 2, 4, 6, 8, 10	1.2	100	800	4	15/22	68	16/22	73	NS
Normal goat	0, 2, 4, 6, 8, 10	1.2	<100	<100	4	16/22	73	17/22	77	NS
Nonimmunized	—	—	—	—	4	16/21	76	17/21	81	—

* Passive immunity to RadLV, a recombinant virus, specifies protection (see Table 1).
† Passive IgG immunity to Gross leukemia virus (GLV) does not provide immunoprotection since it was not prepared against a recombinant virus (note disparate XC titers).
‡ IgG immunity to the C57L xenotropic virus alone does not provide protection.

TABLE 4. *Prevention of 3-methylcholanthrene (3MC) tumors in weanling C3H MTV⁻ mice by passive immunization with antiviral IgG*

Goat IgG used	Days of administration	Total volume administered (ml)	Neutralization titer versus		150 µg 3MC administered on day	Tumor incidence day 190	% Tumors	p value
			AKR	AT124				
RadLV*	0, 2, 4, 6, 8, 10, 14	1.4	1,600	1,600	4	8/30	27	<0.0001
RadLV†	0, 2, 4, 6, 8, 10, 14	1.4	100	200	4	20/30	67	0.03
RLV‡	0, 2, 4, 6, 8, 10, 14	1.4	400	1,600	4	24/27	89	NS
Nonimmunized	—	—	—	—	4	27/29	93	—

* Properties of recombinant virus (see Table 1).
† This low titered neutralization was apparently a partial recombinant.
‡ Rauscher leukemia virus used to make IgG; latter does not show properties of a recombinant virus.

Table 2 illustrates comparable experiments in which two different IgG dosage schedules were employed. The 3MC was given at day 3 in the first experiment and on day 12 in the second. The IgG neutralizing antibody titers directed against the AKR and AT124 viruses were both 1:3,200, thus meeting the specifications of a recombinant. The protection in each experiment was highly significant, $p = 0.006$ and $p = 0.002$. The several experimental groups shown in Table 3 again featured one recombinant RadLV IgG providing highly significant protection ($p = 0.003$ at 250 days). The GLV and C57L antiviral IgGs and the normal goat sera clearly did not meet required specifications as recombinant viruses and did not provide protection.

The experimental groups shown in Table 4 illustrated once again the necessary conditions required for achieving significant protection against 3MC-induced tumors. Immunity to a high-titered RadLV having properties consistent with an antisera to a recombinant virus provided highly significant protection ($p = \ll 0.0001$) during the 190-day period of observation, while RadLV IgG featuring a low titer (100–200) presumed recombinant provided marginal protection ($p = 0.03$). The anti-RLV IgG, despite high levels of antibody to xenotropic virus, did not meet the specifications required of a recombinant virus and provided no protection.

Although these data clearly demonstrated that passive antibodies directed against certain (recombinant) MuLV preparations successfully suppressed 3MC sarcomas, the precise immunological factors involved require considerable analysis. In our view, the RadLV, GLV, and other recombinant viruses used for producing protective IgG clearly must express the transforming proteins of leuk and/or sarc oncogenic sequences, which in the goat IgG specify high level recombinant antibodies capable of suppressing similar expressions of oncogenic sequences (transforming proteins) induced by 3MC in the C3H/f mouse tissues. It should be noted in Tables 2–4 that only high titered recombinant RadLV IgGs produced highly significant protection to 3MC tumors that were essentially free of oncornavirus expressions.

PASSIVE IMMUNITY IN THE MOUSE

It is now clear that the oncogenic oncornaviruses exemplified by sarcoma and leukemia viruses of chickens, mice, rats, and cats in many instances represent recombinants expressing transforming proteins of sarc or leuk oncogenes. This conclusion has been substantiated in a number of elegant molecular studies (Scolnick *et al.* 1976, Stehelin *et al.* 1976, Frankel *et al.* 1976, Roy-Burman and Klement 1975, Duesberg *et al.* 1974). Recently, Hartley *et al.* (1977) and Staal *et al.* (1977) described a new recombinant virus isolated from AKR and other virogenic mouse strains that represent stable recombinants of the endogenous ecotropic and xenotropic viruses. Hartley's recombinant virus, called MCF, begins to develop spontaneously in AKR mice at approximately 200 days after birth; these oncogenic recombinants express leuk and/or sarc genes that can specify accelerated leukemogenesis in AKR and other strains of mice and malignant transformation in mink fibroblasts.

It should be pointed out that some RadLV preparations used in these experiments for immunization of goats, which have the properties of a highly oncogenic recombinant virus, were developed during serial transmissions of the original RadLV in newborn C57BL/6 mice. The resulting virus preparations became highly oncogenic (R. J. Huebner, unpublished observation).

Evidence that sarc gene antigenic expressions specify common tumor antigens and immune protection against chemically induced tumors in mice was also reported by Reiner and Southam (1969) and by Leffell and Coggin (1977).

We deduce from these prevention studies that leuk genes expressed by recombinant RadLV furnished species-specific transforming proteins which provided immunity capable of preventing both leukemia in AKR mice (Huebner *et al.* 1976a, b, c) and 3MC sarcomas in C3H/f mice, as described above.

IMMUNOPREVENTION OF EXPERIMENTALLY INDUCED AND NORMALLY LETHAL TRANSPLANTABLE CANCERS IN RATS

Fischer 344 and Wistar rat systems are similar to the human in that they rarely express type C RNA tumor viruses spontaneously in early life. However, rats do develop lymphomas and other cancers spontaneously with advancing age. Rats regularly respond early in life to administration of chemical carcinogens that result in cancers which are also generally devoid of detectable infectious virus. In addition, F344 normal cells were readily transformed in vitro by chemicals, a process facilitated by prior infection with mouse xenotropic virus or Rauscher leukemia virus (RLV) (Price *et al.* 1971, 1976, 1977). Also, DNA (adenovirus, SV40, and polyoma) virus-induced tumors of Fischer and Wistar rats do not express endogenous RaLV.

The discovery of a tumor antigen held in common by a number of different rat tumors cultured in vitro or transplanted in vivo (Rhim *et al.* 1972a, b) suggested new opportunities for developing transplantation rejection test systems having broad cross-protection in the rat, which might have greater relevance to prevention of environmentally induced cancers occurring in man. The serum antibodies to the common rat tumor antigens were shown to cross-react extensively with rat tumor cells produced by chemicals (4-nitroquinoline-1-oxide [4NQO], dimethylhydrazine [DMH]), by DNA tumor viruses (polyoma and adenovirus), and with rat tumors produced by KiMSV(NP), a nonproducer rat sarcoma virus expressing species-specific transforming proteins of the rat sarc gene (Huebner, in press). The KiMSV-transformed rat cells were therefore particularly interesting since they cross-reacted completely in complement fixation box titrations with common tumor antigens expressed in various rat tumors and tumor cells induced by the diverse methods described and discussed below.

In developing a suitable approach to prevention of cancer in rats, we took advantage of several observations: (1) the isolation and characterization of

Kirsten rat sarcoma virus (Kirsten and Mayer 1967, Klement *et al.* 1971, Rhim *et al.* 1977), (2) demonstration by Scolnick and Parks (1974) of rat sarc genes in the Kirsten and Harvey sarcoma viruses, and (3) the isolation by Rhim *et al.* (1977) of a nonproducer KiMSV(NP) rat sarcoma cell expressing tumor antigens (transforming proteins). Thus, the rat sarcogene specified-antigen expressed by KiMSV(NP) was shown by complement fixation to cross-react with rat tumor antigens held in common with other rat tumors as follows: (1) spontaneously transformed rat cells (Rhim *et al.* 1972b), (2) chemically induced tumors and tumor cells transformed or induced by 3MC, 4NQO, and DMH (Freeman *et al.* 1973, Price *et al.* 1971, Weisburger 1973), and (3) DNA virus-induced tumors and transformed rat cells (adenovirus, SV40, and polyoma) (Huebner *et al.* 1963, Black *et al.* 1963, McAllister *et al.* 1969, Habel and Axelrod 1965, Sjögren 1961). In addition, rat cells transformed by the mouse Moloney sarcoma virus (8613) and by avian sarcoma virus (XC cells) were shown to express the common rat tumor antigen. Thus, each of the tumors listed above having variable modes of induction and expressed as sarcomas and carcinomas were found to express the same rat tumor antigen identified and quantitated by complement fixation and radioimmunoassay tests and shown to have tumor antigens cross-reacting with the antigens held in common by all other known rat tumors serially cultured in vitro and in vivo (Tables 5 and 6). These observations were in themselves unique and significant, since reports by Prehn (1962) and Klein *et al.* (1960) had emphasized that every individual tumor occurring in experimental animals, particularly in mice and rats, possessed individual tumor-specific antigenic determinants, a situation that remains true in studies of immunoprotection of primary tumors using the same tumor as immunogen. However, after serial subcultures and transplantations of the various types of rat tumor cells in syngeneic newborn rats as described above, a common rat tumor antigen was found to be present in all rat tumors when they were tested with antisera generated in rats in which these and various other rat tumors were transplanted (see Tables 5 and 6). It is perhaps important to reemphasize that while the virus-free common rat tumor antigen was shown to be unrelated to the p70's of the specific envelope proteins of the rat or mouse type C virogenes, it was fully cross-reactive with the antigens expressed by the KiMSV(NP) sarcogene-transformed cells* selected for use as the primary immunogen in the transplantation protection studies described below.

---

*S. Rasheed and M. Gardner reported the isolation of rat sarcoma viruses from the 4NQO and polyoma tumor cells described in Tables 5 and 6 and from a transplantable hepatoma tumor from a Buffalo rat. The sarc genes were rescued during cocultivation with infectious rat virus isolated by Rasheed (Rasheed *et al.* 1976). The rat sarc gene was recovered from tissue culture cell lines of these same tumors only when the cells were transplanted and cultured serially in newborn F344 rats (Rasheed *et al.,* in press). This very important discovery of sarcoma gene sequences in tumor cells induced by chemicals, DNA, and RNA tumor viruses supports the postulate that the common tumor antigens reported in these cells several years ago by Rhim and his associates (1972a, b) are also coded by endogenous sarc genes. Thus it appears that the common tumor antigens serve as useful antigen markers for expressions of sarcoma genomes with varying degrees of oncogenic potency.

TABLE 5. *Characterization of the various tumors following serial trocar transplantation in newborn Fischer 344 rats*

Tumor	Presumed transforming agent	Rat origin	Histopathology	EM	Antigen level versus homologous antiserum	Common rat tumor antigen*	Virus expression	
							MuLV	RaLV
KiMSV(NP)	KiMSV	Wistar	Fibrosarcoma	(−)	1:32	1:32	(−)	(−)
KiMSV(P)	KiMSV	Wistar	Sarcoma	+	1:32	1:32	1:8	1:2
KiMSV(Rasheed)	KiMSV & RaLV	344	Fibrosarcoma	+	1:8	1:4	1:16	1:16
4NQO	4NQO	344	Fibrosarcoma	(−)	1:128	1:128	(−)	(−)
PyTRE	Polyoma	344	Fibrosarcoma	(−)	1:32	1:32	(−)	(−)
Colon	Dimethylhydrazine	344	Endocarcinoma	(−)	1:32	1:32	(−)	(−)
8613	M-MSV	344	Sarcoma	+	1:32	1:32	1:32	(−)

Abbreviation: EM, electron microscopy.
* Antibody against 4NQO was used as the standard for detecting the common tumor antigen.

TABLE 6. Cross-reactivity of several nonvirus-expressing rat tumors: Representative reactions

Antigens	Anti-4NQO						Anti-KiMSV(NP)					Anticolon					Anti-PyTRE					
	20	40	80	160	320	640	20	40	80	160	320	20	40	80	160	320	20	40	80	160	320	640
4NQO (sarcoma)																						
2	4	4	4	4	4	1	4	4	4	4	tr	4	4	4	4	4	4	4	4	4	2	1
4	4	4	4	4	4	1	4	4	4	1	tr	4	4	4	4	3	4	4	4	4	2	tr
8	4	4	4	4	4	2	4	4	4	1	tr	4	4	3	1	tr	4	4	4	4	tr	0
16	4	4	4	4	2	1	4	4	2	1	tr	4	1	tr	tr	tr	4	4	4	3	1	0
32	4	4	4	2	1	tr	4	tr	tr	tr	0	tr	tr	0	0	0	4	2	1	1	tr	0
64	1	1	tr	tr	tr	0	2	tr	tr	tr	0	0	0	0	0	0	4	2	tr	tr	0	0
KiMSV(NP) (sarcoma)																						
2	4	4	4	4	4	1	4	4	4	tr	tr	4	4	4	4	1	4	4	4	4	1	tr
4	4	4	4	4	4	1	4	4	4	tr	tr	4	4	3	2	tr	4	4	4	4	1	tr
8	4	4	4	4	4	2	4	4	4	tr	tr	4	3	2	1	tr	4	4	4	4	2	tr
16	4	4	4	4	1	1	4	2	1	3	tr	4	3	2	0	tr	4	4	4	3	2	tr
32	4	tr	3	2	1	tr	1	tr	tr	tr	0	tr	tr	0	0	0	4	4	tr	tr	2	tr
64	1	1	tr	tr	tr	0	1	tr	0	0	0	0	0	0	0	0	4	1	tr	tr	tr	tr
Colon (carcinoma)																						
2	4	4	4	4	4	4	4	4	4	4	4	4	4	4	4	4	4	4	4	4	4	4
4	4	4	4	4	4	4	4	4	4	4	2	4	4	4	4	4	4	4	4	4	4	2
8	4	4	4	4	4	4	4	4	4	4	1	4	4	4	4	3	4	4	4	4	4	2
16	4	4	4	4	4	3	4	4	4	3	tr	4	4	4	2	1	4	4	4	4	4	2
32	4	4	4	3	2	tr	4	3	2	tr	tr	4	3	1	tr	tr	4	4	2	2	1	tr
64	4	4	3	3	2	tr	4	2	tr	tr	tr	2	tr	tr	tr	0	—	—	—	—	—	—
PyTRE (sarcoma)																						
2	4	4	4	4	4	1	4	4	4	1	tr	4	4	4	2	2	4	4	4	4	1	tr
4	4	4	4	4	4	1	4	4	4	1	tr	4	4	4	3	3	4	4	4	4	3	tr
8	4	4	4	4	4	2	4	4	4	1	tr	4	4	4	2	2	4	4	4	4	tr	0
16	4	4	4	4	2	2	4	4	4	1	tr	4	4	tr	2	tr	4	4	4	4	1	0
32	4	4	4	4	2	2	4	3	2	tr	tr	4	3	tr	tr	tr	4	4	4	4	1	0
64	4	4	4	2	1	tr	4	2	2	tr	0	4	tr	tr	0	0	4	4	3	2	tr	0

MATERIALS AND METHODS

Rats

Inbred Fischer 344 rats were obtained either as pregnant females within three to five days of delivery or as three- to five-week-old weanlings of either sex. Animals were obtained from Microbiological Associates and from the Frederick Cancer Research Center. The rats were fed a standard laboratory chow ad libitum. Fluids were provided from feeding fresh apples. Routine examination showed the animals to be free of pathogenic bacteria, endoparasites, ectoparasites, and the following viruses: PVM, Reo 3, GD VII, K, polyoma, Sendai, MVM, KRV, H-1, ectromelia, SV5, M. Ad., MHV, LCM, and RCV.

Origin and History of Rat Tumors in This Study

KiMSV(NP): A nontransformed Wistar rat liver cell line was transformed with KiMSV and cloned. A clone (Cl 17) was isolated which did not produce virus.

KiMSV(P): A nontransformed Wistar rat liver cell line was also transformed by KiMSV and cloned. Of two other clones, Cl 3 produced low levels of virus, while Cl 12 produced high levels as measured by reverse transcriptase activity in the cell culture supernatants, electron microscopic examination of the tumor, and complement fixation tests for the p30 group-specific viral antigens. The KiMSV clones carrying infectious virus were less immunogenic than was KiMSV(NP).

KiMSV(Rasheed): A spontaneously transformed Fischer 344 rat line expressing the endogenous Rasheed rat leukemia virus (Rasheed et al. 1976) was superinfected with a cell-free KiMSV virus. This transformed cell demonstrated high levels of rat type C virus expression when tested by complement fixation.

4NQO: Fischer 344 rat cells in culture were transformed by growth in the presence of 0.1 μg of 4NQO; they were free of virus expression (Price et al. 1977).

PyTRE: Fischer 344 rat embryo cells were transformed by polyoma virus; this tumor cell remains generally free of virus expression (Habel and Axelrod 1965).

Colon: Fischer 344 rats fed dimethylhydrazine developed colon tumors; this tumor was free of virus (Weisburger 1973).

8613: Moloney sarcoma virus (M-MSV) induced tumor cells were transplanted into Fischer 344 rats (Huebner, unpublished observation); subsequently, a cell line (8613) was derived from this tumor (Freeman, personal communication) which continued to produce MuLV. This cell line, like the others above, was used as a transplantable tumor.

Eventually, all the rat tumor cell lines shown in Table 5 were maintained by in vitro tissue culture and passaged serially in newborn rats, developing increasing titers of common rat tumor antigen in the process.

The newborn rats carrying the tumors were observed daily for the development of tumor at the site of injection. When a tumor reached 10–20 mm diameter, the animal was sacrificed, and the tumor was excised and used to prepare (1) a frozen stock in dimethylsulfoxide (DMSO), (2) a 20% (w/v) extract for complement fixation assays, (3) samples for electron microscopy, (4) samples for histology, (5) samples for establishing the line in cell culture, and (6) samples for transplantation.

Frozen stocks from early passages of the tumor were obtained by freezing small sections of the tumor in DMSO (cryoprotective medium [Microbiological Associates] plus 1% veal infusion broth plus 1% penicillin-streptomycin). The tumor was then stored in liquid nitrogen and used to reestablish the tumor fragments at any subsequent time by thawing, washing in Eagle's base, mincing, and implanting by trocar into newborns. Tumor extracts were prepared for complement fixation assays by fine mincing of the tumor in Eagle's minimal essential medium (E-MEM) followed by a three-second exposure to ultrasonic oscillation.

For transplantation, the tumor was minced into 1 cu mm sections (approximately 2×10^8 cells, viability >90%) and injected subcutaneously by trocar transplantation into newborns. After the initial growth, the tumors (3–5 mm) were detectable between days 4 and 9. They were harvested three to six days later, depending on the particular type of tumor required. This procedure generally provided tumors with high complement-fixing antigen titers (up to 1:128) while minimizing anticomplementary activity within the sample. The tumors and tumor-antigen expressions were maintained and often increased in titer by additional consecutive serial transplants into newborn rats.

Antibody Production Versus Tumor

To prepare antibody against the tumor antigens, a 1 cu mm section of tumor from the continuous newborn passage line was injected by trocar into a weanling rat four to six weeks of age. Tumors generally became detectable (3–5 mm) between days 7 and 10 after transplant. The animals were test bled from the retro-orbital sinus plexus for complement-fixing antibody starting on day 21 to 40 after transplant, depending on the tumor system being used. Antibody production started earlier in the virus-transformed tumor systems compared to the chemically or spontaneously transformed tumor systems. When the test bleed result was acceptable (>80 antibody units versus 8 units of antigen), the animal was bled out by decapitation and the sera pooled. Complement-fixing serum titers of 1:320 to 1:640 were achieved and proved very suitable for evaluating common tumor antigens and cross-reactive transforming proteins specified by the KiMSV sarc gene expressions.

Tissue Culture

Cell cultures were established from each of the tumor systems by aseptically mincing the tumor tissue from the newborn animals and growing the cells in RPMI 1640 plus 10% serum and antibiotics. Once established the cells grew equally well in E-MEM. The cultures were routinely monitored for bacteria, yeast, mold, and mycoplasma infection and were found to be free of these contaminants. The cells continued to produce the common rat tumor antigen in culture and maintained their tumorigenic potential.

Passage of Challenge Tumors in Newborn and Weanling Rats

The various challenge tumors were serially passed in newborn rats by trocar transplantation. The results of histopathological examination, electron microscopy, and complement-fixation testing are given in Table 5. These tumors were progressively metastatic and rapidly lethal in the newborns.

Trocar transplantation of these tumors into weanling rats yielded tumors manifesting rapid growth and metastases that eventually killed the rats (20–40 days). Routine postmortem examination, histopathological examination, and complement-fixation tests on various internal organs (especially the lung, thymus, and spleen) showed that the tumors were highly invasive and metastatic.

As shown in Table 5, two of the tumors were used for protective immunization, the allogeneic KiMSV(NP) and the syngeneic KiMSV(Rasheed). On transplantation into weanlings, the tumors generally appeared between days 7 and 9, reached maximum size (10–30 mm) on days 11 to 14, and regressed by days 28–30. All the weanlings developed tumors; however, once the tumor had regressed, none of the rats developed progressive tumors, when observed for over 200 days. Both the low and high passage immunizing sarc-expressing tumors regressed in similar fashion. The only deviation that occurred was when a KiMSV(NP) transplant became a virus producer. This tumor did not regress and killed the weanling rat.

Demonstration of a Common Tumor Antigen

Table 6 shows representative box-type complement fixation test results using tumor extracts as antigens and serum from tumor-bearing rats as antibody. A common cross-reacting antigen-antibody was demonstrated by all tumors studied. In addition to those tumors indicated in the table, the following transplantable tumors showed the presence of the common tumor antigen: KiMSV(NP), KiMSV(Rasheed), Rasheed, 8613, XC cells transformed by avian sarcoma virus, jejunum transformed by DMH, F344 rat embryo cells spontaneously transformed, 3MC sarcomas, KNRK, FeSV-NRK, RL 34 (Wistar) cells transformed by 4NQO, guinea pig herpes virus transformed rat cells, and adeno 12-SV40 hybrid rat tumor cells.

Immunoprevention Tests

Protection against transplantation of otherwise lethal doses of rat tumor cells was primarily accomplished by preimmunizing weanling rats with 10^6 to 10^8 KiMSV(NP) transplantable tumor cells. Although allogeneic, the KiMSV(NP) cells replicated as a subcutaneous tumor that was rejected after two- to three-week intervals. KiMSV(Rasheed), a syngeneic tumor cell vaccine used as immunogen in one experiment, also was rejected.

RESULTS

The KiMSV tumor antigen vaccine(s) induced powerful cell-mediated immunity that suppressed the establishment of other ordinarily highly lethal syngeneic challenge tumor cells and thus provided highly significant protection (Tables 7–10). Four of 15 experiments completed to date are presented in Tables 7–9. In Table 7, 50 weanling rats were immunized by a single trocar implantation of the allogeneic virus-transformed but virus-nonproducing KiMSV(NP) tumor. All rats developed tumors that spontaneously regressed by day 25. On day 39, the rats were challenged by subcutaneous injection of serial log dilutions of either 4NQO or colon tumor cells arising from serial passages in the newborn rats. Highly significant prevention was observed at 10^4 to 10^5 dilutions of challenge cells.

In the experiment shown in Table 8, the rats were immunized by two injections of the KiMSV(NP) cells. All animals developed tumors that regressed by day 27. No tumors developed following the second trocar immunization with KiMSV(NP). The immunized rats were challenged 13 days after the second trocar immunization with 4NQO rat tumors. Significant protection was observed again at 10^4 and 10^5 dilutions.

In the experiment shown in Table 9, two series of immunizations with KiMSV(NP) cells provided extraordinary protection against 10^4, 10^5, and 10^6 challenge cells, thus clearly indicating that rat tumors induced by a DNA tumor virus not only shared common tumor antigens with the KiMSV(NP) immunogen but were prevented from transplanting at all dilution levels. In the preliminary experiment shown in Table 10, the syngeneic KiMSV(Rasheed) tumor cell vaccine also provided protection against lethal 4NQO tumor cells.

CONCLUSIONS

We believe these findings suggest the following conclusions. Within the cells of a given host system (mouse, rat, and perhaps human), there exist sarc and leuk oncogenes which, when induced and expressed, are capable of producing sarcomas in mesenchymal cells, lymphomas in lymphoblastoid cells, and carcinoma in epithelioid cells. The corollary of this suggests the concept that for prevention of various types of cancer in rats and mice, it may only be necessary

TABLE 7. *Rat sarcoma nonproducer (KiMSV[NP]) tumor cells as active immunogen (cell vaccine) to prevent 4NQO and colon transplantable tumors in weanling F344 rats*

	Dose	No. of tumors (day)						p value
		4	10	15	20	25	39 = 0	
Single immunization*		0/50	44/50	50/50	5/50	0/50	0/50	
Challenge†			6	10	17	21		
4NQO sarcoma cells (NB p19)								
Vaccine	10^4		0/10	0/10	0/10	0/10		0.00001
Control	10^4		0/20	9/20	16/20	17/20		
Vaccine	10^5		0/10	0/10	5/10	6/10		0.017
Control	10^5		0/25	17/25	23/25	24/25		
Vaccine	10^6		0/5	4/5	4/5	5/5		NS
Control	10^6		5/5	5/5	5/5	5/5		
DMH colon carcinoma cells (NB p10)								
Vaccine	10^4		0/10	2/10	4/10	—		0.0012
Control	10^4		2/15	13/15	15/15	—		
Vaccine	10^5		0/10	9/10	9/10	—		NS
Control	10^5		3/15	15/15	15/15	—		

* Immunization was by subcutaneous transplantation of approximately 2×10^8 cells NB p5 into the left flank of weanling rats.
† Animals were challenged on day 39 by subcutaneous injection of the indicated cells (>90% viable) into the right flank.

TABLE 8. Rat sarcoma nonproducer (KiMSV[NP]) tumor cells as active immunogen (cell vaccine) to prevent transplantable 4NQO tumors in weanling F344 rats

	Dose	No. of tumors (day)					p value
		7	12	20	34	43 = 0	
Double immunization*		22/25	24/25	17/25	0/25	0/25	0.0048
			0	8	16 = 0		

	Dose	No. of tumors (day)				p value
		10	17	19	21	
Challenge†			0/25	0/25	0/25	
Vaccine	10^4	0/10	0/10	3/10	3/10	0.0048
Control	10^4	9/20	16/20	17/20	17/20	
Vaccine	10^5	1/10	1/10	3/10	4/10	0.0008
Control	10^5	17/25	23/25	24/25	24/25	
Vaccine	10^6	5/5	5/5	5/5	5/5	NS
Control	10^6	5/5	5/5	5/5	5/5	

* Immunization was by subcutaneous trocar transplantation of approximately 2×10^8 cells NB p3 into the left flank of the rats. On day 43, the animals received a second trocar transplant of NB p7 cells. Unimmunized animals that received this trocar material all developed tumors by days 5–8.

† Challenge was by subcutaneous injection of 4 NQO tumor cells (>90% viable) into the right flank of the rats.

TABLE 9. KiMSV(NP) tumor cells as active immunogen (cell vaccine) in weanling F344 rats to prevent transplantable polyoma-induced tumors

Immunization*

	Dose	No. of tumors (day)					p value
	4	**9**	**18**	**27**	**32 = 0**	
	32/40	40/40	14/40	0/40	0/40	
		4	6	13 = 0		

Challenge†

	Dose	No. of tumors (day)				p value
		1	**6**	**13**	**20**	
		0/40	0/40	0/40		
Vaccine	10^3	0/5	0/5	0/5	0/5	NS
Control	10^3	0/10	0/10	0/10	1/10	
Vaccine	10^4	0/10	0/10	0/10	0/10	0.0004
Control	10^4	0/10	0/10	0/10	8/10	
Vaccine	10^5	0/15	0/15	0/15	0/15	0.001
Control	10^5	0/10	0/10	3/10	6/10	
Vaccine	10^6	0/10	0/10	0/10	0/10	<.0001
Control	10^6	0/10	0/10	4/10	10/10	

* Immunization was by subcutaneous transplantation of approximately 2×10^8 cells of NB p9 into the left flank of the rats. On day 32, the animals received a second trocar transplant of 2×10^8 cells NB p8. The unimmunized animals that received this material all developed tumors by day 6.

† Challenge was by subcutaneous injection of polyoma transformed cells NB p7 tumor cells (>90% viable) into the right flank of the animals.

TABLE 10. Use of syngeneic KiMSV (Rasheed) tumor cells as an active immunogen (cell vaccine) in weanling F344 rats to prevent transplantable tumors

Immunization* / Challenge†	16	4	18	15	23	24	29	32 = 0	43	p value
		15/15		15/15		0/15		0/15		
4NQO tissue culture cells, p16										
Vaccine	0/5		0/5		0/5		0/5		0/5	0.004
Control	2/5		4/5		4/5		5/5		5/5	
8613 tissue culture cells, p4‡										
Vaccine	0/5		0/5		0/5		2/5 dead		2/5 dead	NS‖
Control	5/5		5/5		5/5		dead		dead	
Cl 3 tissue culture cells, p15§										
Vaccine	0/5		0/5		0/5		0/5		0/5	NS‖
Control	1/5		3/5		3/5		3/5		3/5	

* Immunization was by subcutaneous trocar transplantation of approximately 2×10^8 cells NB p1 into the left flank of the weanling rats.

† Animals were challenged on day 32 by subcutaneous injection of 10^6 cells (>90% viable) from the indicated tissue culture-grown lines into the right flank of the animal.

‡ 8613: MSV tumor developing in NB F344 rats injected with Moloney leukemia virus (M-MSV) positive leukemia cells. After 26 subcultures, Freeman (unpublished observation) isolated a rat tumor line in tissue culture, 8613. When transplanted into F344 rats, the tumor cells were found to have common rat tumor antigen. Sera from the transplanted rats reacted with the common rat tumor antigen, providing the initial recognition of this antigen.

§ Cl 3: A KiMSV (clone 3) transformed Wistar Furth rat liver cell which contains common rat tumor antigen and xenotropic MuLV (at low levels) (Rhim, unpublished observation).

‖ Significance of 8613 and Cl 3 tests combined: 2/10 versus 8/10 (p = .01).

to immunosuppress expressions of a single endogenous sarc-leuk oncogenic genome postulated to be present in most or all vertebrate cells (Huebner and Todaro 1969). If fully confirmed, such information would simplify various conceptual and operational approaches now being considered in dealing with cause and prevention of cancer. Thus, cancer may not have to be considered in almost hopeless terms, often described as 100 different diseases caused by perhaps thousands of carcinogens.

Future studies increasingly will be focused on investigations of likely sarc-leuk oncogene expressions in human cancers, particularly in those human cancers produced by environmental, physical, or chemical agents.

Our approaches to immunoprevention of human cancer would emphasize a search for and identification of a human sarc oncogene expressing common tumor antigen(s) in a variety of human cancers and/or cancer cells that could then be studied further for common tumor antigens by heterotransplantation in immunosuppressed rats or hamsters. Extensive absorption of suitable reactive antisera acquired from tumor-bearing rats and hamsters conceivably could identify common tumor-specific antigen(s) in human tumors. Such antigen(s), combined with inducers of cell-mediated immunity, could well provide opportunities for immunization of humans at high cancer risk, such as those specified by autosomal dominant genes (i.e., Gardner's syndrome, familial polyposis, Fanconi's syndrome, and telangiectasis). Future immunoprevention studies will focus on identification and amplification of common tumor antigens in human cancers by transplantation methods similar to those that led to the initial isolation of complement-fixing T-antigens of DNA tumor viruses and the common tumor antigens in rats.

Although the T- and common tumor antigens expressed by specified tumors of rats will not be directly applicable for use for protection in human cancer, successful heterotransplantations of human tumors in newborn and weanling ATS-treated rats have been achieved (R. M. McAllister and M. B. Gardner, unpublished observations). Careful selection of sera following extensive absorption will be used to identify antibodies reactive in complement-fixation tests with a variety of human tumor extracts.

We plan also to make use of Kobayashi's general observation that transplantation of allogeneic tumor cells provides effective cell-mediated immunity to a variety of otherwise lethal syngeneic tumor cells, an observation which Kobayashi suggests must imply the presence of a common tumor antigen in his challenge tumors (Kobayashi *et al.* 1974).

REFERENCES

Black, P. H., W. P. Rowe, H. C. Turner, and R. J. Huebner. 1963. A specific complement-fixing antigen present in SV40 tumor and transformed cells. Proc. Natl. Acad. Sci. USA 50:1148–1156.

Duesberg, P., P. K. Vogt, K. Beeman, and M. Lai. 1974. RNA tumor viruses: Mechanisms of recombination and complexity of the genome. Cold Spring Harbor Symp. Quant. Biol. 39:847–848.

Frankel, A. E., R. L. Neubauer, and P. J. Fischinger. 1976. Fractionation of DNA nucleotide transcripts from Moloney sarcoma virus and isolation of sarcoma virus-specific complementary DNA. J. Virol. 18:481–490.

Freeman, A. E., R. V. Gilden, M. L. Vernon, R. G. Wolford, P. E. Hugunin, and R. J. Huebner. 1973. 5-bromo-2'deoxyuridine potentiation of rat embryo cell transformation induced in vitro by 3-methylcholanthrene: Induction of rat leukemia virus gs antigen in transformed cells. Proc. Natl. Acad. Sci. USA 70:2415–2419.

Habel, K., and D. Axelrod. 1965. Continued viral influence in virus-free polyoma tumors, *in* Perspectives in Virology IV. Hoeber Medical Division, Harper and Row, New York, pp. 126–141.

Hartley, J. W., N. K. Wolford, L. J. Old, and W. P. Rowe. 1977. A new class of murine leukemia virus associated with development of spontaneous lymphomas. Proc. Natl. Acad. Sci. USA 74:789–792.

Huebner, R. J. 1978. Immune protection against spontaneous and induced cancers in mice and rats based on virogene and sarcogene specific immunity: A strategy for protection against cancer in man, *in* Tumours of Early Life in Man and Animals (Sixth Perugia Quadrennial International Conference on Cancer, 1977), L. Severi, ed., Division of Cancer Research, Perugia, Italy (In press).

Huebner, R. J., R. V. Gilden, W. T. Lane, R. Toni, R. W. Trimmer, and P. R. Hill. 1976a. Suppression of murine type C RNA virogenes by type specific oncornavirus vaccines: Prospects for prevention of cancer. Proc. Natl. Acad. Sci. USA 73:620–624.

Huebner, R. J., R. V. Gilden, R. Toni, P. R. Hill, and R. W. Trimmer. 1976b. Suppression of endogenous type C murine virogene expressions with virus specific hyperimmune immunoglobulin (IgG), *in* Prevention and Detection of Cancer, Vol. 1, H. E. Nieburgs, ed., Marcel Dekker, Inc., New York and Basel, pp. 483–495.

Huebner, R. J., R. V. Gilden, R. Toni, R. W. Hill, R. W. Trimmer, D. C. Fish, and B. Sass. 1976c. Prevention of spontaneous leukemia in AKR mice by type-specific immunosuppression of endogenous ecotropic virogenes. Proc. Natl. Acad. Sci. USA 73:4633–4635.

Huebner, R. J., W. P. Rowe, H. C. Turner, and W. T. Lane. 1963. Specific adenovirus complement-fixing antigens in virus-free hamster and rat tumors. Proc. Natl. Acad. Sci. USA 50:379–389.

Huebner, R. J., and G. J. Todaro. 1969. Oncogenes of RNA tumor viruses as determinants of cancer. Proc. Natl. Acad. Sci. USA 64:1087–1094.

Igel, H., R. J. Huebner, H. Turner, P. Kotin, and H. L. Falk. 1969. Mouse leukemia virus activation by chemical carcinogens. Science 166:1624–1626.

Kirsten, W. H., and L. A. Mayer. 1967. Morphologic responses to a murine erythroblastosis virus. J. Natl. Cancer Inst. 39:311–335.

Klein, G., H. O. Sjögren, E. Klein, and K. E. Hellstrom. 1960. Demonstration of resistance against methylcholanthrene-induced sarcomas in the primary autochthonous host. Cancer Res. 20:1561–1572.

Klement, V., M. O. Nicolson, and R. J. Huebner. 1971. Rescue of the genome of focus forming virus from rat non-productive lines by 5'-bromodeoxyuridine. Nature New Biol. 234:12–14.

Kobayashi, H., E. Gotohda, N. Kuzumaki, N. Takeichi, M. Hosokawa, and T. Kodama. 1974. Reduced transplantability of syngeneic tumors in rats immunized with allogeneic tumors. Int. J. Cancer 13:522–529.

Leffell, M. S., and J. H. Coggin, Jr. 1977. Common transplantation antigens on methylcholanthrene-induced murine sarcomas detected by three assays of tumor rejection. Cancer Res. 37:4112–4119.

McAllister, R. M., M. O. Nicolson, G. Reed, J. Kern, R. V. Gilden, and R. J. Huebner. 1969. Transformation of rodent cells by adenovirus 19 and other group D adenoviruses. J. Natl. Cancer Inst. 43:917–923.

Prehn, R. T. 1962. Specific antigenicities among chemically induced tumors. Ann. NY Acad. Sci. 101:107–113.

Price, P. J., T. M. Bellew, M. P. King, A. E. Freeman, R. V. Gilden, and R. J. Huebner. 1976. Prevention of viral-chemical co-carcinogenesis in vitro by type-specific anti-viral antibody. Proc. Natl. Acad. Sci. USA 73:152–155.

Price, P. J., A. E. Freeman, W. T. Lane, and R. J. Huebner. 1971. Morphological transformation of rat embryo cells by the combined action of 3-methylcholanthrene and Rauscher leukemia virus. Nature New Biol. 230:144–146.

Price, P. J., W. A. Suk, R. L. Peters, R. V. Gilden, and R. J. Huebner. 1977. Chemical transformation of rat cells infected with xenotropic type C RNA virus and its suppression by virus-specific antiserum. Proc. Natl. Acad. Sci. USA 74:579–581.

Rasheed, S., A. E. Freeman, M. B. Gardner, and R. J. Huebner. 1976. Acceleration of transformation of rat embryo cells by rat type C virus. J. Virol. 18:776–782.

Rasheed, S., M. B. Gardner, and R. J. Huebner. 1978. Isolation of a focus forming rat oncornavirus. Proc. Natl. Acad. Sci. USA (In press).

Reiner, J., and C. M. Southam. 1969. Further evidence of common antigenic properties in chemically induced sarcomas of mice. Cancer Res. 29:1814–1820.

Rhim, J. S., J. M. Kim, T. Okigaki, and R. J. Huebner. 1977. Transformation of rat liver epithelial cells by Kirsten murine sarcoma virus. J. Natl. Cancer Inst. 59:1509–1518.

Rhim, J. S., C. R. Lengel, H. Y. Cho, K. K. Takemoto, H. C. Turner, R. J. Huebner, and R. V. Gilden. 1972a. Expression of a new complement fixing antigen reactive with murine sarcoma virus rat antiserum in rat cells transformed by polyoma virus. Nature New Biol. 235:188–190.

Rhim, J. S., M. L. Vernon, R. J. Huebner, H. C. Turner, W. T. Lane, and R. V. Gilden. 1972b. Spontaneous transformation of rat cells after long-term in vitro cultivation and the "switch-on" of a new complement-fixing antigen. Proc. Soc. Exp. Biol. Med. 140:414–419.

Roy-Burman, P., and V. Klement. 1975. Derivation of mouse sarcoma virus (Kirsten) by acquisition of genes from heterologous host. J. Gen. Virol. 28:193–198.

Scolnick, E. M., R. J. Goldberg, and D. Williams. 1976. Characterization of rat genetic sequences of Kirsten sarcoma virus: Distinct class of endogenous rat type C viral sequences. J. Virol. 18:559–566.

Scolnick, E. M., and W. P. Parks. 1974. Harvey sarcoma virus: A second murine virus with rat genetic information. J. Virol. 13:1211–1219.

Sjögren, H. O. 1961. Further studies on the induced resistance against isotransplantation of polyoma tumors. Virology 15:214–219.

Staal, S. P., J. W. Hartley, and W. P. Rowe. 1977. Isolation of transforming murine leukemia virus from mice with high incidence of spontaneous lymphoma. Proc. Natl. Acad. Sci. USA 74:3065–3067.

Stehelin, D., R. V. Guntaka, H. E. Varmus, and M. Bishop. 1976. Purification of DNA complementary to nucleotide sequences required for neoplastic transformation of fibroblasts by avian sarcoma viruses. J. Mol. Biol. 101:349–365.

Todaro, G. J., and R. J. Huebner. 1972. The viral oncogene hypothesis: New evidence. Proc. Natl. Acad. Sci. USA 69:1009–1015.

Weisburger, J. H. 1973. Chemical carcinogenesis in the gastrointestinal tract, in Seventh National Cancer Conference Proceedings, American Cancer Society, Inc., pp. 465–473.

Whitmire, C. E. 1973. Virus-chemical carcinogenesis: A possible viral immunological influence on 3-methylcholanthrene sarcoma induction. J. Natl. Cancer Inst. 51:473–478.

Whitmire, C. E., and R. J. Huebner. 1972. Inhibition of chemical carcinogenesis by viral vaccines. Science 177:60–61.

Whitmire, C. E., and R. A. Salerno. 1973. Influence of preinfection of C57BL/6 mice with Graffi leukemia virus on 3-methylcholanthrene induced subcutaneous sarcoma. Proc. Soc. Exp. Biol. Med. 144:674–679.

Carcinogens: Identification and Mechanisms
of Action, edited by A. Clark Griffin and
Charles R. Shaw. Raven Press, New York © 1979.

Inhibitors of Carcinogenesis

Lee W. Wattenberg

*Department of Laboratory Medicine and Pathology, University of Minnesota,
Minneapolis, Minnesota 55455*

Cancer is a disease that optimally should be dealt with by prevention. Strategies for preventing cancer can be divided into four categories: (1) identification of cancer-producing agents and their removal from the environment, (2) prevention of the formation of cancer-producing agents in vivo, (3) enhancement of defenses that prevent cancer-producing agents from reaching or reacting with critical target sites, and (4) inhibition of promotion and/or reversal of early stages of neoplasia.

Identification of cancer-producing agents and their removal from the environment is unquestionably the most satisfactory solution to the problem of cancer. This quest should be pursued relentlessly and with all the resources at our command. There are difficulties and uncertainties with this strategy, however. The first is the actual identification of carcinogens that cause cancer in man. Exceedingly few materials have been related to the causation of cancer in large numbers of humans. Most carcinogens for man involve exposures to industrial compounds, with which relatively few persons come in contact. Information relating exposure to defined carcinogens with the occurrence of neoplasia in large human population groups is limited. A second potential problem is suggested by the accumulating data indicating that cancer can be a multistage process and that it may be caused by multiple agents, i.e., initiators, promoters, and cocarcinogens. Thus, in some instances, very small doses of an initiating substance may start the process, and the ultimate appearance of neoplasia could then result from secondary exposures to a variety or combinations of promoting or cocarcinogenic agents, some of which may be in natural products. A further difficulty, and one which at first would seem easily overcome, is in removing cancer-producing agents from the environment once they have been identified. The dramatic situation existing with cigarette smoking illustrates how difficult this is to accomplish. Although difficulties and uncertainties do exist, identification and removal of cancer-producing agents from the environment is a primary goal. However, it is likely that this goal will not be achieved for a considerable period, and therefore backup strategies could be highly important.

The second strategy for prevention of cancer also is directed at control of exposures to cancer-producing agents. However, in this instance, the agents are produced in vivo and include physiological compounds. A dramatic example of prevention of formation of carcinogens in vivo is the inhibition of formation of nitroso compounds in the stomach by ascorbic acid or other agents capable of scavenging nitrites. Mirvish *et al.* (1975) have carried out extensive work relating to this type of inhibition. In recent studies, Varghese *et al.* (1977) showed that human feces contain mutagenic substances. Because there is a high correlation between mutagenicity and carcinogenicity, it is possible that this mutagenic material might be involved in human neoplasia. In further work, these investigators observed that ascorbic acid reduces the amount of the fecal mutagens in human subjects. Conceivably, this could represent a means of reducing the formation of a carcinogenic material in vivo. Potentially, another way of reducing the amounts of cancer-producing agents within organisms resides in dietary manipulation. Diets high in fat, particularly unsaturated fat, have been shown to enhance carcinogenesis (Carroll and Khor 1970, Weisburger *et al.* 1977). Finally, hormonal manipulation may be of value in diminishing neoplasia in hormone-dependent tissues, such as breast, ovaries, and prostate, in persons with hormonal abnormalities or who are at particularly high risk of neoplasia in these tissue sites.

The third strategy, i.e., inhibition of neoplasia by enhancing defenses that prevent cancer-producing agents from reaching or reacting with critical target sites, constitutes the main part of this paper and will be discussed in some detail.

The fourth strategy is to prevent cancer by inhibiting promotion and/or reversing early stages of neoplasia. Extensive work of this nature has been carried out with retinoids by Sporn and his collaborators (1976, 1979, see pages 441 to 453, this volume). Ascorbic acid also may reverse early stages of neoplasia. DeCosse *et al.* (1975) have reported that ascorbic acid reduces the number of polyps in the rectum of persons with multiple polyposis who have undergone ileorectal anastomosis. In addition to pharmacological procedures, immunological techniques for inhibiting the occurrence of neoplasia such as those suggested by Huebner (1979, see pages 277 to 298, this volume) should be considered as a potential constituent of this fourth strategy.

The ranking order of desirability of the four strategies of cancer prevention described is clear. It would be most desirable to prevent exposure to cancer-producing agents. Failing this, it would be advantageous to prevent cancer-producing substances from reaching or exerting their noxious effects on target sites. Inhibition of promotion or reversal of the early phases of neoplasia represents the final protective mechanism against the occurrence of cancer.

INHIBITION OF NEOPLASIA BY ENHANCING DEFENSES THAT PREVENT CANCER-PRODUCING AGENTS FROM REACHING OR REACTING WITH CRITICAL TARGET SITES

An increasing number and diversity of compounds with the capacity to inhibit the occurrence of neoplasia when administered prior to or simultaneously with exposure to cancer-producing agents are being identified. The inhibitors encompass a wide range of chemical stuctures (Figure 1) and include synthetic chemicals as well as compounds that are naturally occurring constituents of food. The quantity of information on these inhibitors is now sufficiently impressive to warrant consideration of two basic questions: What impact do inhibitors

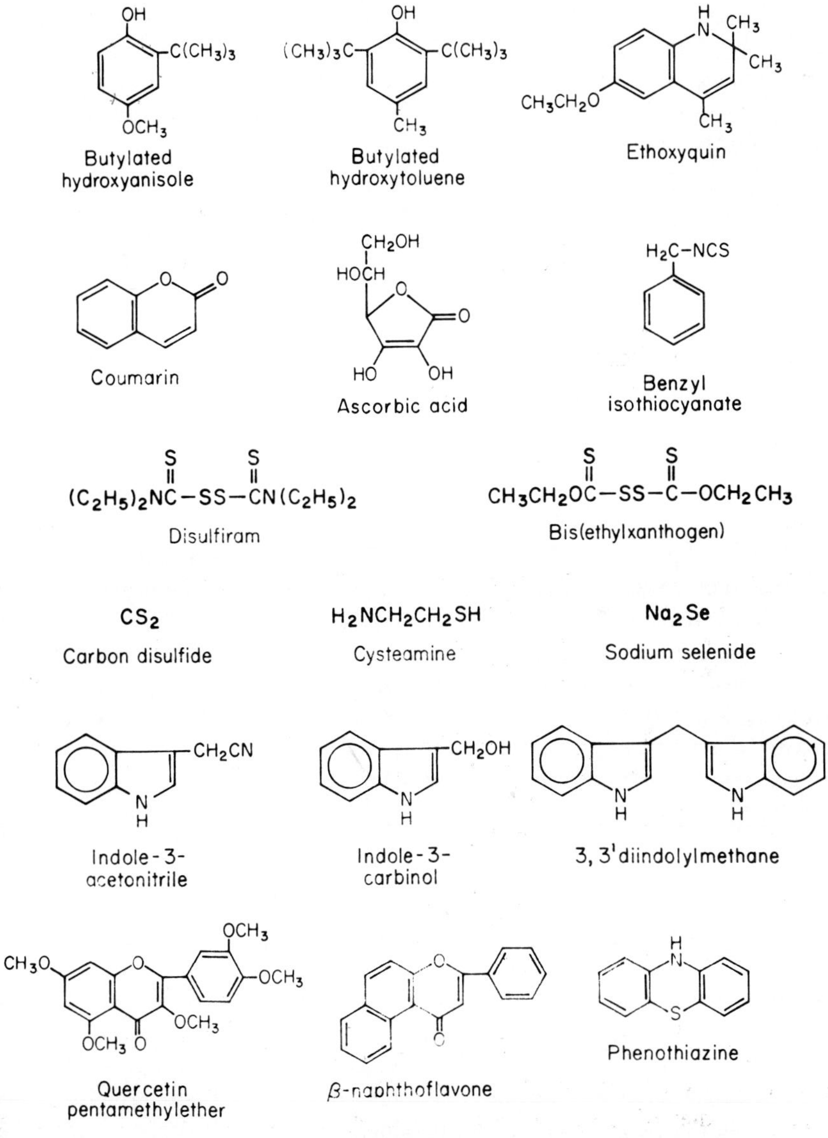

FIG. 1. Some compounds that inhibit chemical carcinogenesis.

already present in the environment have on cancer incidence in human populations and what is the optimal potential of inhibitors for preventing neoplasia? In the following outline, potential mechanisms of inhibition of chemical carcinogenesis are presented. However, much of the actual information on inhibitors has been obtained from empirical studies. Some inhibitors were originally identified as a result of work based on postulated mechanisms of inhibition. Even in these instances, as will become evident, there is frequently doubt about how valid the postulated mechanism really is. Thus, there is a considerable amount of phenomenological data and relatively little solid information on mechanisms of inhibition. As a result, the organization of the presentation of this topic is somewhat arbitrary and is formed around groups of inhibitors having certain common features.

Some Potential Mechanisms for Inhibiting Chemical Carcinogens

---

Alteration of metabolism of the carcinogen by decreased activation, increased detoxification, or both
Scavenging of active molecular species of carcinogens to prevent their reaching critical target sites in the cell
Alteration of permeability or transport
Competitive inhibition

Phenolic Antioxidants and Ethoxyquin

The use of antioxidants as possible inhibitors of chemical carcinogens has been based in general on the concept that the antioxidants may exert a scavenging effect on the reactive species of carcinogens, thus protecting cellular constituents from attack. In early studies, wheat germ oil and alpha-tocopherol were employed. Experiments with positive and negative results have been reported, but confirmatory reports on the positive results have not appeared; thus, the implications of this work are not clear. Results of these investigations as well as our own experience with alpha-tocopherol have been summarized previously (Wattenberg 1972a). In our experience, alpha-tocopherol was not inhibitory; however, it is possible that under some appropriate conditions, an inhibitory effect does occur.

During the past several years, studies have been carried out with other antioxidants. The most extensive work of this type has been done with phenolic compounds, in particular, butylated hydroxyanisole (BHA) and butylated hydroxytoluene (BHT). Inhibition occurs under a variety of experimental conditions and with a broad range of chemical carcinogens, as shown in Table 1. Several nonphenolic antioxidants inhibit chemical carcinogenesis. One of these is ethoxyquin, a widely used antioxidant commonly added to commercial animal feed. Some studies of the mechanism of inhibition of chemical carcinogenesis by BHA and BHT have been carried out. One set has been aimed at determining

TABLE 1. *Inhibition of carcinogen-induced neoplasia by phenols, lactones, and ethoxyquin*

Carcinogen	Antioxidant*	Species	Site of inhibited neoplasm	Reference
Benzo[a]pyrene	BHA	Mouse	Lung	Wattenberg 1973
	Ethoxyquin	Mouse	Lung	Wattenberg, unpublished data
	BHA, BHT	Mouse	Forestomach	Wattenberg 1972a
	Coumarin, α-angelica lactone	Mouse	Forestomach	Wattenberg, unpublished data
7,12-Dimethylbenz[a]anthracene	BHA	Mouse	Lung	Wattenberg 1973
	BHA, ethoxyquin	Mouse	Forestomach	Wattenberg 1972a
	BHA, BHT	Mouse	Skin	Slaga and Bracken 1977
	BHA, BHT, ethoxyquin	Rat	Breast	Wattenberg 1972a
	Coumarin	Rat	Breast	Feuer *et al.* 1976
7-Hydroxymethyl-12-methylbenz[a]anthracene	BHA	Mouse	Lung	Wattenberg 1973
Dibenz[a,h]anthracene	BHA	Mouse	Lung	Wattenberg 1973
Diethylnitrosamine	BHA, ethoxyquin	Mouse	Lung	Wattenberg 1972b
4-Nitroquinoline-N-oxide	BHA, ethoxyquin	Mouse	Lung	Wattenberg 1972b
Uracil mustard	BHA	Mouse	Lung	Wattenberg 1973
Urethane	BHA	Mouse	Lung	Wattenberg 1973
N-2-Fluorenylacetamide	BHT	Rat	Liver	Ulland *et al.* 1973
N-Hydroxy-N-2-fluorenylacetamide	BHT	Rat	Liver, breast	Ulland *et al.* 1973
3-Hydroxyanthranilic acid	Ascorbic acid	Mouse	Urinary bladder	Pipkin *et al.* 1969
4-Dimethylaminoazobenzene	BHT	Rat	Liver	Frankfurt *et al.* 1967
Azoxymethane	BHT	Rat	Large intestine	Weisburger *et al.*, in press
Methylazoxymethanol acetate	BHA	Mouse	Large intestine	Wattenberg, unpublished data
trans-5-Amino-3-[2-(5-nitro-2-furyl)vinyl]-1,2,4-oxadiazole	BHA	Mouse	Forestomach, lung lymphomas	Bueding *et al.*, personal communication

* BHA, butylated hydroxyanisole; BHT, butylated hydroxytoluene.

the mechanism of inhibition of benzo[*a*]pyrene (BP)-induced neoplasia by BHA. BP is metabolized by the microsomal mixed-function oxidase system, which acts on a wide variety of xenobiotic compounds, including polycyclic aromatic hydrocarbons. Reactive metabolites as well as detoxification products are produced. The effects of BHA administration on microsomal metabolism of BP in female A/HeJ mice have been studied under experimental conditions similar to those under which BHA inhibits neoplasia due to this carcinogen. Incubation of BP and DNA with liver microsomes from the BHA-fed mice results in approximately one-half the binding of BP metabolites to DNA as compared with that found with microsomes from control mice (Speier and Wattenberg 1975). Investigations have been undertaken to determine if there are differences in the metabolites of BP that are formed when this carcinogen is incubated with liver microsomes prepared from BHA-fed mice as compared with control mice. Of major interest was the observation of the effects of BHA feeding on BP-oxide formation. Formation of BP-4,5-oxide, which can be measured directly by high-pressure liquid chromatography, was reduced when BP was incubated with microsomes from BHA-fed mice. BP-9,10-oxide and BP-7,8-oxide cannot be measured directly because of instability; however, data based on summation of diols and phenols resulting respectively from the enzymatic and spontaneous conversions of these oxides indicate that they are present in reduced amounts in the incubations of microsomes from BHA-fed mice. 3-Hydroxybenzo[*a*]pyrene (3-HOBP) was the major metabolite in incubations of microsomes from BHA-fed and control mice. This metabolite constituted a significantly higher percentage of the total metabolites formed on incubating BP with microsomes from BHA-fed as compared with control mice. Thus, BHA administration causes two metabolic alterations that could result in its exerting an inhibitory effect on BP-induced carcinogenesis. The first is a decrease in epoxidation, which is an activation process, and the second is an increase in 3-HOBP, a metabolite of detoxification (Lam and Wattenberg 1977).

In studies of the mechanism of inhibition of polycyclic hydrocarbon-induced skin carcinogenesis by phenolic antioxidants (Slaga and Bracken 1977), BHA or BHT was applied topically on mice. Three or 12 hours later, the animals were killed, and the binding of [^{3}H]BP or [^{3}H]7,12-dimethylbenz[*a*]anthracene to DNA was determined in epidermal homogenates. Both carcinogens showed approximately one-half as much binding to DNA in homogenates from mice that had received BHA or BHT three hours before death as in homogenates from control mice. The inhibition of binding was still apparent at 12 hours but was a lesser order of magnitude.

An early investigation aimed at determining the mechanism of inhibition of carcinogenesis of *N*-2-fluorenylacetamide (FAA) and *N*-OH-FAA by BHT was carried out by Grantham *et al.* (1973). These investigators found that administration of BHT in the diet led to increased excretion of each carcinogen in the urine. This higher level of excretion was accounted for chiefly by glucuronic acid conjugates. Animals receiving BHT had lower levels of radioactivity in blood, liver, and in liver DNA 48 hours after injection with labeled carcinogen. Thus, BHA appears to increase detoxification of FAA and *N*-OH-FAA by enhancing conjugation, thereby reducing the pool of metabolites available for activation reactions.

At present, BHA probably is the most versatile and least toxic inhibitor of chemical carcinogenesis that has been identified. BHT also inhibits a variety of carcinogens but unfortunately has some noxious properties, including tumor promotion (Witschi *et al.* 1977). An important difference between the two compounds is the nature of the substitution para to the hydroxyl group (Figure 1). In BHT, this is a methyl group that undergoes oxidation to toxic metabolites. In BHA, a methoxy group is in the para position. If metabolism occurs, it is a hydrolysis. The resultant phenolic group can be conjugated, facilitating the excretion of the compound.

BHA is of interest because it is used extensively as an additive in food for human consumption. Studies in mice have been done in which BHA was added to the diet along with BP, a carcinogen widely encountered in the environment. At a concentration of 5 mg/g diet, BHA inhibits the carcinogenic effect exerted by BP at 1 mg/g diet on the forestomach of the mouse. In the United States, the human consumption of BHA is on the order of several milligrams a day. Assuming that the results of animal experiments hold for man, this amount of the antioxidant could be important in inhibiting the effects of long-term exposure to low doses of carcinogens, the type of exposure that is most likely to occur in human populations.

Disulfiram and Related Compounds

Disulfiram and related compounds are exceedingly interesting in their effects on carcinogen-induced neoplasia of the large intestine (Wattenberg 1975, 1976, Wattenberg *et al.* 1977). When added to the diet, disulfiram, diethyldithiocarbamate, and bisethylxanthogen profoundly inhibit large-bowel neoplasia resulting from subcutaneous administration of symmetrical 1,2-dimethylhydrazine (DMH). Under experimental conditions comparable to those used with DMH, disulfiram also has been found to inhibit neoplasia of the large intestine induced by azoxymethane, an oxidative metabolite of DMH, but to a considerably less extent than with DMH as the carcinogen (Wattenberg *et al.* 1977).

Studies of the mechanism of inhibition of large-bowel neoplasia induced by DMH and azoxymethane have shown that disulfiram inhibits the oxidation of both these carcinogens in vivo (Fiala *et al.* 1976, 1977, Fiala 1977). Investigations bearing on the question of whether the inhibitory function resides in the intact molecule of disulfiram or a metabolite of this compound (Fiala 1977, Fiala *et al.* 1977) have demonstrated that carbon disulfide, a metabolite of disulfiram, inhibits the oxidation of DMH and azoxymethane. Carbon disulfide also has been found to inhibit DMH-induced neoplasia of the large intestine in the mouse (Wattenberg and Fiala 1978). The data obtained suggest that this may be the chemical species responsible for the inhibitory action of disulfiram and related compounds. Results of other studies indicate that incubation of microsomes with carbon disulfide in the presence of NADPH results in covalent binding of the sulfur to the microsomes. There is an accompanying decrease in cytochrome P-450, as measured spectroscopically (DeMatteis 1974, Hunter and Neal 1975). Several thiono-sulfur-containing compounds, including disulfiram and diethyldithiocarbamate, effect a similar decrease in cytochrome P-450 when incubated with microsomes under comparable conditions (Hunter and Neal 1975). This raises the possibility that thiono-sulfur-containing compounds, as a group, may have the potential capacity to modify cytochrome P-450 so as to alter the microsomal metabolism of DMH, azoxymethane, and possibly other carcinogens in a manner that decreases their carcinogenicity.

The carcinogen-inhibiting effects of disulfiram and diethyldithiocarbamate have drawn attention to the possibility that a number of widely used pesticides containing dithiocarbamate or thiocarbamate groups might have similar properties. Several have been tested. Two of these, *S*-propyl dipropylthiocarbamate (Vernolate) and 2-chloroallyl diethyldithiocarbamate, when added to the diet were found to inhibit BP-induced neoplasia of the forestomach of the mouse. An additional pesticide, bisethylxanthogen (Bexide), also was found to exert an inhibitory effect in this test system. Bisethylxanthogen is the only one of these pesticides studied thus far for its effects on DMH-induced neoplasia of the large bowel. Its inhibitory potency is of a similar order of magnitude to that of disulfiram (Wattenberg *et al.* 1977).

Bisethylxanthogen has a feature that makes it of particular interest. The molecule does not contain nitrogen (see Figure 1). Structurally similar dithiocarbamate pesticides have been shown to form nitrosamines, representing a hazard not occurring with bisethylxanthogen. A second relationship between disulfiram and nitrosamines, reported by Schmähl *et al.* (1976), is that disulfiram influences the organotropism of diethylnitrosamine (DENA) and dimethylnitrosamine (DMNA). In the case of DENA, disulfiram added to the diet inhibits liver tumor formation but enhances neoplasia of the esophagus. With DMNA, suppression of neoplasia of the liver again is found, but there is an increase in tumors of the paranasal sinuses.

Experimental studies of the capacity of disulfiram and some related compounds to inhibit chemical carcinogenesis have been carried out with the same experimental models employed for the phenolic antioxidants (Wattenberg 1974). These sulfur-containing compounds are potent inhibitors of BP-induced neoplasia of the forestomach. Work aimed at elucidating the mechanism of disulfiram inhibition has shown that administration of this compound in the diet results in a reduction of binding of [3H]BP and [14C]BP to DNA, RNA, and protein of the forestomach (Borchert and Wattenberg 1976). In these original studies, the whole forestomach was used without separation of the various histological components. When these components are separated by pronase treatment, there is a reduction of binding of BP to the macromolecules of all layers, i.e., keratin, epithelial, and remaining stomach wall. Further work showed that feeding disulfiram reduces the retention (tissue-extractable BP) to a degree parallel to that of macromolecular binding. In in vitro studies, BP was intubated into isolated stomachs from disulfiram-fed mice and corresponding controls post-mortem. The stomachs were incubated aerobically at 37°C and 0°C and also under carbon monoxide. Under all conditions, the BP retention in the tissues of the forestomach was diminished in those mice fed disulfiram previously. These data suggest that the protective effect of disulfiram on BP-induced forestomach cancer is unlikely due to alteration of the metabolism of BP but resides in factors controlling penetration of BP through the keratin barrier (Borchert *et al.* 1978).

Organic Isothiocyanates and Organic Thiocyanates

Along with studies of the inhibitory capacities of sulfur-containing antioxidants, experiments with benzyl isothiocyanate, phenethyl isothiocyanate, and benzyl thiocyanate have been carried out (Wattenberg 1977b). These three compounds are naturally occurring constituents of edible cruciferous plants (Virtanen 1962, Lichtenstein *et al.* 1962). A fourth compound, phenyl isothiocyanate, included in some of the experimental work is synthetic. 1-Naphthylisothiocyanate and 2-naphthylisothiocyanate both have been shown to suppress the neoplastic effects of azo dyes on the liver (Lacassagne *et al.* 1970). Of interest are studies showing that 1-naphthylisothiocyanate alters cytochrome P-450 in a manner comparable to that of thiono-sulfur-containing compounds (DeMatteis 1974).

Coumarins, Ascorbic Acid, and Other Lactones

Coumarins are constituents of a wide variety of plants, including vegetables used for human consumption (Feuer 1973). Administration of coumarin by oral intubation inhibits 7,12-dimethylbenz[*a*]anthracene (DMBA)-induced mammary tumor formation (Feuer *et al.* 1976). With BP-induced neoplasia of the forestomach as the test system, coumarin, 6-nitrocoumarin, and alpha-angelica lactone added to the diet inhibit forestomach tumor formation (Wattenberg, unpublished observation).

Ascorbic acid has been reported to inhibit tumor formation in the urinary bladder implanted with 3-hydroxyanthranilic acid (Pipkin *et al.* 1969). In these studies, ascorbic acid was added to the drinking water of mice whose bladders had been implanted with the carcinogen in cholesterol pellets. In a different type of investigation in human subjects, efforts have been made to relate the chemoluminescence of the urine to occurrence of bladder cancer (Rose and Wallace 1973). Urinary chemoluminescence is higher in normal smokers than in nonsmokers and is higher still in patients with bladder cancer. Oral administration of ascorbic acid reduces urinary chemoluminescence in both normal smokers and nonsmokers. Ascorbic acid has been studied for its inhibitory effects on BP-induced forestomach tumor formation but shows no evidence of suppressing neoplasia (Wattenberg, unpublished data).

Selenium and Selenium Salts

Inhibition of chemical carcinogenesis by selenium salts has been reported. In an initial study, the experimental system consisted of initiation of epidermal neoplasia with DMBA followed by promotion with croton oil. Sodium selenide added to the croton oil suppressed the development of skin tumors (Shamberger 1966). In subsequent work, 3-methylcholanthrene was applied repeatedly to the skin. Again, addition of sodium selenide inhibited epidermal neoplasia. In a further experiment, mice were placed on a selenium-deficient diet (Torula yeast) without supplements or with added sodium selenide or sodium selenite. BP was applied to the skin daily to produce epidermal neoplasia. A slight inhibition was found with both of the selenium salts (Shamberger 1970). Recently it has been shown that addition of sodium selenite to the drinking water will inhibit large-bowel neoplasia in the rat resulting from administration of DMH or methylazoxymethanol acetate (Jacobs *et al.* 1977, Jacobs 1977). In additional work, it was found that selenium reduces mutagenicity of FAA, *N*-OH-FAA, and *N*-OH-FA (N-hydroxyaminofluorene) for the *Salmonella typhimurium* T-1538 histidine mutant (Jacobs 1977). Early epidemiological studies indicated that there was an inverse relationship between the amount of selenium in soil and forage crops and human cancer death rates in the United States and Canada in 1965. Likewise, an inverse relationship between human blood levels of selenium and human cancer death rates in several cities was reported (Shamberger and Willis 1971). Further investigations again have supported the likelihood that an inverse relationship exists between selenium in the environment and cancer mortality (Shamberger *et al.* 1976).

Inducers of Increased Microsomal Mixed-Function Oxidase Activity

A number of studies have demonstrated that it is possible to protect against chemical carcinogens by the administration of inducers of increased microsomal mixed-function oxidase activity (Table 2). The inducers employed have varied from compounds such as polycyclic hydrocarbons, which themselves are noxious agents, to chemicals such as flavones, which have little toxicity (Wattenberg and Leong 1968, 1970, Wattenberg *et al.* 1976). In early studies it was shown that administration of polycyclic hydrocarbon inducers inhibited the occurrence of hepatic cancer resulting from feeding 3′-methyl-4-dimethylaminoazobenzene (Richardson *et al.* 1952, Miller *et al.* 1958). Likewise, it was demonstrated that polycyclic hydrocarbon inducers can substantially reduce the incidence of tumors of the liver, mammary gland, ear duct, and small intestine in rats fed FAA or 7-F1-FAA (Miller *et al.* 1958).

In more recent studies, protection against the carcinogenic effects of a number of other carcinogens has been observed (see Table 2). Considerable work has been done with two polycyclic hydrocarbon carcinogens, DMBA and BP. In the pulmonary adenoma test system in the mouse, flavone inducers will inhibit

TABLE 2. Inhibition of carcinogenesis by inducers of increased microsomal enzyme activity

Carcinogen	Inducer	Species	Organ	References
3'-Methyl-4-dimethylaminoazobenzene	Polycyclic hydrocarbons	Rat	Liver	Richardson et al. 1952
	α-Benzene hexachloride	Rat	Liver	Miller et al. 1958, Thamavit et al. 1974
N-2-Fluorenylacetamide	Polychlorinated biphenyls	Rat	Liver	Makiura et al. 1974
	Polycyclic hydrocarbons	Rat	Liver, breast, small intestine	Miller et al. 1958
	Polychlorinated biphenyls	Rat	Liver, breast, small intestine	Makiura et al. 1974
4-Dimethylaminostilbene	Polycyclic hydrocarbons	Rat	Ear duct	Tawfic 1965
Urethan	Phenobarbital	Mouse	Lung	Adenis et al. 1970, Silva 1967
	β-Naphthoflavone	Mouse	Lung	Wattenberg and Leong 1968
	Chlordane, phenobarbital	Mouse	Lung	Yammamoto et al. 1971
	β-naphthoflavone, quer-citrin pentamethylether	Mouse	Lung	Wattenberg and Leong 1970
Benzo[a]pyrene	β-Naphthoflavone	Mouse	Skin	Wattenberg and Leong 1970
	β-Naphthoflavone	Mouse	Lung	Wattenberg and Leong 1968
7,12-Dimethylbenz[a]anthracene	β-Naphthoflavone	Rat	Breast	Wattenberg and Leong 1968
	Phenothiazines	Rat	Breast	Wattenberg and Leong 1967
	Polycyclic hydrocarbons	Rat	Breast	Huggins et al. 1964
	Indole-3-carbinol, diindolylmethane	Rat	Liver	Wattenberg and Loub, in press
Aflatoxin	Phenobarbital	Rat		McLean and Marshall 1971
Bracken fern carcinogen	Phenobarbital	Rat	Small intestine, bladder	Pamukcu et al. 1971

lung tumor formation resulting from oral administration of these two carcinogens (Wattenberg and Leong 1968, 1970). An experimental model that has been used widely in studies of the effects of inducers of increased mixed-function oxidase activity is mammary tumor formation in rats given DMBA. Several different types of inducers administered prior to DMBA will inhibit tumor formation. These include polycyclic hydrocarbons (Huggins *et al.* 1965, Wheatley 1968), phenothiazines (Wattenberg and Leong 1967), flavones (Wattenberg and Leong 1968), and indoles (Wattenberg and Loub 1978).

Whereas the experiments listed in Table 2 show a protective effect from administration of inducers of increased mixed-function oxidase activity, an apparently conflicting set of data also exists. The microsomal mixed-function oxidase system has been shown to convert many chemical compounds to a proximate carcinogenic form (Miller, E. C., and Miller, J. A. 1974). An initial thought might be that if a compound is activated by an enzyme system to a noxious form, then enhancement of the activity of this system would result in greater damage to the organism. This is true in situations involving a reversible effect, in which there is a substantial threshold. Rapid activation could be important in achieving such a threshold. However, in the case of chemical carcinogenesis, there appears to be either no threshold or a very low threshold (DiPaolo *et al.* 1971). Thus, one might anticipate that slow activation would result in a carcinogenic effect as great as or even greater than that resulting from rapid activation. With slow activation, wastage of activated species of carcinogen from cells due to production of an amount in excess of that most effective for the number of critical binding sites available at a particular time would be less likely. In addition, active carcinogenic species would be present for a longer period and therefore more likely to exist at a critical time or times in the cell cycle.

Another factor that may be important in explaining carcinogen inhibition by induction of increased mixed-function oxidase activity is that in many instances, chemical carcinogens are subjected to detoxification as well as activation reactions by this mechanism. The classic example of this is the aromatic amines. With these compounds, ring hydroxylation results in detoxification, whereas hydroxylation of the nitrogen is an activation reaction (Miller and Miller 1969). Thus, administration of inducers of mixed-function oxidase activity in these instances may result in a relatively greater proportion of the carcinogen being detoxified rather than activated to a carcinogenic metabolite. Changes in proportion of detoxified metabolites to carcinogenic metabolites could be simply the result of relative responses of the two pathways to the inducer. An alternative possibility suggested by the studies with BHA is that a more basic alteration in metabolism may occur, resulting in a changed metabolite pattern. In this instance, the change in metabolite pattern could be independent of the magnitude of induction and, in fact, as in the case of BHA, might occur with no overall increase in mixed-function oxidase activity. Further work is required to ascertain the mechanism of action of compounds that have been shown to have the combined properties of increasing mixed-function oxidase activity and inhibiting chemical carcinogenesis.

Phenobarbital induces increased mixed-function oxidase activity, an increase in endoplasmic reticulum, and liver enlargement. When administered prior to the carcinogen, it has been found to suppress neoplasia (see Table 2). However, if it is given subsequent to the carcinogen, the neoplastic response may be enhanced (Peraino *et al.* 1973). This cocarcinogenic effect represents a hazard that requires evaluation with respect to other inducers.

Inhibitors of Microsomal Mixed-Function Oxidase Activity

If the activity of the microsomal mixed-function oxidase system were totally absent, carcinogens requiring activation by this system would not produce a neoplastic effect. Efforts have been made to achieve inhibition of chemical carcinogenesis by this mechanism. Studies of suppression of polycyclic hydrocarbon-induced neoplasia have been carried out with 7,8-benzoflavone (alpha-naphthoflavone), a potent inhibitor of microsomal mixed-function oxidase activity. In experiments in which DMBA is the carcinogen, epidermal neoplasia has been inhibited (Gelboin *et al.* 1970, Slaga and Bracken 1977). A problem with exploiting inhibition of mixed-function oxidase activity as a means of suppressing chemical carcinogenesis is that it would render the organism more susceptible to the noxious effects of xenobiotic compounds detoxified by this system.

Physiological Trapping Agents

Active forms of chemical carcinogens bind to a wide variety of physiological compounds. Their carcinogenic potential resides in such reactivity occurring at selective sites. However, if the carcinogenic agent is trapped by other cellular nucleophiles, protection might occur. A considerable number of biochemical compounds contain nucleophilic groups. These have been discussed by J. A. Miller and E. C. Miller (1974). The question exists as to whether it might be possible to increase the amount of one or more of such nucleophiles so as to protect against chemical carcinogens. In an experiment of this nature, diets supplemented with cystine or methionine, or containing large amounts of protein (40% casein) were found to inhibit FAA-induced neoplasia of the liver and ear duct glands (Miller and Miller 1972). A compound of particular interest in this regard is glutathione, an excellent trapping agent. However, to increase the level of glutathione by experimental procedures has proved difficult. In contrast, a number of extrinsic factors, particularly administration of toxic compounds, can cause a depletion of glutathione. The levels and control mechanisms of protective cellular nucleophiles could be of great importance in the response to chemical carcinogens. Work aimed at more fully understanding and exploiting this potential defense certainly is warranted.

DISCUSSION

With the knowledge that a wide diversity of inhibitors prevent cancer-producing agents from reaching or reacting with critical target sites, two questions arise. The first relates to the current role that these compounds play in reducing the impact of environmental carcinogens on man. The second is the optimal role that they might have. To assess their current role, additional information is required as to the full spectrum of compounds in the environment that have the capacity to inhibit carcinogens. Figure 1 and Tables 1 and 2 show that compounds with a broad range of chemical structures can inhibit chemical carcinogenesis. The diversity indicates that this capacity to inhibit does not reside in restricted chemical characteristics and suggests that a considerable number of other inhibitors not yet identified almost certainly exist. The quest to identify these inhibitors is important to enable us to correctly take account of their impact. Also of critical importance is full elucidation of the mechanisms of inhibition, which could provide information to assist in identifying compounds in the environment that are inhibitors. In addition, mechanisms of inhibition that entail measurable biochemical parameters could provide a basis for assessing the susceptibility of particular population groups or individuals to neoplasia from chemical carcinogens.

An important aspect of the evaluation of the role of inhibitors is a consideration of toxicity. Inhibitors currently identified have, to a greater or lesser extent, other biological activities. A number have toxic properties. Some are even carcinogens or cocarcinogens. However, noxious properties can be dissected away from the basic mechanisms of inhibition. Thus, among phenolic inhibitors, BHA is considerably less toxic than BHT and is a more effective inhibitor. In early studies in which protection was obtained by inducing increased microsomal mixed-function oxidase activity, the potent carcinogen 3-methylcholanthrene was used. Flavones and phenothiazines cited in Table 2 inhibit by inducing increased mixed-function oxidase activity but are not carcinogens. As more is learned about the basic requirements for inhibition, it is likely that compounds with increasing inhibitory potency and fewer side effects can be found. It is important to stress this point because the inhibitors that currently are available are a first-generation group. Many have been discovered by chance, or if a particular mechanism was being explored, compounds that were readily available were used. With more complete information, it should be possible to design inhibitors in which unnecessary biological activities are peeled away, providing less toxic and more effective compounds.

Considerations of the optimal role of compounds that prevent cancer-producing agents from reaching or reacting with critical target sites entail evaluations of their deliberate use. At present, it would be premature to undertake such measures because we simply do not have an adequate base of information. However, at a future time, when more data are available on mechanisms of inhibition and the diversity of inhibitors and their toxicity, this course of action might be entertained. Accordingly, there would be some value in considering possible criteria that would have to be met prior to deliberate use of inhibitors of chemical carcinogenesis. For any normal group of individuals, a critical restraint is the possibility of an inhibitor's toxicity. To be effective, the inhibitor would have to be taken by individuals for many years; thus, even a low toxicity could outweigh any benefits. However, there are selected situations in which this formidable obstacle might be overcome. One specific instance entails carcinogens within the gastrointestinal tract. In this case, it is conceivable that an inhibitor that would not be absorbed could be designed. Under these conditions, a compound with little or no toxicity might be available. The importance of these types of considerations is made real by recent findings of mutagenic substances in the feces (Varghese *et al.* 1977). If these are, in fact, carcinogens as well as mutagens, efforts at finding effective inhibitors active within the large bowel might be warranted. In other sites, specific situations amenable to selective approaches might exist as well.

A second basis for introduction of an inhibitor into the environment would be the acquisition of favorable data from epidemiological investigations. Such data would include firm evidence that a population group with significant intake of a particular inhibitor has a diminished incidence of one or more neoplasms. Mechanistic data relating the intake of the inhibitor to carcinogen inhibition, e.g., tissues from the particular population group showing an increased capacity to detoxify carcinogens, would be important. In addition, there should be strong evidence that the inhibitor has no toxicity. Under these conditions, consideration of the use of the material bringing about the inhibition would be warranted. This, in essence, is a natural or unplanned type of experiment. Depending on the magnitude of inhibition and the reliability of estimates of adverse side effects, convincing data could be provided for deliberate use of the substance.

There do exist population groups with more exposure to chemical carcinogens. For these people, less rigid requirements for lack of toxicity of inhibitors might be justified. With regard to this possibility, an exceedingly important prohibition is the use of inhibitors as a mechanism for allowing increased exposures to carcinogens or increasing tolerance levels to cancer-producing substances.

ACKNOWLEDGMENTS

Work reported in this paper was supported by U. S. Public Health Service Research Grants CA-14146, CA-09599, and CA-15638 and Contract CP-33364, awarded by the National Cancer Institute.

REFERENCES

Adenis, L., M. N. Valeminck, and J. Driessens. 1970. L'adenome pulmonaire de la souris recevant de l'urethane. VIII. Action du phenobarbital. C. R. Soc. Biol. (Paris) 164:560–562.
Borchert, P., A. Galbraith, and L. W. Wattenberg. 1978. On the mechanism of disulfiram inhibition

of benzo(a)pyrene-induced neoplasia in the mouse forestomach. Proc. Am. Assoc. Cancer Res. 19:61.

Borchert, P., and L. W. Wattenberg. 1976. Inhibition of macromolecular binding of benzo(a)pyrene and inhibition of neoplasia by disulfiram in the mouse forestomach. J. Natl. Cancer Inst. 57:173–179.

Carroll, K. K., and H. T. Khor. 1970. Effects of dietary fat and dose level of 7,12-dimethylbenz(a)anthracene on mammary tumor incidence in rats. Cancer Res. 30:2260–2264.

DeCosse, J. J., M. B. Adams, J. F. Kuzma, P. LoGerfo, and R. Condon. 1975. Effects of ascorbic acid on rectal polyps of patients with familial polyposis. Surgery 78:608–612.

DeMatteis, F. 1974. Covalent binding of sulfur to microsomes and loss of cytochrome P-450 during the oxidative desulfuration of several chemicals. Mol. Pharmacol. 10:849–854.

DiPaolo, J. A., P. J. Donovan, and R. L. Nelson. 1971. In vitro transformation of hamster cells by polycyclic hydrocarbons: Factors influencing the number of cells transformed. Nature New Biol. 230:240–242.

Feuer, G. 1973. The metabolism and biological action of coumarins. Prog. Med. Chem. 10:85–157.

Feuer, G., J. A. Kellen, and K. Kovacs. 1976. Suppression of 7,12-dimethylbenz(a)anthracene induced carcinoma by coumarin in the rat. Oncology 33:35–39.

Fiala, E. S. 1977. Investigations into the metabolism and mode of action of the colon carcinogens 1,2-dimethylhydrazine and azoxymethane. Cancer 40:2436–2445.

Fiala, E. S., G. Bobotas, C. Kulakis, L. W. Wattenberg, and J. H. Weisburger. 1977. The effects of disulfiram and related compounds on the in vivo metabolism of the colon carcinogen 1,2-dimethylhydrazine. Biochem. Pharmacol. 26:1763–1768.

Fiala, E. S., G. Bobotas, C. Kulakis, and J. H. Weisburger. 1976. Inhibition of 1,2-dimethylhydrazine metabolism by disulfiram. Xenobiotica 7:5–9.

Frankfurt, O. S., L. P. Lipchina, T. V. Bunto, and N. M. Emanuel. 1967. The influence of 4-methyl-2,6-tertbutylphenol (Ionol) on the development of hepatic tumors in rats. Bull. Exp. Biol. Med. 8:86–88.

Gelboin, H. V., F. Wiebel, and L. Diamond. 1970. Dimethylbenzanthracene tumorigenesis and aryl hydroxylase in mouse skin: Inhibition by 7,8-benzoflavone. Science 170:169–171.

Grantham, P. H., J. H. Weisburger, and E. K. Weisburger. 1973. Effect of the antioxidant butylated hydroxytoluene on the metabolism of the carcinogens N-2-fluorenylacetamide and N-hydroxy-N-2-fluorenylacetamide. Food Cosmet. Toxicol. 11:209–217.

Huebner, R. J., and D. C. Fish. 1979. Sarc and leuk oncogene-transforming proteins as antigenic determinants of cause and prevention of cancer in Mice and Rats, *in* Carcinogens: Identification and Mechanisms of Action (The University of Texas System Cancer Center 31st Annual Symposium on Fundamental Cancer Research, 1978), A. C. Griffin and C. R. Shaw, eds., Raven Press, New York, pp. 277–298.

Huggins, C., G. Lorraine, and R. Fukunishi. 1964. Aromatic influences on the yields of mammary cancers following administration of 7,12-dimethylbenz(a)anthracene. Proc. Natl. Acad. Sci. USA 51:737–742.

Hunter, A. L., and R. A. Neal. 1975. Inhibition of hepatic mixed-function oxidase activity in vitro and in vivo by various thiono-sulfur-containing compounds. Biochem. Pharmacol. 24:2199–2205.

Jacobs, M. N. 1977. Inhibitory effects of selenium on 1,2-dimethylhydrazine and methylazoxymethanol colon carcinogenesis. Cancer 40:2557–2564.

Jacobs, M. N., B. Jansson, and A. C. Griffin. 1977. Inhibitory effects of selenium on 1,2-dimethylhydrazine and methylazoxymethanol acetate induction of colon tumors. Cancer Lett. 2:133–138.

Lacassagne, A., L. Hurst, and M. D. Xuong. 1970. Inhibition par deux naphthoisothiocyanates de l'hépatocancérogenèse produite, chez le rat par le p-diméthylamino-azobenzène (DAB). C. R. Soc. Biol. (Paris) 164:230–233.

Lam, L. K. T., and L. W. Wattenberg. 1977. Effects of butylated hydroxyanisole on the metabolism of benzo(a)pyrene by mouse liver microsomes. J. Natl. Cancer Inst. 58:413–417.

Lichtenstein, E. P., F. M. Strong, and D. G. Borgan. 1962. Identification of 2-phenylisothiocyanate as an insecticide occurring naturally in edible parts of turnips. Agricult. Food Chem. 10:30–33.

Makiura, S. H., S. Aoe, S. Sigihara, K. Hirao, A. Masayuki, and N. Ito. 1974. Inhibitory effect of polychlorinated biphenyls on liver turmorigenesis in rats treated with 3'-methyl-4-dimethylaminoazobenzene, N-2-fluorenylacetamide, and diethylnitrosamine. J. Natl. Cancer Inst. 53:1253–1257.

McLean, A. E., and A. Marshall, 1971. Reduced carcinogenic effects of aflatoxin in rats given phenobarbitone. Br. J. Exp. Pathol. 52:322–329.

Miller, E. C., and J. A. Miller. 1972. Approaches to the mechanisms and control of chemical carcinogenesis, *in* Environment and Cancer (The University of Texas System Cancer Center 24th Annual Symposium on Fundamental Cancer Research, 1971), Williams and Wilkins Co., Baltimore, pp. 5–39.

Miller, E. C., and J. A. Miller. 1974. Biochemical mechanisms of chemical carcinogenesis, *in* The Molecular Biology of Cancer, H. Busch, ed., Academic Press, New York, pp. 337–342.

Miller, E. C., J. A. Miller, R. R. Brown, and J. MacDonald. 1958. On the protective action of certain polycyclic aromatic hydrocarbons against carcinogenesis by aminoazo dyes and 2-acetyl-aminofluorene. Cancer Res. 18:469–477.

Miller, J. A., and E. C. Miller. 1969. The metabolic activation of carcinogenic aromatic amines and amides. Prog. Exp. Tumor Res. 11:273–301.

Miller, J. A., and E. C. Miller. 1974. Some current thresholds of research in chemical carcinogenesis, *in* Chemical Carcinogenesis, P. O. Ts'o and J. A. DiPaolo, eds., Marcel Dekker Inc., New York, pp. 61–86.

Mirvish, S. S., A. Cardesa, L. Wallcave, and P. Shubik. 1975. Induction of mouse lung adenomas by amines or urea plus nitrite and by N-nitroso compounds: Effects of ascorbate, gallic acid, thiocyanate, and caffeine. J. Natl. Cancer Inst. 55:633–636.

Pamukcu, A. M., L. W. Wattenberg, J. M. Price, and G. T. Bryan. 1971. Phenothiazine inhibition of intestinal and urinary bladder tumors induced in rats by bracken fern. J. Natl. Cancer Inst. 47:155–159.

Peraino, C., R. J. Fry, E. Staffeldt, and W. D. Kisieleski. 1973. Effects of varying exposure to phenobarbital on its enhancement of 2-acetylaminofluorene-induced hepatic tumorigenesis in the rat. J. Natl. Cancer Inst. 33:2701–2705.

Pipkin, G. E., J. U. Schlegel, R. Nishimura, and G. N. Schultz. 1969. Inhibitory effect of L-ascorbate on tumor formation in urinary bladders implanted with 3-hydroxyanthranilic acid. Proc. Soc. Exp. Biol. Med. 131:522–524.

Richardson, H. L., A. R. Stein, and E. Borson-Nacht-Nebel. 1952. Tumor inhibition and adrenal histologic responses in rats in which 3-methyl-4-dimethyl-aminoazobenzene and 2-methylcholan-threne were simultaneously administered. Cancer Res. 12:356–371.

Rose, G. A., and D. M. Wallace. 1973. Observations on urinary chemiluminescence of normal smokers and nonsmokers and of patients with bladder cancer. Br. J. Urol. 45:520–533.

Schmähl, D., F. W. Krüger, M. Habs, and B. Diehl. 1976. Influence of disulfiram on the organotropy of the carcinogenic effect of dimethylnitrosamine and diethylnitrosamine in rats. Z. Krebsforsch. 85:271–276.

Shamberger, R. J. 1966. Protection against cocarcinogenesis by antioxidants. Experientia 22:116.

Shamberger, R. J. 1970. Relationship of selenium to cancer. I. Inhibitory effect of selenium on carcinogenesis. J. Natl. Cancer Inst. 44:931–936.

Shamberger, R. J., S. A. Tytko, and C. E. Willis. 1976. Antioxidants and cancer. VI. Selenium and age-adjusted human cancer mortality. Arch. Environ. Health 31:231–235.

Shamberger, R., and C. Willis. 1971. Selenium distribution and human cancer mortality. Clin. Lab. Sci. 2:211–221.

Silva, E. A. 1967. Da acaō inhibitória do pretratamento com fenobarbital sōbre a atividade carcinoge-nica pulmonar da uretana etilica em camundongos. Hospital Rio de Janeiro 71:1483–1493.

Slaga, T. J., and W. M. Bracken. 1977. The effects of antioxidants on skin tumor initiation and aryl hydrocarbon hydroxylase. Cancer Res. 37:1631–1635.

Speier, J. L., and L. W. Wattenberg. 1975. Alterations in microsomal metabolism of benzo(a)pyrene in mice fed butylated hydroxyanisole. J. Natl. Cancer Inst. 55:469–472.

Sporn, M. B., N. M. Dunlop, D. L. Newton, and J. M. Smith. 1976. Prevention of chemical carcinogenesis by vitamin A and its synthetic analogs (retinoids). Fed. Proc. 35:1332–1338.

Sporn, M. B., D. L. Newton, J. M. Smith, N. Acton, A. E. Jacobson, and A. Brossi. 1979. Retinoids and cancer prevention: The importance of the terminal group of the retinoid molecule in modifying activity and toxicity, *in* Carcinogens: Identification and Mechanisms of Action (The University of Texas System Cancer Center 31st Annual Symposium on Fundamental Cancer Research, 1978), Raven Press, New York, pp. 441–453.

Tawfic, H. N. 1965. Studies on ear duct tumors in rats. II. Inhibitory effects of methylcholanthrene and 1,2-benzanthracene on tumor formation by 4-dimethylaminostilbene. Acta Pathol. Jpn. 15:255–260.

Thamavit, W., Y. Hiawa, N. Ito, and N. Phamarapravati. 1974. The inhibitory effects of α-benzene hexachloride on 3′-methyl-4-dimethylaminoazobenzene and DL-ethioline carcinogenesis in rats. Cancer Res. 34:337–340.

Ulland, B. M., J. H. Weisburger, R. S. Yammamoto, and E. K. Weisburger. 1973. Antioxidants and carcinogenesis: Butylated hydroxytoluene, but not diphenyl-p-phenylene-diamine, inhibits cancer induction by N-2-fluorenylacetamide and by N-hydroxy-N-2-fluorenylacetamide in rats. Food Cosmet. Toxicol. 11:199–207.

Varghese, A. J., P. Land, R. Furrer, and W. R. Bruce. 1977. Evidence for the formation of mutagenic N-nitroso compounds in the human body. (Abstract) Proc. Am. Assoc. Cancer Res. 18:80.

Virtanen, A. I. 1962. Some organic sulfur compounds in vegetables and fodder plants and their significance in human nutrition. Angew. Chem. [Engl.] 1:299–306.

Wattenberg, L. W. 1972a. Inhibition of carcinogenic and toxic effects of polycyclic hydrocarbons by phenolic antioxidants and ethoxyquin. J. Natl. Cancer Inst. 48:1425–1430.

Wattenberg, L. W. 1972b. Inhibition of carcinogenic effects of diethylnitrosamine and 4-nitroquino-line-N-oxide by antioxidants. Fed. Proc. 31:633.

Wattenberg, L. W. 1973. Inhibition of chemical carcinogen-induced pulmonary neoplasia by buty-lated hydroxyanisole. J. Natl. Cancer Inst. 50:1541–1544.

Wattenberg, L. W. 1974. Inhibition of carcinogenic and toxic effects of polycyclic hydrocarbons by several sulfur-containing compounds. J. Natl. Cancer Inst. 52:1583–1587.

Wattenberg, L. W. 1975. Inhibition of dimethylhydrazine-induced neoplasia of the large intestine by disulfiram. J. Natl. Cancer Inst. 54:1005–1006.

Wattenberg, L. W. 1976. Inhibition of chemical carcinogenesis by antioxidants and some additional compounds, *in* Fundamentals of Cancer Prevention (Proceedings of the Sixth International Symposium of the Princess Takamatsu Cancer Research Fund), P. N. Magee, S. Takayama, T. Sugimura, and T. Matsushima, eds., University Park Press, Baltimore, pp. 153–166.

Wattenberg, L. W. 1977a. Inhibitors of chemical carcinogenesis, *in* Origins of Human Cancer (Cold Spring Harbor Symposium), H. H. Hiatt, J. D. Watson, and J. A. Winsten, eds., American Book-Stratford Press, Inc., Saddle Brook, New Jersey, pp. 785–799.

Wattenberg, L. W. 1977b. Inhibition of carcinogenic effects of polycyclic hydrocarbons by benzyl isothiocyanate and related compounds. J. Natl. Cancer Inst. 58:395–398.

Wattenberg, L. W., and E. Fiala. 1978. Inhibition of DMH-induced neoplasia of the large bowel by carbon disulfide. J. Natl. Cancer Inst. 60:1515–1517.

Wattenberg, L. W., L. K. T. Lam, A. Fladmoe, and P. Borchert, 1977. Inhibitors of colon carcinogenesis. Cancer 40:2432–2435.

Wattenberg, L. W., and J. L. Leong. 1967. Inhibition of 9,10-dimethylbenzanthracene (DMBA) induced mammary tumorigenesis by phenothiazines. Fed. Proc. 26:692.

Wattenberg, L. W., and J. L. Leong. 1968. Inhibition of the carcinogenic action of 7,12-dimethyl-benz(a)anthracene by beta-naphthoflavone. Proc. Soc. Exp. Biol. Med. 128:940–943.

Wattenberg, L. W., and J. L. Leong. 1970. Inhibition of the carcinogenic action of benzo(a)pyrene by flavones. Cancer Res. 30:1922–1925.

Wattenberg, L. W., and W. D. Loub. 1978. Inhibition of polycyclic hydrocarbon-induced neoplasia by naturally occurring indoles. Cancer Res. 38:1410–1413.

Wattenberg, L. W., W. D. Loub, L. K. T. Lam, and J. L. Speier. 1976. Dietary constituents altering the responses to chemical carcinogens. Fed. Proc. 35:1327–1331.

Weisburger, E. K., R. P. Evarts, and M. L. Wenk. 1978. Inhibitory effect of butylated hydroxytoluene (BHT) on intestinal carcinogenesis in rats by azoxymethane. Food Cosmet. Toxicol. (In press)

Weisburger, J. H., B. S. Reddy, and E. L. Wynder. 1977. Colon cancer: Its epidemiology and experimental production. Cancer 40:2414–2420.

Wheatley, D. N. 1968. Enhancement and inhibition of the induction by 7,12-dimethylbenz(a)anthra-cene of mammary tumors in female Sprague-Dawley rats. Br. J. Cancer 22:787–792.

Witschi, H., D. Williamson, and S. Lock. 1977. Enhancement of urethan tumorigenesis in mouse lung by butylated hydroxytoluene. J. Natl. Cancer Inst. 58:301–305.

Yammamoto, R. S., J. H. Weisburger, and E. K. Weisburger.1971. Controlling factors in urethan carcinogenesis in mice: Effects of enzyme inducers and metabolic inhibitors. Cancer Res. 31:483–486.

Cellular and Molecular Markers of the Carcinogenic Process

Carcinogens: Identification and Mechanisms of Action, edited by A. Clark Griffin and Charles R. Shaw. Raven Press, New York © 1979.

Physiological and Molecular Markers during Carcinogenesis

Emmanuel Farber, Ross G. Cameron, Brian Laishes, Jung-Chung Lin, Alan Medline, Katsuhiro Ogawa, and Dennis B. Solt

Department of Pathology, University of Toronto, Toronto, Ontario, Canada

It is now clearly evident that the development of cancer in many, if not all epithelial tissues as well as in some connective tissue and other mesodermal and nonepithelial ectodermal cells and tissues, is a multistep process. In this process, new cell populations appear that have altered phenotypic properties, and at least some of these new cell types appear to participate as steps in a sequence of events leading to cancer (malignant neoplasia). These collections of new cells are often highlights in the process. The identification and characterization of these various cells and the delineation of their role in the development of cancer remains a major challenge, not only as essential components in evolving an understanding of the nature of a malignant neoplasm but also as a basis for new approaches to the early diagnosis of preneoplasia and neoplasia and to the interruption of the carcinogenic process.

Fundamental to the success of this approach is the discovery of markers for each selective population of cells. Such markers could be structural and architectural, physiological, biochemical, enzymatic, and molecular and genetic. Each type would add an element of versatility to the analysis of the neoplastic process such that each key piece could be placed in its appropriate position in the jigsaw puzzle we call carcinogenesis.

Many phenotypic alterations have been described in numerous cancers in humans and in experimental animals. It would take pages just to enumerate them. Yet, it is evident that their use in the analysis of cancer and cancer development remains doubtful in most instances because of one major uncertainty—with what step in the carcinogenic process are they associated? To date, we have no models from which each major property of preneoplastic and neoplastic cell populations can be separated and isolated and thus related to a marker. Structural, as well as functional or biochemical changes in virtually every cell organelle (Svoboda and Reddy 1975), have been described in one or more systems (Robbins and Nicolson 1975). However, it is virtually impossible to assign any role, either trivial or essential, to these alterations since we have no way of dissecting the behavior patterns of the altered cells involved in cancer development. In view of this, it would appear to be more appropriate in this presentation to concentrate on one system, rather than attempting any type of systematic coverage of possible markers in carcinogenesis.

We have been concentrating our efforts exclusively on one system, the development of liver cancer with some chemicals, in the hope of laying a foundation that might be a guide in other less well-developed models. The validity of this approach is based on two assumptions: (a) that cancer development in any single organ, such as the liver, has a basic similarity in principle to the developmental process of cancer in many other organs or tissues, and (b) that the components responsible for the behavior pattern of any type of malignant neoplasm are most easily dissected and identified by an historical approach, that is by developing a model that will allow a sequential analysis of the steps essential for cancer development, beginning with a quiescent cell population, such as the vast majority of hepatocytes in a mature liver.

LIVER CARCINOGENESIS

Figure 1 illustrates our current view of the major steps in liver carcinogenesis initiated by chemicals, including an approximate estimate of the relative time scale of these steps in the process. We think that the preneoplastic phase, including initiation, takes up well over 50% of the whole process in the liver, and this fits well with what we know in many other organs or tissues, including some in humans (lung, skin, liver, urinary bladder, etc.). Initiation is quite rapid and consists of at least two steps—the induction of some one or more molecular alterations as the first step, and a round of cell replication for "fixation" as the second step. A delay in the time of occurrence of the second step may favor the reversibility of the first step by repair processes. This is followed by a long period dominated by selection and growth of the putative initiated cells and the progressive differentiation of these cells. In the first step in this differentiation process, which we call *neodifferentiation* (Farber, in press), the hepatocytes in the focal aggregates of proliferating initiated cells undergo progressive enlargement, characterized by a large accumulation of smooth endoplasmic reticulum and other changes to be discussed below. The majority of these aggregates then slowly mature or differentiate into normal-appearing liver, while a small minority fail to mature. These collections of altered hepatocytes, which have an apparent block in their maturation or differentiation option, are the site for the occurrence of "rare event number 2," that is, the first step in the neoplastic process. It is at this step that the first acquisition of autonomy or independence is expressed. The subsequent steps are much less clear but seem to consist of at least one and probably more than one additional event leading to malignant neoplasia. "Nodules within nodules" (Popper *et al.* 1960, Popper 1977) are characteristic of this later phase of carcinogenesis and probably indicate the selection of few newly altered cells within a larger population of cells at the immediately preceding step in the process. These rare events are probably clonal

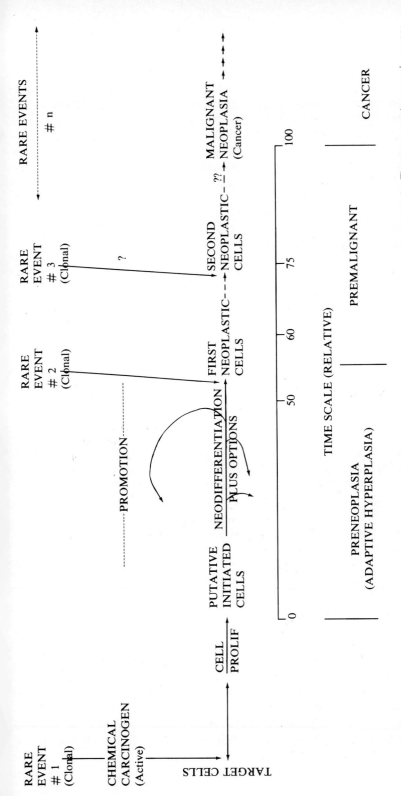

FIG. 1. Diagrammatic representation of our current concept of the steps in the development of liver cancer with chemicals. The rare events occur in a very small number of cells in a much larger population and therefore are analogous to a mutation-like phenomenon. In contrast, the steps between the rare events involve essentially the whole of that population. As indicated, the rare events are probably clonal in origin.

in origin. Whether these later "rare events" are built into the initiation process but require time to be expressed or are induced by components in the endogenous or exogenous environment are provocative questions to be explored. Ultimately, the overall process leads to the appearance of one or a few foci of malignant neoplasia that invade, metastasize, and eventually kill the host (Solt *et al.* 1977b). Obviously, major improvements in our models must be made if we are to discover markers for each discrete step. This remains a major challenge for the future.

Despite this deficiency, it is now possible to relate some markers to some of the steps in the process and to derive new insights into some aspects of this important area. This is the subject of the remainder of this presentation, including architectural and vascular, biochemical, enzymatic and molecular, cytological, and, finally, physiological markers.

Architectural and Vascular Markers

The first recognizable, altered cell population induced by a carcinogen, the putative initiated cells (see Figure 1), grow in a pattern distinctly different from that of a normal mature liver. Hepatocytes in the mature liver of most mammalian species are arranged predominantly as single cell plates, separated by the blood sinusoids. The apparently rare random cell that appears after even brief exposure to an hepatocarcinogen grows as a collection of hepatocytes arranged in sheets or plates, two or more cells thick, and in glands (Farber 1976b). This pattern persists throughout the preneoplastic phase of liver carcinogenesis and is seen in a modified form in the premalignant lesions and in virtually every cancer. In the latter, the details in the architectural arrangement of the malignant hepatocytes may show some variation, but a "normal" pattern is rarely, if ever, seen.

Accompanying these new cell-to-cell arrangements is an obvious change in the mix of arterial and portal blood supply. By the use of radiolabeled microspheres, it has been shown that preneoplastic nodules are supplied much more by arterial blood and much less by portal venous blood (Solt *et al.* 1977a). Hepatomas appear to be supplied predominantly or exclusively with arterial blood (Breedis and Young 1954, Solt *et al.* 1977a). The differences between the blood supply of normal mature liver and of nodules and hepatomas have been confirmed recently by perfusion techniques in the arterial and portal vascular systems using appropriate colored resins (H. Tsuda and E. Farber, unpublished observations). The significance of these alterations in such an important physiological parameter as blood supply is not understood. However, this change might be related to the appearance of a biochemical marker, γ-glutamyl transferase (GGT), in hepatocytes following portocaval anastomosis (Müller *et al.* 1974) and in very early preneoplastic hepatocytes, as discussed below.

The architectural arrangement of the preneoplastic hepatocytes in early foci and nodules is not fixed and absolute but often undergoes a progressive return to a normal-appearing pattern in nodules that mature or differentiate (Farber 1976b). As mentioned above, the majority of hyperplastic nodules undergo remodeling to a normal-like liver. This remodeling is accompanied by the gain of negative markers and loss of some positive ones and is considered to be a form of differentiation or maturation (Farber 1973, 1974, Farber *et al.* 1975, Kitagawa and Pitot 1975, Becker *et al.* 1971). During the remodeling and maturation, the hepatocytes in the nodules become reorganized into single-cell plates. Presumably, the vascular pattern also becomes more normal, but this has not yet been studied.

Biochemical and Enzymatic Markers

The very early new hepatocyte populations, the preneoplastic putative initiated cells, rapidly acquire many quite reproducible biochemical or enzymatic alterations that are useful as markers (see Farber 1973, for references to early work). Some are negative, that is, appear as a decrease or loss of some property, and some are positive.

Negative Markers

Until very recently, the negative ones have been most used. Among these are the decrease or loss of activities of glucose-6-phosphatase, nucleotide polyphosphatase, glucuronidase, serine dehydratase, and glycogen phosphorylase (see Farber 1976a for references) and ribonucleases and deoxyribonucleases (Daoust 1963, Fontaniere and Daoust 1973). Some of these markers have proved useful in the histochemical analysis of early events in liver carcinogenesis with at least three models (Kitagawa 1971, Kitagawa and Pitot 1975, Scherer and Emmelot 1975, 1976, Pugh and Goldfarb 1977, Pitot *et al.* 1978, K. Ogawa, D. B. Solt and E. Farber, unpublished experiments). To date, almost all their use has been restricted to histochemical studies in tissue slices at the light and, occasionally, at the electron microscopic level.

Despite their usefulness, it is difficult to pursue negative markers to any great depth in a mechanistic sense. Also, since they represent a heterogeneous collection with respect to fine intracellular localization, there seems to be no physiologic or behavioral changes in the affected cells that can be related to any of the negative markers discovered to date. Hopefully, as the biochemical basis for cell function begins to attract more attention, a meaningful physiologic pattern may become evident from the available data. It should be pointed out that these markers appear relatively early in carcinogenesis, long before the advent of any indications of neoplastic behavior. This important aspect will be discussed more fully below.

Positive Markers

Alpha-Fetoprotein

This was the first positive marker to be described (Abelev 1971). It has received considerable attention as a possible marker during carcinogenesis. Unfortunately, its life history and significance as an indicator for a cancer precursor cell remain controversial. Some studies show that brief exposure to many hepatotoxins without the development of cancer and also liver regeneration following partial hepatectomy are associated with an increase in liver and serum alpha-fetoprotein (AFP) (Sell and Wepsic 1975, Uriel 1975). Alpha-fetoprotein was localized predominantly to hyperplastic nodules during liver carcinogenesis with 2-acetylaminofluorene (2-AAF) using an immunofluorescent technique (Okita *et al.* 1974). Other studies indicate the presence of AFP in ductal cells that often proliferate during carcinogenesis (Kitagawa *et al.* 1972, Uriel *et al.* 1973, Tchipysheva *et al.* 1977). It must be pointed out that the majority of these studies induce liver carcinogenesis with 4-dimethylaminoazobenzene ("butter yellow") or a derivative and that this group of carcinogens induces a special series of changes in duct cells, which favors their conversion to hepatocytes and possibly hepatocellular carcinoma (Farber 1976b). Clearly, there is need for a basic clarification of the relationship of AFP to possible cancer precursor cells before this interesting marker can be of mechanistic use in the characterization and analysis of the carcinogenic process.

Preneoplastic Antigen

An antigenic component in the endoplasmic reticulum of hyperplastic nodules induced by either 2-AAF or ethionine has been described (Okita and Farber 1975, Okita *et al.* 1975, Lin *et al.* 1977). This was tentatively called preneoplastic antigen (PN antigen). It is present in the smooth endoplasmic reticulum (SER) of hyperplastic nodules and of hepatomas induced by one of five different carcinogens. It appears to be exclusively localized in the ER and to be a marker for abnormal ER that appears in preneoplastic cells during liver carcinogenesis (Lin *et al.* 1977).

This preneoplastic antigen has recently been purified by Griffin and Kizer (1978) and by Lin and Farber (unpublished results). Using the purified material as immunogen, it has been found to be present to a small degree in a masked form in normal, rough ER (RER) (Lin and Farber 1977). It is present in normal ER in about one-fifth to one-tenth the concentration in SER of nodules but is completely masked under normal circumstances. If the membranes are stripped of their ribosomes, the antigen appears.

The antigen from hyperplastic nodules is a dimer of a molecular weight of about 140,000 daltons. The subunits are identical, have serine as their N-terminal amino acid, and contain carbohydrate (J-C. Lin and E. Farber, unpublished work). Whether this protein is the same in SER of hyperplastic nodules and in RER of normal liver remains to be established.

The PN antigen appears in virtually every hyperplastic nodule and remains positive by immunofluorescence in persistent nodules and in hepatomas. The nodules that undergo maturation to normal-like liver show a progressive loss of their staining capacity for this protein. Thus, the PN antigen, like many of the negative markers (see above) and some positive ones (see below), is characteristic of a relatively early preneoplastic phase of liver carcinogenesis. Thus, it is more a marker of preneoplasia than of neoplasia.

Gamma-Glutamyl Transferase

One of the most useful markers for preneoplastic cells is γ-glutamyl transferase (GGT). This was first described by Fiala and co-workers (1972, 1976) in quantitative studies using experimental hepatomas and liver during cancer development. Subsequent histochemical studies showed the enzyme to be present in proliferating ductular cells (bile ducts, oval cells) as well as in hyperplastic nodules (Kalengayi *et al.* 1975, Harada *et al.* 1976) induced by two different carcinogens, N-hydroxy-2-AAF (N-OH-2-AAF) and aflatoxin B_1. Also, primary tumors of liver induced by aflatoxin B_1, 3'-methyl-4-dimethylaminoazobenzene (3'-me-DAB), N-OH-2-AAF, and 2-AAF and whole liver during carcinogenesis had elevated levels of activity (Taniguchi *et al.* 1974, Harada *et al.* 1976).

Quantitative and histochemical study of putative initiated hepatocytes during the development of liver cancer with a new model (Solt and Farber 1976, Solt *et al.* 1977b) has shown that GGT is "turned on" very rapidly and is one of the best markers for preneoplastic hepatocytes (Ogawa 1977, Cameron *et al.* 1978). The enzyme appears in both the SER and the bile canaliculus, with the greatest apparent concentration in the latter site. GGT activity is also high in fetal liver, again in the bile canaliculus. Ninety to ninety-five percent of the early preneoplastic foci and nodules stain positively for GGT, in contrast to the decrease in glucose-6-phosphatase and ATPase that occurs in only 60 to 70% of such lesions (K. Ogawa, D. B. Solt and E. Farber, unpublished results).

The enzyme activity, as judged histochemically, is similar to many of the negative enzyme markers and to PN antigen in that it reflects the presence and persistence of some change in the altered liver cells related to their apparent role in carcinogenesis. For example, on remodeling and maturation of the nodules that appear during preneoplasia, the enzyme activity progressively disappears. It remains very active in those nodules that persist and in many but not all hepatomas.

It is present in isolated cells from some transplantable hepatomas including the HTC hepatoma, which grows well in suspension in tissue culture (Laishes *et al.* 1978a). In these cells, as well as in individual hepatocytes isolated from hyperplastic nodules and from some primary hepatocellular carcinomas (induced by 2-AAF or by diethylnitrosamine [DEN]), the enzyme appears to stain only a portion of the surface membrane. Conceivably, this could be a specialized area that is related to the original bile canaliculus in nonneoplastic hepatocytes.

As mentioned above, GGT "appears" in hepatocytes when portal blood is shunted to the inferior vena cava (Müller *et al.* 1974). Since this vascular pattern resembles that of foci and nodules, it is tempting to consider that the appearance of GGT in hepatocytes in early preneoplastic foci and nodules might be a reflection of the change in balance between arterial and portal venous blood. Thus, this marker might be one for altered blood supply and not for some other change associated with preneoplasia.

D-T Diaphorase

A new, interesting marker for early preneoplastic hepatocytes is D-T diaphorase. This soluble oxido-reductase has been known for a long time as being capable of oxidizing reduced pyridine nucleotides (NADH and NADPH), being stimulated by vitamin K and inhibited by dicumarol. It was found to be elevated in some hepatomas (Schor and Morris 1977) and in Leydig cell tumors of the rat testis (Schor *et al.* 1976).

It was recently found to be elevated four to six times over normal liver in early and late hyperplastic nodules, as measured quantitatively, and to be high in very early preneoplastic hepatocytes when viewed histochemically (N. A. Schor, K. Ogawa, G. Lee, and E. Farber, unpublished experiments). Like GGT, 90 to 95% of the early preneoplastic foci and nodules stain positively for elevated D-T diaphorase. Also, like GGT and other positive and negative markers, D-T diaphorase returns to a more "normal" level in hepatocytes that are present in remodeling and maturing nodules.

An interesting facet of the D-T diaphorase results concerns the activation of carcinogens. As discussed below under "Physiological Markers," preneoplastic hepatocytes are resistant to the toxic effects of many chemical carcinogens. The basis for this resides no doubt in part in the deficiency of activating enzyme activity in the ER for several types of carcinogens.

The elevation in D-T diaphorase introduces a new insight into this aspect of carcinogenesis. At least two types of carcinogens, nitroquinolines and nitrofurans (Matsushima and Sugimura 1971, Weisburger and Williams 1975) are probably enzymatically reduced to hydroxyamino compounds as part of the activation pattern. D-T diaphorase may play an important role in this pathway, and an elevated level could make the preneoplastic hepatocytes not only less resistant but actually more susceptible to these carcinogens.

Chorionic Gonadotropin

An interesting marker that has recently been found in early and late preneoplastic hepatocyte populations is a component that reacts with antibodies to the β-subunit of human chorionic gonadotropin (Malkin *et al.* 1977). The provocative finding of a trophoblast hormone in preneoplastic rat liver lesions must await careful and complete purification of rat and human proteins and their subunits and the preparation of monospecific antibodies before this observation can be considered as established. However, antibodies to human prolactin and growth hormone do not show a positive immunofluorescent reaction in these lesions. It should be recalled that McManus *et al.* (1976) reported that 25 of 28 human malignant neoplasms stained positively for the β-chain of human chorionic gonadotropin. Most of the tumors had no obvious anatomical or physiological relationship to trophoblast or sites where trophoblast can occur. The implications of the possible presence of chorionic gonadotropin in early preneoplastic liver lesions are interesting and point to a need for more emphasis on trophoblastic components in carcinogenesis.

Cytologic Markers

Nuclei

The vast majority if not all preneoplastic hepatocytes at the earliest stage in development show a characteristic change in the appearance of nuclei on light microscopic examination. The putative initiated hepatocytes contain nuclei that are slightly larger in diameter than nuclei in normal hepatocytes. The chromatin is loose and very poorly stained, and the nucleolus is almost always very large and single (Solt *et al.* 1977b). The nucleus resembles closely that seen at the height of regeneration of hepatocytes. However, with normal regeneration, the nuclei return to a normal appearance within a few days. In the preneoplastic hepatocytes, the nuclei remain in the open loose form with large nucleoli virtually throughout carcinogenesis, even when the nodules become remodeled to a normal-appearing architecture. Thus, it appears that, so far, the only marker that seems to be relatively permanent is the nuclear appearance.

The loose chromatin structure and large nucleoli are usually associated with an activated RNA metabolism in cells that have been stimulated to enter the active cell cycle (Harris 1974). It should be emphasized that the preneoplastic hepatocytes undergo at most only very slow cell proliferation unless stimulated by an appropriate environmental perturbation (Farber 1973, Solt *et al.* 1977b, Williams *et al.* 1977).

Endoplasmic Reticulum

One of the most characteristic cytological changes during neodifferentiation is the acquisition of abundant SER (Farber 1973). This occurs after the earliest growth of the putative initiated cells and dominates the cytology of preneoplasia. This alteration is characteristic of hepatocytes in nodules that persist and become the precursor for the next step, neoplasia (see Figure 1). Like many of the biochemical and architectural markers, the abundant SER disappears as the nodules undergo remodeling during maturation to normal-appearing liver. The abundant SER is associated with a decrease in activity of some of the key components in the mixed function mono-oxygenase (MFO) system (see next section) and may play an important role in the development of resistance to carcinogen cytotoxicity by the preneoplastic hepatocytes (Gravela *et al.* 1975, Cameron *et al.* 1976). Also, the increased concentration of PN antigen in the SER, compared to a masking of the activity in normal ER, suggests a possible basic rearrangement in the organizational pattern of the ER membranes in the preneoplastic hepatocytes (Lin and Farber 1977).

There is a remarkable resemblance of the "ground glass" appearance of the preneoplastic hepatocyte with abundant SER to the Shikata cell containing similarly abundant SER and also hepatitis B surface antigen in hepatitis B carriers (Farber, in press). The possible relationship of these two types of cells as potential precursors for hepatocellular carcinoma has been discussed briefly (Farber, in press).

Plasma Membrane

Recent studies in our laboratory (K. Ogawa, H. Tsuda, and A. Medline, unpublished observations) indicate that a striking change in the cell-to-cell arrangements occurs early in preneoplasia. The bile canaliculi become very dilated and distorted with abnormal microvilli, and the remainder of the plasma membrane shows separation from neighbors with the appearance of long irregular microvilli. This change occurs long before there is any evidence of neoplastic behavior, such as any autonomy of growth (Williams *et al.* 1977).

Thus, obvious, reproducible alterations in the structure of the nucleus, the ER, and the plasma membrane characterize the early preneoplastic hepatocytes well before any objective evidence of independence of growth or other criteria of neoplastic behavior can be seen.

Physiological Markers

Resistance to Carcinogen-Induced Cytotoxicity

In any analysis of markers for the various hepatocyte populations that are steps in the development of cancer, the most important markers are those that either generate new insight into our understanding of some phase of the process or suggest new practical approaches for diagnosis or therapy or for the assay of carcinogens. This marker does both and is without a doubt the most useful analytical tool in liver carcinogenesis in our research.

The physiological marker is expressed in a variety of ways. The most clearcut is the ability to respond to a growth stimulus such as partial hepatectomy or liver cell necrosis in the presence of a concentration of a carcinogen, such as 2-AAF, that is strongly inhibitory to cell proliferation. Under such circumstances, hepatocytes altered by prior exposure to a carcinogen can respond vigorously by cell proliferation such that visible foci and even nodules of 1 to 2 mm in diameter appear within seven to ten days (Solt and Farber 1976, Solt *et al.* 1977b).

This resistance is also seen as a failure to undergo cell death or necrosis when exposed to a necrogenic dose of carbon tetrachloride (CCl_4) or dimethylnitrosamine (DMN) (Farber *et al.* 1976). Also, isolated liver cells from livers containing foci or nodules or from hyperplastic nodules per se show a resistance to the lethal effects of aflatoxin B_1. At concentrations of aflatoxin of 10^{-5} M, all hepatocytes from normal livers die within 48 to 72 hours. In livers from the carcinogen-treated animals (2-AAF, DEN, etc.), up to 50% of the hepatocytes are completely resistant to aflatoxin at a concentration of 10^{-4} M (Laishes *et al.* 1978b).

Thus, by at least three criteria—growth, cell death in vivo, and cell death in vitro, and with several different hepatotoxins and hepatocarcinogens, carcinogen-induced putative initiated and preneoplastic hepatocytes are quite able to survive and function well in concentrations of carcinogens that kill or inhibit cell proliferation of normal or uninitiated hepatocytes.

Some appreciation is available for the possible biochemical basis for such resistance. With one carcinogen, 2-AAF, the resistant cells do not take it up very much. They show about 90% inhibition of uptake (Farber *et al.* 1976). With DMN, the resistant cells show more than a 50% decrease in the ability to activate the carcinogen and to have it interact covalently with DNA, RNA, and protein (Farber *et al.* 1976). Consistent with this is a large decrease in the concentration of cytochrome P-450 and in aryl hydrocarbon hydroxylase activity in the ER of the resistant cells (Cameron *et al.* 1976). Thus, they have acquired some change in uptake ability, presumably a change in the plasma membrane, and a change in the MFO system in the ER. This is most easily interpreted as a package—an interference with some regulatory gene or gene product that controls response to hepatotoxins at two membrane levels.

We consider the resistance as one type of alteration, akin to a somatic mutation, induced by carcinogens that initiate the carcinogenic process. In Figure 1, this would be one type of biological consequence of "rare event number 1." The induction of this marker, we think, could be a major determinant of whether a carcinogen will or will not initiate carcinogenesis. Parenthetically, we do not consider that this marker has any relationship to growth control. We think the resistant cell has the normal pattern and degree of growth control; it simply can respond to a mitogenic stimulus under adverse conditions.

Naturally, it now becomes possible to measure for two properties of carcinogens—the ability to induce resistant hepatocytes, initiation, and the ability to create an inhibitory environment that will favor the selection or growth of the resistant cell in the presence of a suitable stimulus for cell proliferation, such as cell removal, cell death (e.g., CCl_4) or even a mitogen (e.g., alphahexachlorocyclohexane). In fact, the second property, which can be broadly considered as a phenomenon of promotion, has been used already as a possible short-term screen for hepatocarcinogens (Tatematsu *et al.* 1977).

Work in our laboratory indicates that this approach can be used also as a rapid or short-term assay for carcinogens generally. Compounds such as 3-methylcholanthrene, N-methyl-N′-nitro-N-nitrosoguanidine (MNNG), N-methyl-nitrosourea, and 7,12-dimethyl-benzanthracene, compounds not normally carcinogenic for the liver, are positive using this new approach when coupled with a round of cell proliferation.

Lack of Iron Accumulation

Hepatocytes, as well as Kupffer cells, take up considerable amounts of iron under appropriate circumstances of iron exposure. Hepatocytes in hyperplastic nodules as well as in malignant neoplasms of liver fail to do so (Williams and Yamamoto 1972). Subsequent work has shown this to be a property of very early preneoplastic lesions as well (Williams *et al.* 1976). This property might prove to be useful in identifying exceptionally small early foci of preneoplastic cells.

GENERAL CONSIDERATIONS

This brief outline of some interesting markers of populations of hepatocytes that appear during the development of liver cell cancer clearly points to the need for many more markers, especially for the more discrete and later steps. However, despite this obvious deficiency, it appears that some tentative generalizations might be entertained. These relate to the use of markers for distinguishing early diversity of origin, the diagnosis of preneoplasia, the use of physiological markers as "driving forces" for progression from one step to another before a considerable degree of autonomy or independence for growth occurs, the possible occurrence of posttranslational controls for some markers, and the possible importance of differential markers between initiated and uninitiated surrounding cells in the development of cancer.

Diversity or Uniformity

It might appear that the common occurrence of many positive and negative markers in early and later preneoplastic and neoplastic hepatocyte populations suggests a uniformity of hepatocytes, a phenomenon in apparent conflict with the clonal nature of many neoplasms and the uniqueness of early cancer. Pugh and Goldfarb (1977) and Pitot *et al.* (1978) have shown that late hyperplastic nodules show a diversity with respect to several histochemical markers—GGT, glucose-6-phosphatase, and "ATPase." While many nodules have all three markers, significant numbers have only one or two, the commonest being GGT. Hepatomas are even more diverse with respect to these markers.

Unfortunately, both groups failed to consider the possibility that at least some of the diversity could be related to different rates of reappearance of two negative markers and of loss of GGT during remodeling. Such a selective differentiation of individual markers could account for the observations.

Work in our laboratory (K. Ogawa and D. B. Solt, unpublished results) has examined the same question but at a time *before* any remodeling has occurred. Under these conditions, 90 to 95% of early foci were positive for GGT and D-T diaphorase, while the percentage of foci that showed loss of either glucose-6-phosphatase or nucleotide polyphosphatase was considerably less. These data indicate that the diversity seen in hepatomas could appear at the time of initiation. They would also suggest that these biochemical markers are not essential for carcinogenesis. They could be near but not adjacent to critical, affected genes, if the step is at the gene level, or could be reflections of the altered blood supply or other local physiological modulations that characterize the preneoplastic as well as the neoplastic hepatocyte populations.

Markers for Preneoplasia

All the work on the markers during liver carcinogenesis strongly suggests that many alterations ostensibly related to cancer are in fact markers or indicators for preneoplasia. The very early appearance of positive markers including some embryonic or fetal ones during liver carcinogenesis indicates a high probability that similar types of markers may be associated with the early development of preneoplasia in other organs. A search for enzyme or other types of markers that could be used in cytologic examination would almost certainly open up the whole area of early postinitiation steps for diagnosis. Such a development could conceivably have important applications for cancers in several sites, such as bronchus, urinary bladder, and colon. Also, the stimulation to secrete a discrete marker, such as a chorionic gonadotropin or other specialized markers, could lead to early diagnosis of preneoplasia by blood examination.

Posttranslational Control for Some Markers

One of the most intriguing aspects of the study of markers in carcinogenesis is the suggestion that posttranslational control may play a role in determining the altered behavior patterns of neoplasms. It is generally considered on mainly theoretical grounds that many phenotypic alterations, especially so-called "important ones," are a reflection of an alteration in "gene expression," that is, are controlled at the level of transcription. Our data on PN antigen and other data indicate that some manifestations of new cell populations during the development of cancer may be controlled predominantly at the posttranslational level. The obvious control of the expression of a protein in the ER by the state of the ribosomes could be an important control point, especially in view of the major changes in ER in many of its properties.

Physiologic Markers as Driving Forces

There is no positive evidence and accumulating negative evidence for the generally accepted thesis that all new cell populations, including those appearing during initiation, have some defect or alteration in growth control. Our data on the liver fail to support this thesis (e.g., Williams *et al.* 1977). Instead, our data suggest that we must look for other ways to account for the growth of preneoplastic cells before their acquisition of some autonomy of growth.

The importance of resistance as a marker is clearly shown in its role as a "handle" to create a driving force by the imposition of an appropriate selection pressure. While resistance to toxins and carcinogens is appropriate for the liver, other tissues or organs could very well have other physiological markers as their type of initiation. For skin, some differential response or resistance to ultraviolet light might be appropriate. For breast or uterus or ovary, a differential response or resistance to some effect of a hormone would seem to be appropriate. For urinary bladder, a differential response or resistance to some urinary component would seem to be appropriate. Thus each site for carcinogenesis might have a different physiological marker as the "handle" by which a presumptive initiated cell could be selectively encouraged to grow.

This differential effect appears to be an important aspect of carcinogenesis. Virtually all carcinogenic processes involve the focal growth, that is, the growth of a few altered cells. Something in the local natural or artificial environment could be exerting an influence that allows presumptive initiated cells to respond somewhat differently, either quantitatively or qualitatively, as compared to the surrounding uninitiated majority. According to this formulation, one of the important challenges becomes the identification of the nature of the physiological marker in the initiated cell that allows it to be selected and the appropriate stimulus in the environment that creates the selection pressure.

ACKNOWLEDGMENTS

The investigations included in this report were supported in part by research grants from the National Cancer Institute of Canada, the Medical Research Council of Canada, by Grant CA-21157 and by a contract CP-75879 from the National Cancer Institute, Department of Health, Education and Welfare, and by a grant from the Connaught Fund of the University of Toronto. We would like to express our thanks to Mrs. Sandra Leon for her assistance in the preparation of this manuscript.

REFERENCES

Abelev, G. I. 1971. Alpha-fetoprotein in ontogenesis and its association with malignant tumors. Adv. Cancer Res. 14:295–358.

Becker, F. F., R. A. Fox, K. M. Klein, and S. R. Wolman. 1971. Chromosome patterns in rat hepatocytes during N-2-fluorenyl acetamide carcinogenesis. J. Natl. Cancer Inst. 46:1261–1269.

Breedis, C., and G. Young. 1954. The blood supply of neoplasms in the liver. Am. J. Pathol. 30:969–985.

Cameron, R., G. D. Sweeney, K. Jones, G. Lee, and E. Farber. 1976. A relative deficiency of cytochrome P-450 and aryl hydrocarbon (benzo[a]pyrene) hydroxylase in hyperplastic nodules induced by 2-acetylaminofluorene in rat liver. Cancer Res. 36:3888–3893.

Cameron, R., G. Kellen, A. Kolin, A. Malkin, and E. Farber. 1978. Gamma-glutamyl transferase in putative premalignant liver cell populations during hepatocarcinogenesis. Cancer Res. 38:823–829.

Daoust, R. 1963. Cellular populations and nucleic acid metabolism in rat liver parenchyma during azo dye carcinogenesis. Can. Cancer Conf. 5:225–239.

Farber, E. 1973. Hyperplastic liver nodules, in Methods in Cancer Research, H. Busch, ed., Vol. 7, Academic Press, New York, pp. 345–375.

Farber, E. 1974. Pathogenesis of liver cancer. Arch. Pathol. 98:145–148.

Farber, E. 1976a. Hyperplastic areas, hyperplastic nodules and hyperbasophilic areas as putative precursor lesions. Cancer Res. 36:2532–2533.

Farber, E. 1976b. The pathology of experimental liver cell cancer, in Liver Cell Cancer, H. M. Cameron, D. A. Linsell, and G. P. Warwick, eds., Elsevier/North-Holland Biomedical Press, Amsterdam, pp. 243–277.

Farber, E. 1978. Response of liver to carcinogens—A new analytical approach, in Toxic Liver Injury, E. Farber and M. M. Fisher, eds., Marcel Dekker, New York (In press).

Farber, E., S. Hartman, and D. Solt. 1975. Interruption of differentiation ("blocked ontogeny") during induction of liver cancer by hepatocarcinogens. Proc. Am. Assoc. Cancer Res. 16:3.

Farber, E., S. Parker, and M. Gruenstein. 1976. The resistance of putative premalignant liver cell populations, hyperplastic nodules, to the acute cytotoxic effects of some hepatocarcinogens. Cancer Res. 36:3879–3887.

Fiala, S., A. E. Fiala, and B. Dixon. 1972. Gamma-glutamyl transpeptidase in transplantable, chemically induced rat hepatomas and "spontaneous" mouse hepatomas. J. Natl. Cancer Inst. 48:1393–1401.

Fiala, S., A. Monhindru, W. G. Kettering, A. E. Fiala, and H. P. Morris. 1976. Glutathione and gamma-glutamyl transpeptidase in rat liver during chemical carcinogenesis. J. Natl. Cancer Inst. 57:591–598.

Fontanière, B., and R. Daoust. 1973. Histochemical studies on nuclease activity and neoplastic transformation in rat liver during diethylnitrosamine carcinogenesis. Cancer Res. 33:3108–3111.

Gravela, E., F. Feo, R. A. Canuto, R. Garcea, and L. Gabriel. 1975. Functional and structural alterations of liver ergastoplasmic membranes during DL-ethionine hepatocarcinogenesis. Cancer Res. 35:3041–3047.

Griffin, M. J., and D. E. Kizer. 1978. Purification and quantitation of preneoplastic antigen from hyperplastic nodules in normal liver. Cancer Res. 38:1136–1141.

Harada, M., K. Okabe, K. Shibata, H. Masuda, K. Miyota, and M. Enomoto. 1976. Histochemical demonstration of increased activity of gamma-glutamyl transpeptidase in rat liver during hepato-carcinogenesis. Acta Histochem. Cytochem. 9:168–179.

Harris, H. 1974. Nucleus and Cytoplasm. 3rd ed. Oxford University Press, London.

Kalengayi, M. M. R., G. Ronchi, and V. J. Desmet. 1975. Histochemistry of gamma-glutamyl transpeptidase in rat liver during aflatoxin B_1-induced carcinogenesis. J. Natl. Cancer Inst. 55:579–588.

Kitagawa, T. 1971. Histochemical analysis of hyperplastic lesions and hepatomas of the liver of rats fed 2-fluorenylacetamide. Gann 62:207–216.

Kitagawa, T., and H. C. Pitot. 1975. The regulation of serine dehydratase and glucose-6-phosphatase in hyperplastic nodules of rat liver during diethylnitrosamine and N-2-fluorenylacetamide feeding. Cancer Res. 35:1075–1084.

Kitagawa, T., T. Yokochi, and H. Sugano. 1972. Alpha-fetoprotein and hepatocarcinogenesis in rats fed 3'-methyl-4-dimethylamino-azobenzene or N-2-fluorenylacetamide. Int. J. Cancer 10:368–381.

Laishes, B. A., K. Ogawa, E. Roberts, and E. Farber. 1978a. Gamma-glutamyl transpeptidase: A positive marker for cultured rat liver cells derived from putative premalignant and malignant lesions. J. Natl. Cancer Inst. 60:1009–1016.

Laishes, B. A., E. Roberts, and E. Farber. 1978b. In vitro measurement of carcinogen-resistant liver cells during hepatocarcinogenesis. Int. J. Cancer 21:186–193.

Lin, J-C., and E. Farber. 1977. Effect of ribosome stripping procedures on antigenicity and confirmation of endoplasmic reticulum membrane. Biochem. Biophys. Res. Commun. 76:1247–1252.

Lin, J-C., Y. Hiasa, and E. Farber. 1977. Preneoplastic antigen as a marker for endoplasmic reticulum of putative premalignant hepatocytes during liver carcinogenesis. Cancer Res. 37:1972–1981.

Malkin, A., J. A. Kellen, A. Kolin, R. Cameron, and E. Farber. 1977. The immunochemical detection of chorionic gonadotropin in experimental rat hepatomas. International Research Group for Carcinoembryonic Proteins—5th Meeting (Aug. 6–9) (Abstract), p. 59.

Matsushima, T., and T. Sugimura. 1971. Metabolism. Recent Results Cancer Res. 34:53–60.

McManus, L. M., M. A. Naughten, and A. Martinez-Hernandez. 1976. Human chorionic gonadotropin in human neoplastic cells. Cancer Res. 36:3476–3481.

Müller, E., J. P. Colombo, E. Peheim, and J. Bircher. 1974. Histochemical demonstration of gamma-glutamyl transpeptidase in rat liver after portacaval anastomosis. Experientia 30:1128–1129.

Ogawa, K. 1977. Gamma-glutamyl transpeptidase (GGT) as a very early marker of putative preneo-plastic cells in liver carcinogenesis. Proc. Am. Assoc. Cancer Res. 18:158.

Okita, K., M. Gruenstein, M. Klaiber, and E. Farber. 1974. Localization of alpha-fetoprotein by immunofluorescence in hyperplastic nodules during hepatocarcinogenesis induced by 2-acetylami-nofluorene. Cancer Res. 34:2758–2763.

Okita, K., and E. Farber. 1975. An antigen common to preneoplastic hepatocyte populations and liver cancer induced by N-2-fluorenylacetamide, ethionine or other hepatocarcinogens. Gann Monogr. Cancer Res. 17:283–299.

Okita, K., L. H. Kligman, and E. Farber. 1975. A new common marker for premalignant and malignant hepatocytes induced in the rat by chemical carcinogens. J. Natl. Cancer Inst. 54:199–202.

Pitot, H. C., L. Barsness, T. Goldsworthy, and T. Kitagawa. 1978. Biochemical characterization of stages of hepatocarcinogenesis after a single dose of diethylnitrosamine. Nature 271:456–458.

Popper, H. 1977. Pathologic aspects of cirrhosis. A review. Am. J. Pathol. 87:228–264.

Popper, H., S. S. Sternberg, B. L. Oser, and M. Oser. 1960. The carcinogenic effect of aramite in rats. A study of hepatic nodules. Cancer 13:1035–1046.

Pugh, T., and S. Goldfarb. 1977. Quantitative histochemical and autoradiographic studies of 2-acetaminofluorene (2-AAF) carcinogenesis. Proc. Am. Assoc. Cancer Res. 18:130.

Robbins, J. C., and L. G. Nicolson. 1975. Surfaces of normal and transformed cells, *in* Cancer—A Comprehensive Treatise, F. F. Becker, ed., Vol. 4, Plenum Press, New York, pp. 3–40.

Scherer, E., and P. Emmelot. 1975. Foci of altered liver cells induced by a single dose of diethylnitro-samine and partial hepatectomy: Their contribution to hepatocarcinogenesis in the rat. Eur. J. Cancer 11:145–154.

Scherer, E., and P. Emmelot. 1976. Kinetics of induction and growth of enzyme-deficient islands involved in hepatocarcinogenesis. Cancer Res. 36:2544–2554.

Schor, N. A., B. F. Rice, and R. F. Huseby. 1976. Dehydrogenation of reduced pyridine nucleotide by Leydig cell tumours of the rat testis. Proc. Soc. Exp. Biol. Med. 151:418–421.

Schor, N. A., and H. P. Morris. 1977. The activity of the D-T diaphorase in experimental hepatomas. Cancer Biochem. Biophys. 2:5–9.

Sell, S., and H. T. Wepsic. 1975. Alpha-fetoprotein, *in* The Liver: Normal and Abnormal Functions, F. F. Becker, ed., Part B, Marcel Dekker, New York, pp. 773–820.

Solt, D. B., and E. Farber. 1976. A new principle for the sequential analysis of chemical carcinogenesis, including a quantitative assay for initiation in liver. Nature 263:701–703.

Solt, D. B., J. B. Hay, and E. Farber. 1977a. Comparison of the blood supply to dimethylnitrosamine-induced hyperplastic nodules and hepatomas and to the surrounding liver. Cancer Res. 37:1686–1691.

Solt, D. B., A. Medline, and E. Farber. 1977b. Rapid emergence of carcinogen-induced hyperplastic lesions in a new model for the sequential analysis of liver carcinogenesis. Am. J. Pathol. 88:595–618.

Svoboda, D., and J. Reddy. 1975. Some effects of chemical carcinogens on cell organelles, *in* Cancer—A Comprehensive Treatise, F. F. Becker, ed., Vol. 1, Plenum Press, New York, pp. 289–322.

Tatematsu, M., T. Shirai, H. Tsuda, Y. Miyota, Y. Shinohara, and N. Ito. 1977. Rapid production of hyperplastic liver nodules in rats treated with carcinogenic chemicals in a new approach for an in vivo short term screening test for hepatocarcinogens. Gann 68:499–507.

Tchipysheva, T. A., V. I. Guelstein, and G. A. Bonnikov. 1977. Alpha-fetoprotein containing cells in the early stages of liver carcinogenesis induced by 3'-methyl-4-dimethylaminoazobenzene and 2-acetylaminofluorene. Int. J. Cancer. 20:388–393.

Taniguchi, N., Y. Tsukada, K. Mukuo, and H. Hirai. 1974. Effect of hepatocarcinogenic azo dyes on glutathione and related enzymes in rat liver. Gann 65:381–387.

Uriel, J., C. Aussel, D. Bouillon, B. de Nechaud, and F. Louillier. 1973. Localization of rat liver alpha-fetoprotein by cell affinity labelling with tritiated aestrogens. Nature 244:190–192.

Uriel, J. 1975. Fetal characteristics of cancer, *in* Cancer—A Comprehensive Treatise, F. F. Becker, ed., Vol. 3, Plenum Press, New York, pp. 21–56.

Weisburger, J. H., and G. R. Williams. 1975. Metabolism of chemical carcinogens, *in* Cancer—A Comprehensive Treatise, F. F. Becker, ed., Vol. 1, Plenum Press, New York, pp. 185–234.

Williams, G. M., M. Klaiber, and E. Farber. 1977. Differences in growth of transplants of liver, liver hyperplastic nodules and hepatocellular carcinomas in the mammary fat pad. Am. J. Pathol. 89:379–390.

Williams, G. M., M. Klaiber, S. E. Parker, and E. Farber. 1976. Nature of early-appearing, carcinogen-induced liver lesions resistant to iron accumulation. J. Natl. Cancer Inst. 57:157–165.

Williams, G. M., and R. S. Yamamoto. 1972. Absence of stainable iron from preneoplastic and neoplastic lesions in rat liver with 8-hydroxyquinoline-induced siderosis. J. Natl. Cancer Inst. 49:685–692.

Carcinogens: Identification and Mechanisms
of Action, edited by A. Clark Griffin and
Charles R. Shaw. Raven Press, New York © 1979.

Multihit Kinetics of Tumor Cell Formation and Risk Assessment of Low Doses of Carcinogen

E. Scherer and P. Emmelot

Division of Chemical Carcinogenesis, Antoni Van Leeuwenhoek-Huis, The Netherlands Cancer Institute, Amsterdam, The Netherlands

Tumors in man apparently result mainly from the action of carcinogenic agents present in his environment; these agents consist predominantly of chemical compounds, natural as well as those resulting from human activities. Thus, in principle, cancer is preventable, and prevention by way of reducing man's exposure to such agents should obviously be a primary aim in fighting cancer.

The first step in cancer prevention is the detection of the carcinogenic agents in our air, water, and food supplies. The next step is to decrease human exposure to the recognized carcinogens by means of regulatory decisions and educational programs.

Our paper seeks to answer the problem of whether a scientific basis may be formulated on which regulatory decisions can be founded. This problem can be reduced to the following question: If a chemical is recognized in animal experiments as carcinogenic, what is the expected tumor risk at much lower dose-rates than that at which tumors are obtained experimentally? This problem of extrapolation cannot be avoided in risk assessment in large populations because of the impossibility of conducting experiments using the necessarily very large number of animals.

In the past, various answers have been adduced to this question. The most conservative is that our knowledge of the processes leading to tumor formation is too limited to allow any risk assessment at all. A practical example of this view is the Delaney clause, i.e., a substance recognized as carcinogenic in animals or man cannot be allowed as a food additive.

However, even if this clause is strictly enforced, it only provides a partial solution to the problem of the relationship between food intake and tumor formation—not to mention the risk problem at large involving other exposures. The Delaney clause can be affixed to nonessential additions, but what about economically essential additives (nitrite), naturally occurring substances in food (secondary amines that in our body react with nitrite to form the carcinogenic N-nitrosamines, preformed N-nitrosamines, aflatoxins, etc.), or other ubiquitous precursors which, by pyrolytic treatment both in the home (Nagao et al. 1977) and by industry (benzo[a]pyrene in double-roasted coffee beans, etc.), yield carcinogens and/or mutagens? Here, at least, in the case of preformed carcinogens, if an outright ban cannot be imposed (which is apparently often the case and in reality may actually be impossible), a decision must be made about acceptable levels. This involves risk assessment, and consequently a reliable extrapolation method and knowledge about the mechanism of action of the carcinogens involved.

The term carcinogen(ic) is frequently used, such as in the Delaney clause, without further qualification as to (1) the type of end-effect obtained, i.e., that the significance and predictability of the animal test model is not taken into consideration and (2) the mechanism of action of the carcinogen in question (as if this were not important). First, in our opinion, the end-effect should be properly defined, *viz.* malignant tumor. Second, the mechanism of carcinogenic action should be known, in view of the problem of threshold versus nonthreshold types of effects.

For reversible-acting substances (such as most hormones, cocarcinogens, promoters, DNA-repair inhibitors, etc.) a threshold will in all probability exist. (Note that inclusion of these agents under the operational notion of the term carcinogen implies the likelihood that in test animals and man spontaneous (endogenous) or background (exogenous) carcinogenic stimuli may act together with these substances to yield a malignant tumor.)

In contrast, irreversible-acting carcinogenic substances, *viz.* complete carcinogens and initiators, leave a permanent imprint in somatic cells. In this situation, nonthreshold kinetics of effect is indicated. Our discussion is concerned with this latter category of carcinogens. The further problem of whether complete carcinogens and initiators, which are active in animals, behave qualitatively and quantitatively similarly in man, will not be dealt with here.

Thus we address ourselves to the problem of extrapolation per se: Which method may be considered as the most reliable? Since low-dose risk assessment cannot be made by direct experiments, the answer to this question remains, per force, a reasoned choice between several alternative procedures. To prepare for that choice, we discuss the kinetics of tumor cell formation in some length, taking both human and animal data into consideration. First of all, however, we seek to establish a model of carcinogenesis that may serve as the framework for interpretation.

THE STOCHASTIC, MULTIHIT CONCEPT OF CARCINOGENESIS

Any view on the matter of risk assessment must incorporate and comply with the results of both experimental and human carcinogenesis. Thus, biology rather than pure statistics, should guide us—or at least statistical parameters should be reasonably interpretable as biologically meaningful parameters. Hence we are in need of a model of carcinogenesis that incorporates the existing knowledge best, to serve as the framework for further discussion. This model is based on the following findings.

—Precancerous cells causally involved in the carcinogenic process as intermediaries or tumor-cell precursors have been widely recognized.

—Progression, as defined by Foulds (1969), operates from the very onset of the carcinogenic process as "stepwise" changes expressed in cell phenotypes, if not in karyotypes. These changes leading to variant cells with a selective advantage occur randomly.

—Carcinogenesis is a relatively rare event considering the number of cells that are relevantly affected by carcinogen in a target tissue.

—With few exceptions, tumors are irreversible biological entities.

—The changes relevant for the carcinogenic process, which are produced by carcinogens, have a lasting effect on the cell and subsequent cell lines even in the absence of carcinogen. This irreversible effect of carcinogenic action has variously been designated as a hit-and-run effect, self-replicating or memory effect, or as a genetic (hereditary) imprint left by a carcinogen.

—A close correlation exists between the carcinogenic and mutagenic properties of chemical compounds, i.e., their capacity to interact with and change DNA and to produce cytogenetic changes.

—Furthermore, carcinogenesis starts in single cells, and the resulting tumor is of clonal origin.

From the involvement of precancerous cells in the carcinogenic process it may be concluded that a tumor cell generally does not arise from a normal cell by way of a one-step mechanism, i.e., the tumor cell does not represent the first cell stage in carcinogenesis. Moreover, the very possibility of detecting precancerous cells means that these cells are capable of proliferating to reach observable populations. They have apparently acquired a selective growth advantage as compared with their unchanged parent cells. Actually it has been demonstrated that the first phenotypic cell stage (islands) causally involved in rat liver carcinogenesis has the inherent capacity of growing in the absence of carcinogen and, thus, represents an irreversible hyperplasia (Scherer *et al.* 1972). Further local change and selective proliferation occurring in these islands is evidence for focal progression (Scherer and Emmelot 1975b, Kitagawa 1976).

The steps causally involved in carcinogenesis are considered to lead to discrete changes, which are variously expressed phenotypically, and may or may not be discernible by the detection methods employed. The conversion of a normal cell into a tumor cell requires a certain number of these discrete changes or relevant effects to occur. The relevant effects are brought about by a carcinogen in cellular components critically involved in the carcinogenic process. The target molecules to be hit are sometimes referred to as "cancer control centers" and the hits (and their relevant effects) as discrete events. This model is known as the multihit (multistep, multievent; multi ≥ 2) concept of tumor cell formation. It is now widely assumed that the critical components with which carcinogens react irreversibly are DNA molecules and that the discrete changes represent somatic mutations. (To the dissenters of this view it has been pointed out previously [Emmelot and Scherer 1977] that for a quantitative interpretation of carci-

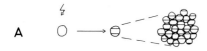

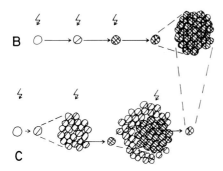

FIG. 1. Kinetic models of tumor cell formation. A, one-hit process; B, multihit process and resting precancerous cells; C, multihit process and proliferating precancerous cells. (The thunderbolt arrow denotes a relevant hit.)

nogenesis, the quality of the target molecules does not, however, matter, provided the effect of a hit becomes a hereditary property.)

The most likely sequence of the carcinogenic process is schematically illus-trated in Figure 1C for a moderately effective dose rate. It features an assumed number of three discrete alterations brought about sequentially in a cell line by a similar number of carcinogenic hits, in each case followed by selective growth of the relevantly changed cells. Accordingly, in carcinogenesis the malig-nant attributes are acquired stepwise, proliferation being the first significant attribute. Different tumors or different stages of cancer expression may require a different number of hits for their induction.

The one-hit character of the individual steps has been demonstrated for the first step in liver carcinogenesis consisting of island cell formation (Scherer and Emmelot 1975b, and following) and is also theoretically indicated.

Less likely sequences in carcinogenesis are the one-step/one-hit process (Figure 1A) and hits scored sequentially in resting cells (Figure 1B). Historically, mode B was used first by Nordling (1953), Armitage and Doll (1954), and others for the kinetic interpretation of epidemiological data, later to be replaced by model C (Armitage and Doll 1957, Fisher 1958).

A further property of the hit theory is that hits are randomly distributed in and over target cells with a low probability (*cf.* Emmelot and Scherer 1977 *fn.* 8; Shimkin and Stoner 1975) to provoke the discrete events that are relevant for the development of the carcinogenic process. Hits occur independently of each other, i.e., a relevant hit scored in a cell does not predispose that cell for a second hit by carcinogen (but see Table 2, no. 2). Very particular sites must be hit in order to bear relevance, and other nonrelevant, but also randomly occurring interactions, do predominate. According to this view, carcinogenesis is a stochastic process.

Now, it is immediately apparent that an increase in relevantly altered cells, i.e., the tumor cell precursors, by proliferation of these cells will markedly enhance the probability of further conversion. First, increasing the number of cells at risk to be further converted will increase the probability that the next hit will be scored. Second, proliferation, DNA synthesis occurring before DNA repair takes place or faulty DNA repair during DNA synthesis, may fix a single-strand change in DNA (produced by one hit) as a hereditary property in one of the two daughter cells following mitosis.

KINETICS OF TUMOR FORMATION

Definitions

Two important notions that are used in human cancer epidemiology and bear directly on our discussion are the age-specific cancer incidence rate and the cumulative cancer incidence.

The age-specific incidence rate is a measure of the number of persons of a given age group (say from 40 to 44 years) that contract (morbidity) or die from (mortality) a given tumor per 10^5 persons; this is abbreviated as I_t.

The cumulative tumor incidence, $P(t)$, designated sometimes as $I(t)$ in the literature, represents I_t integrated over the time:

$$P(t) = \int_o^t I_t \cdot dt \text{ and } I_t = dP(t)/dt.$$

P thus represents the calculated fraction of all individuals developing a given cancer until age t. (It is assumed for the calculation that people dying from unrelated causes would have had the same chance for developing cancer as the surviving population.)

Human patients usually contract only one tumor of a kind, but in the experimental situation multiple tumors may arise in a given tissue in response to the carcinogen administered. Thus, the further distinction must be made between (1) the number of tumors per individual at risk until time t (by being subject to a certain carcinogenic load that is fixed in the animal experiment but is supposedly constant for the average human during his whole life-span), henceforward to be designated as I; and (2) the probability, P, that confronts an individual (see above) to contract a certain cancer, irrespective of the number of tumors per site, until time (age) t. P may vary from 0 to 1; in the latter case each individual gets that particular cancer. The age-specific cancer incidence rate, I_t, is thus the age-specific probability density dP/dt or P'.

Hence, whereas in human carcinogenesis I is virtually identical with P, in experimental carcinogenesis I is larger than P. In order to make the two situations comparable for kinetic and mathematical analysis, the relationship between $I(t)$ and $P(t)$ needs to be known.

We assume that the multiplicity of tumors in a given tissue results from stochastic processes so that the tumors are distributed independently of each other over the population, i.e., the chance of getting a second tumor is not being influenced by the occurrence of first tumor. In that case, the Poisson distribution holds (and Poisson probability paper can be used for plotting the data).

The relation between I and P then reads:

$$P = (1 - e^{-I})$$

and P can be converted via Poisson statistics to I. (This conversion is required for experimental cases in which I, as defined, has not been established [only I having been listed] or cannot be measured. The formula should be adapted to the expected number of tumors per animal at time t of the diagnosis [cf. fn 5, Emmelot and Scherer 1977]).

The Time-Response Relation

The age-specific incidence rate of a given cancer in man, I_t, covers a very broad range from about 0.1 (at young age) to several hundreds (at old age) per 10^5 persons per year. If P, the tumor probability as a function of time, is calculated from I_t (Saffiotti et al. 1972), P extends over a range from 10^{-5} to 0.1–0.2.

For many human cancer types, the tumor probability seems to fit, over the whole reported age range, a relationship of the form:

$$P \sim (1 - e^{-kt^r}).$$

According to this formula, P increases proportional to t^r from very low to the relatively low value of P = 0.1.

Experimentally, if a constant dose rate (d) of carcinogen is applied continuously until tumors arise, the tumor probability as a function of time may reach the value P = 1, yielding a sigmoid curve in a linear plot. Plotted in this way, the curve merely registers the biological response. However, when the relationship is interpreted, different procedures are used, and authors plot their data on different kinds of probability paper.

First, if the sigmoid character is interpreted in terms of biological variation of the cancer induction time, the probit-log time is used (Bryan and Shimkin 1941, Druckrey 1967, Albert and Altshuler 1973). (A proportion is correlated via the normal probability function to the corresponding probit value [Bliss 1935]. In practice, a table for probit analysis is used [Pierson and Hartley 1970]. In case the time required for tumor formation (time-to-tumor) is log-normally distributed in the animal population, a straight line is obtained. The inverse of the slope represents the standard deviation, σ, of the tumor induction time.

Second, if carcinogenesis is understood as a stochastic process, the number of tumors per animal, I, is related to the tumor probability, P, by the Poisson distribution. In that case, the data are plotted on Poisson probability paper (log I *vs.* log t). (Note that the Poisson probability scale for **P** [ordinate] is equivalent to the log scale of I.) A straight line illustrates that the increase of tumor number per animal with time is given by the formula:

$$I(t) \sim t^r.$$

(For influence of variation, see section, Magnitude of Variations, following.)

Experimental data are generally limited to the relatively high tumor probability range of $P = 0.1$ to $P = 1$. (Thus, where the human data stop [large populations] the animal data [small populations] are just beginning to emerge.) Therefore, one should be careful to draw kinetic conclusions from the animal tumor probability data, because they do not include the lower range of **P**'s observed for man. Now, whether plotted as probit-log t or log I-log t functions, the experimental data fit straight lines (Figure 2). The experimental data do not favor one

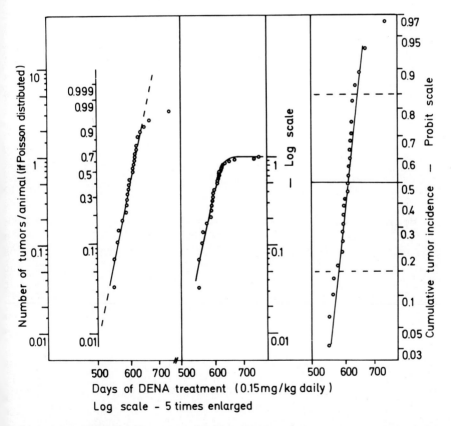

FIG. 2. Experimental tumor probability data plotted versus log time (constructed from data in Druckrey *et al.* 1963). Left: P plotted on Poisson probability paper and corresponding number of tumors per animal (log scale). Middle: P plotted on a log scale. Right: P plotted as probits. (DENA, diethylnitrosamine.)

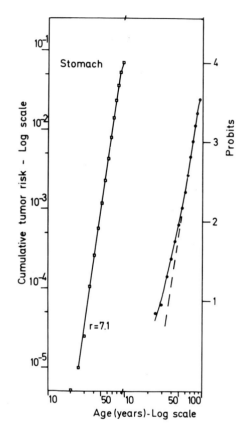

FIG. 3. Human tumor probability data plotted versus log time (constructed from data in Waterhouse *et al.* 1976, for Swedish males, 1966–1970). Left: P plotted on Poisson probability paper. Right: P plotted as probits.

or the other procedure c.q. interpretation. (The effect of a given dose rate is implicitly considered to be the same for all animals if they were identical, the observed differences in response being attributed to differences in the individual's susceptibility, vs. all animals of the population are equally susceptible, the differences in response resulting from the stochastic nature of the process.)

However, when the two procedures are applied to the low human tumor probability data, they may result in different curves. As shown in Figure 3, for stomach cancer, the use of Poisson probability paper yields a straight line for the whole range of P's (same result in the classical log P-log t plot, since I is about similar to P). In the probit-log t plot, however, the data fit a straight line only in the upper part of the curve and deviate from linearity in the lower part. Accordingly, if experimental carcinogenesis data are extrapolated to low tumor probabilities via the straight line of the probit-log time plot, the curve may deviate from the t^r relationship that holds for many human cancers at a much lower range of P's than obtainable in the experiment. Therefore, the Poisson distribution is advocated for extrapolation of experimental data.

If the number of tumors per animal at risk, I, instead of P, is taken as the incidence parameter, i.e., the mean number of tumors per animal as expected from Poisson statistics, r can be obtained from the log I-log t plot being the slope of that straight line. The straight lines obtained on the Poisson probability paper indicate that one type of function, $I \sim t^r$, describes both the high experimental and the low human tumor incidences.

Formula $I(t) \sim t^r$, which relates the increase of the tumor incidence to a power of time, is basically different from pure statistical considerations such as those underlying the "probit method." The latter does not consider the factors nor the mechanisms that determine the induction time.

The $I \sim t^r$ relation, on the other hand, can be interpreted in terms of hits and the time that is needed for scoring the number of hits required for tumor cell formation (time from first exposure to carcinogen until the time at which the tumor cell arises = induction time; the latency period, then, is the time required for the tumor cell to grow out into a detectable tumor, the latter time being generally much smaller than the former).

Originally (see Figure 1B) the exponent r was equated to m, the number of hits required for tumor formation in resting cells. Accordingly, neither the time of exposure nor the dose rate but rather the total dose received ($D = d \times t$) was considered as the real variable: $I \sim D^m$.

This would be true if a time factor were not involved in carcinogenesis.

The Time Factor in Carcinogenesis. Estimation of the Number of Hits Required for Tumor Cell Formation

Druckrey *et al.* (1963, 1967) in now classical experiments established a relationship between different dose rates applied to groups of animals and the corresponding times of administration of carcinogen, t, required to yield the same tumor probability in all the animals. This relation reads:

$$dt^n = K \text{ (a constant).}$$

Since the power of time in this formula amounted to $n > 1$, mainly between 2 and 4, it was concluded that time exerts an "autonomous" enhancing effect on the carcinogenic process—the *time factor*. Although any endogenous process that in the passage of time accelerates the carcinogenic process will contribute to the factor n, we suggested, on the basis of pertinent experiments (Scherer and Emmelot 1975a, 1975b, 1976), that the rate of proliferation of the precancerous clones involved in the carcinogenic process is the main factor determining the time effect.

Furthermore, we derived the formula $r = m \cdot n$, where r is the power of time in the time-incidence relation, and m is the number of hits required for tumor cell formation (Emmelot and Scherer 1977; Table 1 and Figure 4). With this formula it becomes possible to calculate m, if r is known and n is estimated or experimentally established; examples are given in Emmelot and Scherer (1977).

Parenthetically, for a real one-hit process of tumor cell formation both m

TABLE 1. *Summary of experimental procedures, graphical analyses, and relations obtained between dose rate (d), time of exposure (t) and tumor incidence (I). Derivation of the relation between the factors r, m, and n.*

d	t	I	Plot	Formula
fix	vary	measure	$\longrightarrow$ log I-log t	:	$I(t) \sim t^r$ ....(1)
			set d constant		
			set I		
vary	vary	measure	$\longrightarrow$ log d-log t constant	:	$dt^n = a$ constant .....(2)
			set t constant		
vary	fix	measure	$\longrightarrow$ log I-log d	:	$I(d) \sim d^m$ ....(3)
			Combine (1) and (3)	:	$I(d,t) \sim d^m t^r$ ....(4)
			Set I(d,t) in (4) constant, Combine with (2)	:	$r = m \cdot n$ ....(5)

and r are equal to 1 and thus also n = 1; in this case, no proliferating intermediary cell population can be involved.

The time factor generally operates in carcinogenesis, as shown by Druckrey (1967) for various chemical carcinogens and rat tumors and by Blum (1959) for UV-carcinogenesis in mice; other examples are cited by Jones and Grendon (1975). Thus, in all these cases multihit kinetics ($m \geq 2$) is indicated.

According to the formula $dt^n = a$ constant, carcinogenesis is far more dependent on time than on dose rate. From this it can be considered that if each of the relevant steps were to follow multiorder kinetics, n would be smaller than 1. Since for the multihit process of carcinogenesis, covering all separate relevant steps, n is always greater than 1, these separate steps should follow first-order kinetics ($m = 1$).

An estimation of m for late-onset cancers in man by formula $m = r/n$, with $r = 7$ (derived from epidemiological data) and n estimated as 2 to 3, shows that two to three hits are instrumental in the induction of these tumor cells. This result is similar to that obtained some 20 years ago by Armitage and Doll (1957) and Fisher (1958) on the basis of assumed rates of proliferation

---

FIG. 4. Idealized experiment in which the tumor number per animal for various dose rates is determined as a function of time. This figure is of a composite nature. The log I-log t plots are drawn in the left lower portion, A, of the figure. For a constant response level (I), the induction time as a function of dose rate is plotted in part B (log d-log t). For a constant induction time, the tumor incidence as a function of dose rate is plotted at C (log I-log d). Parameters chosen were r = 10 and n = 2. Extrapolation to low dose rates, discussed in the text, is by the dashed arrow running from the log d-log t plot in B to the induction time expected for a chosen "low" dose rate. After that time, the exposure to the "low" dose rate would have led to the constant response level chosen in A, provided the animals lived long enough. From that level one may extrapolate according to the slope observed in A, as given by D,

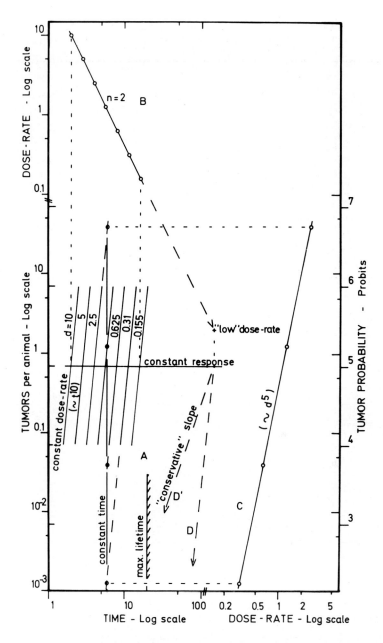

or to a less steep "conservative" slope (D'). Intersection of these straight lines with the time during which exposure is considered to take place, i.e., maximum lifetime, gives the tumor incidence for the "low" dose rate at maximum lifetime. Note that if the increase in tumor incidence with time is interpreted in terms of biological variation of the tumor induction time, and therefore P is plotted in probits (scale at the right), the same arguments apply but for a tumor probability in probits instead of tumor number per animal.

of the precancerous cell clones. However, formula m = r/n is a general one (but Fisher's formula can also be generalized to yield such a result [see Emmelot and Scherer 1977, *fn.* 4]) and, furthermore, contains the experimentally accessible factor n as a measure of the proliferation rates.

If the results of experiments of the type performed by Druckrey, as illustrated in Figure 4 in idealized form, serve for the derivation of kinetic parameters, the following conditions should be met.

1. The log I-log t plots (A in Figure 4) for the various dose rates applied should be straight lines.

2. The slope (tang.) of these plots should amount to +r for all dose rates, provided that the tumor type remains the same, i.e., r is independent of dose rate.

3. Log d-log t should be a straight line (B) with slope -n, in order that the condition dt^n = a constant is satisfied.

4. The tumor incidence I, not the tumor probability P, should be measured, or P should be converted to I (see above); n should be calculated for a fixed number of tumors per animal.

If these conditions are satisfied (Emmelot and Scherer 1977, Charts 1 and 2), the factors r and n can be derived (see Table 1). In addition it is possible by upward and downward extrapolation of the various log I-log t plots belonging to the various doses and fixing an arbitrary time, t, to obtain (C) the dose-response relation, log I-log d, the slope of which denotes the number of hits, m, required for tumor cell formation. By the latter procedure it can be determined that for rat liver carcinogenesis by diethylnitrosamine, m amounts to 7. This is the graphical illustration of the calculation of m by formula m = r/n, where r is obtained from the log I-log t plot (r = 12) and n from the log d-log t plot (n = 1.8) to yield m = 7.

The same procedure has been followed for analyzing the epidemiological data on lung cancer formation in smokers (Emmelot and Scherer 1977). Graphically it was derived that n amounts to 5. This value is also obtained by inserting the known values of r = 5 and m = 1 (with respect to smoke dose) of this process in formula r = m·n. However, as argued previously, the values r =

TABLE 2. *Background carcinogenic stimuli instrumental in spontaneous carcinogenesis, which may act additively with extra carcinogen*

1. Physiological processes that very seldom make a spontaneous mistake relevant to carcinogenesis, e.g., faulty base-pairing during DNA synthesis as a natural noise.
2. Processes to a similar effect, induced by a previous somatic hit, e.g., an infidel DNA polymerase.
3. *Ditto* processes due to a hit present in the genome *ab initio*—a germinal hit.
4. Possible endogenous carcinogenic stimuli: virus and metabolites.
5. Environmental carcinogens, which, next to extra carcinogen (applied in the experiment or considered for analysis in the human situation), have access to the population examined.
Note: The latter category of carcinogenic stimuli is especially important for the risk assessment of extra carcinogen confronting man.

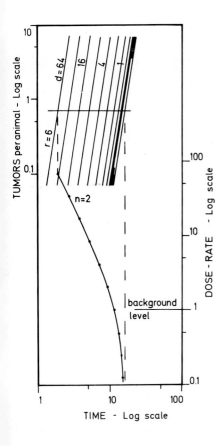

FIG. 5. Idealized experiment in which for various dose rates of extra carcinogen and a constant level of background carcinogen, tumor number per animal is measured as a function of time (log I-log t), and the factor n is determined. The most right-hand straight line of the succession of plots represents the tumor response for d = 0 with respect to extra carcinogen (= spontaneous tumors due to background carcinogen). Parameters chosen: 3-hit process, r = 6, n = 2, and background level equals dose rate 1 in effectiveness. The log d-log t plot is given by the downward curve and shows a slope of −2 for the high dose range of extra carcinogen, tending towards −∞ for d → 0.

5, m = 1, and n = 5 are mutually incompatible, because for a one-hit process of tumor cell formation r = m = n = 1. This paradox can, however, be easily solved by assuming that at least one other background hit (Table 2) operates in the process of lung tumor cell formation.

An unnoticed background hit contributing to a carcinogenic process developing through the action of a low-effective dose rate of carcinogen enhances this process and thus would formally fall into the category of the time effect and, thereby, increase the value of n. This is apparently the case for lung cancer formation by smoking.

In the schematic representation in Figure 5 it is shown that if background stimuli have access to the system, the straight lines of the log I-log t plots converge with decreasing dose rates of extra carcinogen towards the log I-log t plot for spontaneous tumor formation. As a consequence the log d-log t plot deflects from linearity, and in the very low dose region its slope tends to −∞, i.e., n → ∞ for d → 0.

For kinetic analysis the contribution of background processes to n should be eliminated, and thus we arrive at the formula

$$(m_{ex} + m_b)n = r$$

where m_{ex} and m_b stand for the number of hits produced by applied (extra) carcinogen and background carcinogenic stimuli, respectively.

The Dose-Response Relation

This section briefly deals with the dose-response relationship as obtained by administration of different dose rates of carcinogen to groups of animals and then measurement of the tumor incidence at a *fixed* time. The latter condition is sometimes not observed (e.g., Cornfield 1977) in which case one obtains meaningless results. Ideally, log I plotted versus log d yields a straight line with slope $+m$. In case $m = 1$, the process follows one-hit kinetics. For values of $m \geqslant 2$, multihit kinetics is operating, $m = 2$, two-hit kinetics, etc.

Experimental data on dose-response relations in the literature are very scarce. One-hit kinetics has been established for
—lung adenoma formation in strain A mice by urethane, respectively $1:2:5:6$ dibenzanthracene (Henshaw and Meyer 1945, Heston and Schneiderman 1953);
—transformation of fibroblast-like cells by various chemical carcinogens or X-rays (Huberman and Sachs 1966, Takano *et al.* 1972, Borek and Hall 1973);
—the transforming step leading to enhanced colony-forming activity in semisolid medium of human cells by N-methyl-N'-nitro-N-nitrosoguanidine (MNNG) (Freedman and Shin 1977);
—the initiating step of skin tumor formation by β-propiolactone (Colburn and Boutwell 1966);
—the first step in rat liver carcinogenesis by diethylnitrosamine (Scherer and Emmelot 1975b, Solt and Farber 1976).

Two-hit kinetics has been reported for
—induction of skin tumors by benzo[a]pyrene (Peto *et al.* 1975);
—transformation of a particular clone of a hamster cell line by three different carcinogens or ultraviolet radiation (Ishii *et al.* 1977).

It may not be astonishing that tumor formation by a process of more than two hits, as measured by these dose-response experiments, has not been reported. Higher order kinetics is very difficult to establish by this method due to (1) the strong dependence of the response on the dose (for $m = 3$, a difference of a factor 10 in dose rate would give a difference of a factor 10^3 in the response) and (2) the narrow range of experimentally observable tumor incidences due to the infeasibility of working with large numbers of animals, this along with other conditions that hamper the execution of kinetically meaningful experiments (Wollman 1955, Emmelot and Scherer 1977). Higher order kinetics may, however, be established by using the formula $r = m \cdot n$ (Emmelot and Scherer 1977).

It should be further noted that lung adenoma formation is a particular case since the mice are genetically disposed to a high spontaneous incidence and their lungs are, in a sense, already in a precancerous state. Chemical transformation in vitro appears to cover one or sometimes two steps in a process that is already ongoing or brought to completion spontaneously (Ishii *et al.* 1977).

Moreover, the direct measurement of the dose-response relation yields only the number of hits contributed by the carcinogen applied and does not include the background hits (see previous section). Thus for dose rates high enough to outweigh any background processes that may also produce relevant alteration, m represents the number of hits required for the development of a tumor from a normal cell(line) by the carcinogen applied (m_{ex}). However, at low dose rates, some of the necessary steps will be performed by background processes (m_b).

Apart from lung cancer and perhaps some cases of industrially caused cancer, epidemiological data on dose-response relations are not available. The occurrence of marked geographical differences in tumor incidences suggests that effective dose rates or particular chemicals adding up to the dose may vary considerably in the various environments.

The epidemiological data do, however, indicate that for a given tumor, the basic parameter r of the time-response relation is independent of the frequency of that tumor in the various countries (Burch 1976). Thus, though the straight line of the log P-log t plot may be shifted along the t abscissa, its slope r remains the same. Hence one may conclude that r is not dependent on dose rate; the experiments of Druckrey (see previous section) have also shown that.

Magnitude of Variations That May Affect the Time-Response Relationship of Human Carcinogenesis

The use of epidemiological data for deriving kinetic mechanisms of tumor development may be criticized because of the possibility that a large variation in the relevant parameters (individual susceptibilities or dose rates received) would obscure the basic time-response relationship. Therefore, the influence of variation on the kinetics of tumor induction according to a multihit process has been determined by calculating time-response curves using different values for the standard deviation, σ, of the transformation probability constant, K, using the basic formula (*cf.* Table 1 and Figure 7):

$$I \sim (K \cdot d)^m t^{m \cdot n}$$

(K contains a factor for the potency of effect of carcinogen as well as one for individual susceptibility). The latter is assumed to be log-normally distributed in the population at risk; furthermore, in any individual the value of K is taken as constant for all hits involved in the carcinogenic process.

Figure 6 illustrates the curves obtained (for the assumed values of m = 3 and n = 2) in a log P-log t plot (left side), respectively a probit-log t plot (right side). For $\sigma = 0$, i.e., no interference by variation, as expected, a straight line with slope 6 is obtained in the log P-log t plot, except for the upper portion in which the curve has to deflect toward the horizontal line of P = 1. In the

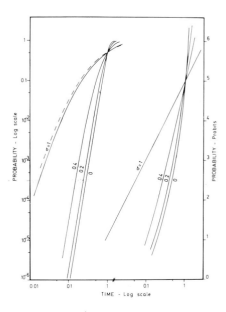

FIG. 6. Log P-log t plots, respectively, probit-log t plots for a 3-hit process and n = 2, and various values for the variation in tumor susceptibility, σ. (See text.) Formula used:

$$P = \int_{K=0}^{\infty} (1 - \exp - A(K(d_b + d_{ex}))^m \cdot t^{m \cdot n}) \cdot$$

$$\frac{1}{\sqrt{2\pi}\,\sigma} \cdot \exp - \frac{1}{2} \left(\frac{(\log K - \log K_m)}{\sigma} \right)^2 dK$$

probit-log t plot, a curve is obtained that is concave upward over the whole range.

The curves for $\sigma = 0.2$ and 0.4 both yield in the main part of the log P-log t plot straight lines with slope 6. In the probit-log t plot the curves deflect from linearity in their lower part; whereas in the upper part, the influence of the variation predominates, leading to a straight part of the curve. For $\sigma = 1$, the curve (log P-log t) is more or less completely determined by the variation of the transformation probability constant K. In this case there is little difference between the curves calculated for a two-hit and a three-hit process (solid and dashed lines, respectively).

The probability-time relation for human stomach cancer (see Figure 3) shows the same principal form as the curves constructed for $\sigma = 0.2$ and 0.4 in Figure 6: a straight line in the lower, i.e., main portion of the log P-log t plot and deviation from linearity in the lower part of the probit-log t plot. This example and others (Burch 1976) indicate that human cancer data are influenced by some variation in dose rate and susceptibility but that in general, variation is not of such magnitude that the curve would be dominated by the variation such as the case for the curve constructed for $\sigma = 1$ (see Figure 6, left).

Calculation of log P-log t curves expected for higher values of m and r (m = 7, r = 14) and various σ values has shown (not illustrated) that a σ of 0.4 already has an overwhelming influence. The curve in the log P-log t plot had no straight part at all, and the tangent constructed at the curve between P = 10^{-5} and P = 10^{-4} reached a slope of only 7.3 instead of the expected 14. At $\sigma = 0.2$, however, the kinetics of the multihit process predominated again, the largest part of the log P-log t plot fitting a straight line with slope 14.

Accordingly, if human tumor probability data fit a straight line in at least the lower part of a log P-log t plot, its slope being r, it is indicated that the variation of relevant parameters, such as susceptibility and dose rate, does not predominate the kinetics of tumor formation and thus leaves the factor r as a kinetically meaningful parameter.

In the general population, susceptibility for cancer is not dependent on any single parameter, such as one enzyme, but results from the interplay of many biological functions, enhancing (carcinogen-activating enzymes, cell proliferation) as well as reducing ones (detoxifying enzymes, DNA repair, etc.). Furthermore, many carcinogens and a multitude of agents modifying the carcinogenic response are likely to contribute. The probability of the end-effect is therefore the sum of all processes and factors involved. The high number of parameters thus resulting may imply that within an individual the variation of one parameter, diverging from the population mean into one direction of effect (facilitating), may be more or less counteracted by another parameter deviating from the

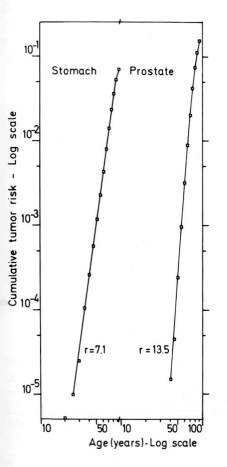

FIG. 7. Tumor probability (= cumulative tumor risk) as a function of age for stomach and prostate cancer. (For data see Figure 3.)

mean in the opposite direction (inhibiting). According to this view, the overall biological variation may be limited and especially so the more the various, variable parameters are specific for different carcinogens and different steps of the carcinogenic process and the larger the number of steps required for tumor cell formation. However, in case these parameters are not carcinogen and step specific, they would act in the whole course of the process; this, and a cancer process requiring only a small number of hits for completion, tend toward higher degrees of biological variation. Also, the mean daily carcinogenic load for individuals in a population with similar feeding habits may be fairly equal when their whole life-spans are considered; special cases, of course, excepted.

Granted that individual susceptibilities and dose rates received do not vary greatly for individuals in a given population at risk, as is apparently so in quite a number of cases, in view of the straight log P-log t plots obtained (Figure 7), why, then, do people not contract cancer in a more narrow time (age) span? The answer here, as well as for spontaneous and induced cancer formation in a highly inbred animal strain (subjected to a profound degree of standarization), is that carcinogenesis is a stochastic process. The outcome is determined by the probability of whether the number of hits required for tumor cell formation are scored in a given time period of exposure.

LOW-DOSE EXTRAPOLATION MODELS

The following procedures have been proposed:

1. Extrapolation to the low-dose range according to the dose-response relation actually obtained experimentally.

2. Extrapolation with a "conservative" slope being shallower than the one to be expected for human carcinogenesis.

3. Extrapolation according to the dose-response relationship that is expected to hold in the low-dose range because of deductions made from models of carcinogenesis.

Each one will be discussed briefly.

Extrapolation According to the Dose-Response Relationship Derived from Experiments

The fundamental question here is if this dose-response relationship correctly describes the tumor probability at dose rates far below the experimentally measurable range. If no other factors act additively with the carcinogen under consideration (background carcinogen being of minor importance within the high experimental dose range), the extrapolation of the tumor probability to low values via an experimentally derived dose-response relationship seems acceptable for the experimental situation. Such a method, using the Druckrey relation $d \cdot t^n =$ constant, has been proposed by Albert and Altshuler (1973); this method will be discussed below under "Conservative Methods."

Extrapolation without assumptions about the biological processes governing tumor induction by means of purely mathematical procedures has been recently proposed. If tumor incidence data are experimentally available for different dose rates, a suitable function, polynome with nonnegative coefficients (Crump *et al.* 1976, Guess and Crump 1976, Guess *et al.* 1977, Hartley and Sielkin 1977), is fitted to the data, and its coefficients are calculated by means of a computer procedure called maximum likelihood estimation. The resulting formula has been considered as suitable for extrapolation to low doses (Hartley and Sielkin 1977).

However, extrapolation with observed slopes was criticized as early as 1961 by Mantel and Bryan. They stated: "These methods, however, are based on the assumption that the relationship observed between tumor occurrence and dose at the levels tested will continue to apply in the regions to which extrapolation is being made. The validity of such an assumption cannot be tested." As will be argued below, this criticism is justified by the influence that background carcinogens are expected to have on the dose-response relationship for added risk. The significance of an observed or derived dose-response relationship is thus limited to the aspect of kinetics of tumor formation in the experimental dose range. Another point of criticism is that even the best experimental data, leading to a good estimate of the extrapolation curve, can only be valuable for that experimental situation. In man, the tumor type induced by the carcinogen may be different from the one obtained in the experiment, and therefore the dose-response relation of its induction can also differ.

Although the direct extrapolation with the dose-response relation obtained from experiments is a questionable procedure, the mathematical approach of Guess *et al.* (1977) nevertheless revealed that in the low dose range, the upper confidence level of induced tumor risk, which is the relevant curve for a safe extrapolation, becomes linear in the dose. This approach leads to a type of extrapolation which is favored as a conservative method (see below), and which also follows from the consideration that background carcinogenic stimuli are facing man.

Conservative Methods of Extrapolation

The Unit-Probit Slope and Related Rules

A method of extrapolation is termed conservative if it yields in the low dose range a higher response than the one that is expected to occur on the basis of the proposed mechanism. Mantel and Bryan (1961) proposed a method (updated by Mantel *et al.* 1975, and discussed by Mantel and Schneiderman 1975) which is based on the assumption that tumor development depends on individual threshold doses—a tumor developing only if the dose of carcinogen ingested within the lifetime exceeds the individual threshold dose. The logarithm of the individual threshold doses was assumed to be distributed normally in the population. In a probit-log dose plot, tumor probability versus dose (time constant) under these assumptions is given by a straight line with the slope 1/ standard deviation. For extrapolation, a slope of 1 has been proposed to be conservative enough not to underestimate the carcinogenic risk at low dose rates.

Using a somewhat different approach, Albert and Altshuler (1973) came to the same type of function. According to the time-tumor incidence analyses of Blum (1959) and Druckrey (1967), the log of the tumor induction time (constant dose rate) was assumed to be normally distributed in the population, the occurrence of tumors in a group of animals continuously fed carcinogen being given by a straight line in a probit-log time plot (see Figure 4). Furthermore, the relationship between the dose rate (d) and the mean tumor induction time (t_{50}), $d \times t_{50}^n = $ constant (Druckrey 1967), was used by Albert and Altshuler (1973) for the derivation of the dose-response relationship. (By the use of Druckrey's time factor, this method resembles our approach for deriving the dose-response relationship in the scope of the multihit concept of carcinogenesis [*cf.* preceding section, "The Time Factor in Carcinogenesis"].) According to $d_1 \times t_{50,1}^n = d_2 \times t_{50,2}^n$, the mean induction time t_{50} expected for low dose rates was calculated (becoming much larger than the mean life-span), and via the tumor incidence-time relationship (straight line in a probit-log time plot), which is assumed to hold also in the low incidence range, the lifetime tumor incidence was determined. As a conservative component, Albert and Altshuler (1973) proposed the use of a slope shallower than that found experimentally, such as a slope derived from human time-tumor incidence data. Such a slope generally will be greater than one, the method therefore being less conservative than the one proposed by Mantel and Bryan (1961).

Both methods can be criticized in that they assume that the kinetics of tumor formation is mainly determined by the distribution of susceptibility in the population at risk and not by the process leading to the cancer cell. The analysis, presented in the preceding section, of the kinetics of human tumor risk together with the discussion of the influence that biological variation of the relevant parameters may be expected to exert on the kinetics of tumor incidence, indicates, however, that the main part of the human tumor incidence-time relationship ($I \sim t^r$) is but moderately influenced by biological variation. Therefore, an approach that takes into account the process determining the tumor induction time, such as the multihit hypothesis, is, in our opinion, more likely to describe correctly the cancer risk in the low dose range.

Linear Extrapolation: The One-Hit Rule

If chemical carcinogens are assumed to act in a stochastic manner (and there is ample evidence from the induction by chemical carcinogens of mutations, precancerous lesions, or transformed cell clones in vitro), with several hits being necessary to alter a normal cell into a cancer cell, the most conservative process that leads to tumor cell formation is by one-hit kinetics leading to the linear or one-hit extrapolation rule. For radiation hazard in man, which is certainly based on stochastic processes, the linear, nonthreshold concept of dose-response relationship has recently been adopted by The Environmental Protection Agency for the estimation of genetic and carcinogenic risks (EPA 75, as cited by Brown 1976). The problem, i.e., whether linearity overestimates the risk of low doses/ dose rates of radiation, is discussed by Brown (1976). His conclusion is that there is even some doubt as to whether the risk is not underestimated.

The appreciation of the influence that background carcinogen has on the relevance of action of low dose rates of extra carcinogen to the biological end-effect adds further support to the linear extrapolation model (see below).

Spontaneous Carcinogenesis and One-Hit Kinetics of Extrapolation

Man, whose extra cancer risk due to extra carcinogen has to be estimated, is exposed continuously to exogenous (and endogenous) carcinogens. These agents, together with spontaneous biochemical accidents, are believed to be responsible for most cancers occurring in the human population. What is the influence of these background carcinogens on the effect of small doses of extra carcinogen?

A simple calculation (Crump *et al.* 1976) shows what happens: If the extra carcinogen is considered to act additively with carcinogenic principles already present, the total dose rate can be written as $d = d_b + d_{ex}$. The tumor probability $P(d,t)$ at a fixed time t is $P(d)$. If d_{ex} is small, as compared to d_b, it follows that $P(d) = P(d_b + d_{ex}) \approx P(d_b) + P'(d_b) \cdot d_{ex}$ and the extra tumor risk $\Delta P = P(d) - P(d_b)$ therefore becomes $\Delta P \approx P'(d_b) \cdot d_{ex} \sim d_{ex}$.

Accordingly, irrespective of what the formula $P(d)$ for the tumor probability actually portrays, the extra risk is proportional to the dose rate of extra carcinogen, provided the latter is small as compared to d_b and that $P'(d_b) > 0$.

Independently, Albert and Altshuler (1976) and Emmelot and Scherer (1977), considering the special case of a log-normally distributed cancer induction time, respectively, the multihit model (Figure 8), came to the same result of low-dose linearity.

The probability for the most frequent tumors in man is about 10% at the end of life, and therefore the level of background carcinogenic activity facing him is about similar to the lowest levels of carcinogenic activity in animal experiments. The condition of $d_{ex} \ll d_b$ is thus a reasonable assumption for the largest part of the extrapolation range.

For a special carcinogen under consideration, we do not know if its effect is additive to that of the carcinogens already present. In view of their large number, it is reasonable to assume that some background carcinogens are acting additively with new ones. The fraction of background carcinogens doing so cannot be determined. In order to be conservative, one therefore has to assume that virtually all background carcinogens act additively with the extra carcino-

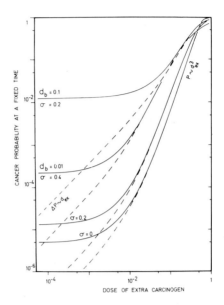

FIG. 8. Tumor formation in the presence of background carcinogenic stimuli. Tumor probability as a function of the dose of extra carcinogen (log P — log d_{ex}) is calculated for a three-hit process ($m = 3$ and $n = 2$), with different values for the background carcinogenic activity (expressed as dose equivalents of extra carcinogen) and the variation (σ) of the transformation probability constant K. Solid lines: tumor probability P; upper curve—dose equivalent of background carcinogen $d_b = 0.1$, $\sigma = 0.2$. The three lower solid lines represent curves for $d_b = 0.01$, and σ values of 0.4, 0.2, and 0. Dashed lines: increment of tumor probability above background, $\Delta P = P(d_{ex} + d_b) - P(d_b)$. ΔP becomes proportional to the dose of extra carcinogen if the latter is small as compared with the dose equivalent of background carcinogen. For low levels of spontaneous cancer risk ($d_b = 0.01$, $\sigma = 0$, 0.2, and 0.4) a considerable (upper) part of the ΔP curve is quite steep (slopes between 2 and 3), and linear extrapolation from the range of experimental tumor probability ($P \approx 0.1$) would considerably overestimate the real cancer risk at low doses of extra carcinogen. For a higher spontaneous cancer risk ($d_b = 0.1$, $\sigma = 0.2$: $P(d_b) \approx 0.01$), however, ΔP is proportional to the dose of extra carcinogen over almost the whole range of d_{ex}, linear extrapolation from experimental values now yielding a good estimate of the real extra risk at low doses of extra carcinogen.

gen. The linear method of extrapolation from experimental data to expected human cancer risk seems therefore unavoidable.

THE THRESHOLD PROBLEM—MECHANISTIC VERSUS PROBABILISTIC INTERPRETATIONS

A threshold in the effect of every carcinogen can be obtained in any experiment in which the dose rate applied is low enough. A "no-effect" level of carcinogen, the daily dose at which no tumors arise, further depends on the number of animals in the assay and the time during which carcinogen is administered. This time is limited by the natural life-span of the animals. From the summation of the effects found for daily doses to the lowest ones tested by Druckrey (1967), the conclusion can be drawn that a given, even lower dose than the lowest one tested, which would have no effect in the animal during his whole life-span, still could produce an effect if it were possible to administer the carcinogen over a longer period than that covered by the natural life-span. (The irreversibility of the relevant changes produced by carcinogen is another conclusion.) In this respect the life-span can be considered as the factor limiting the effect of a low dose rate in a given population at risk. Though the occurrence of an experimental (or practical) threshold is a fact, there is, according to this view, no reason to suppose that an absolute (or theoretical) threshold would exist; in other words, the first cannot be a reason for postulating the second.

A similar conclusion is indicated if the number of animals in the assay is considered; when the probability that a given dose rate produces a tumor is low, an effect would rather appear in a 1000- than in a 100-sized population.

For the risk assessment of carcinogenic action in a large population, such as formed by man, the problem of whether the theoretical threshold exists is important. Its existence or nonexistence cannot be proved experimentally because of the impossibility of carrying out experiments with very large numbers of animals and of lengthening the life-span of the animals.

In the above discussion, the term "effect" means the end-effect of carcinogenic action: the appearance of cancer. However, carcinogenesis in general is a multi-step process. A very low continuous dose may still carry out at least one relevant step in a very considerable part of the population at risk, although not being capable of inducing the entire process in that part of the population. (Note that the possibility exists, in view of the stochastic nature of the carcinogenic process, that even this very low dose may induce cancer in some individuals—the larger the population at risk, the greater the number of individuals suffering this fate.) Thus, with respect to the bulk of the population, a "no-effect"—with tumor as the criterion—does not mean that with respect to a step of the process no effect has been scored at low dose rates. On the contrary, the partial action of sub-carcinogenic doses has been well illustrated by experiments (e.g., Schmähl 1976, Yokoro *et al.* 1977). An illustrative case in point that has been quantitated is the induction of precancerous island cells in rat liver by a subcarcinogenic dose of carcinogen. Furthermore, the direct proportion between number of islands induced and the low doses of diethylnitrosamine applied, as well as between these doses, and DNA-ethylation products has been demonstrated (Scherer and Emmelot 1975b, 1976; Scherer *et al.* 1977).

A threshold in the partial or complete action (number of necessary steps considered) of a carcinogen must mean that a threshold exists in the molecular mechanism of carcinogenic action. Such a threshold might be set by the following two conditions:

1. The critical molecular effect produced by carcinogen disappears with time. For instance, the relevantly altered cells have only a limited life expectancy and die if they do not receive the next hit in time (this is a variant of the model of Jones and Grendon 1975).

2. The critical molecular effect will not be produced at very low dose rates because in the low to very low dose range a disproportionality arises in the molecular fate of the carcinogenic molecules as compared with the situation at higher doses. For instance, at low to very low doses the detoxification of carcinogen and repair of DNA-carcinogen adducts would increase by percentage relative to the metabolic activation of carcinogen, DNA-carcinogen interaction, and genetic fixation of the DNA lesion; hence, a threshold would be reached at very low doses. In this model, an absolute protective "filter" is introduced along which the carcinogen has to pass before the filter would be saturated by higher doses, whether toxic or not.

Ad 1. This possibility does not receive experimental support. On the contrary, the initiated stage of skin cells remains for long periods in the absence of further treatment (Berenblum and Shubik 1949, Boutwell 1964). The foci of precancerous liver cells referred to above (Scherer and Emmelot 1975a,b) continue to grow in the absence of carcinogen and remain detectable during the whole life-span of the rats. Cervical carcinoma in situ and genetically determined preneoplastic intestinal polyps, which ultimately are converted into carcinomas, have a long existence. Recently it has been shown that precancerous cells in rat mamma produced by a subcarcinogenic dose of N-nitroso-N-butylurea may persist for at least seven months (Yokoro *et al.* 1977).

Ad 2. The introduction of an absolute, protective filter is based on a nonstochastic argument. From this model it would follow that if the carcinogen concentration is fixed at a certain dose and the number of protective entities (the capacity of the filter) were to be varied, the interaction between carcinogen and the protective entities would be relatively more pronounced (at the disproportional expense of interaction with relevant molecules, i.e., DNA) the lower the number of protective entities. An analogous reasoning has been applied previously when it was thought that a given concentration of drug (in excess, including drugs that act by the same type of mechanism as do chemical carcinogens) would kill a progressively greater percentage of cells, the smaller the number of the cells. However, since then it has been shown that this is not the case and that the same percentage of cells is killed irrespective of cell number—the principle of constant fractional kill (Skipper *et al.* 1964, 1965).

Because of the stochastic concept of carcinogenesis (which we favor), the fate of the carcinogen in the nontoxic dose range will be proportional to its concentration; according to this view, a constant fractional interaction with relevant (and irrelevant) molecules, independent of dose, will take place in the nontoxic region. Computer simulations of metabolic reactions involving carcinogens have indeed shown that the ratio between dose and DNA-carcinogen adducts (and nongenetic RNA and protein adducts for that matter) is constant at low doses (Gehring 1977).

Very recently a model was introduced (Cornfield 1977) that leads to a threshold (disproportionality) in the action of carcinogen. Along with the above arguments, we disagree (Scherer and Emmelot, in press) with this model and its analysis, particularly on the following three points: (a) the choice of the reversible conditions of the metabolic processes in which the carcinogen participates, (b) the fact that the mathematical analysis of the model is based on steady-state conditions, and (c) the quantitative comparison of the predicted outcome of the model with certain published data on carcinogenesis that cannot be used to this end because they were derived from experiments in which the dose rate was varied but the time at which the response was recorded was not fixed (see above).

We have argued that the carcinogenically relevant cellular response does increase linearly in the low to very low dose range. But at the higher concentrations of carcinogen where toxicity ensues, the increase of the DNA-carcinogen adduct formation will be steeper than that due to overwhelming of, *inter alia,* the DNA repair processes (Gehring 1977). However, if DNA-adduct formation increases beyond a certain proportion of free DNA sites, cell death will result, leading to a loss of carcinogenically relevant genetic change from the system and to a decrease of tumor or precursor cell yield (Scherer and Emmelot 1975b). Accordingly, as has been pointed out previously (Wolmann 1955, Emmelot and Scherer 1977) dose-response curves in the toxic dose range cannot and should not be used for analysis of the kinetics of tumor cell formation nor for extrapolation purposes. Neither can such curves serve as argument for the existence of a threshold.

Metaphors have been used to describe (Gehring 1977, Fig. 3) as well as to criticize the threshold model. In the latter case the existence of a threshold per se is not denied, but it is argued that the threshold has no effect in man, when the many background stimuli facing him are considered. These stimuli together with a very low dose of carcinogen would readily pass the threshold ("sea-sweeps-over-dike" metaphor). The nonstochastic, threshold concept does not reckon with the background stimuli; however, even if a threshold should exist, nonthreshold kinetics applies to man if these stimuli are taken into account. In the speculations on the threshold, protective entities in the cell are featured as such (*cf.* above). Only if these are saturated (by background + extra carcinogenic stimuli) would the extra carcinogen be capable of carrying out its relevant reaction.

This view is contrary to that of the stochastic, nonthreshold concept. According to the latter, the background stimuli per se do not affect the probability of whether a given dose of carcinogen, even the lowest, may score a relevant hit in *a cell.* That dose per se may do so, also in the absence of background stimuli. However, the background stimuli, by initiating steps of the process followed by proliferation of the precancerous cells, increase the chance that extra carcinogen may score a hit in *a tissue thus affected* (increase of target cells). Accordingly, the background stimuli do not "carry" the very low dose of extra carcinogen "over" the threshold, in the process of which both suffer loss, but the former allow the carcinogen to contribute to the sequence of steps leading to a cancer cell. (This is the reason why, as discussed previously, the linear model of extrapolation is preferred, although carcinogenesis is a multistep process.)

Thus, a fraction of even the lowest dose may in principle reach and react with its relevant target by a kind of "tunnel effect." Actually the stochastic, nonthreshold model uses a quantum mechanical type of argument, whereas the nonstochastic, threshold model follows the principles of classical mechanics. We believe that molecular toxicology, especially if it is concerned with irreversible reactions and small numbers of molecules, is based on stochastic principles and kinetic probabilities but not on steady-states. Some possibility that a relevant interaction occurs will always exist, no matter how small the dose and how large the number of protective entities, including irrelevant reactions, may be.

ACKNOWLEDGMENTS

The authors' work has been partially supported by the Scientific Council on Smoking and Health. The authors are much indebted to Miss I. H. Haighton for her dedicated assistance in the preparation of the manuscript.

REFERENCES

Albert, R. E., and B. Altshuler. 1973. Considerations relating to the formulation of limits for unavoidable population exposure to environmental carcinogens, *in* Radionucleotide Carcinogenesis, C. L. Saunders, R. H. Bush, J. E. Ballou, and D. D. Mahium, eds, (AEC Symposium Series, CONF-72050, Springfield Va.), U.S. Atomic Energy Commission Office of Information Services, Washington, D. C., pp. 233–253.

Albert, R. E., and B. Altshuler. 1976. Assessment of environmental carcinogen risk in terms of life shortening. Environmental Health Perspectives 13:91–94.

Armitage, P., and R. Doll. 1954. The age distribution of cancer and a multi-stage theory of carcinogenesis. Br. J. Cancer 8:1–12.

Armitage, P., and R. Doll. 1957. A two-stage theory of carcinogenesis in relation to the age distribution of human cancer. Br. J. Cancer 11:161–169.

Berenblum, I., and P. Shubik. 1949. The persistence of latent tumor cells induced in the mouse's skin by a single application of 9,10-dimethyl-1,2-benzanthracene. Br. J. Cancer 3:384–386.

Bliss, C. I. 1935. The comparison of dosage-mortality data. Ann. Appl. Biol. 22:307–333.

Blum, H. F. 1959. Carcinogenesis by Ultraviolet Light. Princeton University Press, Princeton, N.J.

Borek, C., and E. J. Hall. 1973. Transformation of mammalian cells in vitro by low doses of X-rays. Nature 243:450–453.

Boutwell, R. K. 1964. Some biological aspects of skin carcinogenesis. Prog. Exp. Tumor Res. 4:207–250.

Brown, J. M. 1976. Linearity *vs.* non-linearity of dose response for radiation carcinogenesis. Health Phys. 31:231–245.

Bryan, W. R., and M. B. Shimkin. 1941. Quantitative analysis of dose-response data obtained with carcinogenic hydrocarbons. J. Natl. Cancer Inst. 1:807–833.

Burch, P. R. J. 1976. The Biology of Cancer. A New Approach. Medical and Technical Press Ltd., Lancaster, England.

Colburn, N. H., and R. K. Boutwell. 1966. The binding of β-propiolactone to mouse skin DNA in vivo; its correlation with tumor-initiating activity. Cancer Res. 26:1701–1706.

Cornfield, J. 1977. Carcinogenic risk assessment. Science 198:693–699.

Crump, K. S., D. G. Hoel, C. H. Langley, and R. Peto. 1976. Fundamental carcinogenic processes and their implications for low dose risk assessment. Cancer Res. 36:2973–2979.

Druckrey, H. 1967. Quantitative aspects in chemical carcinogenesis, *in* Potential Carcinogenic Hazards from Drugs, R. Truhaut, ed., U.I.C.C. Monograph Ser. 7, pp. 60–78.

Druckrey, H., A. Schildbach, D. Schmähl, R. Preussmann, and S. Ivankovic. 1963. Quantitative Analyse der carcinogenen Wirkung von Diäthylnitrosamin. Arzneimittel-Forsch. 13:841–851.

Emmelot, P., and E. Scherer. 1977. Multi-hit kinetics of transformation with special reference to experimental liver and human lung carcinogenesis and some general conclusions. Cancer Res. 37:1702–1706.

Environmental Protection Agency. 1975. Relationship between Radiation Dose and Effect, Policy Statement Issued by the Office of Radiation Programs. U.S. Environmental Protection Agency, Washington, D.C.

Fisher, J. C. 1958. Multiple-mutation theory of carcinogenesis. Nature 181:651–652.

Foulds, L. 1969. Neoplastic Development. Vol. I. Academic Press, New York.

Freedman, V. H., and S-il. Shin. 1977. Isolation of human diploid cell variants with enhanced colony-forming efficiency in semisolid medium after a single-step chemical mutagenesis. J. Natl. Cancer Inst. 58:1873–1875.

Gehring, P. 1977. The risk equations. The threshold controversy. New Scientist 426–428.

Guess, H. A., and K. S. Crump. 1976. Low-dose-rate extrapolation of data from animal carcinogenicity experiments—Analysis of a new statistical technique. Mathematical Biosci. 32:15–36.

Guess, H., K. Crump, and R. Peto. 1977. Uncertainty estimates for low-dose-rate extrapolation of animal carcinogenicity data. Cancer Res. 37:3475–3483.

Hartley, H. O., and R. L. Sielken, Jr. 1977. Estimation of "safe doses" in carcinogenic experiments. Biometrics 33:1–30.

Henshaw, P. S., and H. L. Meyer, 1945. Further studies on urethane-induced pulmonary tumors. J. Natl. Cancer Inst. 5:415–417.

Heston, W. E., and M. A. Schneiderman. 1953. Analysis of dose-response in relation to mechanism of pulmonary tumor induction in mice. Science 117:109–111.

Huberman, E., and L. Sachs. 1966. Cell susceptibility to transformation and cytotoxicity by the carcinogenic hydrocarbon benzo(a)pyrene. Proc. Natl. Acad. Sci. USA 56:1123–1129.

Ishii, Y., J. A. Elliott, N. K. Mishra, and M. W. Lieberman. 1977. Quantitative studies of transformation by chemical carcinogens and ultraviolet radiation using a subclone of BHK_{21} clone 13 Syrian hamster cells. Cancer Res. 37:2023–2029.

Jones, H. B., and A. Grendon. 1975. Environmental factors in the origin of cancer, and estimation of the possible hazard to man. Food Cosmet. Toxicol. 13:251–268.

Kitagawa, T. 1976. Sequential phenotypic changes in hyperplastic areas during hepatocarcinogenesis in the rat. Cancer Res. 36:2534–2539.

Mantel, N., N. R. Bohidar, C. C. Brown, J. L. Ciminera, and J. W. Tukey. 1975. An improved Mantel-Bryan procedure for "safety" testing of carcinogens. Cancer Res. 35:865–872.

Mantel, N., and W. R. Bryan. 1961. "Safety" testing of carcinogenic agents. J. Natl. Cancer Inst. 27:455–470.

Mantel, N., and M. A. Schneiderman. 1975. Estimating "safe" levels, a hazardous undertaking. Cancer Res. 35:1379–1386.

Nagao, M., M. Honda, Y. Seino, T. Yahaga, and T. Sugimura. 1977. Mutagenicities of smoke condensates and the charred surface of fish and meat. Cancer Letters 2:221–226.

Nordling, C. O. 1953. A new theory on the cancer-inducing mechanism. Br. J. Cancer 7:68–72.

Pierson, E. S., and H. O. Hartley, eds. 1970. Biometrica Tables for Statisticians. Vol. 1. Cambridge University Press, London.

Peto, R., F. J. C. Roe, P. N. Lee, L. Levy, and J. Clack. 1975. Cancer and ageing in mice and men. Br. J. Cancer 32:411–426.

Saffiotti, U., R. Montesano, A. R. Sellakumar, F. Cefis, and D. G. Kaufman. 1972. Respiratory tract carcinogenesis in hamsters induced by different numbers of administrations of benzo(a)pyrene and ferric oxide. Cancer Res. 32:1073–1081.

Scherer, E., and P. Emmelot. 1975a. Foci of altered liver cells induced by a single dose of diethylnitrosamine and partial hepatectomy: Their contribution to hepatocarcinogenesis in the rat. Eur. J. Cancer 11:145–154.

Scherer, E., and P. Emmelot. 1975b. Kinetics of induction and growth of precancerous liver-cell foci, and liver tumour formation by diethylnitrosamine in the rat. Eur. J. Cancer 11:689–696.

Scherer, E., and P. Emmelot. 1976. Kinetics of induction and growth of enzyme-deficient islands involved in hepatocarcinogenesis. Cancer Res. 36:2544–2554.

Scherer, E., and P. Emmelot. 1978. Comment on Cornfield. Science (In press).

Scherer, E., M. Hoffmann, P. Emmelot, and H. Friedrich-Freksa. 1972. Quantitative study on foci of altered liver cells induced in the rat by a single dose of diethylnitrosamine and partial hepatectomy. J. Natl. Cancer Inst. 49:93–106.

Scherer, E., A. P. Steward, and P. Emmelot. 1977. Kinetics of formation of O^6-ethylguanine in, and its removal from liver DNA of rats receiving diethylnitrosamine. Chem.-Biol. Interact. 19:1–11.

Schmähl, D. 1976. Combination effects in chemical carcinogenesis (Experimental results). Oncology 33:73–76.

Shimkin, M. B., and G. D. Stoner. 1975. Lung tumors in mice: Application to carcinogenesis bioassay. Adv. Cancer Res. 21:1–57.

Skipper, H. E., F. M. Schabel, Jr., and W. S. Wilcox. 1964. Experimental evaluation of potential anticancer agents. XIII. On the criteria and kinetics associated with "curability" of experimental leukemias. Cancer Chemother. Rep. 35:1–111.

Skipper, H. E., F. M. Schabel, Jr., and W. S. Wilcox. 1965. Experimental evaluation of potential anticancer agents. XIV. Further study of certain basic concepts underlying chemotherapy of leukemia. Cancer Chemother. Rep. 45:5–29.

Solt, D., and E. Farber. 1976. New principle for the analysis of chemical carcinogenesis. Nature 263:701–703.

Takano, K., L. P. Balough, N. S. Merkel, and J. A. DiPaolo. 1972. Quantitation of chemically induced neoplastic transformation of BALB/3T3 cloned cell lines. (Abstract) Fed. Proc. 31:633(2360).

Waterhouse, J., C. Muir, P. Correa, and J. Powell, eds. 1976. Cancer Incidence in Five Continents. Vol. III. IARC Scientific Publications No. 15, International Agency for Research on Cancer, Lyon, p. 370.

Wollman, S. H. 1955. Comments on the analysis of dose-response data in experimental carcinogenesis. J. Natl. Cancer Inst. 16:195–204.

Yokoro, K., M. Nakano, A. Ito, K. Nagao, Y. Kodama, and K. Hamada. 1977. Role of prolactin in rat mammary carcinogenesis: Detection of carcinogenicity of low doses of carcinogens and of persisting dormant cancer cells. J. Natl. Cancer Inst. 58:1777–1783.

Carcinogens: Identification and Mechanisms of Action, edited by A. Clark Griffin and Charles R. Shaw. Raven Press, New York © 1979.

Neoantigens in Chemical Carcinogenesis

Robert W. Baldwin, Michael J. Embleton, and Malcolm V. Pimm

Cancer Research Campaign Laboratories, University of Nottingham, Nottingham NG7 2RD England

Neoplastic transformation by chemical carcinogens leads to the expression in the transformed cell of neoantigens that are not present on normal cells, at least in the adult host (reviewed by Baldwin 1973, Baldwin and Price 1975). This has been established in many experiments demonstrating that immunity to carcinogen-induced tumors transplanted into syngeneic hosts can be induced by pretreatment of the recipients with tumor cells prevented from progressive growth, e.g., by radiation treatment (Sjögren 1965). The neoantigens responsible for these tumor-rejection responses have been termed tumor-specific transplanta-tion antigens (TSTA), and with most chemically induced tumors, these are distinctive and stable characteristics of each individual tumor. Immunization against an individual carcinogen-induced tumor, therefore, confers no protection against challenge with a second tumor, even if histologically identical and induced by the same carcinogen (Basombrio 1970, Baldwin 1973).

Neoantigens expressed at the tumor cell surface with identical specificities to the TSTAs can be demonstrated on chemically induced tumors by their reaction in vitro with sensitized lymphocytes or serum antibody from tumor immune donors (Hellström and Hellström 1974, Price and Baldwin 1975, Ting and Herberman 1976). These tumor-specific cell surface antigens (TSCSA) are invaluable as cell surface markers for neoplastic cells, although there is no formal proof that these are the same tumor products as the TSTAs functioning to produce tumor rejection.

In addition to the tumor-specific antigens (TSTA, TSCSA), carcinogen-in-duced tumors may also express a variety of common antigenic determinants, such as oncodevelopmental antigens (Coggin and Anderson 1974, Rees *et al.,* in press). These tumor-associated antigens are detectable by reaction of tumor cells in vitro with serum or sensitized lymphoid cells from multiparous female donors, the concept being that these antigens as expressed on developing embryos elicit responses during multiple pregnancies.

Many of the tumor-associated antigens may be considered as targets for immu-nosurveillance so that the host responses to these tumor products may influence the carcinogenic process. More pertinent in the present context is the view that these tumor cell products, especially the tumor-specific components, may be used to characterize cellular events involved in chemical carcinogenesis.

TUMOR-SPECIFIC ANTIGEN EXPRESSION

Tumor-specific antigens have been identified on many types of chemically induced tumors including polycyclic hydrocarbon-induced sarcomas and hepatocellular carcinomas induced by aminoazo dyes and alkylnitrosamines (reviewed by Baldwin and Price 1975). Cells transformed in vitro by chemical carcinogens, e.g., mouse embryo and prostate cells treated with 3-methylcholanthrene (MCA) (Mondal *et al.* 1970, Embleton and Heidelberger 1975), also exhibit tumor-specific antigens, defined by their capacity to induce immunity against tumors growing from transformed cells injected into syngeneic mice or by in vitro reactions with sensitized lymphoid cells or serum antibody.

Without doubt the most significant characteristic of the tumor-specific antigens, whether defined by in vivo tumor rejection tests or by in vitro reactions with sensitized lymphoid cells or antibody, is their high degree of polymorphism. This is illustrated by studies showing that immunity elicited against individual MCA-induced murine sarcomas was directed only against the immunizing tumor (Basombrio 1970). While it was not practical to evaluate large populations of tumors by this approach, these investigations did indicate that none of 25 sarcomas tested reproducibly exhibited cross-reacting rejection antigens. This point has been investigated in considerable detail with both MCA-induced sarcomas and DAB-induced (4-dimethylaminoazobenzene) hepatomas in the rat where tumor-specific cell surface antigens were typed by membrane immunofluorescence reactions of syngeneic tumor-immune antisera with panels of viable tumor cells (Baldwin *et al.* 1972). For example, with antisera raised against seven individual MCA-induced sarcomas, each reacted with cells of the immunizing tumor, but only 1/121 cross-tests was positive (Table 1). At the present time there are no other studies on large populations of tumors to define with any degree of certainty how frequently cross-reacting tumor-specific antigens occur on chemically induced tumors. These in vitro approaches, moreover, are rendered more difficult with murine tumors in which common, cross-reacting antigens, probably reflecting viral products, are frequently expressed (Forbes *et al.* 1975, Fritze *et al.* 1976, Leffell and Coggin 1977). With these tumors, therefore, it has generally been necessary to use the tumor rejection assay to detect tumor-specific antigens, since the common neoantigens do not elicit immune responses capable of producing tumor rejection. These assays are tedious, however, and are difficult to control when studying large groups of tumors.

The data currently available do indicate that tumor-specific antigens are highly polymorphic, and the estimate of greater than 100 specificities from the studies on MCA-induced rat sarcomas may be of the correct order.

Antigenic Differences between Primary and Secondary
MCA-Induced Rat Sarcomas

The individually distinct neoantigens on carcinogen-induced tumors provide convenient markers for studying the characteristics of tumor cell populations

TABLE 1. *Membrane immunofluorescence cross-tests with 3-methylcholanthrene-induced rat sarcomas**

Fluorescence indices against target cells of sarcoma

Serum from rats immune to sarcoma	Mc3	Mc4	Mc5	Mc7	Mc10	Mc14	Mc15	Mc16	Mc21	Mc26	Mc30	Mc31	Mc32	Mc33	Mc35	Mc37	Mc38	Mc39	Mc40	Mc42	Mc46	Mc49	Mc50	Mc54	Mc57	Mc58
Mc4	0.02	*0.60 ± 0.17*	0.04 (†)	0.07	—	—	—	0.13	0.06	0.00	—	0.01	0.15	0.00	0.12	0.00	0.11	0.00	0.01	0.00	0.00	0.25 0.03	0.00	0.00	0.00 0.07	0.00
Mc5	0.22 0.01	0.00	*0.58 ± 0.08*	0.09	0.19	—	0.25 0.05	0.00	0.10	0.20 0.10	0.10	0.27 0.11	*0.46 ± 0.09*	—	—	—	—	—	—	0.01	—	0.03	—	—	0.07	—
Mc7	0.20 0.01	0.00	0.09	*0.65 ± 0.02*	0.00	0.00 0.05	0.05	0.09	0.09 0.00	0.02	0.01	0.00	—	—	—	—	—	—	—	—	—	—	—	—	—	—
Mc10	0.00 0.18	0.00	0.03	0.00	*0.49 ± 0.05*	—	0.09	0.00	0.12	0.00	0.01	0.00 0.12	0.00	—	0.01	—	0.00 0.00	0.15	0.03	0.00	0.00	0.00	—	—	0.01 0.00	0.00
Mc16	0.00	0.00	0.03	0.21	0.00	0.21 0.01	0.05	*0.54 ± 0.07*	0.11 0.07	0.08	0.08	0.01	0.06 0.06	0.12	0.04	0.04	0.27	0.25	0.00	0.00	0.00	0.14	0.01	0.07	0.19 0.06	0.00
Mc21	0.01	0.02	0.08	0.23 0.04	0.00	0.18 0.00	0.06	0.11 0.07	*0.57 ± 0.06*	0.00	0.05	0.01	0.00 0.14	—	—	—	—	—	—	—	—	0.00	—	—	—	—
Mc26	—	—	—	0.04	—	—	0.07	—	—	*0.59 ± 0.06*	—	—	—	—	—	—	—	—	—	—	—	—	—	—	—	—
Mc39	0.00 0.00	0.13	0.08	0.00	—	—	—	0.00	0.00	0.07	—	0.15	0.06	0.00	0.03	0.00	0.00	*0.60 ± 0.50*	0.19	0.00 0.00	0.00	0.00	0.00	0.00	0.26 0.03	0.00

* Rats immunized by graft excision and repeated viable challenges, or repeated implantation of irradiated sarcoma tissue.
† Mean ± standard deviation. Fluorescence index ≥ 0.30 regarded as significant reaction.

arising during carcinogenesis. This is exemplified by recent studies designed to investigate the immunological characteristics of rat sarcomas induced by MCA (Pimm and Baldwin 1977).

Primary sarcomas induced by subcutaneous injection of MCA were surgically removed and established as tumor lines by transplantation into syngeneic recipients (Figure 1). The surgically treated rats were then kept until second tumors developed at the site of the primary, and these were also established as transplanted tumor lines (Figure 2). Several primary and secondary tumor lines established from individual rats were evaluated for immunogenicity, and in each case it was established that they exhibited different tumor rejection antigens. This is exemplified by the data in Table 2 showing that induction of immunity to primary sarcoma Mc40 provided no protection to the second tumor, Mc40A, arising at the site of the initial neoplasm, and vice versa. These studies suggest that in each case the primary and secondary sarcomas arose by clonal amplification of separate populations of MCA-transformed cells and not simply by expansion of residual tumor that remained following resection of the primary. This latter proposal cannot be completely ruled out, but in ongoing studies it has been possible in only one of four cases to select antigenically different tumor lines by transplanting to normal syngeneic rats tissue taken from opposite poles of primary MCA-induced sarcomas. Similar tests also established that selection of tumor lines differing in tumor-antigen specificity by transplanting opposite poles from primary MCA-induced murine sarcomas was only successful with one of nine tumors (Prehn 1970).

One interpretation of these findings is that treatment with MCA affects many cells either simultaneously or sequentially through exposure to persisting carcinogen, but the resulting tumor represents the progeny of a single cell or, at most, a few cells. This is consistent with the view that tumors are frequently mono-

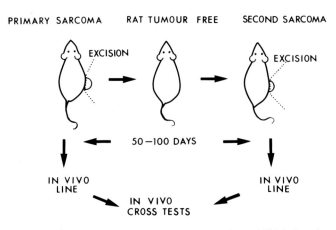

FIG. 1. Establishment of in vivo transplant lines from a primary MCA-induced sarcoma and the second tumor developing at the site of surgical removal of the primary.

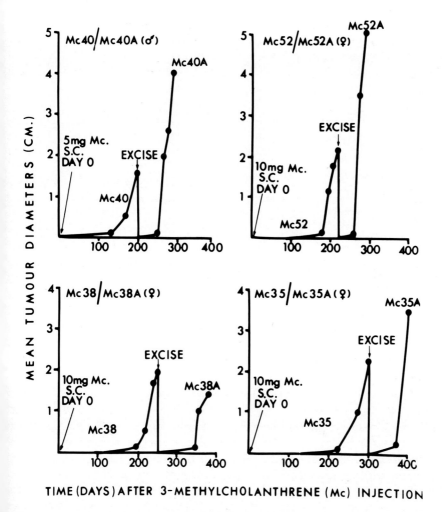

TIME (DAYS) AFTER 3-METHYLCHOLANTHRENE (Mc) INJECTION

FIG. 2. Development of primary sarcomas in rats injected with 3-methylcholanthrene and the growth of second tumors following surgical removal of the primaries.

clonal, as defined by several approaches to tumor cell characterization such as cytogenetic and isoenzyme studies (Nowell 1976, Burnet 1977). The present immunological studies also suggest that other transformed cells are present but remain dormant during the growth of the primary sarcoma and only develop when this is removed. The possibility that further transformation by residual carcinogen occurs after removal of the primary tumor cannot be excluded, but this is less likely in view of the rapid growth of the second tumor. This rapid growth of the second tumor from dormant transformed cells may simply reflect the influence of trauma resulting from surgical removal of the primary or the considerable immunosuppressive effects of even simple surgical manipulation

TABLE 2. *Cross-challenge tests with sarcomas Mc40 and Mc40A* *

| Immunization | | Challenge | | Tumor takes | |
Tumor	Method	Tumor	No. of cells	Test	Controls
Mc40	IR graft†	Mc40	5×10^5	0/4	5/5
		Mc40A	5×10^5	3/5	3/4
Mc40	Excision‡	Mc40	5×10^5	0/5	5/5
		Mc40A	5×10^5	5/5	4/4
Mc40A	Excision	Mc40	5×10^5	10/10	10/10
		Mc40A	5×10^5	0/10	10/10

* Sarcoma Mc40 was excised 200 days after subcutaneous injection of 3-methylcholanthrene (5 mg) in trioctanoin. This tumor was removed intact in the subcutaneous tissue capsule, and it was determined that the excision site was free of visibly detectable tumor. The second tumor Mc40A arose at the site of the original tumor 80 days following its resection.
† Four weekly implants of 15,000R irradiated tumor tissue.
‡ Surgical excision of subcutaneously growing tumor graft.

(Haddow 1974). It cannot be discounted, however, that tumor-host or tumor cell–tumor cell interactions, which are not necessarily of an immunological nature, may influence the capacity of neoplastic cells to progress and so develop into frank tumors.

CARCINOGEN INTERACTIONS AND TUMOR-SPECIFIC ANTIGEN EXPRESSION IN IN VIVO STUDIES

In considering the relationship between tumor-specific antigen expression and neoplastic transformation, it has to be recognized that within some systems, e.g., MCA-induced murine sarcomas, there may be considerable variability in tumor immunogenicity. For example, some MCA-induced murine sarcomas may be highly immunogenic as defined by the maximum tumor cell challenge rejected by immunized mice compared to the minimum cell inoculum required for progressive tumor growth in controls, while others may lack demonstrable immunogenicity (Bartlett 1972, Prehn 1975). Also, there may be considerable differences between the immunogenicities of tumors of similar histogenic types but induced by different carcinogens. This is exemplified by the reproducible demonstration of tumor rejection antigens on hepatic tumors induced in rats by aminoazo dyes, while those induced by N-2-fluorenylacetamide only infrequently are immunogenic (Baldwin and Barker 1967, Baldwin and Embleton 1971). Because of the complex immunological reactions involved in the induction of tumor rejection responses (Baldwin and Robins 1977, Byers and Baldwin, in press), it is not possible to conclusively establish that so-called "nonimmunogenic" tumors do not still express tumor-specific antigens at levels too low to be detected by the rejection-type assays. But, these studies do point to a wide variability, at least quantitatively, in tumor-specific antigen expression; and this, as has been suggested from studies on MCA-induced murine sarcomas, may be related to the dose of carcinogen used for tumor induction (Prehn 1975). With MCA induced rat sarcomas, however, it has not been found that tumor immunogenicity correlated with the dose of carcinogen administered. This is illustrated in Figure 3, showing the incidence of immunogenic sarcomas induced by a single subcutaneous injection of MCA in trioctanoin at doses ranging from 100 μg to 10 mg. In this particular series, none of the rats receiving 100 μg MCA developed progressively growing tumors over a 300-day observation period. Sarcomas arose in almost all of the rats receiving a dose of MCA of 1 mg or greater, but the proportion of immunogenic tumors induced with each dose of carcinogen was approximately the same. In these studies, the immunogenicity of a tumor was defined by its capacity to induce immunity to transplanted tumor cells in preimmunized rats. Although it is difficult to quantitate this, an indication of relative reactivities can be obtained from the *tumor rejection index,* i.e., the maximum tumor cell challenge rejected in preimmunized hosts compared to the minimum tumor cell inoculum needed for progressive tumor growth in untreated controls. By this criterion, there were no detectable differences between the immunogenicities of sarcomas induced by different doses of MCA. For example, tumors induced following injection of either 1 or 5 mg MCA produced a variable immune rejection response so that in both groups immunity to challenge with up to 20 times the minimum tumor cell challenge for growth in controls was obtained.

In comparison with these studies on MCA-induced sarcomas, it has been shown that the frequency of immunogenic tumors in a population of naturally occurring rat sarcomas was low, and in some cases, the maximum tumor cell inoculum rejected by immunized rats was only slightly greater than that needed to produce progressive tumor growth in nonimmunized controls (Baldwin and Embleton 1974). These so-called "spontaneous tumors" arise in low frequency and, therefore, only limited numbers have been investigated. Nevertheless, few

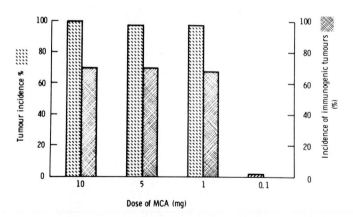

FIG. 3. Induction of primary sarcomas in rats by subcutaneous injection of 3-methylcholanthrene and the immunogenicity of syngeneic transplant lines established from primary tumors.

tumors of this type, including rat and murine sarcomas, rat mammary carcinomas, and a variety of other tumor types, have been reported as immunogenic (Prehn and Main 1957, Hammond *et al.* 1967, Baldwin and Embleton 1969, Hewitt *et al.* 1976); and it is generally recognized that spontaneous tumors only infrequently express tumor-rejection antigens (Klein and Klein 1977).

This comparison between the immunogenic characteristics of MCA-induced and spontaneous rat sarcomas supports the view that the expression of a tumor-specific rejection antigen is associated with changes mediated by carcinogen interaction within cells undergoing neoplastic change. Nevertheless, the observation that a proportion of the tumors induced in rats exposed to doses of MCA as great as 10 mg are not immunogenic indicates that carcinogen-induced transformation does not necessarily lead to the expression of new cell surface components recognized as tumor-rejection antigens. This could arise, for example, if there are multiple cellular sites for carcinogen interaction that lead to neoplastic change, but only some of these produce alterations coding for cell surface proteins, or more probably glycoproteins that function as tumor-specific antigens.

In Vitro Studies

Cells transformed in vitro by carcinogenic polycyclic hydrocarbons, e.g., MCA or 7,12-dimethylbenz[*a*]anthracene (DMBA) may also express surface-associated neoantigens not found on nontransformed control cells which can be identified as TSTA by in vivo rejection tests or as TSCSA by in vitro reactions of transformed cells with lymphocytes or serum from immunized syngeneic animals (Mondal *et al.* 1970, 1971, Embleton and Heidelberger 1972, 1975). For example, a total of 19/22 chemically transformed lines derived from cloned mouse prostate cells and 8/8 derived from 10T½ murine embryo cells were shown to express neoantigens (Table 3). Exhaustive cross-tests using in vitro assays detecting reactiv-

TABLE 3. *Neoantigens on murine cells transformed by chemical carcinogens in vitro*

Origin of cells	Status	Carcinogen	No. of cell lines with neoantigens demonstrable by	
			Cell-mediated cytotoxicity	Membrane immunofluorescence
Prostate	Nontransformed control	None	0/4	0/4
Embryo	Nontransformed control	None	0/3	0/3
Prostate	Transformed	MCA*	13/16	11/16
Prostate	Transformed	MCA-epoxide†	6/6	4/6
Embryo	Transformed	MCA	4/4	4/4
Embryo	Transformed	DMBA‡	4/4	3/4

* 3-methylcholanthrene
† K-region epoxide of 3-methylcholanthrene
‡ 7,12-dimethylbenz[*a*]anthracene

ity of sera or lymphoid cells from syngeneic mice immunized with transformed cells showed that these neoantigens, like the TSCSA of tumors induced in vivo by chemical carcinogens, were generally unique for individual cell lines (Embleton and Heidelberger 1972, 1975). Moreover, since the cross-tested transformed cells were the progeny of single parent control clones, the neoantigens arose as a consequence of specific interactions between cells and the carcinogen and not as a result of amplification of pre-existing antigenically aberrant clones or clones with a high concentration of a normal antigen that would otherwise pass unnoticed (Burnet 1970). In these studies, the acquisition of neoantigens was closely associated with the neoplastic state, since MCA-treated cells that did not transform showed no evidence of antigenicity in the syngeneic host. Also, antigenic neoplastic cells undergoing reversion to a stage showing less abnormal growth characteristics showed diminished immunogenicity (Mondal *et al.* 1971). However, these investigations also suggest that the expression of detectable tumor-specific antigens is not a necessary concomitant of neoplastic transformation since some MCA-transformed cell lines had no detectable neoantigens. This is further emphasized by the observation that spontaneous transformants generally did not express tumor-specific antigens (Embleton and Heidelberger 1972, 1975). These findings are comparable to the studies already discussed showing that sarcomas induced in vivo by MCA are frequently immunogenic, whereas spontaneous sarcomas usually are not, and further reinforce the view that tumor-specific antigen expression is a carcinogen-related event.

NEOANTIGEN EXPRESSION DURING EARLY STAGES OF MCA-CARCINOGENESIS

In order to investigate further the role of carcinogen-cell interactions in the expression of tumor-specific antigens, antigenic changes have been investigated in cells undergoing short-term treatment with MCA. The primary objective of these studies is to establish whether neoantigens with the same specificities as those expressed on MCA-induced rat sarcomas can be identified at an early stage of the carcinogenesis process, even before neoplastic transformation has occurred, that is, to determine whether neoantigen expression in cells results from cellular events following interaction of carcinogen metabolites with cellular macromolecules but at a stage prior to the acquisition of neoplastic characteristics.

In the experimental approach adopted, freshly suspended 17- to 19-day-old rat embryo cells were exposed in culture to MCA dissolved in DMSO (0.5% DMSO and 10 μg MCA/ml culture medium) for 18 hours. The MCA-treated embryo cells, as well as cells treated with DMSO to serve as controls, were washed six times and used to immunize syngeneic rats. In each experiment, rats were immunized four times at 10-day intervals using freshly prepared batches of MCA-treated embryo cells (10^8 cells), and the sera from these animals were tested for antibody reacting against a range of tumors including sarcomas induced in vivo with MCA (Table 4). In the first experiment, antibody was detected against cells from two MCA-induced sarcomas, Mc7 and Mc97P, as well as one DAB-induced hepatoma, D192A. In the second experiment, anti-MCA embryo cell serum reacted with two MCA-sarcomas, Mc97P and Mc103C. These reactions were reproducible and specific for the reacting tumor cells, while anti-sera against DMSO-treated embryo cells were uniformly negative with all the tumor cells tested.

The reactivity of the sera in these studies suggested (a) that multiple neoantigens were induced by MCA treatment of the rat embryo cells, and (b) that at least some of these were expressed upon tumor cells that have been tested. The status of the MCA-treated embryo cells regarding transformation is not yet known, but in view of the short time between initial treatment with MCA and use of these cells for immunization under conditions in which long-term survival in vivo would not be expected, it was considered unlikely that they were neoplastic. Since, however, their period of survival when injected into syngeneic rats is unknown, it cannot be excluded that they may have undergone

TABLE 4. *Tumor-associated antibody in serum from rats immunized with 3-methylcholanthrene-treated embryo cells*

| | Fluorescence indices* with serum from | | | |
| | Experiment 1 | | Experiment 2 | |
Target cells	DMSO-treated	MCA-treated	DMSO-treated	MCA-treated
Rat embryo (18-day)	0.00	0.00	NT"	NT
Mammary carcinoma:†				
Sp4	0.02	0.05	0.00	0.06
Hepatoma:‡				
D23	0.05	0.06	0.00	0.06
D30	0.01	0.01	NT	NT
D192A	0.03	*0.37*	0.00	0.04
Sarcoma:§				
Mc4	0.04	0.12	0.00	0.00
Mc7	0.13	*0.43*	0.07	0.05
Mc40A	0.00	0.00	0.03	0.00
Mc57	0.17	0.11	0.03	0.01
Mc96A	0.08	0.00	0.00	0.00
Mc97G	NT	NT	0.00	0.00
Mc97P	0.00	*0.34*	0.00	0.36
Mc102A	0.11	0.04	0.00	0.00
Mc103B	0.00	0.10	0.00	*0.56*
Mc103C	0.01	0.00	0.20	0.03
Mc104	0.00	0.00	0.00	0.00
Mc110B	0.00	0.00	0.00	0.00

* Fluorescence indices ⩾0.30 are positive.
† Spontaneously arising
‡ 4-dimethylaminoazobenzene-induced
§ 3-methylcholanthrene-induced
" NT: Not tested

in vivo neoplastic change. It is doubtful that sufficient carcinogen would have been transferred with the embryo cells to effect in vivo transformation of other host cells. Notwithstanding these as yet unanswered questions, the studies suggest that the individually specific type of neoantigens of chemically induced tumors can be expressed on nontransformed cells. Verification of this hypothesis is clearly of considerable importance because this implies that the tumor-specific-type neoantigens reflect changes induced in cells by carcinogens, even though they are not specifically related to neoplastic change.

DISCUSSION

Of the neoantigens arising in cells transformed by chemical carcinogens, the tumor-specific antigens (TSTA, TSCSA) are of particular interest, since these cell surface components probably reflect carcinogen-induced derangements. The expression of tumor-specific antigens is not a necessary concomitant of neoplastic change, however, as tumors can be induced with carcinogens such as MCA in which this type of neoantigen may or may not be expressed (Prehn 1975, cf. Figure 3). Conversely, expression of tumor-specific antigens appears to be related to carcinogen exposure, since they are less frequently detected upon spontaneous tumors (Baldwin and Embleton 1974, Klein and Klein 1977). These findings can be interpreted to indicate that the tumor-specific antigens arise as a consequence of cellular interactions with carcinogen metabolities, but these changes are not in themselves necessarily involved in the neoplastic process. Alternatively, it may be that multiple carcinogen interactions can occur within the cell, which result in transformation. But not all of these code for cell surface-expressed products which, when modified in the transformed cell, appear as tumor-specific antigens.

Further consideration of these hypotheses is limited by the paucity of knowledge about the nature of the cell surface components on tumor cells which function as tumor-specific antigens. It is generally recognized, however, that these antigens are intimately associated with the tumor cell surface, since many of the in vitro methods used for their detection, e.g., complement-mediated antibody lysis of tumor cells, involve interaction with components on intact tumor cells. Furthermore, extensive studies with several types of rat tumors, including DAB-induced hepatomas and MCA-induced sarcomas, have established that tumor-specific antigen is associated with membrane preparations from tumor homogenates but is not contained in soluble fractions (Baldwin et al. 1973, Price and Baldwin 1974, 1977). Also, the product detected at the tumor cell surface is intimately associated with the plasma membrane since tumor antigen is only released by degradative treatments such as papain digestion or extraction with chaotropic agents, e.g., 3M KCl or detergent solubilization with agents such as sodium deoxycholate (reviewed by Price and Baldwin 1977). Chemical characterization of tumor-specific antigens following their release from tumor cells and solubilization is now in progress in several laboratories and generally has reached the stage where chemically homogenous preparations are being defined. With the DAB-induced rat hepatoma D23, for example, a homogenous product retaining tumor-specific antigen activity has been isolated with molecular weight of approximately 50 to 60 K daltons (Harris *et al.* 1973, Price and Baldwin 1977).

Although these biochemical approaches are providing well-characterized tumor antigens, the goal of isolating material of sufficient purity in terms of tumor-specific antigen is still far from being attained, so that compositional analyses are not yet feasible. Increasing attention is being given, therefore, to the possibility that tumor-specific antigens are modified macromolecular components present on normal cells. One proposal, that they are modified normal alloantigens, arose from studies indicating a reciprocal relationship between tumor-specific and H-2 antigen expression on murine MCA-induced tumors (Haywood and McKhann 1971). Also, MCA-induced murine sarcomas express H-2 and/or non-H-2 histocompatibility antigens foreign to the strain in which the tumor arose (Invernizzi and Parmiani 1975, Meschini *et al.* 1977). This concept has not been substantiated, however, since other investigators have questioned the relationship between tumor antigen and H-2 expression (Sikora and Lachmann, unpublished findings), while the hypothesis that TSTA is an alien H-2 antigen is unresolved (Carbone *et al.* 1978). Furthermore, analysis of hybrid cells derived from fusion of the TA3Ha mammary carcinoma (H-2^a) and an MCA-induced sarcoma (H-2^s) with elimination of chromosome 17 of one strain or another by selective passage in the opposite parental strain did not result in the loss of TSTA (Klein and Klein 1975, Klein 1975). This argues against the possibility that the TSTA on the MCA-induced sarcoma is a modified form of H-2. In similar studies with DAB-induced hepatoma D23, it was found that the tumor-specific antigen could be isolated by binding to immunoabsorbent containing insolubilized alloantibody (Bowen and Baldwin 1975). It has subsequently been established, however, that the tumor-specific antigen does not have any association with β2-microglobulin (Bowen and Baldwin, unpublished findings), so that it is not related to antigens of the major histocompatibility locus in the rat (RT1). This suggests that the D23 tumor antigen is related to minor alloantigens such as differentiation antigens (Williams 1977), but no further characteristics of the normal cell component are yet available.

While the precise nature of tumor-specific antigens remains unidentified, the concept that these products represent normal cell products modified by carcinogen interaction is of considerable importance in understanding the carcinogenic process. As already indicated, the major characteristic of these tumor cell components is their high degree of polymorphism. The related question, therefore, is, does this polymorphism represent alterations in a wide array of different normal cell surface proteins, or is it due to variable charges in a single protein or small group of proteins? Related to this, it has still to be established more conclusively whether tumor-specific antigens are induced in cells at a stage prior to neoplastic transformation. This could occur, for example, if exposure of cells to carcinogen led to the expression of neoantigens showing a wide diversity of specificity. In this case it would be necessary to have clonal amplification of an individual cell after it undergoes neoplastic transformation in order for a particular antigen to be detected, and so defined as a tumor-specific antigen. In this context, the preliminary studies presented indicate that it is possible, by treating rat embryo cells with MCA for a period of 18 hours, to induce the expression of an abnormal antigen cross-reacting with tumor-specific antigen on MCA-induced sarcomas (Table 4). It should also be noted that "abnormal" antigens were detected in rat liver membrane and cytosol fractions during the early stages of DAB-carcinogenesis, and some of these antigens were identified as normal liver components modified by covalent interaction with carcinogen metabolites (Baldwin 1965). These early studies were not concerned with identifying neoantigens expressed on hepatic tumor cells, but further investigation of this relationship is clearly warranted. Whatever the stage in carcinogenesis at which tumor-specific antigens become expressed, it has to be recognized that in general these are stable characteristics of the transformed cell. As such, therefore, they must be considered as products of genetic or epigenetic changes within the cell progressing to the neoplastic state.

ACKNOWLEDGMENTS

This work was supported by a grant from the Cancer Research Campaign.

REFERENCES

Baldwin, R. W. 1965. Abnormal cell antigens in aminoazodye induced rat liver tumours. Br. J. Cancer 19:894–902.

Baldwin, R. W. 1973. Immunological aspects of chemical carcinogenesis. Adv. Cancer Res. 18:1–75.

Baldwin, R. W., and C. R. Barker. 1967. Tumour-specific antigenicity of aminoazodye-induced rat hepatomas. Int. J. Cancer 2:355–364.

Baldwin, R. W., and M. J. Embleton. 1969. Immunology of spontaneously arising rat mammary adenocarcinomas. Int. J. Cancer 4:430–439.

Baldwin, R. W., and M. J. Embleton. 1971. Tumor-specific antigens in 2-acetylaminofluorene-induced rat hepatomas and related tumors. Isr. J. Med. Sci. 7:144–153.

Baldwin, R. W., and M. J. Embleton. 1974. Neoantigens on spontaneous and carcinogen-induced rat tumours defined by *in vitro* lymphocytotoxicity. Int. J. Cancer 13:433–443.

Baldwin, R. W., M. J. Embleton, and M. Moore. 1973. Immunogenicity of rat hepatomata membrane fractions. Br. J. Cancer 28:389–399.

Baldwin, R. W., D. Glaves, M. V. Pimm, and B. M. Vose. 1972. Tumour specific and embryonic antigen expression on chemically induced rat tumours. Ann. Inst. Pasteur (Paris) 122:715–728.

Baldwin, R. W., and M. R. Price. 1975. Neoantigen expression in chemical carcinogenesis, *in* Cancer—A Comprehensive Treatise, F. F. Becker, ed., Vol. 1. Plenum Press, New York, pp. 353–459.

Baldwin, R. W., and R. A. Robins. 1977. Induction of tumor-immune responses and their interaction with the developing tumor. Contemp. Top. Mol. Immunol. 6:177–207.

Bartlett, G. 1972. Effect of host immunity on the antigenic strength of primary tumours. J. Natl. Cancer Inst. 49:493–504.

Basombrio, M. A. 1970. Search for common antigenicities among twenty-five sarcomas induced by methylcholanthrene. Cancer Res. 30:2458–2462.

Bowen, J. G., and R. W. Baldwin. 1975. Tumour-specific antigen related to rat histocompatibility antigens. Nature 258:75–76.

Burnet, F. M. 1970. A certain symmetry: Histocompatibility antigens compared with immunocyte receptors. Nature 226:123–126.

Burnet, F. M. 1977. Morphogenesis and cancer. Med. J. Aust. 1:5–9.

Byers, V. S., and R. W. Baldwin. 1978. Tumor immunology, *in* Basic and Clinical Immunology, H. H. Fudenberg, D. P. Stites, J. L. Caldwell, and J. V. Wells, eds., Lange, Los Altos, California (In press).

Carbone, G., G. Invernizzi, A. Meschini, and G. Parmiani. 1978. In vitro and in vivo expression of original and foreign H-2 antigens and of the tumor-associated transplantation antigen of a murine fibrosarcoma. Int. J. Cancer 21:85–93.

Coggin, J. H., and N. G. Anderson. 1974. Cancer, differentiation and embryonic antigens: Some central problems. Adv. Cancer Res. 19:105–165.

Embleton, M. J., and C. Heidelberger. 1972. Antigenicity of clones of mouse prostate cells transformed in vitro. Int. J. Cancer 9:8–18.

Embleton, M. J., and C. Heidelberger. 1975. Neoantigens on chemically transformed cloned C3H mouse embryo cells. Cancer Res. 35:2049–2055.

Forbes, J. T., Y. Nakao, and R. T. Smith. 1975. Tumor specific immunity to chemically induced tumors. Evidence for immunologic specific and shared antigenicity in lymphocyte responses to soluble tumor antigens. J. Exp. Med. 141:1181–1200.

Fritze, D., D. H. Kern, J. A. Hume, C. R. Drogmuller, and Y. H. Pilch. 1976. Detection of private and common tumor-associated antigens in murine sarcomas induced by different chemical carcinogens. Int. J. Cancer 17:138–147.

Haddow, A. 1974. Molecular repair, wound healing and carcinogenesis: Tumor production, a possible overhealing. Adv. Cancer Res. 16:181–234.

Hammond, W. G., J. C. Fisher, and R. J. Rolley. 1967. Tumor-specific transplantation immunity to spontaneous mouse tumors. Surgery 62:124–133.

Harris, J. R., M. R. Price, and R. W. Baldwin. 1973. The purification of membrane-associated tumour antigens by preparative polyacrylamide gel electrophoresis. Biochim. Biophys. Acta 311:600–614.

Haywood, G. R., and C. F. McKhann. 1971. Antigenic specificities on murine sarcoma cells. J. Exp. Med. 133:1171–1187.

Hellström, K. E., and I. Hellström. 1974. Lymphocyte-mediated cytotoxicity and serum activity to tumor antigens. Adv. Immunol. 18:209–277.

Hewitt, H. B., E. R. Blake, and A. S. Walder. 1976. A critique of the evidence for active host defence against cancer, based on personal studies of 27 murine tumours of spontaneous origin. Br. J. Cancer 33:241–259.

Invernizzi, G., and G. Parmiani. 1975. Tumour-associated transplantation antigens of chemically induced sacromata cross reacting with allogenic histocompatability antigens. Nature 254:713–714.

Klein, G. 1975. Tumor-associated antigens in H-2 hemizygous isoantigenic variants of a somatic cell hybrid, derived from the fusion of a 3-methylcholanthrene-induced sarcoma and a mammary carcinoma. J. Natl. Cancer Inst. 58:383–386.

Klein, G., and E. Klein. 1975. Are methylcholanthrene-induced sarcoma-associated, rejection inducing (TSTA) antigens, modified forms of H-2 or linked determinants? Int. J. Cancer 15:879–887.

Klein, G., and E. Klein. 1977. Rejectability of virus-induced tumours and nonrejectability of spontaneous tumours—A lesson in contrasts. Transplant. Proc. 15:666–676.

Leffell, M. S., and J. H. Coggin. 1977. Common transplantation antigens on methylcholanthrene-induced murine sarcomas detected by three assays of tumor rejection. Cancer Res. 37:4112–4119.

Meschini, A., G. Invernizzi, and G. Parmiani. 1977. Expression of alien H-2 specificities on a chemically induced BALB/c fibrosarcoma. Int. J. Cancer 20:271–283.

Mondal, S., P.T. Iype, L. Griesbach, and C. Heidelberger. 1970. Antigenicity of cells derived from mouse prostate cells after malignant transformation in vitro by carcinogenic hydrocarbons. Cancer Res. 30:1593–1597.

Mondal, S., M. J. Embleton, H. Marquardt, and C. Heidelberger. 1971. Production of variants of decreased malignancy and antigenicity from clones transformed in vitro by methylcholanthrene. Int. J. Cancer 8:410–420.

Nowell, P. C. 1976. The clonal evolution of tumor cell populations. Science 194:23–28.
Pimm, M. V., and R. W. Baldwin. 1977. Antigenic differences between primary methylcholanthrene-induced rat sarcomas and postsurgical recurrences. Int. J. Cancer 20:37–43.
Prehn, R. T. 1970. Analysis of antigenic heterogeneity within individual 3-methylcholanthrene-induced mouse sarcomas. J. Natl. Cancer Inst. 45:1039–1045.
Prehn, R. T. 1975. Relationship of tumor immunogenicity to concentration of the oncogen. J. Natl. Cancer Inst. 55:189–190.
Prehn, R. T., and J. M. Main. 1957. Immunity to methylcholanthrene-induced sarcomas. J. Natl. Cancer Inst. 18:769–778.
Price, M. R., and R. W. Baldwin. 1974. Preparation of aminoazo dye induced rat hepatoma membrane fractions retaining tumour specific antigen. Br. J. Cancer 30:382–393.
Price, M. R., and R. W. Baldwin. 1975. Immunobiology of chemically induced tumors, in Cancer: A Comprehensive Treatise, F. F. Becker, ed. Vol. 4. Plenum Press, New York, pp. 209–236.
Price, M. R., and R. W. Baldwin. 1977. Shedding of tumor cell surface antigens, in Dynamic Aspects of Cell Surface Organisation. G. Poste and G. L. Nicolson, eds., Elsevier/North-Holland Biomedical Press, Amsterdam, pp. 423–471.
Rees, R. C., M. R. Price, and R. W. Baldwin. 1978. Oncodevelopmental antigen expression in chemical carcinogenesis, in Methods in Cancer Research—XV, H. Busch and W. H. Fishman, eds., Academic Press, New York (In press).
Sjögren, H. O. 1965. Transplantation methods as a tool for detection of tumor-specific antigens. Prog. Exp. Tumor Res. 6:289–322.
Ting, C-C, and R. B. Herberman. 1976. Humoral host defense mechanisms against tumors. Int. Rev. Exp. Pathol. 15:93–152.
Williams, A. F. 1977. Differentiation antigens of the lymphocyte cell surface. Contemp. Top. Mol. Immunol. 6:83–116.

Carcinogens: Identification and Mechanisms
of Action, edited by A. Clark Griffin and
Charles R. Shaw. Raven Press, New York © 1979.

Plasma Membrane Alterations during Carcinogenesis

Earl F. Walborg, Jr., James J. Starling,* Edward M. Davis,†
Douglas C. Hixson, and James P. Allison

*The University of Texas System Cancer Center Science Park, Research Division, Smithville,
Texas 78957; *Department of Biochemistry, University of Florida, Gainesville, Florida
32610; †Biology Department, Yale University, New Haven, Connecticut 06520*

The carcinogenic potential of an increasing number of natural and synthetic chemicals is being documented (Weisburger and Williams 1975, Miller and Miller 1976), and epidemiological studies are implicating a number of these chemicals in the etiology of human cancers (Higginson and Muir 1977). These cancers occur predominantly in those epithelial tissues that interface with the environment, e.g., skin, tracheobronchial tree, gastrointestinal tract, and bladder (Miller and Miller 1974). If the incidence of cancer is to be reduced, more emphasis must be placed on prevention through reduction of man's exposure to environmental carcinogens and on development of methods to inhibit or reverse early events in the carcinogenic process. Clearly, a more effective approach to cancer prevention requires a better understanding of the cellular and molecular mechanisms operative during carcinogenesis in epithelial tissues.

Elucidation of the mechanisms of carcinogenesis requires additional research on three aspects of the problem: First, delineation of the mechanisms whereby carcinogens alter the content or expression of genetic information; second, identification of the crucial phenotypic alterations that result in the escape of cells from the normal constraints on cellular proliferation and positional order; and third, clarification of the selective processes responsible for cellular evolution to the malignant state. Phenotypic alterations involving the surface properties of cells are clearly relevant to the latter two aspects of the carcinogenesis problem. The following statement by Leslie Foulds (1969) offers considerable insight into the problem of carcinogenesis:

> The central problem of neoplasia is not merely one of growth but also one of morphological pattern. The central . . . problem is one of biological organization in space and time.

Indeed, a hallmark of early events during carcinogenesis in epithelial tissues is the progressive loss of normal tissue architecture or morphological pattern (Farber 1976). Local invasion of surrounding normal tissue is an early indication of malignancy—a distinct breach in normal tissue architecture (Prehn and Prehn 1975). Morphological pattern results from the specific association of cells into multicellular units, a process that presumably involves spatial and temporal programming of recognitive macromolecules located at the cell periphery (Lilien 1969, Roth 1973, Balsamo and Lilien 1975); thus, it is not surprising that cancer has been considered a disorder of cell-cell interactions, evolving from alterations in the composition, structure, topography, and/or dynamics of the plasma membrane and associated structures (Abercrombie and Ambrose 1962, Wallach 1968, Burger 1971, Holley 1972, Emmelot 1973, Nicolson 1976b, Smith and Walborg 1977).

Conceptual advances concerning the structure of biological membranes have greatly influenced research on the role of the plasma membrane in carcinogenesis. The formulation of the fluid mosaic model of membrane structure (Singer and Nicolson 1972) stimulated research on the dynamic interactions of membrane proteins and lipids, including lipid fluidity, the mobility of membrane proteins, phase transitions, and cooperativity of protein-lipid and protein-protein interactions (Inbar *et al.* 1973b, Shinitzky and Inbar 1974a, Nicolson 1974, McConnell 1975, and Wallach 1976). The demonstration that the plasma membrane is associated with cytoskeletal elements, particularly the interaction of membrane protein with microfilaments, has provided a structural and functional link between the cellular environment and the cytoplasm (Nicolson 1976a).

ALTERATIONS OF CELL-SURFACE MICROANATOMY

The loss of positional order in cells undergoing carcinogenesis is accompanied by alterations in the cell-surface microanatomy, alterations that affect intercellular adhesion and communication. More than 20 years ago, Coman (1953) demonstrated that malignant epithelial cells exhibited decreased mutual adhesiveness and suggested that this alteration facilitated invasion and metastasis. Coman's original observations have been confirmed by more reproducible and sophisticated techniques (Modjanova and Malenkov 1973, Tjernberg and Zajicek 1965). In many cases, this defective mutual adhesiveness of malignant cells is associated with a decrease in junctional specializations. Reductions in the number of tight, gap, and desmosomal junctions have been observed following malignant transformation of a variety of epithelial tissues, and, furthermore, these reductions in junctional membranes may be correlated with invasiveness or the severity of the architectural abnormality of malignant tissues (Weinstein *et al.* 1975). Tight junctions serve as permeability seals around epithelial cells and may be important in maintaining the functional segregation of membrane macromolecules. Attenuation of tight junctions, which is a common occurrence during carcinogenesis, may result in disruption of the extracellular microenvironment, allowing direct exposure of basal cell layers to carcinogens (Weinstein *et al.* 1975).

In addition to their role in cellular adhesion, specialized intercellular junctions are also involved in cell-to-cell communication (McNutt and Weinstein 1973,

Loewenstein 1975, Weinstein *et al.* 1975). Gap junctions function as low-resistance pathways for the intercellular exchange of ions and low molecular weight metabolites; consequently, the loss of these junctions during malignant transformation results in the insulation of malignant cells from the growth-controlling influences of their normal neighbors. The formation of desmosomes may represent a complex form of intercellular cooperativity since these junctions are almost always symmetric, with a contribution of one cell matched by that of the other.

Although it seems certain that intercellular junctions play an important role in mutual cellular adhesiveness, the relative contribution of each type of cell junction to the adhesive process is largely unexplored. Mutual cellular adhesiveness is clearly a multifactorial process that does not necessarily involve junctional specializations (Revel *et al.* 1978); indeed, junction formation may be a late event in the adhesive process. Early events, involving glycosyltransferase ectoenzyme systems (Bosmann 1977), serum factors (Grinnell 1976), and sulfhydryl residues of cell-surface proteins (George and Rao 1975), may lead to physical adherence of cells without formation of specialized junctions. Subsequent reorganization of the plasma membrane, involving cytoskeletal elements (McNutt and Weinstein 1973, Revel *et al.* 1978) and/or membrane glycoproteins such as large external transformation-sensitive (LETS) protein (Hynes *et al.* 1978), may stabilize these initial contacts and ultimately lead to membrane specialization and assembly of intercellular junctions.

Recent investigations suggest that certain cell-surface properties may be modulated by submembranous arrays of microfilaments and microtubules (Nicolson 1976a). These surface modulating assemblies (Edelman 1976) have been postulated to control the mobility and topographical arrangement of cell-surface macromolecules and to regulate and transmit environmental stimuli from the cell surface to the cell interior (McClain and Edelman 1978). Indirect evidence for this concept has been obtained by observing the effects of cytoskeleton-disrupting drugs on the topographical distribution and mobility of cell-surface macromolecules (Edelman 1976, McClain and Edelman 1978). More direct evidence for transmembrane interactions has been reported by Ash and Singer (1976), who observed a close relationship between the distributions of surface-bound concanavalin A and linear arrays of intracellular myosin-containing filaments.

Currently, there is conflicting evidence concerning the role of cytoskeletal systems in malignant transformation. Initial immunofluorescence studies with antibodies directed against actin and tubulin, the major structural proteins of microfilaments and microtubules, suggested that microfilament and microtubule arrays were greatly reduced following malignant transformation by oncogenic viruses (Weber *et al.* 1974, Brinkley *et al.* 1975). Similar observations were also reported for primary cultures established from chemically induced putative premalignant lesions and carcinomas from murine mammary glands (Asch *et al.* 1977). Subsequent studies, however, have indicated that transformed cells contain significant numbers of microtubules (Osborn and Weber 1977). Furthermore, alterations of microfilament systems appear to be more closely related to adhesiveness to substrate than to acquisition of the malignant phenotype (Willingham et al. 1977).

Elucidation of the molecular mechanisms involved in intercellular adhesion and communication will require a better understanding of the complex interactions between cell-surface macromolecules and the role of the cytoskeletal systems in determining the character and extent of these interactions. In this respect, it is important to note that experimentation, to date, has utilized primarily in vitro model systems. Although such systems have contributed greatly to our understanding of the cellular and molecular events involved in the adhesive process, it remains to be determined whether adhesive interactions involved in the attachment of cells to artificial substrates are representative of those involved in cellular interactions in vivo.

ALTERATION OF PLASMA MEMBRANE LIPIDS

Studies of plasma membrane lipids relevant to carcinogenesis in vivo have focused on the content of cholesterol and the structure of the glycolipids. Cholesterol is a major determinant of the physical properties of cellular membranes, serving as a "fluidity buffer" by increasing the fluidity of the acyl moieties of phospholipids and reducing the cooperativity of gel/liquid crystal transitions (Wallach 1975); thus, alterations of cholesterol content can be expected to modify the functional properties of the plasma membrane. Hepatocellular carcinomas and leukemia cells exhibit aberrant regulation of cholesterol biosynthesis (Siperstein 1970, Heiniger et al. 1976). Exogenous cholesterol inhibits cholesterol biosynthesis in normal tissues, whereas this feedback control is lost by malignant cells. In the case of murine hepatocellular carcinoma cells, the loss of feedback control of cholesterol biosynthesis is accompanied by a significant increase in the cholesterol content of the plasma membrane (van Hoeven and Emmelot 1973). A similar correlation is not seen for the plasma membrane of leukemic cells, which, in fact, exhibit a lower cholesterol content (Inbar and Shinitzky 1974). This latter finding may be explained by an alteration in the rate of exchange of cholesterol between the plasma membrane of leukemic cells and serum lipoproteins (Inbar and Shinitzky 1974). Regardless of the mechanism or direction of the cholesterol alteration, it is clear that alterations of this magnitude significantly affect the fluidity of membrane lipid (Shinitzky and Inbar 1974a), as well as the rotational mobility (Shinitzky and Inbar 1974b) and perhaps the vertical displacement (Shinitzky and Rivnay 1977) of integral membrane proteins.

Hakomori (1975) demonstrated that malignant transformation in vitro was accompanied by compositional or structural alterations of membrane glycolipids. At confluency, nontransformed cells were able to add monosaccharides to the nonreducing termini of oligosaccharide moieties of precursor glycolipids, a process that presumably involves specific glycosyltransferases present at the cell surface (Hakomori *et al.* 1975). In contrast, transformed cells showed defective oligosaccharide chain extension with consequent accumulation of precursor glycolipids. These in vitro studies have now been extended to cells transformed in vivo, e.g., murine hepatocellular carcinomas, including minimal deviation types (Siddiqui and Hakomori 1970), murine mammary carcinoma (Keenan and Morré 1973), human renal carcinoma (Karlsson *et al.* 1974), and human leukemic cells (Hildebrand *et al.* 1972). Although there is considerable compositional variation in the glycolipids isolated from these diverse types of cancer, simplification of their oligosaccharide moieties has remained a consistent feature.

ALTERATIONS OF CELL-SURFACE ANTIGENS

The concept that the tumor cell surface differs antigenically from its normal cell counterpart has become well established since the pioneering studies of Foley (1953), Baldwin (1955), Prehn and Main (1957), and Klein *et al.* (1960). These classic studies demonstrated that tumor cells expressed neoantigens capable of inducing specific protective immune responses in syngeneic animals or in the autochthonous host. Antigens defined by such in vivo immunoprotection assays are best described as tumor-associated rejection antigens (TARA). The TARA of chemically induced tumors show extreme individual specificity even among tumors of the same histological origin induced by the same chemical agent (Gordon 1965, Baldwin and Barker 1967, Baldwin and Price 1976). Individually specific TARA have been demonstrated even among multiple tumors induced in the same host (Ishidate 1970). Physicochemical studies of the TARA of an azo-dye-induced rat hepatocellular carcinoma suggests that TARA, like histocompatibility antigens, are glycoproteins firmly embedded in the lipid bilayer of the plasma membrane (Baldwin and Glaves 1972a, Baldwin *et al.* 1973, Baldwin *et al.* 1974). However, TARA may also be found in soluble form or as immune complexes in the circulation (Bowen and Baldwin 1976, Rao and Bonavida 1977, and Price and Baldwin 1977). The elaboration of TARA by tumor cells can, as a result of the immune reponses evoked in the host, have profound effects on tumor formation, growth, and metastasis.

With the advent of sophisticated immunochemical techniques, it has become apparent that alteration of the tumor cell surface may be quite extensive and may include expression of additional antigens that are not necessarily capable of inducing protective immune responses. For example, retrodifferentiation processes associated with neoplastic transformation may result in the re-expression of fetal components. Two nonmembrane bound fetal products, α-fetoprotein (Abelev 1971) and carcinoembryonic antigen (Gold and Freedman 1965), have proved to be of some predictive value in human neoplasia (Freedman 1976). In animal models, azo-dye- and N-2-fluorenylacetamide-induced tumors as well as spontaneous tumors have been shown to express cross-reactive embryonic antigens showing tissue specificity (Baldwin *et al.* 1972, Baldwin and Vose 1974). Prehn (1972) has proposed that these cross-reactive embryonic antigens might play a role in normal cell communication and growth regulation during ontogeny; thus, inappropriate expression of embryonic cell-surface antigens in adult tissue might play a central role in determining the aberrant behavior of tumor cells. In addition to expressing normal antigens displaced in time, chemically induced tumors also exhibit altered expression of normal adult antigens. A loss of normal tissue antigens was first reported by Weiler (1959) who showed that azo-dye-induced rat hepatocellular carcinomas lacked normal liver antigens. These studies were confirmed and extended to other chemically induced tumors (Fel and Tsikarishvili 1964, Carruthers and Baumler 1965, Baldwin and Glaves 1972b). Especially interesting is the report by Muller and Sutherland (1971) who demonstrated that loss of normal epidermal antigens was most evident at the invading edge of a squamous cell carcinoma. This provocative finding suggests that alteration of the normal mosaic of surface antigens may free neoplastic cells from the constraints on positional control and lead to accelerated growth.

Equally provocative are the many reports of altered expression of histocompatibility antigens. Garrido *et al.* (1976) reported that virus-induced tumors of mice expressed H-2 antigens of foreign allotype as a result of de-repression of silent genes. Codington (1975) found that the histocompatibility antigens present on the surface of TA3 mouse mammary carcinoma cells were masked by a certain plasma membrane glycoprotein termed epiglycanin. Tsakraklides *et al.* (1974) and Haywood and McKhann (1971) found an inverse relationship between expression of tumor-associated antigens and H-2 antigens on chemically and virally induced tumors. Callahan and Allison (1978) have reported that the apparent absence of serologically detectable H-2 antigens from the surface of a murine lymphoma might be a result of masking of the H-2 antigens by intimate association with tumor antigens. Since the ubiquitous histocompatibility antigens are involved in cell communication and self-recognition (Zinkernagel and Doherty 1974, and Schrader *et al.* 1975), their modification may have profound effects both on the immune response of the host and on the growth of the tumor cells.

Collectively, these cell-surface antigenic alterations represent valuable molecular markers for cellular events associated with carcinogenesis in epithelial tissues. Available immunochemical techniques provide a sophisticated means for analyzing changes in the antigenic mosaic of the cell surface and thereby identifying plasma membrane alterations that influence cellular proliferation and positional order.

ALTERATIONS OF PLASMA MEMBRANE GLYCOPROTEINS

Many of the phenotypic alterations of cells undergoing carcinogenesis may be explained by alterations that affect the composition, structure, and/or dynamics of plasma membrane proteins (Wallach 1976). Considerable emphasis has been placed on the delineation of qualitative or quantitative alterations of glycoproteins associated with the cell periphery, e.g., the numerous antigenic alterations that involve plasma membrane glycoproteins have been discussed in the previous section. Other investigators have utilized controlled peptidolysis (Wallach 1972) of intact cells to obtain information concerning alterations of plasma membrane glycoproteins relevant to malignant transformation. Fucopeptides, cleaved from the surface of intact cells by trypsin and reduced to their limit glycopeptides by exhaustive digestion with pronase, exhibit alterations following malignant transformation in vitro (Warren *et al.* 1973). Similar results were obtained when this approach was extended to epithelial cells, e.g., normal and malignant rat liver cells (Smets *et al.* 1975). Peptidolysis of malignantly transformed cells yielded limit fucopeptides enriched in a class of glycopeptides of higher molecular weight, an alteration that may result from increased sialylation of the cell-surface glycopeptides (Warren *et al.* 1974) or from differences in the branching of their heterosaccharide moieties (Ogata *et al.* 1976).

Lectins, sugar-binding proteins, have been widely used to detect alterations of plasma membrane glycoproteins relevant to malignant transformation (Burger 1973, Smith and Walborg 1977). Interest in lectins as molecular markers for malignant transformation was stimulated by the observation that fibroblasts, propagated and transformed in vitro, acquired increased agglutinability by concanavalin A (ConA) and wheat germ agglutinin (WGA) (Inbar and Sachs 1969, Burger and Goldberg 1967). These early studies led to an explosion of experimentation to delineate the molecular basis for the altered lectin-induced agglutination of malignantly transformed cells (Nicolson 1974, Smith and Walborg 1977). It was soon apparent that lectin-induced cytoagglutination was an extremely complex reaction, dependent on many factors relating to the properties of the lectin receptors and plasma membrane. Variable properties of the lectin include saccharide specificity, valency, and molecular size and shape. The properties of the plasma membrane receptors that affect the agglutination reaction include their number, topography, binding affinity, valency, steric presentation, and lateral mobility within the membrane matrix. Recent evidence indicates that the cytoskeleton may also play a role in lectin-induced cytoagglutination by anchoring certain lectin receptors and thereby restricting their lateral mobility within the membrane matrix (Nicolson 1976a,b). Properties of the plasma membrane that affect lectin-induced cytoagglutination include its morphology, deformability, and surface charge; also to be considered are certain cellular properties, including metabolic state and phase of the cell cycle. Several hypotheses have been proposed to explain the altered lectin-induced agglutinability of malignantly transformed cells, including alterations in the expression (Burger 1969, Inbar and Sachs 1969), number (Noonan and Burger 1973), structure (Burger 1973, Smith and Walborg 1977), topography (Nicolson 1971), or dynamics (Nicolson 1973, Inbar *et al.* 1973a) of the cell-surface lectin receptors. Although no unifying hypothesis to explain the increased agglutinability of malignantly transformed cells has emerged, considerable new information concerning the surface of normal and malignant cells has been gained.

Most of the investigations regarding lectin-induced cytoagglutination have utilized cells propagated and transformed in vitro. It is essential that these studies be extended to epithelial cells undergoing carcinogenesis in vivo. The efforts of this laboratory have been devoted to this problem and have focused on the interaction of lectins with normal and malignant rat liver cells.

CONCANAVALIN A AS A MOLECULAR PROBE OF THE SURFACE PROPERTIES OF NORMAL AND MALIGNANT RAT LIVER CELLS

Experimental Model

This laboratory has extended the use of lectins to the investigation of normal and malignant rat liver cells, a cell system that serves as a model for carcinogenesis in epithelial tissues. This paper summarizes some of our recent studies on the interaction of ConA with rat hepatocytes and Novikoff ascites hepatocellular carcinoma cells (Novikoff 1957) and suggests directions for future research on the role of the plasma membrane in carcinogenesis.

Suspensions of rat hepatocytes were isolated by perfusion of the intact liver by an adaptation (Starling et al. 1977) of the method of Bonney (1974). Bovine serum albumin was added to the collagenase-containing perfusion medium to minimize the action of proteases derived from lysed cells or present as contaminants in the enzyme preparation. Hepatocytes prepared by this procedure were 78% viable, as determined by dye exclusion, and exhibited excellent morphology and ultrastructural integrity (Starling et al. 1977). Novikoff ascites tumor cells were prepared as described previously (Starling et al. 1977).

Concanavalin A-Induced Agglutination of Hepatocytes and Novikoff Hepatoma Cells

Lectin-induced cytoagglutination was measured by a quantitative assay (Davis et al. 1976) adapted from the method of Oppenheimer and Odencrantz (1972). This assay measures the degree of agglutination as a function of the disappearance of single cells from a cell suspension containing varying concentrations of lectin. With this method, it was possible to assess accurately the concentration of lectin necessary for 5% agglutination (threshold agglutination) or 50% agglutination (half-maximal agglutination). The ConA-induced agglutination of Novikoff cells and hepatocytes was compared by this assay (Table 1). Direct quantitative comparison between the agglutination reactions of the two cell types is not possible because of inherent differences between the cell systems, including differences in cell size and the presence of some cell doublets and higher aggregates in suspensions of hepatocytes (Starling et al. 1977). This latter factor decreases the sensitivity of the agglutination assay with hepatocytes. An important fact remains, i.e., both Novikoff cells and hepatocytes are agglutinated by low concentrations of ConA; thus, unlike in vitro fibroblast model systems, ConA-induced agglutination cannot be used as a molecular marker for malignant transformation of rat liver cells. This observation differs from that of Becker (1974) who reported

TABLE 1. *Concanavalin A-induced agglutination of hepatocytes and Novikoff tumor cells*

	Lectin concentration (μg/ml) required for agglutination	
Cells and treatment	Threshold	Half maximal
Hepatocytes		
Untreated	2.5	23
Incubated control*	3.4	23
Papain-digested	0.78	6.4
Novikoff cells		
Untreated	0.97	4.5
Incubated control*	0.93	5.3
Papain-digested	1.7	8.5

* Incubated under the conditions of papain digestion but without enzyme.
(Adapted from Starling *et al.* [1977] and used with permission of Academic Press.)

that collagenase-dispersed adult hepatocytes were not agglutinated by high concentrations of ConA. Becker (1974), however, used an isolation technique that did not employ perfusion of the liver in situ, and such techniques have been shown to yield cells of low viability (Schreiber and Schreiber 1972).

Binding of Concanavalin A to the Surface of Normal and Malignant Rat Liver Cells

The binding of lectin to the surface of hepatocytes and Novikoff cells was investigated using ^{125}I-labeled ConA (Davis *et al.* 1977). The method of Steck and Wallach (1965) was used to calculate the amount of ConA bound per cell (Table 2). In addition, the density of surface-bound ConA was calculated,

TABLE 2. *Binding of ConA to the surface of hepatocytes and Novikoff tumor cells*

Cells and treatment	Molecules bound per cell ($\times 10^{-6}$)	Molecules bound per μm^{-2} ($\times 10^{-3}$)
Hepatocytes		
Untreated	180	130
Incubated control*	110	80
Papain-digested	96	69
Novikoff cells		
Untreated	64	72
Incubated control*	140	160
Papain-digested	17	19

* Incubated under the conditions of papain digestion but without enzyme.
(Adapted from Starling *et al.* [1977] and used with permission of Academic Press.)

assuming the cells to be perfect spheres. Considering the errors inherent in estimating the surface area of cells (Collard and Temmink 1975), it is clear that the average densities of surface-bound ConA were similar for hepatocytes and Novikoff cells. Since binding studies on intact cells did not reveal significant differences between normal and malignant rat liver cells, another experimental approach was pursued.

Plasma membrane glycoproteins can be degraded by proteases (Wallach 1972); therefore, the effect of papain digestion on the binding of ConA to hepatocytes and Novikoff cells was investigated (see Table 2). Proteolysis conditions were chosen such that maximal release of cell-surface sialic acid was obtained with minimal cell lysis, i.e., incubation with 0.02% papain for 40 minutes at 37°C (Starling *et al.* 1977). Two differences in the surface properties of hepatocytes and Novikoff cells were noted: First, the buffer used for papain digestion had a differential effect on the binding of ConA to the two cell types, increasing binding to Novikoff cells and decreasing binding to hepatocytes. Although this difference has not been explored in any depth, it may reflect the removal of peripheral proteins that mask cell-surface ConA receptor or the removal of peripheral glycoproteins possessing ConA receptor activity. Second, there is a marked reduction in the binding of ConA to papain-digested Novikoff cells. Comparison of ConA binding to papain-digested cells and their incubated controls revealed that controlled proteolysis resulted in an 88% reduction in the amount of ConA bound to Novikoff cells, but only a 13% reduction in the amount of ConA bound to hepatocytes.

Isolation of Glycopeptides Cleaved from the Surface of Hepatocytes and Novikoff Cells by Papain

The results of the ConA binding studies predict that more glycopeptides bearing ConA receptor activity should be released from the surface of Novikoff cells than from hepatocytes. Nondialyzable cell-surface glycopeptides were prepared, and subjected to gel filtration on Sephadex G-50 (Starling *et al.* 1977). Papain digestion released equivalent amounts of cell-surface glycopeptides from both hepatocytes and Novikoff cells (Starling *et al.* 1977).

The elution profiles of the glycopeptides from Sephadex G-50 are shown in Figure 1. The upper panel shows the elution profile of glycopeptides cleaved from the surface of Novikoff cells. Two distinct glycopeptide fractions were present: a fraction excluded from the gel, designated crude sialoglycopeptide fraction A (C-SGP-A), and a lower molecular weight fraction partially accessible to the gel matrix (C-SGP-C). An intermediate fraction, C-SGP-B, was also pooled. The elution profile of the glycopeptides cleaved from the surface of hepatocytes was markedly different. Little sialic acid was excluded from the gel; rather, 90% of the sialic acid was contained in glycopeptides partially accessible to the gel matrix. The exclusion limit of the Sephadex G-50, calibrated with oligosaccharides and glycopeptide standards, is 4,200 daltons (Bhatti and

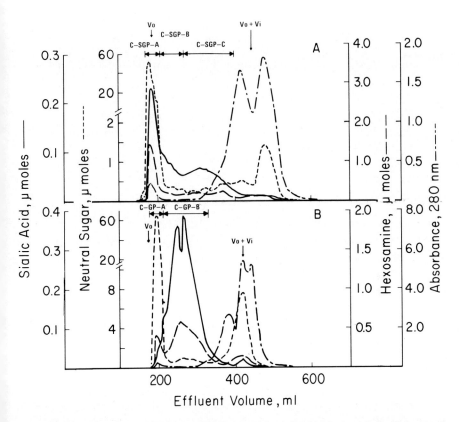

FIG. 1. Gel filtration of the cell-surface glycopeptides from A, Novikoff tumor cells; B, enzymatically dispersed hepatocytes. The column (2.5 × 90 cm) of Sephadex G-50 was equilibrated and eluted with 0.1 N acetic acid at a flow rate of 20 ml/hr at 23°C. The samples were applied in 3 ml; fraction size was 5 ml. The column effluent was analyzed as described previously (Starling *et al.* 1977). Sugar concentrations are expressed as μmole/fraction. C-SGP was isolated from 56 ml of packed Novikoff tumor cells, while C-GP was isolated from 65 ml of packed enzymatically dispersed hepatocytes. The volume outside the gel matrix (V_o) was determined with Blue Dextran 2,000 (Pharmacia). The sum of the volumes inside and outside the gel matrix ($V_o + V_i$) was determined with Cl⁻ as detected by precipitation with Ag⁺. (Reproduced from Starling *et al.* 1977, with permission of Academic Press.)

Clamp 1968); consequently, the hepatocyte sialoglycopeptides have molecular weights between 2,600 and 4,200 daltons. Two glycopeptide fractions were pooled from this column, C-GP-A, crude glycopeptide fraction A, and the major sialoglycopeptide fraction, C-GP-B.

ConA Receptor Activity of Glycopeptides Cleaved from the Surface of Hepatocytes and Novikoff Cells by Papain

The ConA receptor activity of cell-surface glycopeptides from hepatocytes and Novikoff cells was assayed by a hemagglutination inhibition assay (Smith

TABLE 3. *ConA receptor activity of cell-surface glycopeptides from hepatocytes and Novikoff cells*

Glycopeptide fraction	Yield (mg/100 mg glycopeptide)	Specific ConA receptor activity (HAIU/mg)*
Hepatocyte		
C–GP–A	17	<70
C–GP–B	83	<70
Novikoff cells		
C–SGP–A	26	2,500
C–SGP–B	29	710
C–SGP–C	45	250
Ovalbumin glycopeptide		2,200

* Receptor activities are expressed as hemagglutination inhibition units (HAIU), as described by Smith and Walborg (1976).
(Adapted from Starling *et al.* [1977] and used with permission of Academic Press.)

and Walborg 1976). This semiquantitative method measures the ability of glycopeptides to inhibit ConA-induced agglutination of guinea pig erythrocytes. Consistent with the binding studies, the glycopeptide fractions from hepatocytes possessed no detectable ConA receptor activity, whereas the sialoglycopeptide fractions from Novikoff cells possessed potent ConA receptor activity (Table 3). Furthermore, in terms of recovery, the macrosialoglycopeptide fraction (C-SGP-A) contained > 80% of the total ConA receptor activity of the papain-released glycopeptides. Little or no macrosialoglycopeptides were released from rat hepatocytes.

CONCLUSIONS

These investigations demonstrate the utility of lectins as molecular probes for detecting cell-surface alterations relevant to carcinogenesis of epithelial tissues. Comparative studies on rat hepatocytes and Novikoff ascites hepatocellular carcinoma cells revealed no significant differences in the ConA-induced cytoagglutination or in the average density of surface-bound ConA on hepatocytes and Novikoff cells. Differences were noted, however, in the susceptibility of cell-surface ConA receptors to cleavage by protease, the cell-surface ConA receptors of Novikoff cells being more labile to cleavage by papain. Furthermore, qualitative differences in the glycopeptides cleaved from the cell surface were demonstrated by gel filtration and assay of their ConA-receptor activity. These observations indicate the existence of qualitative differences in the plasma membrane glycoproteins for normal and malignant rat liver cells, differences that may provide an objective marker for malignant transformation of hepatocytes in vivo.

Direction for Future Research

If we are to understand cancer causation in human populations, increasing emphasis must be given to the investigation of carcinogenesis in epithelial tissues. Our present knowledge concerning the role of the plasma membrane in malignant transformation relies heavily on data obtained using nonepithelial cell models, such as mammalian fibroblasts propagated and transformed in vitro and cells of lymphoid origin. Although these systems will continue to yield valuable data concerning the plasma membranes of normal and malignantly transformed cells, extrapolation of this information to epithelial cells is fraught with difficulty. Our studies on the ConA-induced agglutination rat hepatocytes and hepatocellular carcinoma cells clearly demonstrate that it is not possible to generalize observations made in the fibroblast models to the in vivo situation involving epithelial cells. In addition, the in vitro fibroblast cell models possess several serious disadvantages: (1) long-term culture in vitro selects for cells with specialized surface properties, making any extrapolation to the in vivo situation of questionable value, and (2) the in vitro models do not adequately address the process of cellular selection, a crucial aspect of carcinogenesis in epithelial tissues.

Many investigations, including those reported herein, have compared the surface properties of normal cells to those of transplantable tumor cells. Such studies cannot easily distinguish between alterations induced during malignant transformation and those that occur during progression of the tumor to a more malignant state. Future research should focus on epithelial cell models that yield identifiable cell populations, representing various stages of cellular evolution to malignancy. Several epithelial cell systems are available for such studies, e.g., chemically induced carcinogenesis of rat liver (Newberne 1976) or mouse mammary (Medina 1976) cells. Putative premalignant lesions have been identified in both these epithelial tissues. In the case of N-2-fluorenylacetamide-induced hepatocarcinogenesis in the rat, reversible and irreversible putative premalignant lesions have been partially resolved (Teebor and Becker 1972). Only by studying such systems will it be possible to correlate plasma membrane alterations with early events in the carcinogenic process, malignant transformation, and progression of a tumor to a more malignant state.

ACKNOWLEDGMENTS

The original research reported herein was supported by grants from the National Cancer Institute (CA-11710 and CA-18829), the Paul and Mary Haas Foundation, and the George and Mary Josephine Hamman Foundation. J. J. S. was the recipient of a Rosalie B. Hite predoctoral fellowship in cancer research. E. M. D. was the recipient of a predoctoral fellowship from the American Legion Auxiliary.

REFERENCES

Abelev, G. I. 1971. Alpha-fetoprotein in oncogenesis and its association with malignant tumors. Adv. Cancer Res. 14:295–358.

Abercrombie, M., and E. J. Ambrose. 1962. The surface properties of cancer cells. A review. Cancer Res. 22:525–548.

Asch, B. B., D. Medina, and B. R. Brinkley. 1977. Cytoskeletal changes during neoplastic progression of mouse mammary epithelial cells. J. Cell Biol. 75:292a.

Ash, J. F., and S. J. Singer. 1976. Concanavalin A-induced transmembrane linkage of concanavalin A surface receptors to intracellular myosin-containing filaments. Proc. Natl. Acad. Sci. USA 73:4575–4579.

Baldwin, R. W. 1955. Immunity to methylcholanthrene-induced tumours in inbred rats following atrophy and regression of the implanted tumours. Br. J. Cancer 9:652–657.

Baldwin, R. W., and C. R. Barker. 1967. Demonstration of tumour-specific humoral antibody against aminoazo dye-induced rat hepatoma. Br. J. Cancer 21:793–800.

Baldwin, R. W., J. G. Bowen, and M. R. Price. 1974. Solubilization of membrane associated tumor specific antigen by β-glucosidase. Biochim. Biophys. Acta 367:47–58.

Baldwin, R. W., and D. Glaves. 1972a. Solubilization of tumor specific antigen from plasma membrane of an aminoazo-dye induced rat hepatoma. Clin. Exp. Immunol. 11:51–56.

Baldwin, R. W., and D. Glaves. 1972b. Deletion of liver-cell surface membrane components from aminoazo-dye-induced rat hepatomas. Int. J. Cancer 9:76–85.

Baldwin, R. W., D. Glaves, and R. W. Vose. 1972. Embryonic antigen expression in chemically induced rat hepatomas and sarcomas. Int. J. Cancer 10:233–243.

Baldwin, R. W., J. R. Harris, and M. R. Price. 1973. Fractionation of plasma membrane associated tumor specific antigen from aminoazo-dye induced rat hepatomas. Int. J. Cancer 11:385–397.

Baldwin, R. W., and M. R. Price. 1976. Cell membrane associated antigens in chemical carcinogenesis, *in* Biomembranes, L. A. Manson, ed., Vol. 8, Plenum Press, New York, pp. 89–129.

Baldwin, R. W., and B. M. Vose. 1974. Embryonic antigen expression on 2-acetylaminofluorene induced and spontaneously arising rat tumours. Br. J. Cancer 30:209–214.

Balsamo, J., and J. E. Lilien. 1975. The binding of tissue-specific adhesive molecules to the cell surface. A molecular basis for specificity. Biochemistry 14:167–171.

Becker, F. F. 1974. Differential lectin-induced agglutination of fetal, dividing-postnatal, and malignant hepatocytes. Proc. Natl. Acad. Sci. USA 71:4307–4311.

Bhatti, T., and J. R. Clamp. 1968. Determination of molecular weight of glycopeptides by exclusion chromatography. Biochim. Biophys. Acta 170:206–208.

Bonney, R. J. 1974. Adult liver parenchymal cells in primary culture. Characteristics and cell recognition standards in vitro. In Vitro 10:130–142.

Bosmann, H. B. 1977. Cell surface enzymes. Effects on mitotic activity and cell adhesion. Int. Rev. Cytol. 50:1–23.

Bowen, J. G., and R. W. Baldwin. 1976. Isolation and characterization of tumour-specific antigen from the serum of rats bearing transplanted aminoazo dye-induced hepatomas. Transplantation 21:213–219.

Brinkley, B. R., G. M. Fuller, and D. P. Highfield. 1975. Cytoplasmic microtubules in normal and transformed cells in culture. Analysis by tubulin antibody immunofluorescence. Proc. Natl. Acad. Sci. USA 72:4981–4985.

Burger, M. M. 1969. A difference in the architecture of the surface membrane of normal and virally transformed cells. Proc. Natl. Acad. Sci. USA 62:994–1001.

Burger, M. M. 1971. Cell surfaces in neoplastic transformation. Curr. Top. Cell. Regul. 3:35–93.

Burger, M. M. 1973. Surface changes in transformed cells detected by lectins. Fed. Proc. 32:91–101.

Burger, M. M., and A. R. Goldberg. 1967. Identification of a tumor-specific determinant on neoplastic cell surfaces. Proc. Natl. Acad. Sci. USA 57:359–366.

Callahan, G. N., and J. P. Allison. 1978. H-2 antigens on a murine lymphoma are associated with additional proteins. Nature 271:165–167.

Carruthers, C., and A. Baumler. 1965. Immunochemical staining with fluorescein-labeled antibodies as an aid in the study of skin cancer formation. J. Natl. Cancer Inst. 34:191–200.

Codington, J. R. 1975. Masking of cell-surface antigens on cancer cells, *in* Cellular Membranes and Tumor Cell Behavior (The University of Texas System Cancer Center 28th Annual Symposium on Fundamental Cancer Research, 1975), Williams and Wilkins Co., Baltimore, pp. 399–419.

Collard, J. G., and J. H. M. Temmink. 1975. Differences in density of concanavalin A-binding sites due to differences in surface morphology of suspended normal and transformal 3T3 fibroblasts. J. Cell Sci. 19:21–32.

Coman, D. R. 1953. Mechanism responsible for the origin and distribution of blood borne tumor metastases. A review. Cancer Res. 13:397–410.

Davis, E. M., J. J. Starling, and E. F. Walborg, Jr. 1976. A microquantitative method to characterize lectin-induced cytoagglutination. Exp. Cell Res. 99:37–46.

Davis, E. M., D. D. Tsay, M. Schlamowitz, and E. F. Walborg, Jr. 1977. A device to simplify the assay of ligand binding to cell surfaces. Anal. Biochem. 80:416–419.

Edelman, G. M. 1976. Surface modulation in cell recognition and cell growth. Science 192:218–226.

Emmelot, P. 1973. Biochemical properties of normal and neoplastic cell surfaces. A review. Eur. J. Cancer 9:319–333.

Farber, E. 1976. Putative precursor lesions. Summary and some analytical considerations. Cancer Res. 36:2703–2705.

Fel, V. J., and T. N. Tsikarishvili. 1964. Reduction of normal muscle antigens in rat tumors of muscle origin induced by intramuscular injection of methylcholanthrene. Cancer Res. 24:1675–1677.

Foley, E. J. 1953. Antigenic properties of methycholanthrene-induced tumors in mice of the strain of origin. Cancer Res. 13:835–837.

Foulds, L. 1969. Neoplastic Development. Vol. 1. Academic Press, New York, p. 224.

Freedman, S. O. 1976. Antigens in tumors, *in* Scientific Foundations of Oncology, T. Symington and R. L. Carter, eds., Year Book Medical Publishers, Chicago, pp. 505–514.

Garrido, F., V. Schirrmacher, and H. Festenstein. 1976. H-2-like specificities of foreign haplotypes appearing on a mouse sarcoma after vaccinia virus infection. Nature 259:228–230.

George, J. V., and K. V. Rao. 1975. The role of sulfhydryl groups in cellular adhesiveness. J. Cell. Physiol. 85:547–556.

Gold, P., and S. O. Freedman. 1965. Demonstration of tumor specific antigens in human colonic carcinomata by immunological tolerance and absorption techniques. J. Exp. Med. 121:439–462.

Gordon, J. 1965. Isoantigenicity of liver tumours induced by an azo dye. Br. J. Cancer 19:387–391.

Grinnell, F. 1976. Biochemical analysis of cell adhesion to a substratum and its possible relevance to cell metastasis, *in* Membranes and Neoplasia. New Approaches and Strategies, V. T. Marchesi, ed., Alan L. Liss, Inc., New York, pp. 227–236.

Hakomori, S. 1975. Structure and organization of cell surface glycolipids. Dependency on cell growth and malignant transformation. Biochim. Biophys. Acta 417:55–89.

Hakomori, S., C. G. Gahmberg, R. A. Laine, and G. Yogeeswaran. 1975. Organization and modification of membrane glycolipids and glycoproteins, *in* Cellular Membranes and Tumor Cell Behavior (The University of Texas System Cancer Center 28th Annual Symposium on Fundamental Cancer Research, 1975), Williams and Wilkins Co., Baltimore, pp. 289–308.

Haywood, G. R., and C. F. McKhann. 1971. Antigenic specificities on tumor cells. Reciprocal relationship between normal transplantation antigens (H-2) and tumor-specific immunogenicity. J. Exp. Med. 133:1171–1187.

Heiniger, H. J., H. W. Chan, O. L. Applegate, Jr., L. P. Schacter, B. Z. Schacter, and P. N. Anderson. 1976. Elevated synthesis of cholesterol in human leukemic cells. J. Mol. Med. 1:109–116.

Higginson, J., and C. S. Muir. 1977. The role of epidemiology in elucidating the importance of environmental factors in human cancer. Bull. Cancer 64:365–384.

Hildebrand, J., P. A. Stryckmans, and J. Vanhouche. 1972. Gangliosides in leukemic and non-leukemic human leukocytes. Biochim. Biophys. Acta 260:272–278.

Holley, R. 1972. A unifying hypothesis concerning the nature of malignant growth. Proc. Natl. Acad. Sci. USA 69:2840–2841.

Hynes, R. O., I. V. Ali, V. M. Mautner, and A. Destree. 1978. LETS glycoprotein. Arrangement and function at the cell surface, *in* The Molecular Basis of Cell-Cell Interactions, R. A. Lerner and D. Bergsma, eds., Alan L. Liss, Inc., New York, pp. 139–153.

Inbar, M., C. Huet, A. R. Oseroff, and H. Ben-Bassat. 1973a. Inhibition of lectin agglutinability by fixation of the surface membrane. Biochim. Biophys. Acta 311:594–599.

Inbar, M., and L. Sachs. 1969. Interaction of the carbohydrate-binding protein concanavalin A with normal and transformed cells. Proc. Natl. Acad. Sci. USA 63:1418–1425.

Inbar, M., and M. Shinitzky. 1974. Cholesterol as a bioregulator in the development and inhibition of leukemia. Proc. Natl. Acad. Sci. USA 71:4229–4231.

Inbar, M., M. Shinitzky, and L. Sachs. 1973b. Rotational relaxation time of concanavalin A bound to the surface membrane of normal and malignant transformal cells. J. Mol. Biol. 81:245–253.

Ishidate, M. 1970. Antigenic specificity of hepatoma cell lines derived from a single rat. (Abstract) 10th International Cancer Congress, p. 227.

Karlsson, K. A., B. E. Sammuelsson, T. Scherstén, G. O. Steen, and L. Wahlquist. 1974. The sphingolipid composition of human renal carcinoma. Biochim. Biophys. Acta 337:349–355.

Keenan, T. W., and D. J. Morré. 1973. Mammary carcinoma. Enzymatic block in disialoganglioside biosynthesis. Science 182:935–937.

Klein, G., H. O. Sjögren, E. Klein, and K. E. Hellstrom. 1960. Demonstration of resistance against methylcholanthrene-induced sarcomas in the primary autochthonous host. Cancer Res. 20:1561–1572.

Lilien, J. E. 1969. Toward a molecular explanation for specific cell adhesion. Curr. Top. Dev. Biol. 4:169–195.

Loewenstein, W. R. 1975. Intercellular communication in normal and neoplastic cells, *in* Cellular Membranes and Tumor Cell Behavior (The University of Texas System Cancer Center 28th Annual Symposium on Fundamental Cancer Research, 1975), Williams and Wilkins Co., Baltimore, pp. 239–248.

McClain, D. A., and G. M. Edelman. 1978. Surface modulation and transmembrane control, *in* The Molecular Basis of Cell-Cell Interactions, R. A. Lerner and D. Bergsma, eds., Alan L. Liss, Inc., New York, pp. 1–28.

McConnell, H. M. 1975. Role of lipid in membrane structure and function, *in* Cellular Membranes and Tumor Cell Behavior (The University of Texas System Cancer Center 28th Annual Symposium on Fundamental Cancer Research 1975), Williams and Wilkins Co., Baltimore, pp. 61–80.

McNutt, S., and R. S. Weinstein. 1973. Membrane ultrastructure at mammalian intercellular junctions. Prog. Biophys. Mol. Biol. 26:47–101.

Medina, D. 1976. Preneoplastic lesions in murine mammary cancer. Cancer Res. 36:2589–2595.

Miller, J. A., and E. C. Miller. 1974. Some current thresholds of research in chemical carcinogenesis, *in* Chemical Carcinogenesis, P. O. P. Ts'o and J. DiPaola, eds., Marcel Dekker, New York, pp. 62–64.

Miller, J. A., and E. C. Miller. 1976. Carcinogens occurring naturally in foods. Fed. Proc. 35:1316–1321.

Modjanova, E., and A. Malenkov. 1973. Alteration of properties of cell contacts during progression of hepatomas. Exp. Cell Res. 76:305–314.

Muller, H. K., and R. C. Sutherland. 1971. Epidermal antigens in cutaneous dysplasia and neoplasia. Nature 220:384–385.

Newberne, P. M. 1976. Experimental hepatocellular carcinogenesis. Cancer Res. 36:2573–2578.

Nicolson, G. L. 1971. Difference in topology of normal and tumor cell membranes shown by different surface distributions of ferritin-conjugated concanavalin A. Nature New Biol. 233:244–246.

Nicolson, G. L. 1973. Temperature-dependent mobility of concanavalin A sites on tumor cell surfaces. Nature New Biol. 243:218–220.

Nicolson, G. L. 1974. The interactions of lectins with animal cell surfaces. Int. Rev. Cytol. 39:89–190.

Nicolson, G. L. 1976a. Transmembrane control of the receptors on normal and tumor cells. I. Cytoplasmic influence over cell surface components. Biochim. Biophys. Acta 457:57–108.

Nicolson, G. L. 1976b. Transmembrane control of the receptors on normal and tumor cells. II. Surface changes associated with transformation and malignancy. Biochim. Biophys. Acta 458:1–72.

Noonan, K. D., and M. M. Burger. 1973. The relationship of concanavalin A binding to lectin-initiated cell agglutination. J. Cell. Biol. 59:134–142.

Novikoff, A. G. 1957. A transplantable rat liver tumor induced by 4-dimethyl-aminoazobenzene. Cancer Res. 17:1010–1027.

Ogata, S. I., T. Muramatsu, and A. Kobata. 1976. New structural characteristics of the large glycopeptides from transformed cells. Nature 259:580–582.

Oppenheimer, S. B., and J. Odencrantz. 1972. A quantitative assay for measuring cell agglutination. Agglutination of sea urchin embryo and mouse teratoma cells by concanavalin A. Exp. Cell Res. 73:475–480.

Osborn, M., and K. Weber. 1977. The display of microtubules in transformed cells. Cell 12:561–571.

Prehn, R. T. 1972. Summary of the tumor antigens session, *in* Cellular Antigens, A. Nowotny, ed., Springer-Verlag, New York, pp. 320–323.

Prehn, R. T., and J. M. Main. 1957. Immunity to methylcholanthrene-induced sarcomas. J. Natl. Cancer Inst. 18:769–778.

Prehn, R. T., and L. M. Prehn. 1975. Pathobiology of neoplasia. A teaching monograph. Am. J. Pathol. 80:529–550.

Price, M. R., and R. W. Baldwin. 1977. Shedding of tumor cell-surface antigens, *in* Dynamic Aspects of Cell Surface Organization, G. Poste and G. L. Nicolson, eds., Elsevier/North Holland Biomedical Press, Amsterdam, pp. 423–471.

Rao, V. S., and B. Bonavida. 1977. Detection of soluble tumor-associated antigens in serum of tumor-bearing rats and their immunological role in vivo. Cancer Res. 37:3385–3389.

Revel, J. P., G. Parr, E. B. Griepp, R. Johnson, and M. M. Miller. 1978. Cell movement and intercellular contact formation, *in* The Molecular Basis of Cell-Cell Interactions, R. A. Lerner and D. Bergsma, eds., Alan L. Liss, Inc., New York, pp. 67–81.

Roth, S. 1973. A molecular model for cell interaction. Q. Rev. Biol. 48:541–563.

Schrader, J. W., B. H. Cummingham, and G. M. Edelman. 1975. Functional interactions of viral and histocompatibility antigens at tumor cell surfaces. Proc. Natl. Acad. Sci. USA 72:5066–5070.

Schreiber, G., and M. Schreiber. 1972. The preparation of single cell suspensions from liver and their use for the study of protein synthesis. Subcell. Biochem. 2:321–383.

Shinitzky, M., and M. Inbar. 1974a. Difference in microviscosity induced by different cholesterol levels in the surface membrane lipid of normal lymphocytes and malignant lymphoma cells. J. Mol. Biol. 85:603–615.

Shinitzky, M., and M. Inbar. 1974b. Rotational diffusion of lectins bound to the surface membrane of normal lymphocytes. FEBS Lett. 34:247–250.

Shinitzky, M., and B. Rivnay. 1977. Degree of exposure of membrane proteins determined by fluorescence quenching. Biochemistry 16:982–986.

Siddiqui, B., and S. Hakomori. 1970. Change of glycolipid pattern in Morris hepatomas 5123 and 7800. Cancer Res. 30:2930–2936.

Singer, S. J., and G. L. Nicolson. 1972. The fluid mosaic model of the structure of cell membranes. Science 175:720–731.

Siperstein, M. D. 1970. Regulation of cholesterol biosynthesis in normal and malignant tissues. Curr. Top. Cell. Regul. 2:65–100.

Smets, L. A., W. P. van Beek, J. G. Collard, H. Temmink, B. van Gils, and P. Emmelot. 1975. Comparative evaluation of plasma membrane alterations associated with neoplasia, *in* Cellular Membranes and Tumor Cell Behavior (The University of Texas System Cancer Center 28th Annual Symposium on Fundamental Cancer Research, 1975), Williams and Wilkins Co., Baltimore, pp. 269–287.

Smith, D. F., and E. F. Walborg, Jr. 1976. A microhemagglutination inhibition assay for concanavalin A receptor activity, *in* Concanavalin as a Tool, H. Bittiger and H. P. Schnebli, eds., John Wiley and Sons, New York, pp. 271–277.

Smith, D. F., and E. F. Walborg, Jr. 1977. The tumor cell periphery. Carbohydrate components, *in* Mammalian Cell Membranes, G. A. Jamieson and D. M. Robinson, eds. Vol. 3. Butterworths, Boston, pp. 115–146.

Starling, J. J., S. C. Capetillo, G. Neri, and E. F. Walborg, Jr. 1977. Surface properties of normal and neoplastic rat liver cells. Lectin-induced cytoagglutination and lectin receptor activity of cell-surface glycopeptides. Exp. Cell Res. 104:177–190.

Steck, T. L., and D. F. H. Wallach. 1965. The binding of kidney-bean phytohemagglutinin by Ehrlich ascites carcinoma. Biochim. Biophys. Acta 97:510–522.

Teebor, G. W., and F. F. Becker. 1972. Regression and persistence of hyperplastic hepatic nodules induced by N-2-fluorenylacetamide and their relationship to hepatocarcinogenesis. Cancer Res. 31:1–3.

Tjernberg, B., and J. Zajicek. 1965. Cannulation of lymphatics leaving cancerous nodes in studies on tumor spread. Acta Cytol. 9:197–202.

Tsakraklides, E., C. Smith, J. H. Kersey, and R. A. Good. 1974. Transplantation antigens (H-2) on virally and chemically transformed BALB/3T3 fibroblasts in culture. J. Natl. Cancer Inst. 52:1499–1504.

van Hoeven, R. P., and P. Emmelot. 1973. Plasma membrane lipids of normal and neoplastic tissues, *in* Tumor Lipids: Biochemistry and Metabolism, R. Wood, ed., American Oil Chemists Society, Champaign, Illinois, pp. 126–138.

Wallach, D. F. H. 1968. Cellular membranes and tumor behavior. A new hypothesis. Proc. Natl. Acad. Sci. USA 61:868–874.

Wallach, D. F. H. 1972. The disposition of proteins in the plasma membrane of animal cells. Analytical approaches using controlled peptidolysis and protein labels. Biochim. Biophys. Acta 265:61–83.

Wallach, D. F. H. 1975. Closing remarks—Membrane aberrations in neoplasia. Relevance to the malignant process, *in* Cellular Membranes and Tumor Cell Behavior (The University of Texas System Cancer Center 28th Annual Symposium on Fundamental Cancer Research, 1975), Williams and Wilkins Co., Baltimore, pp. 549–567.

Wallach, D. F. H. 1976. Membrane anomalies of neoplastic cells. Med. Hypotheses 2:241–256.

Warren, L., J. P. Fuhrer, and C. A. Buck. 1973. Surface glycoproteins of cells before and after transformation by oncogenic viruses. Fed. Proc. 32:80–85.

Weber, K., E. Lazarides, R. D. Goldman, A. Vogel, and R. Pollack. 1974. Localization and distribution of actin fibers in normal, transformed and revertant cells. Cold Spring Harbor Symp. Quant. Biol. 39:363–369.

Weiler, E. 1959. Loss of specific cell antigen in relation to carcinogenesis, *in* Ciba Foundation Symposium on Carcinogenesis. Mechanism of Action, G. E. W. Wolstenholme and M. O'Conner, eds., J. and A. Churchill, Ltd., London, pp. 155–178.

Weinstein, R. S., F. B. Merk, and J. Alroy. 1975. The structure and function of intercellular junctions in cancer. Adv. Cancer Res. 20:23–89.

Weisburger, J. H., and G. M. Williams. 1975. Metabolism of chemical carcinogens, *in* Cancer: A Comprehensive Treatise, F. F. Becker, ed. Vol. 1. Plenum Press, New York, pp. 185–234.

Willingham, M. C., K. M. Yamada, S. S. Yamada, J. Pouyssegur, and I. Pastan. 1977. Microfilament bundles and cell shape are related to adhesiveness to substratum and are dissociable from growth control in cultured fibroblasts. Cell 10:375–380.

Zinkernagel, R. M., and P. C. Doherty. 1974. Immunological surveillance against altered self components by sensitized T lymphocytes in lymphocytic choriomeningitis. Nature 251:547–548.

Carcinogens: Identification and Mechanisms of Action, edited by A. Clark Griffin and Charles R. Shaw. Raven Press, New York © 1979.

Molecular and Cellular Events Associated with the Action of Initiating Carcinogens and Tumor Promoters

I. Bernard Weinstein, Hiroshi Yamasaki, Michael Wigler, Lih-Syng Lee, Paul B. Fisher, Alan Jeffrey, and Dezider Grunberger

Division of Environmental Sciences and Institute of Cancer Research, Columbia University, College of Physicians and Surgeons, New York, New York 10032

The preceding papers in this Symposium have emphasized that the carcinogenic process is multifactor in its causation and multistep in its evolution. Indeed, the presentation of this year's Bertner award to Drs. Isaac Berenblum and Philippe Shubik recognizes their fundamental contributions to this concept. The two-stage mouse skin carcinogenesis system developed by these and other investigators most clearly demonstrates at least two qualitatively different phases of the carcinogenic process and indicates that these two phases are elicited by two distinctly separate classes of chemical agents—initiating agents and promoters (for reviews see Van Duuren 1969, Boutwell 1974, Hecker 1975, Berenblum 1975). This paper will briefly review the available information on the molecular events in the action of a rather classic initiating agent, benzo[*a*]pyrene, and then summarize recent studies that provide clues to the biologic action of the phorbol ester class of tumor promoters. We shall then attempt to combine these two areas of information into a unified theory of initiation and promotion.

MOLECULAR EVENTS IN INITIATION

It is now an axiom in cancer research that many (and perhaps all) carcinogens yield electrophiles, either spontaneously or via metabolic activation, that form covalent adducts with nucleophilic residues in DNA and other cellular macromolecules. There is also considerable evidence that these reactions represent the initial events in the encounter between cells and chemical carcinogens (see Miller 1978, Weinstein 1977, 1978). The first part of this paper will briefly review the molecular details of such events recently elucidated with the carcinogen benzo[*a*]pyrene (BP), contrast these findings with those obtained with an aromatic amine carcinogen, N-2-acetylaminofluorene (AAF), and then make some speculative comments about how these molecular events relate to the initiation phase of the carcinogenic process.

Recent studies from laboratories in England and the United States indicate that the major metabolite of BP responsible for its mutagenic and carcinogenic activity is a dihydrodiol-epoxide derivative, 7,8-dihydroxy-9,10-epoxy-7,8,9,10 tetrahydro benzo[*a*]pyrene (BPDE). (For a general review of this subject see Gelboin and Ts'o, in press.) Our group at Columbia University, in collaboration with the laboratory of Dr. Koji Nakanishi in the Chemistry Department at Columbia University and with Dr. Ronald Harvey's group at the University of Chicago, elucidated the complete chemical structure and stereochemistry of the major adduct formed between BPDE and cellular RNA and DNA (Weinstein *et al.* 1976, Jeffrey *et al.* 1977). As shown in Figure 1, it consists of a guanine residue linked via its 2-amino group to the 10 position of BP.

Although the structure depicted in Figure 1 represents the major BPDE-nucleoside adduct, the modification of nucleic acids by BPDE is considerably more complicated. This results from the fact that there are several isomers of BPDE and that both *cis* and *trans* addition of nucleoside to the epoxide ring could occur. In addition, adenine and cytosine bases as well as the phosphate residues of the nucleic acid backbone could be modified (Jennette *et al.* 1977, Weinstein *et al.* 1978a, Moore *et al.* 1977, Straub *et al.* 1977). Studies in progress suggest that the extent to which these different factors prevail depends on the cell type in which metabolism occurs (Ivanovic *et al.* 1978) as well as the reaction conditions and the physical state of the DNA (Leffler *et al.* 1978, and unpublished studies).

Because of the existence of DNA repair enzymes, the modification of DNA by BPDE and other carcinogens is not a *fait accompli*. Preliminary evidence suggests that the different deoxynucleoside adducts formed by BPDE undergo differential rates of excision during DNA repair (Shinohara and Cerutti 1977, Ivanovic *et al.* 1978). There is precedent for this as earlier studies indicated that the N^2 and C-8 adducts of N-2-acetylaminofluorene (AAF) (Kriek 1972, Westra *et al.* 1976, Yamasaki *et al.* 1977c), and the O^6 and N^7 adducts of methylating agents (for review see Goth-Goldstein 1977) are removed from the DNA at markedly different rates. The ability of specific DNA adducts to elude DNA repair mechanisms may be an important determinate of carcinogen potency.

To gain insight into the structural changes in DNA resulting from covalent modification by bulky carcinogen residues we have studied the orientation of the BPDE residue when it is covalently attached to double-stranded DNA (Pul-

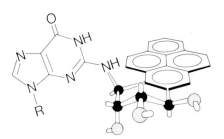

FIG. 1. Structure of BP-guanine adduct formed by the reaction of (±)7β,8α-di-hydroxy-9α, 10α-epoxy-7,8,9,10-tetrahydro-benzo(a)-pyrene (BPDE) with nucleic acids. The 2 amino group of guanine is linked to the 10 position of BP. (Reproduced from Weinstein *et al.* 1976, with permission of Science.)

krabek *et al.* 1977) and contrasted this conformation with that previously elucidated for covalently bound AAF residues (Weinstein and Grunberger 1974, Grunberger and Weinstein, in press). These results are summarized in Table 1. AAF modification is associated with appreciable localized denaturation of the DNA helix at sites of modification, and the AAF residue is oriented almost perpendicularly to the DNA helix axis. We refer to this conformation as "base displacement," and supporting evidence from our laboratory and from studies by Fuchs and co-workers (1976) has been reviewed in detail elsewhere (Grunberger and Weinstein 1976). In contrast, BPDE modification of native calf thymus DNA results in very little denaturation of the DNA helix (Pulkrabek *et al.* 1977). In collaborative studies with N. Geacintov's laboratory we have obtained evidence from electric dichroism studies that the covalently bound BPDE residue is oriented at about 35°, rather than 90°, with respect to the helix axis (Geacintov *et al.,* in press). In addition, fluorescence quenching studies indicate that the BPDE residue is exposed on the exterior of the DNA helix, rather than inserted into the DNA helix via intercalation (Prusik *et al.,* in press). These results, together with model building studies, suggest that the convalently bound BPDE residue lies in the minor groove of the DNA helix. This model is shown in Figure 2 and is contrasted with that of intercalative-type binding.

Much work remains to be done in terms of the functional consequences of the above-described changes in DNA structure induced by AAF and BP. In vitro studies indicate that DNA modified by AAF or BPDE is impaired in its template activity both with respect to replication (Hsu *et al.* 1977) and transcription (Yamasaki *et al.* 1977b, Leffler *et al.* 1978), and in bacterial systems, AAF and BP can induce frame-shift mutations (McAnn *et al.* 1975). Thus far we have been unable to detect an affect of DNA modification by these carcinogens on gross aspects of nucleosome structures (Yamasaki *et al.* 1977b, Yamasaki *et al.* 1978b, in press); but it seems likely that more subtle aspects of chromatin structure and function may be altered, and this remains to be assessed.

TABLE 1. *Comparative effects of modification of native DNA with activated forms of AAF or BP**

	AAF	BP
Decrease in T_m	1.1°	0.75°
Formaldehyde unwinding:		
Relative fraction open base plates	0.172†	0.023
Average number open base		
plates/modified base	12–13†	0–1
S_1 nuclease digestion	15%	0–1%
Orientation of carcinogen		
with respect to helix axis	~90%	~35%
Conformation	base	minor groove
	displacement	modification

* Extrapolated to a 1% modification of the total bases.
† From data of Fuchs *et al.* 1976. For sources of other data, see text.

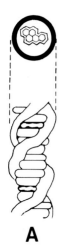 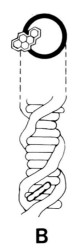

FIG. 2. Schematic representations of a DNA double helix containing benzo(*a*)pyrene physically bound by intercalation (A) and covalently bound benzo(*a*)pyrene diol epoxide residue lying in the minor groove of the helix (B). (Reproduced from Grunberger and Weinstein et al. 1978a, with permission of Academic Press.)

A   B

At this point we would like to speculate about how covalent binding of carcinogens to DNA might result in the initiation phase of carcinogenesis (Table 2). There has been a tendency to think of this event as a simple random-point mutation resulting from errors in replicating the damaged DNA. Certain aspects of the carcinogenic process, particularly the apparently high efficiency of initiation and the long latent period required for expression, however, are not consistent with this simple notion (Weinstein 1976).

A modified form of the random mutation theory is that carcinogens do not act simply by producing errors in DNA replication at the sites at which they damage DNA. In bacteria, physical and chemical agents that damage DNA, including chemical carcinogens, or other factors that interfere with DNA replication, induce a highly pleiotropic response called "SOS functions" (Witkin 1976, Radman *et al.* 1977, Moreau *et al.* 1976). These functions include induction of lysogenic phage, filamentous growth, and mutagenesis. The mutagenesis appears to result from the induction of an error-prone DNA synthesis mechanism that can mutagenize even undamaged DNAs. It is thought to have a positive function because it allows the replication mechanism to read through a damaged

TABLE 2. *Possible molecular mechanisms of initiation of the carcinogenic process*

A. *With Permanent Changes in DNA Sequence*
   1. Point mutations
      a. Direct: base substitution, frame shift, deletion-in structural or regulatory gene.
      b. Indirect: induction of "SOS-type" error-prone DNA synthesis.
   2. Aberrations at the DNA level in genetic mechanisms that *may* normally control differentiation: mobile genes, insertion sequences, other sequence changes.
B. *Without Permanent Changes in DNA Sequence*
   Aberrations in epigenetic mechanisms of differentiation: altered chromatin structure, altered feedback loops, DNA methylation, etc.

region of DNA and thus permit cell survival. It is not yet clear that similar inducible responses to DNA damage occur in eukaryotic cells, although recent experiments support this possibility (D'Ambrosio and Setlow 1976, Sarasin and Hanawalt 1978, DasGupta and Summers 1978). In *Escherichia coli,* the induction of phage synthesis and mutagenesis following damage to DNA appears to involve the action of a protease (Meyn *et al.* 1977) that destroys repressor protein(s). In this regard, it is of interest that the carcinogenic process also appears to be frequently associated with increased synthesis of the protease plasminogen activator, and perhaps other proteases. (For a review of this subject, see Reich *et al.* 1975, and later sections of this paper.) Further studies are required to determine the possible role in the carcinogenic process of inducible DNA repair and error-prone DNA synthesis mechanisms, and the significance of protease induction.

An entirely different hypothesis to explain initiation relates to recent studies indicating that the linear arrangement of coding sequences in DNA may be more complex and also more plastic than previously envisioned. These results provide support for the hypothesis put forward by McClintock a number of years ago that, during the normal course of development and differentiation of eukaryotic organisms, ordered and highly specific rearrangements of genes occur within the chromosomes, and these rearrangements control states of gene expression (see Finchman and Sastry 1974). Once established in a somatic cell line, these rearrangements could be preserved during the course of cell division and thus transmitted to progeny cells of that lineage. In this way, a specific program of gene expression could be maintained and could account for stable patterns of cellular determination and differentiation. Specific mechanisms might also exist by which such rearrangements in DNA sequence are reversed, thus returning the genome to its "basal" state. This aspect would account for those cases in which differentiated tissues demonstrate pleuripotency. It is of interest that a simple "flip-flop" inversion of a specific phage gene controls its expression in *Salmonella* (Zieg *et al.* 1977, Kamp *et al.* 1978). Brack and Tonegawa (1977) have found that the synthesis of a specific mouse immunoglobulin is associated with somatic rearrangements of immunoglobulin genes coding for the variable and constant regions. Although at the present time this is the only known case in mammalian cells, it is possible that genome rearrangements will be found to underlie other aspects of development and differentiation in mammalian systems.

Rather complex and delicate biochemical mechanisms must underlie the above-described specific rearrangements in DNA sequence, and it would not be surprising if chemical modification of the DNA by carcinogens disrupted these mechanisms. By scrambling an otherwise orderly process of genome rearrangements, carcinogens could produce major distortions in the control of gene expression and differentiation and thus initiate the carcinogenic process. Table 2 also lists possible epigenetic mechanisms (i.e., not involving heritable alterations in DNA sequence) for initiation of carcinogenesis. These assume that normal differentiation proceeds via epigenetic mechanisms such as alterations in chromatin structure, DNA methylation, positive feedback loops or other stabilized and heritable programs of gene expression.

The recent finding of spacer sequences ("introns" or "insertion sequences") within several eukaryotic genes, sequences that are not actually translated into amino acid sequences in the related protein, is revolutionizing our concepts concerning the organization of the genome, the mechanisms underlying mRNA processing, and the control of gene expression (for review see Gilbert 1978). It is too early to predict the possible implications of carcinogen attack on nucleic acids in terms of disruptions of these aspects of gene structure and expression.

Powerful techniques are now available for analyzing the fine structure and function of mammalian DNA. It is, for example, now possible to transfer (or "transfect") specific genes into mammalian cells (Wigler *et al.* 1978). The application of these techniques to carcinogenesis research should provide direct information relating to the theories listed in Table 2 and may reveal entirely unanticipated mechanisms.

CELLULAR EFFECTS OF TUMOR PROMOTERS

The existence of a distinct phase of carcinogenesis termed "promotion" has been well defined in studies on mouse skin carcinogenesis (Berenblum 1975). There is also abundant evidence that in other tissues the carcinogenic process is multistep (Foulds 1969) and that a phase analogous to promotion occurs in tissues other than skin (Peraino *et al.* 1978).

Although, as discussed above, major gaps exist in our understanding of the process of initiation, even less is known at the biochemical level in terms of the action of tumor promoters. Table 3 contrasts the known biologic properties of carcinogens and tumor promoters, based largely on mouse skin carcinogenesis studies (also see Weinstein *et al.* 1978b). We want to stress that although carcinogens bind covalently to DNA, are mutagenic and generally produce irreversible

TABLE 3. *A comparison of biologic properties of initiating agents and promoting agents*

Initiating Agents	Promoting Agents
1. Carcinogenic by themselves—"solitary carcinogens"	1. Not carcinogenic alone
2. Must be given *before* promoting agent	2. Must be given *after* the initiating agent
3. Single exposure is sufficient	3. Require prolonged exposure
4. Action is irreversible and additive	4. Action is reversible (at early stage) and not additive
5. No apparent threshold	5. Probable threshold
6. Yield electrophiles that bind covalently to cell macromolecules	6. No evidence of covalent binding
7. Mutagenic	7. Not mutagenic

Reproduced from Weinstein *et al.* 1978b, with permission of Raven Press.

effects, these characteristics do not apply to tumor promoters. Thus, tumor promoters must act by an entirely separate mechanism and one that is likely to involve epigenetic events.

Induction of Plasminogen Activator

A few years ago we became interested in utilizing cell culture systems to study the biologic effects of the phorbol ester tumor promoters. Because W Troll and his colleagues had obtained evidence that proteases were involved in the promotion phase of mouse skin carcinogenesis (Troll *et al.* 1975) and because E. Reich's laboratory had shown that cell transformation was often associated with a marked increase in the synthesis of the protease plasminogen activator (P.A.) (Reich *et al.* 1975), we studied the effects of tumor promoters on the expression of the latter enzyme in cell culture. M. Wigler, in our group, found that 12-O-tetradecanoyl-phorbol-13-acetate (TPA) and several related macrocyclic plant diterpenes were extremely potent inducers of P.A. synthesis in both chick embryo fibroblasts (CEF) and HeLa cultures (Wigler and Weinstein 1976, Weinstein *et al.* 1976, Wigler *et al.* 1978). The structures of some of these compounds are shown in Figure 3, and the induction effect is illustrated in Figure 4. The major features of this induction process are summarized in Table 4. It is apparent that the effect is highly specific, that it involves de novo macromolecular synthesis, and that it correlates with the tumor promoting potency of a series of phorbol ester analogs.

A particularly intriguing aspect was the finding that TPA causes a further increase of P.A. synthesis in transformed cells that are already synthesizing high levels of P.A. (Wigler and Weinstein 1976, Weinstein *et al.* 1977). We refer to this phenomenon as "enhancement." Studies with chick embryo fibroblasts transformed by a temperature-sensitive mutant of Rous sarcoma virus (RSV) showed that enhancement of TPA-induced P.A. synthesis required continuous expression of the sarcoma gene of RSV (Weinstein *et al.* 1977, Weinstein *et al.* 1978b). Other examples of an enhanced response to TPA by transformed cells have now been seen in terms of morphological changes (Wigler and Weinstein 1976, Weinstein *et al.* 1977), ornithine decarboxylase (ODC) induction (O'Brien and Diamond 1978), and prostaglandin synthesis (Levine and Hassid 1977). In addition, TPA enhances the appearance of transformed foci in cells infected with an adenovirus (Fisher *et al.* 1978). The phenomenon of enhancement may be a useful model for understanding tumor promotion and progression because it provides examples in which previous changes in a cell type alter its subsequent response to a tumor-promoting agent.

Mimicry of Transformation

In view of the results obtained with P.A., it was natural to ask the question of whether TPA and related compounds also enhanced the expression of other

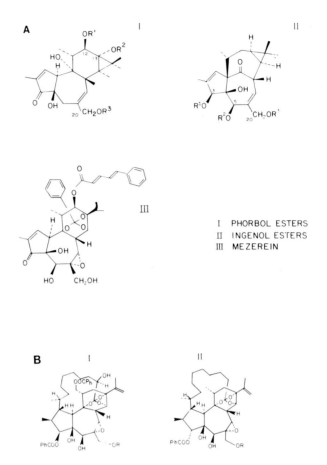

I   PHORBOL ESTERS
II INGENOL ESTERS
III MEZEREIN

I - GNIDIMACRIN
II - GNILATIMACRIN
III - GNIDILATIN

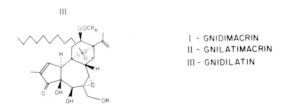

FIG. 3. Structures of some macrocyclic plant diterpenes derived from the families Euphorbia-ceae (A-I and A-II) and Thymelaeaceae (A-III and B). (Reproduced from Weinstein *et al.* 1978b, with permission of Raven Press.)

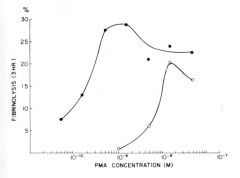

FIG. 4. Dose-response curve of HeLa and CEF to TPA. Replicate, subconfluent plates of HeLa (●——●) and CEF (O——O) were exposed to varying concentrations of TPA in medium containing serum for 24 hours and lysates prepared and assayed as described previously (Wigler and Weinstein 1976).

biologic markers frequently associated with transformation and tumorigenicity. Data from several laboratories are summarized in Table 5 indicating that indeed TPA induces several phenotypic properties in normal cells that mimic those often seen in transformed cells. This mimicry includes changes in cell morphology, growth properties, cell surface properties, and specific enzymes. I must stress, however, two aspects of the effects obtained when normal cells not previously exposed to an initiating carcinogen are incubated with TPA: (1) TPA-treated cells do not mimic all of the properties of fully transformed tumorigenic cells, of particular importance is that they do not acquire the capacity for growth in agar; and (2) in contrast to fully malignant cells, the maintenance of transformation properties in normal cells is dependent on the continuous presence of the promoting agent, and the cells revert to normal when the agent is removed from the medium. In mouse skin previously exposed to a carcinogen, the repeated application of TPA, however, can lead to "autonomous" malignant tumors. TPA can also enhance the stable transformation of fibroblast cultures previously exposed to a chemical carcinogen, UV- or X-irradiation (Mondal *et al.* 1976, Mondal and Heidelberger 1976, Kennedy *et al.* 1978). The latter results suggest

TABLE 4. *General characteristics of induction of plasminogen activator (P.A.) by TPA and related macrocyclic diterpenes*

1. Induction occurs with concentrations in the range of 10^{-8} M to 10^{-10} M.
2. Induction is detectable within one hour, plateaus at 24 to 48 hours and is reversed when the agent is removed from the medium.
3. Cells from a variety of species and tissues respond, although many cell cultures are not inducible.
4. Induction is blocked by inhibitors of RNA and protein synthesis.
5. The structural requirements for induction of P.A. parallel those for tumor promotion and the other biologic effects of these compounds.
6. In transformed cells already synthesizing high levels of P.A., these compounds can further enhance P.A. synthesis.

For details, see Wigler and Weinstein 1976, Weinstein *et al.* 1977, Weinstein *et al.* 1978b, and Wigler *et al.* 1978.

TABLE 5. *Effects of TPA on the phenotype of cell cultures*

	References
Cell Surface and Membrane Changes	
Altered Na/K ATPase	Sivak and Van Duuren 1967
Altered morphology	Wigler and Weinstein 1976, Driedger and Blumberg 1977
Increased phospholipid synthesis	Suss *et al.* 1972
Altered fucose-glycopeptides	Weinstein *et al.* 1978b
Decreased LETS protein	Blumberg *et al.* 1976
Increased uptake ^{32}P, ^{86}Rb, deoxyglucose	Moroney *et al.* 1978, Driedger and Blumberg 1977
Altered receptors	Lee and Weinstein 1978c, Grimm and Marks 1974, Mufson *et al.* 1977
Altered fluorescence polarization	Fisher, Flamm, Schachter, and Weinstein, unpublished studies
Growth Properties	
Increased saturation density	For review, see Weinstein *et al.* 1978b
Altered cell-cell orientation	Driedger and Blumberg 1977
Decreased serum requirement	Fisher and Weinstein, unpublished studies
Enzymatic	
Increased plasminogen activator synthesis	Wigler and Weinstein 1976, Wigler *et al.* 1978, Loskutoff and Edgington 1977, Vassalli *et al.* 1977
Increased ornithine decarboxylase	Yuspa *et al.* 1976, O'Brien and Diamond 1978
Increased prostaglandin synthesis	Levine and Hassid 1977, Mufson, Laskin, and Weinstein, unpublished studies

that initiated cells have a qualitatively different response to TPA than completely normal cells. We shall discuss possible reasons for this difference at the end of this paper.

Inhibition of Terminal Differentiation

Because it is likely that carcinogenesis involves major disturbances in differentiation it was of interest to determine if TPA would affect the differentiation of certain well-defined tissue culture systems. Table 6 summarizes examples from our own laboratory and from the literature which indicate that TPA is a highly potent inhibitor of terminal differentiation in a variety of cell culture systems (see also Weinstein and Wigler 1977). This inhibitory effect is extremely specific, is not simply a consequence of toxicity or growth inhibition, and, in certain cases, is reversed when TPA is removed from the culture. Nor is the effect limited to a specific program of differentiation (Table 6). As with the phenomenon of mimicry of transformation, evidence has shown that the relative potencies of a series of phorbol ester analogs as inhibitors of differentiation correlates with their potencies as promoters on mouse skin (Yamasaki *et al.* 1977a).

TABLE 6. *Examples of TPA inhibition of differentiation in cell culture*

Cell culture system	Type of differentiation	References
Murine erythroleukemia	Erythroid	Yamasaki *et al.* 1977a, Rovera *et al.* 1977
Chicken embryo myoblasts	Myogenesis	Cohen *et al.* 1977
Chicken embryo chondroblasts	Chondrogenesis	Pacifici and Holtzer 1977
Murine 3T3	Lipocytes	Diamond *et al.* 1977
Murine neuroblastoma	Neurite	Ishii *et al.* 1978
Murine melanoma	Melanogenesis	Mufson *et al.* 1978

The Cell Surface Membrane as the Primary Target of TPA Action

Early studies on the effects of TPA in cell culture suggested that the cell surface membrane might be the major target of TPA action, and more recent studies have reinforced this hypothesis (for a list of effects of TPA on cell surfaces and membranes, see Table 5).

Lih-Syng Lee in our laboratory recently studied the uptake of ^{3}H-TPA by cells in culture (Lee and Weinstein 1978a). During these studies he found it necessary to repurify the ^{3}H-TPA by high pressure liquid chromatography (HPLC), because material that appears to be pure by thin-layer chromatography can show considerable contamination when examined by HPLC. Figure 5 indicates that total uptake is linear across a wide range of ^{3}H-TPA concentration and does not appear to be saturable. We have been unable to demonstrate a distinct high affinity saturable receptor, although we are still pursuing this aspect.

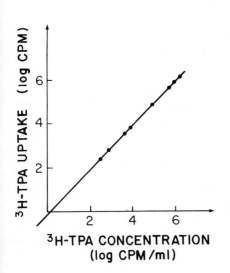

FIG. 5. Uptake of ^{3}H-TPA by HeLa cell cultures. A suspension of HeLa cells in Dulbecco's modified Eagle's medium lacking serum was incubated with increasing amounts of a ^{3}H-TPA-albumin complex (1:55 molar ratio) at 37°C for 60 minutes, with frequent shaking. The cells were then pelleted and washed by membrane filtration with PBS containing 1 mg/ml albumin and the amount of cell-associated radioactivity determined. For additional details, see Lee and Weinstein 1978a, in press.

Cell fractionation studies indicate that the uptake is almost entirely into the membranous fractions of the cell and appears to be a simple partitioning of the highly hydrophobic compound into the lipid phase of the membrane. Uptake by the nucleus was extremely low. Cellular uptake was not inhibited by a large excess of nonradioactive TPA, inhibitors of energy metabolism, inhibitors of macromolecular synthesis, or cytochalasin B. There was no evidence of covalent binding to cellular macromolecules, and almost all of the cell-associated ^{3}H-TPA was released when the cells were placed in serum containing medium lacking TPA or when cells were extracted with lipid solvents.

In view of the evidence that TPA is concentrated largely in the lipid phase of cell membranes, in collaboration with D. Schachter's laboratory at Columbia University, we have looked for evidence of a change in the physical properties of cell membranes by studying the fluorescence polarization of an asymmetric chromophore, 1,6-diphenyl-1,3,5-hexatriene (DPH) (Fisher, Flamm, Schachter, and Weinstein, unpublished studies). This highly fluorescent compound concentrates in cellular lipids, and its rotational freedom, which can be monitored by fluorescence polarization, is a function of membrane fluidity or microviscosity (Schachter and Shinitsky 1977). We found that concentrations of TPA as low as 0.1 ng/ml (10^{-10} M) produced a reproducible decrease in fluorescence polarization of DPH (Figure 6). The change was detected within one to two hours and was not blocked by cycloheximide or actinomycin D. Other phorbol esters having tumor-promoting activity (PDD and PDB) also exerted this effect, whereas the compounds phorbol and 4αPDD, which lack tumor-promoting activity, were inactive. These results indicate that TPA produces a rather gross change in the physical properties of the lipid phase of cellular membranes and that this effect appears to be a direct one which does not require macromolecular synthesis. The most likely interpretation is that TPA induces physical or biochemical changes in the lipid phase which result in increased membrane fluidity, although other interpretations have not been excluded.

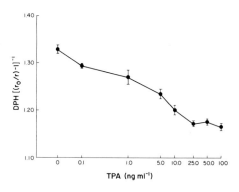

FIG. 6. Effect of TPA on the fluorescence polarization of 1,6-diphenyl-1,3,5-hexatriene (DPH). Confluent rat embryo cultures (∼5 × 10^6 cells per 9 cm dish) were re-fed cell culture medium plus 2% fetal calf serum and exposed to the indicated concentrations of TPA for four hours. Cells were dispersed with trypsin, washed three times with PBS, resuspended in 1 ml of PBS and incubated for two hours with 10^{-6}M DPH. Fluorescence polarization of DPH was then determined and expressed as $[(r_0/r)-1]^{-1}$ (Schachter and Shinitsky 1977). Values are means ± SE for four determinations on each sample. TPA O refers to dimethyl sulfoxide (DMSO) (0.01%)-treated RE cells.

MODELS OF TPA ACTION AND THEIR RELEVANCE TO TUMOR PROMOTION

Figure 7 is a schematic representation in which we attempt to integrate the various cellular effects of TPA into a comprehensive model. As discussed above, the primary action of TPA appears to be at the cell surface membrane. Changes in cell surface morphology, cellular adhesion, and an apparent increase in membrane lipid fluidity provide evidence that TPA produces a generalized change in cell membrane structure. These early effects do not appear to require de novo RNA and protein synthesis, but their physical and biochemical basis remains to be elucidated. These structural changes presumably account for several effects of TPA on membrane function, including an alteration in membrane-associated Na/K ATPase, increased transport of ^{86}Rb, ^{32}P, and 2-deoxyglucose and enhanced phospholipid synthesis (see Table 5). The function of β-adrenergic receptors (Grimm and Marks 1974, Mufson *et al.* 1977, Belman, Troll, and Garte, personal communication), the receptor for epithelial growth factor (Lee and Weinstein, 1978b, in press), and perhaps other receptors involved in growth control is also altered. The ability of retinoids to antagonize certain actions of TPA and to inhibit tumor promotion (Sporn *et al.* 1979, see pages 441 to 453, this volume) may be due to reciprocal effects of the retinoids at the membrane level. Elsewhere (Weinstein *et al.* 1977) we have speculated that since a number of the effects of TPA resemble those of hormonal agents, it is possible that TPA acts by usurping the function of a cellular receptor system normally used by an endogenous growth regulatory substance.

Following the above-mentioned early effects of TPA on cell membranes there are a series of secondary cellular responses that require RNA and protein synthesis and, therefore, probably reflect the action of "transmembrane signals" on nuclear and cytoplasmic functions. As in the case of certain polypeptide hormones and mitogens that exert their primary effects at the cell surface, the

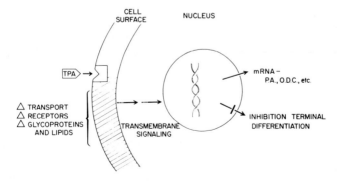

FIG. 7. A schematic model of the primary action of TPA on the cell surface, with secondary effects on nuclear function. For a detailed description, see text.

nature of these transmembrane signals is not understood at the present time. The secondary responses to TPA include induction of P.A. and ODC synthesis, inhibition or stimulation of DNA synthesis, increased lipolysis and prostaglandin synthesis, altered cell surface glycoproteins, and inhibition of the expression of pre-existent programs of terminal differentiation (see Tables 5 and 6).

We must emphasize that cell types differ considerably in terms of which aspects of the above responses will be elicited by TPA. Thus, TPA does not induce P.A. in certain cell types, yet these same cells may show other responses to TPA. Analogous variations in responses to the same hormone by different target cells are well known in endocrinology. Clonal variants of Friend erythroleukemia cells that are resistant to TPA inhibition of terminal differentiation have recently been isolated (Yamasaki et al. 1978b, in press), and these may prove useful in dissecting out the diverse actions of TPA. Since the transformation process itself leads to changes in cell surface structure and function, one might anticipate that cells previously altered by exposure to a chemical or viral carcinogen would have quantitatively and/or qualitatively different responses to TPA when compared to completely normal cells. This aspect could explain the phenomenon of "enhancement" observed when transformed cells are exposed to TPA. Mechanisms involving sequential alterations in the response of the same cell type to tumor promoters and growth-controlling substances may underlie the stepwise process of tumor promotion and progression.

A number of years ago, Berenblum (1954) postulated that tumor promoters act by inducing disturbances in differentiation, and several observations on mouse skin provided indirect support for this hypothesis (Raick 1974, Yuspa et al. 1976a,b, Colburn et al. 1975). The results in cell culture systems provide direct evidence that the phorbol esters are potent inhibitors of terminal differentiation (see Table 6). This effect may be an important clue to the ability of the phorbol esters to act as tumor promoters on mouse skin. A possible model is illustrated schematically in Figure 8. The stem cells in the epidermis are continually dividing; yet the tissue as a whole is in a state of balanced growth, and a stable stem cell pool size is maintained. This is probably achieved by a regular asymmetric division of the stem cell. One daughter cell becomes a stem cell, and the other daughter cell is committed to keratinize and terminally differentiate, irreversibly losing its growth potential. If an "initiated" stem cell were restrained to the stem cell mode of division, it could not increase its proportion in the stem cell pool. If, however, the stem cell division mode were interrupted by the action of a promoting agent, the initiated cell could undergo exponential division, thus yielding a clone of similar cells. Since TPA can also induce phenotypic changes in cells that mimic those of transformed cells, the microenvironment of a clone of such cells might itself enhance their further outgrowth and development into a tumor.

Although the above speculations provide plausible models for thinking about mechanisms by which the phorbol esters enhance the induction of papillomas on mouse skin previously exposed to an initiating agent, they do not readily

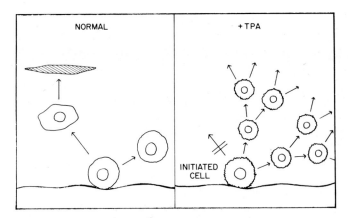

FIG. 8. Schematic representation of the normal mode of asymmetric stem cell division in epidermis and of the hypothesis that TPA induces exponential growth of an initiated stem cell thus yielding a clone of such cells from which tumors can arise. For a detailed description, see text.

explain why repeated applications of these agents to mouse skin eventually result in the formation of malignant tumors that do not regress, even after application of TPA has been stopped. Stated in other terms, the question is this: how is a cellular response mechanism that is normally inductive converted to one which is constitutive or autonomous? This remains one of the major dilemmas in carcinogenesis. It seems likely that the answer to this question relates to the nature of the irreversible change in cells produced by the initiating carcinogen. Earlier in this paper we raised the question of whether the latter lesion is a simple random-point mutation or a more complex change in genome structure related to normal mechanisms of cellular differentiation. One hypothesis of two-stage carcinogenesis is that the initiating agent results in the acquisition of an aberrant program of differentiation (by one of the mechanisms listed in Table 2), and this program remains dormant until expression of the related genes is induced by the promoting agent. With repeated induction, the expression of this program becomes "locked-in" by mechanisms (yet to be discovered) similar to those that provide stability to normal states of differentiation (Weinstein *et al.* 1978b).

   An alternative theory is that a late and irreversible step in the formation of a fully malignant tumor involves a further change in the cellular genome induced by the tumor promoter. Kinsella and Radman (personal communication) have recently found that TPA induces sister chromatid exchanges (SCE) in cell culture, perhaps by inducing enzymes related to chromosomal rearrangements. They have speculated that the initiating agent results in a cell carrying a recessive mutation and that tumor promoters, by enhancing chromosomal rearrangements, increase the likelihood that progeny clones will arise, by segregation or other mechanisms, that have become homozygous for this mutant gene and thus express the malignant cell phenotype. It is not yet clear, however, whether SCE is a side effect of TPA or is closely related to its action as a tumor promoter.

Although the above hypotheses relating to the action of carcinogens and tumor promoters are highly speculative, a number of cell culture systems, genetic approaches, and molecular techniques are now available for specifically testing these and other theories. It seems likely, therefore, that an understanding of the multistage mechanism of carcinogenesis is amenable to solution within the near future. This understanding will not only profoundly influence our approaches to cancer prevention and treatment but will also provide insights into mechanisms underlying normal cellular growth control, development, and differentiation.

ACKNOWLEDGMENTS

The authors wish to acknowledge the valuable contributions made to these studies by Drs. Peter Pulkrabek, Steven Leffler, Vesna Ivanovic, Koji Nakanishi, Ronald Harvey, Curtis Harris, Nicholas Geacintov, Steven Blobstein, Karen Jennette, Allan Mufson, and D. Schachter. They are also grateful to Drs. W. Troll, J. Cairns, and M. Radman for helpful discussions on the action of tumor promoters.

This investigation was supported by Grant CA-21111–02, and Contract NO-1-CP-2-3234 awarded by the National Cancer Institute, Department of Health, Education, and Welfare, and Grant EPA-R-805482010, awarded by the Environmental Protection Agency.

REFERENCES

Berenblum, I. 1954. Carcinogenesis and tumor pathogenesis. Adv. Cancer Res. 2:129–175.

Berenblum, I. 1975. Sequential aspects of chemical carcinogenesis: Skin, in Cancer: A Comprehensive Treatise, F. F. Becker, ed., Vol. 1. Plenum Press, New York, pp. 323–344.

Blumberg, P. M., P. E. Driedger, and P. W. Rossow. 1976. Effect of a phorbol ester on transformation-sensitive surface protein of chick fibroblasts. Nature 264:446–447.

Boutwell, R. K. 1974. The function and mechanism of promoters of carcinogenesis. CRC Crit. Rev. Toxicol. 2:419–443.

Brack, C., and S. Tonegawa. 1977. Variable and constant parts of the immunoglobulin light chain gene of a mouse myeloma cell are 1250 nontranslated bases apart. Proc. Natl. Acad. Sci. USA. 74:5652–5656.

Cerutti, P. 1978. ICN-UCLA Winter Conference on DNA Repair Mechanisms. Repairable damage in DNA. (In press).

Cohen, R., M. Pacifici, N. Rubenstein, J. Biehl, and H. Holtzer. 1977. Effect of a tumor promoter on myogenesis. Nature 266:538–540.

Colburn, N. H., S. Lau, and R. Head. 1975. Decrease of epidermal histidase activity by tumor-promoting phorbol esters. Cancer Res. 35:3154–3159.

DasGupta, U. B., and W. C. Summers. 1978. Ultraviolet reactivation of herpes simplex virus is mutagenic and inducible in mammalian cells. Proc. Natl. Acad. Sci. USA 75:2378–2381.

D'Ambrosio, S. M., and R. B. Setlow. 1976. Enhancement of postreplication repair in Chinese hamster cells. Proc. Natl. Acad. Sci. USA 73:2396–2400.

Diamond, L., T. G. O'Brien, and G. Rovera. 1977. Inhibition of adipose conversion of 3T3 fibroblasts by tumour promoters. Nature 269:247–248.

Driedger, P. E., and P. M. Blumberg. 1977. The effect of phorbol diesters on chicken embryo fibroblasts. Cancer Res. 37:3257–3265.

Finchman, J. R. S., and G. R. K. Sastry. 1974. Controlling elements in maize. Ann. Rev. Genet. 8:15–50.

Fisher, P. B., I. B. Weinstein, D. Eisenberg, and H. S. Ginsberg. 1978. Interactions between adenovirus, a tumor promoter, and chemical carcinogens in transformation of rat embryo cell cultures. Proc. Natl. Acad. Sci. USA 75:2311–2314.

Foulds, L. 1969. Neoplastic Development. Academic Press, New York.

Fuchs, R. P. P., J. F. Lefevre, J. Pouyet, and M. P. Daune. 1976. Orientation of the fluorene residue in native DNA modified by N-acetoxy-N-2-acetylaminofluorene and two 7-halogen derivatives. Biochemistery 15:3347–3351.

Geacintov, N. E., A. Gagliano, V. Ivanovic, and I. B. Weinstein. 1978. Electric linear dichroism study on the orientation of benzo(a)pyrene-7,8-dihydrodiol 9,10-oxide covalently bound to DNA. Biochemistry (In press).

Gelboin, H. V. and P. O. P. Ts'o, eds. 1978. Polycyclic Hydrocarbons and Cancer: Environment, Chemistry, Molecular and Cell Biology. Academic Press. (In press).

Gilbert, W. 1978. Why genes in pieces? Nature 271:501.

Goth-Goldstein, R. 1977. Repair of DNA damaged by alkylating carcinogens is defective in xeroderma pigmentosum-derived fibroblasts. Nature 267:81–82.

Grimm, W., and F. Marks. 1974. Effect of tumor-promoting phorbol esters on the normal and the isoproterenol-elevated level of adenosine $3',5'$-cyclic monophosphate in mouse epidermis *in vivo.* Cancer Res. 34:3128–3134.

Grunberger, D., and I. B. Weinstein. 1976. The base displacement model: An explanation for the conformational and functional changes in nucleic acids modified by chemical carcinogens, *in* Biology of Radiation Carcinogenesis, J. M. Yuhas, R. W. Tennant and J. D. Regan, eds., Raven Press, New York, pp. 175–187.

Grunberger, D., and I. B. Weinstein. 1978. Conformational changes in nucleic acids modified by chemical carcinogens, *in* Chemical Carcinogens in DNA, CRC Press, Cleveland (In press).

Hecker, E. 1975. Cocarcinogens and cocarcinogenesis, *in* Handbuch der Allgemeinen Pathologie, Vol. IV/6, Geschwulste, Tumors, II, E. Grundmann, ed., Springer-Verlag, Berlin-Heidelberg, pp. 651–676.

Hsu, W. T., E. J. S. Lin, R. G. Harvey, and S. B. Weiss. 1977. Mechanism of phage φX174 DNA inactivation by benzo(a)pyrene-7,8-dihydrodiol-9,10-epoxide. Proc. Natl. Acad. Sci. USA 74:3335.

Ishii, D. N., E. Fibach, H. Yamasaki, and I. B. Weinstein. 1978. Tumor promoters inhibit morphological differentiation in cultured mouse neuroblastoma cells. Science 200:556–559.

Ivanovic, V., N. Geacintov, H. Yamasaki, and I. B. Weinstein. 1978. DNA and RNA adducts formed in hamster embryo cell cultures exposed to benzo(a)pyrene. Biochemistry 17:1597–1603.

Jeffrey, A. M., I. B. Weinstein, K. W. Jennette, K. Grzeskowiak, K. Nakanishi, R. G. Harvey, H. Autrup, and C. Harris. 1977. Structures of benzo(a)pyrene-nucleic acid adducts formed in human and bovine bronchial explants. Nature 269:348–350.

Jennette, K. W., A. M. Jeffrey, S. H. Blobstein, F. Beland, R. G. Harvey, and I. B. Weinstein. 1977. Characterization of nucleoside adducts from the *in vitro* reaction of benzo(a)pyrene-4,5-oxide with nucleic acids. Biochemistry 16:932–938.

Kamp, D., R. Kahmann, D. Zipser, T. R. Broker, and L. T. Chow. 1977. Inversion of the G DNA segment of phage Mu controls phage infectivity. Nature 271:577–580.

Kennedy, A., S. Mondal, C. Heidelberger, and J. B. Little. 1978. Enhancement of x-radiation transformation by a phorbol ester using C3H/10T½ Cl 8 mouse embryo fibroblasts. Cancer Res. 38:439–443.

Kriek, E. 1972. Persistent binding of a new reaction product of the carcinogen N-hydroxy-N-2-acetylaminofluorene with guanine in rat liver DNA *in vivo*. Cancer Res. 32:2042–2048.

Lee, L. S., and I. B. Weinstein. 1978a. Uptake of the tumor promoting agent 12-0-tetradecanoyl-phorbol 13-acetate by HeLa cells. J. Environ. Pathol. Toxicol. 1:627–639.

Lee, L. S. and I. B. Weinstein. 1978b. Epidermal growth factor, like tumor promoting phorbol esters, induces plasminogen activator in HeLa cells. Nature 274:696–697.

Lee, L. S., and I. B. Weinstein. 1978c. Tumor promoting phorbol esters inhibit binding of epidermal growth factor to cellular receptors. Science (In press).

Leffler, S., P. Pulkrabek, D. Grunberger, and I. B. Weinstein. 1977. Template activity of calf thymus DNA modified by a dihydrodiol epoxide derivative of benzo(a)pyrene. Biochemistry 16:3133–3136.

Leffler, S., P. Pulkrabek, D. Grunberger, and I. B. Weinstein. 1978. Structural and functional changes in plasmid and phage DNA modified by a diol epoxide derivative of benzo(a)pyrene (BP). (Abstract) Fed. Proc. 37:1383.

Levine, L., and A. Hassid. 1977. Effects of phorbol-12,13-diesters on prostaglandin production and phospholipase activity in canine kidney (MDCK) cells. Biochem. Biophys. Res. Commun. 79:477–483.

Loskutoff, D. J., and T. S. Edgington. 1977. Synthesis of a fibrinolytic activator and inhibitor by endothelial cells. Proc. Natl. Acad. Sci. USA 74:3903–3907.

McAnn, J., E. Choie, E. Yamasaki, and B. N. Ames. 1975. Detection of carcinogens as mutagens in the Salmonella/microsome test: Assay of 300 chemicals. Proc. Natl. Acad. Sci. USA 72:5,135.

Meyn, M. S., T. Rossman, and W. Troll. 1977. A protease inhibitor blocks SOS functions in *Escherichia coli:* Antipain prevents lambda repressor inactivation, ultraviolet mutagenesis, and filamentous growth. Proc. Natl. Acad. Sci. USA 74:1152.

Miller, E. C. 1978. Some current perspectives on chemical carcinogenesis in human and experimental animals: Presidential Address. Cancer Res. 38:1479–1496.

Mondal, S., and C. Heidelberger. 1976. Transformation of C3H/10T½ CL8 mouse embryo fibroblasts by ultraviolet irradiation and a phorbol ester. Nature 260:710–711.

Mondal, S., D. W. Brankow, and C. Heidelberger. 1976. Two-stage chemical oncogenesis in cultures of C3H/10T½ cells. Cancer Res. 36:2254–2260.

Moore, P. D., M. Koreeda, P. G. Wislocki, W. Levin, A. H. Conney, H. Yagi, and D. M. Jerina. 1977. *In vitro* reactions of the diastereomeric 9,10-epoxides of (+) and (−)-*trans*-7,8-dihydroxy-7,8-dihydrobenzo(a)pyrene with polyguanylic acid and evidence for formation of an enantiomer of each diastereomeric 9,10-epoxide from benzo(a)pyrene in mouse skin. Am. Chem. Soc. Symp. Series 44:127.

Moreau, P., A. Bailone, and R. Devoret. 1976. Prophage λ induction in *E. coli* K12 envA uvrB: A highly sensitive test for potential carcinogens. Proc. Natl. Acad. Sci. USA 73:3700–3704.

Moroney, J., A. Smith, L. D. Tomel, and C. E. Wenner. 1978. Stimulation of $^{86}Rb^+$ and ^{32}Pi movements in 3T3 cells by prostaglandins and phorbol esters. J. Cell. Physiol. 95:287–294.

Mufson, R. A., R. C. Simsiman, and R. K. Boutwell. 1977. The effects of phorbol ester tumor promoters on the basal and catecholamine stimulated levels of adenosine $3':5'$-monophosphate in mouse skin and epidermis in vivo. Cancer Res. 37:665–699.

Mufson, R. A., P. B. Fisher, and I. B. Weinstein. 1978. Phorbol esters produce a delay in the expression of melanogenesis by B-16 cells. (Abstract) Proc. Am. Assoc. Cancer Res. 19:183.

O'Brien, T. G., and L. Diamond. 1978. Ornithine decarboxylase, polyamines and tumor promoters, *in* Carcinogenesis Vol. 2. Mechanisms of Tumor Promotion and Cocarcinogenesis, T. J. Slaga, A. Sivak, and R. K. Boutwell, eds., Raven Press, New York, pp. 273–287.

Pacifici, M., and H. Holtzer. 1977. Effects of a tumor-promoting agent on chondrogenesis. Am. J. Anat. 150:207–212.

Peraino, C., R. J. M. Fry, and D. D. Grube. 1978. Drug-induced enhancement of hepatic tumorigenesis, *in* Carcinogenesis Vol. 2. Mechanisms of Tumor Promotion and Cocarcinogenesis, T. J. Slaga, A. Sivak, and R. K. Boutwell, eds., Raven Press, New York, pp. 421–432.

Prusik, T., N. E. Geacintov, C. Tobiasz, V. Ivanovic, and I. B. Weinstein. 1978. Fluorescence study of the physicochemical properties of a benzo(a)pyrene 7,8-dihydrodiol 9,10-oxide derivative bound covalently to DNA. Photochem. Photobiol. (In press).

Pulkrabek, P., S. Leffler, I. B. Weinstein, and D. Grunberger. 1977. Conformation of DNA modified with a dihydrodiol epoxide derivative of benzo(a)pyrene. Biochemistry 16:3127–3132.

Radman, M., G. Villani, S. Boiteux, M. Defais, and P. Caillet-Fauquet. 1977. On the mechanism and genetic control of mutagenesis induced by carcinogenic mutagens, *in* Origins of Human Cancer, Cold Spring Harbor Conferences on Cell Proliferation Vol. 4, H. H. Hiatt, J. D. Watson, and J. A. Winsten, eds., Cold Spring Harbor Laboratory, Cold Spring Harbor, New York, pp. 903–922.

Raick, A. N. 1974. Cell differentiation and tumor promoting action in skin carcinogenesis. Cancer Res. 34:2915–2925.

Reich, E., D. B. Rifkind, and E. Shaw. eds. 1975. Proteases and Biological Controls, Cold Spring Harbor Laboratory, Cold Spring Harbor, New York.

Rovera, G., T. A. O'Brien, and L. Diamond. 1977. Tumor promoters inhibit spontaneous differentiation of Friend erythroleukemia cells in culture. Proc. Natl. Acad. Sci. USA 74:2894–2898.

Sarasin, A. R., and P. C. Hanawalt. 1978. Carcinogens enhance survival of UV-irradiated simian virus 40 in treated monkey kidney cells: Induction of a recovery pathway. Proc. Natl. Acad. Sci. USA 75:346–350.

Schachter, D., and M. Shinitsky. 1977. Fluorescence polarization studies of rat intestinal microvillus membranes. J. Clin. Invest. 59:536–548.

Shinohara, K., and P. A. Cerutti. 1977. Excision repair of BP-deoxyguanosine adducts in baby hamster kidney cells and in secondary mouse embryo fibroblasts. Proc. Natl. Acad. Sci. USA 74:979–983.

Sivak, A., and B. L. Van Duuren. 1967. Phenotypic expression of transformation: Induction in cell culture by a phorbol ester. Science 157:1443–1444.

Sporn, M. B., D. L. Newton, J. M. Smith, N. Acton, A. E. Jacobson, and A. Brossi. 1979. Retinoids and cancer prevention: The importance of the terminal group of the retinoid molecule in modifying activity and toxicity, *in* Carcinogens: Identification and Mechanisms of Action (The University of Texas System Cancer Center 31st Annual Symposium on Fundamental Cancer Research, 1978), A. C. Griffin and C. R. Shaw, eds., Raven Press, New York, pp. 441–453.

Straub, K. M., T. Meehan, A. L. Burlingame, and M. Calvin. 1977. Identification of the major adducts formed by reaction of benzo(a)pyrene diol epoxide with DNA *in vitro*. Proc. Natl. Acad. Sci. USA 74:5285–5289.

Suss, R., G. Kreibich, and V. Kinzel. 1972. Phorbol esters as a tool in cell research. Eur. J. Cancer 8:299–304.

Troll, W., T. Rossman, J. Katz, M. Levitz, and T. Sugimura. 1975. Proteases in tumor promotion and hormone action, *in* Proteases and Biological Controls, E. Reich, D. B. Rifkin, and E. Shaw, eds., Cold Spring Harbor Laboratory, Cold Spring Harbor, New York, pp. 977–987.

Van Duuren, B. L. 1969. Tumor promoting agents in two-stage carcinogenesis. Prog. Exp. Tumor Res. 11:31–68.

Vassalli, J. D., J. Hamilton, and E. Reich. 1977. Macrophage plasminogen activator: Modulation of enzyme production by anti-inflammatory steroids, mitotic inhibitors, and cyclic nucleotides. Cell 8:271–281.

Weinstein, I. B. 1976. Molecular events in chemical carcinogenesis, *in* Advances in Pathobiology, Vol. 4, Cancer Biology II, Etiology and Therapy, M. Fenoglio and D. W. King, eds., Stratton Intercontinental Medical Book Corp., New York, New York, pp. 106–117.

Weinstein, I. B. 1977. Types of interaction between carcinogens and nucleic acids, *in* Mechanismes D'Alteration et de Reparation du DNA, Relations avec la Mutagenese et la Cancerogenese-Chimique. Colloques Internationaux du C.N.R.S. No. 256. Centre National de la Recherche Scientifique, Paris, France, pp. 2–40.

Weinstein, I. B. 1978. Current concepts on mechanisms of chemical carcinogenesis. Bull. NY Acad. Sci. 54:366–383.

Weinstein, I. B., and D. Grunberger. 1974. Structural and functional changes in nucleic acids modified by chemical carcinogens, *in* Chemical Carcinogenesis, Part A., P. Ts'o and J. DiPaolo, eds., Marcel Dekker, New York, pp. 217–235.

Weinstein, I. B., A. M. Jeffrey, K. W. Jennette, S. H. Blobstein, R. G. Harvey, C. Harris, H. Autrup, H. Kasai, and K. Nakanishi. 1976. Benzo(a)pyrene diol-epoxides as intermediates in nucleic acid binding *in vitro* and *in vivo*. Science 193:592–595.

Weinstein, I. B., A. M. Jeffrey, S. Leffler, P. Pulkrabek, H. Yamasaki, and D. Grunberger. 1978a. Interactions between polycyclic aromatic hydrocarbons and cellular macromolecules, *in* Polycyclic Hydrocarbons and Cancer: Environment, Chemistry, Molecular and Cell Biology, H. V. Gelboin and P. O. P. Ts'o, eds. Vol. 2. Academic Press, New York, pp. 3–36.

Weinstein, I. B., and M. Wigler. 1977. Cell culture studies provide new information on tumour promoters. Nature 270:659–661.

Weinstein, I. B., M. Wigler, and C. Pietropaolo. 1977. The action of tumor-promoting agents in cell culture, *in* Origins of Human Cancer, Cold Spring Harbor Conferences on Cell Proliferation. Vol. 4. H. H. Hiatt, J. D. Watson, and J. A. Winsten, eds. Cold Spring Harbor Laboratory, Cold Spring Harbor, New York, pp. 751–752.

Weinstein, I. B., M. Wigler, P. Fisher, E. Sisskin, and C. Pietropaolo. 1978b. Cell culture studies on the biologic effects of tumor promoters, *in* Carcinogenesis, Vol. 2., Mechanisms of Tumor Promotion and Cocarcinogenesis, T. J. Slaga, A. Sivak, and R. K. Boutwell, eds., Raven Press, New York, pp. 313–333.

Westra, J. G., E. Kriek, and H. Hittenhausen. 1976. Identification of the persistently bound form of the carcinogen N-acetyl-2-aminofluorene to rat liver DNA in vivo. Chem. Biol. Interact. 15:149–164.

Wigler, M., D. DeFeo, and I. B. Weinstein. 1978. Induction of plasminogen activator in cultured cells by macrocyclic plant diterpene esters and other agents related to tumor promotion. Cancer Res. 38:1434–1437.

Wigler, M., S. Silverstein, L. S. Lee, A. Pellicer, Y. C. Cheng, and R. Axel. 1977. Transfer of purified Herpes virus thymidine kinase gene to cultured mouse cells. Cell 11:223–232.

Wigler, M., and I. B. Weinstein. 1976. Tumour promoter induces plasminogen activator. Nature 259:232–233.

Witkin, E. M. 1976. Ultraviolet mutagenesis and inducible DNA repair in *Escherichia coli.* Bacteriol. Rev. 40:869–907.

Yamasaki, H., E. Fibach, U. Nudel, I. B. Weinstein, R. A. Rifkind, and P. A. Marks. 1977a. Tumor promoters inhibit spontaneous and induced differentiation of murine erythroleukemia cells in culture. Proc. Natl. Acad. Sci. USA 74:3451–3455.

Yamasaki, H., E. Fibach, I. B. Weinstein, U. Nudel, R. A. Rifkind, and P. A. Marks. 1978a. Inhibition of Friend leukemia cell differentiation by tumor promoters, *in* Oncogenic Viruses and Host Cell Genes, Oji International Seminar on Friend Virus and Friend Cells, Yoji Ikawa, ed., Academic Press, New York. (In press).

Yamasaki, H., S. Leffler, and I. B. Weinstein. 1977b. Effect of N-2-acetyl-aminofluorene modification on the structure and template activity of DNA and reconstituted chromatin. Cancer Res. 37:684–691.

Yamasaki, H., P. Pulkrabek, D. Grunberger, and I. B. Weinstein. 1977c. Differential excision from DNA of the C-8 and N^2 guanosine adducts of N-acetyl-2-aminofluorene by single strand-specific endonucleases. Cancer Res. 37:3756–3760.

Yamasaki, H., T. W. Roush, and I. B. Weinstein. 1978b. Benzo(a)pyrene 7,8-dyhydrodiol 9,10-oxide modification of DNA: Relation to chromatin structure and reconstitution. Chem. Biol. Interact. (In press).

Yuspa, S. H., T. Ben, E. Patterson, D. Michael, K. Elgjo, and H. Hennings. 1976a. Stimulated DNA synthesis in mouse epidermal cell cultures treated with 12-0-tetradecanoyl-phorbol-13-acetate. Cancer Res. 36:4062–4068.

Yuspa, S. H., U. Lichti, T. Ben, E. Patterson, H. Hennings, T. J. Slaga, N. Colburn, and W. Kelsey. 1976b. Phorbol esters stimulate DNA synthesis and ornithine decarboxylase activity in mouse epidermal cell cultures. Nature 262:402–404.

Zieg, J., M. Silverman, M. Hilmen, and M. Simon. 1977. Recombinant switch for gene expression. Science 196:170–172.

Carcinogens: Identification and Mechanisms of
Action, edited by A. Clark Griffin and
Charles R. Shaw. Raven Press, New York © 1979.

Effects of Carcinogens on Nuclear Protein Composition and Metabolism

Alterations in Chromatin Structure and Activity as Related to Postsynthetic Modification of Histones and to Disposition of DNA-Binding Proteins

Vincent G. Allfrey, Lidia C. Boffa, and Giorgio Vidali

Rockefeller University, New York, New York 10021

The experiments to be described deal with changes in nuclear protein composition and rates of synthesis during the induction of tumors of the intestinal epithelium by the alkylating carcinogen, 1,2-dimethylhydrazine (DMH). A particular subset of nuclear nonhistone proteins of molecular weight 43,000–45,000 daltons (designated TNP_1) is synthesized selectively at early stages in carcinogenesis. Some of these are DNA-binding proteins that can be separated by affinity chromatography on DNA covalently linked to solid supports. Some of the TNP_1 proteins appear to be localized on actively transcribing regions of the chromatin, as judged by their preferential release during limited digestions of the tumor nuclei with DNase I under conditions known to selectively degrade the active genes in a variety of nuclear types.

The structural basis for the selective degradation of transcriptionally active DNA sequences by DNase I has been investigated by experimentally raising the level of acetylation of nucleosomal histones H3 and H4 in intact HeLa cells. We find that DNA associated with highly acetylated histones is preferentially degraded and that the most highly acetylated forms of histone H4 are released at very early times during DNase I digestion, as would be expected if the modified histones were localized in regions of the chromatin that had been activated for transcription. The role of histone acetylation and deacetylation in the control of chromatin structure and in the hepatic response to carinogens such as aflatoxin B_1 is discussed.

CHANGES IN NUCLEAR PROTEINS DURING CARCINOGENESIS

Aberrant patterns of transcription in tumor cells—often evident in the activation of "embryonic genes" and in the production of "tumor-specific" antigens—strongly suggest changes in the interactions between DNA and those associated chromosomal proteins that regulate chromatin structure and control the specificity, timing, and extent of RNA synthesis in the nucleus. The nonhistone nuclear proteins, which have been strongly implicated in transcriptional control mechanisms, are known to be altered in a variety of carcinogen-induced tumors (Boffa et al. 1975, Gronow and Thackrah 1974a,b, Yeoman et al. 1974) and transplantable tumor lines (Arnold et al. 1973, Chae et al. 1974, Orrick et al. 1973, Stein et al. 1974).

The significance of such changes in the expression of the malignant phenotype is difficult to assess for several reasons. Changes in the proportions of nuclear nonhistone proteins are commonly observed in normal differentiative processes (Boffa et al. 1975, Teng et al. 1971), in liver regeneration (Garrard and Bonner 1974), in the maturation of erythrocytes (Ruiz-Carrillo et al. 1974), and in lymphocyte activation (Johnson et al. 1974), and they need not indicate aberrant genetic control. A second difficulty in interpreting most of the observed differences between normal and tumor nuclear proteins is the complexity of the cell populations examined. Many established tumor lines have different numbers of chromosomes and thus would be expected to vary in their chromosomal protein contents. Normal tissues and tumors in situ generally include a variety of cell types programmed for different functions. Nuclei from different cell types of normal tissues such as brain, liver, or intestinal epithelium are known to differ in their nonhistone protein complement (Austoker et al. 1972, Boffa et al. 1976, Gonzales-Mujica et al. 1973, Wilson et al. 1975), and the same is true for different nuclear classes from Morris hepatomas (Wilson et al. 1975) and colonic adenocarcinomas (Boffa and Allfrey 1976). Such differences in protein composition among different classes of nuclei in both normal tissues and tumors complicate interpretations of quantitative or qualitative differences between the normal and malignant states.

In an attempt to improve the resolution and simplify the analysis of chromosomal protein changes in malignant transformation, we have combined a study of tumor induction by the chemical carcinogen DMH with procedures for the separation of more homogeneous populations of nuclei from normal and tumor tissues. The results point to a striking correlation between the appearance of a "new" class of DNA-binding proteins and the onset of malignancy in colonic epithelial cells.

Preparation of Nuclei from DMH-Induced Tumors

The induction of colonic adenocarcinomas by the administration of 1,2-dimethylhydrazine to rodents provides a model of chemical carcinogenesis with the advantages of organ specificity, reproducible timing, and high tumor incidence (Druckrey 1970, Druckrey et al. 1967, Martin et al. 1973). The normal patterns of cell proliferation and differentiation in the crypts of the intestinal epithelium are modified, and aberrations in nucleic acid synthesis become evident soon after DMH-treatment is begun (Hawks et al. 1974, Thunherr et al. 1973). Previous studies of cell kinetics in the intestinal mucosa have shown that there is a gradient of DNA-synthetic activity at different levels of the crypts (Chang and Leblond 1970, Lipkin and Quastler 1962). In normal epithelium the cells proliferate in the lower and middle levels of the crypts, migrate toward the lumen of the intestine, and are gradually extruded from the surface. Autoradiographic studies have shown that ^{3}H-thymidine incorporation into DNA is mainly restricted to cells in the lower one third of the crypts. DNA-synthesizing cells are much less common in the mid-regions of the crypts, and they are usually absent from the upper region. In colonic tumors, however, the distribution of DNA-synthesizing cells is significantly altered; the gradient of DNA-synthetic activity is much less pronounced in established adenocarcinomas and in premalignant growths due to the presence of many more dividing cells in the upper levels of the crypts (Deschner *et al.* 1963, 1966, Lipkin 1974). In tumors induced by DMH, cells close to the luminal surface were found to incorporate ^{3}H-thymidine, in contrast to the inactivity of the corresponding cells in normal colonic epithelium (Thunherr *et al.* 1973).

Given such complexity in cell kinetics and the fact that the dividing cell population of the tumor represents its potential for invasive growth, we have developed methods for the fractionation of colonic tumor nuclei to yield subsets that differ in their capacity for DNA synthesis (Boffa *et al.* 1976, Boffa and Allfrey 1976). The method is applicable to both normal and malignant tissues and depends on the differences in buoyant density between various nuclear classes at different stages in the cell cycle. This makes it possible to compare nuclear protein compositions as a function of cell type and stage in differentiation (Boffa *et al.* 1976) and to determine which proteins are associated with the dividing cell populations of normal and malignant tissues.

In the experiments to be described, tumors were induced in CFN-Wistar male rats by weekly s.c. injections of DMH at a dosage of 20 mg/kg body weight. By the 21st week, more than 98% of the treated animals had multiple tumors of the colon (Boffa *et al.* 1975). The excised tumor tissue was homogenized, and a purified nuclear fraction was isolated by centrifugation through a 2.2 M sucrose density barrier. This fraction, representing all of the cell types present in the tumor, was suspended in 2.5 M sucrose and used as a component of a discontinuous density gradient ranging in sucrose concentration from 2.30 M to 2.70 M. After centrifugation at $75,000 \times g$ for 90 minutes, fractions were collected from the gradient, and the nuclei in each fraction were characterized (Boffa *et al.* 1976). The procedure separates tumor nuclei that differ in buoyant density and size, as shown in Figure 1. Measurements of DNA-specific activity in each nuclear subset after labeling with ^{3}H-thymidine in vivo show that the most radioactive nuclei are distributed within the gradient in a manner which parallels the distribution of their cells of origin in the crypts (Boffa *et al.* 1976, Boffa and Allfrey 1976). In general, the DNA-synthetic activity of the nucleus decreases as the nuclei enlarge and their buoyant density decreases. For example, in fractionations of nuclei from normal colonic epithelium after pulse-labeling with ^{3}H-thymidine, the specific activity of the DNA in nuclei

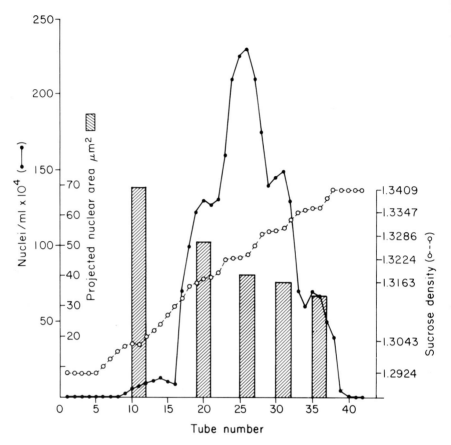

FIG. 1. Separation of different subsets of nuclei from DMH-induced colonic tumors by centrifugation in a discontinuous sucrose density gradient. The number of nuclei at different levels of the gradient is shown by the solid line. The histogram indicates the average nuclear cross-sectional area in sq μm for nuclei at the indicated buoyant densities.

banding at the bottom of the gradient is six times greater than that of nuclei at the top of the gradient, in accordance with the autoradiographic evidence that most of the dividing cells occur at the base of the crypts. Moreover, the widening of the proliferative zone in neoplastic mucosa (Deschner *et al.* 1963, 1966, Lipkin 1974, Thunherr *et al.* 1973) is matched by a broader dispersion of ^{3}H-labeled tumor nuclei in the sucrose gradient (Boffa and Allfrey 1976).

Nuclear Proteins of DMH-Induced Tumors

Tumor nuclei recovered from different levels of the density gradient differ markedly in their total protein/DNA ratios; from 2.6/1.0 at the bottom of the gradient to 3.9/1.0 at the top of the gradient. These differences are due entirely to changes in the nuclear content of nonhistone proteins. The histone/ DNA ratios remain constant across the gradient. Electrophoretic analyses, using unidirectional sodium dodecyl sulfate (SDS)-polyacrylamide gels (Laemmli 1970) and two-dimensional gels that separate nuclear proteins according to charge and molecular weight (O'Farrell 1975), show great complexity in the nonhistone protein complement. The electrophoretic profiles are clearly different for tumor nuclei at different levels of the gradient (Boffa and Allfrey 1976). The differences are likely to be significant and not artefactual because the extraction procedure employed (6 M urea, 0.4 M guanidine-HCl, 0.1 M Na_2HPO_4, 0.1% 2-mercapto-ethanol) permits recovery of $87 \pm 2\%$ of the total nonhistone protein, thus minimizing the possibility that the observed, and often extreme, differences in protein complements in different nuclear subsets might simply be due to variations in protein extractability.

Earlier electrophoretic comparisons of the nonhistone nuclear proteins of normal colonic epithelial nuclei and DMH-induced colonic tumor nuclei have indicated a characteristic shift in protein complement during carcinogenesis, with a striking increase in the concentrations of two classes of acidic proteins of molecular weight ca. 44,000 daltons (TNP_1) and ca. 62,000 daltons (TNP_2) (Boffa et al. 1975). These proteins eventually dominate the electrophoretic profile of the tumor nuclear proteins, as shown in the top two panels of Figure 2. Fractionation of the tumor nuclei in discontinuous sucrose gradients, as shown in Figure 1, followed by electrophoretic analysis of the proteins in each nuclear subset, indicated that the TNP_1 protein class was selectively localized in the DNA-synthesizing nuclei of the dividing cell population and was virtually absent from the nondividing cells of the tumor mass (Boffa and Allfrey 1976). It is noteworthy that proteins resembling TNP_1 have been detected in human adeno-carcinomas and in malignant cell lines derived from human adenocarcinomas (such as HT-29)(Boffa and Allfrey 1976), but they were not observed in normal colonic epithelium or in nonmalignant hyperplastic growths (Boffa and Allfrey 1977).

In the induction of colonic tumors by DMH, TNP_1 and TNP_2 both accumulate progressively. Quantitation of TNP_1 and TNP_2 levels at biweekly intervals showed a continuing increase from the 7th to the 21st week, when over 98% of the animals have multiple tumor foci (Boffa et al. 1975). At that time, TNP_1 and TNP_2 each comprise about 15% of the total protein remaining in dehiston-ized colonic tumor nuclei.

Isotopic labeling experiments, using radioactive amino acids, have shown that the progressive accumulation of these nuclear proteins in DMH-treated animals is due to an early and selective increase in their rates of synthesis. The change in synthetic rate becomes evident within the first four weeks of DMH treatment (Boffa et al. 1975); this is long before pathological indications of malignancy appear.

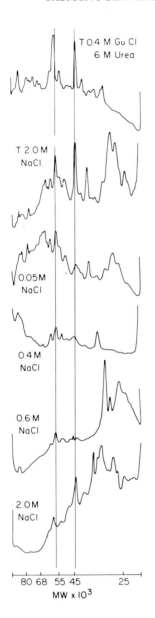

FIG. 2. DNA-affinity chromatography of tumor proteins. The upper panel shows the electrophoretic profile of the proteins extracted in 6 M urea, 0.4 M guanidine-HC1, 0.1 M Na_2HPO_4, 0.1% 2-mercaptoethanol. Beneath it is the corresponding electrophoretic profile of the nuclear proteins extractable in 2 M NaCl. Both profiles show the characteristic peaks at ca. 44,000 daltons (TNP_1) and ca. 62,000 daltons (TNP_2). The proteins of the 2 M NaCl extract were applied to a column of DNA covalently bound to Sephadex G-25 and eluted by stepwise increments in the NaCl concentration of the eluting buffer, as indicated on the right of the corresponding electrophoretic profile. Note that the tumor nuclear protein fraction of molecular weight ca. 44,000 daltons (TNP_1) is not displaced from the DNA at low ionic strengths but requires 2 M NaCl for its elution. Most of the TNP_2 peak is released from the DNA column at low ionic strengths.

Characterization of Tumor-Associated Nonhistone Nuclear Proteins

TNP_1 and TNP_2 were isolated from the nuclei of DMH-induced tumors by preparative gel electrophoresis. The amino acid compositions of both fractions was determined. TNP_1 and TNP_2 showed a strong predominance of glutamic and aspartic acids over the basic amino acids lysine, arginine, and histidine.

Both fractions were lacking in cysteine, methionine, and proline (Boffa *et al.* 1975).

The banding patterns of the nuclear nonhistone proteins, as separated by unidirectional electrophoresis in SDS-polyacrylamide gels, do not adequately depict the complexity of the tumor nuclear-protein complement. A better indication of size and charge heterogeneity is provided by two-dimensional gel electrophoretic separations that combine isoelectric focusing in the first dimension, with size separations in the second dimension. We have modified the procedure of O'Farrell (1975) to permit higher recoveries of proteins in the isoelectric focusing step (Boffa and Allfrey 1977). Subsequent separations in SDS-polyacrylamide gels (at 90°C to the original direction of charge-dependent migration) provided a two-dimensional display of the nuclear proteins of DMH-induced adenocarcinomas. As described previously (Boffa and Allfrey 1977), the narrow bands in the 44,000 dalton range (TNP_1) and 62,000 dalton range (TNP_2) show considerable complexity in two-dimensional gels. Both TNP_1 and TNP_2 have isoelectric points in the acidic range, in agreement with the predominance of aspartic and glutamic acids in the overall amino acid compositions. TNP_2 shows a major subgroup of proteins of molecular weight ca. 61,000 with pI's ranging from 5.6 to 6.5, and another group of molecular weight ca. 63,000 with pI's between 6.2 and 6.8. The TNP_1 class appears to be simpler, and it is more acidic; its major components focus over the pH range 4.85 to 5.25, but a single component has a pI of 6.5. It is known that many of the tumor nonhistone nuclear proteins are phosphorylated, and some of the charge heterogeneity observed in isoelectric focusing experiments may reflect different levels of phosphorylation of the same polypeptide chains.

We have recently described the application of raster-scanning microdensitometry and computer-assisted graphics to the analysis of the complex images provided by two-dimensional gel electrophoresis of nuclear proteins (Allfrey *et al.*, in press). The computer plots not only indicate the molecular weight and isoelectric point coordinates for each protein but also reveal subtle heterogeneities in size and charge. This can be particularly useful in the study of postsynthetic modifications of nuclear proteins which alter their charge (phosphorylation, acetylation, ADP-ribosylation, etc.), especially when combined with autoradiographic techniques and raster-scanning microdensitometry of the radiographs.

DNA-Binding by Tumor Nuclear Proteins

In order to investigate the DNA-binding properties of the tumor-associated proteins, the usual extraction procedure was modified to avoid denaturing agents such as urea and guanidinium chloride. Instead, the nuclear proteins were extracted in 2 M NaCl at pH 8.0, and the clarified extract was mixed with double-stranded rat DNA covalently bound to Sephadex G-25 (Allfrey *et al.* 1974, Allfrey and Inoue 1977). After a series of dialysis steps to reduce the NaCl concentration to 50 mM, the DNA-Sephadex/protein mixture was poured into a chromatographic column, and the proteins were eluted by stepwise increments in the ionic strength of the eluting buffer. This chromatographic procedure has been previously shown to reproducibly separate sets of nuclear proteins differing in DNA affinity and to detect proteins that selectively interact with DNA sequences of different C_0t values (Allfrey *et al.* 1974, Allfrey and Inoue 1977).

DNA-affinity chromatography of the tumor nuclear proteins soluble in 2M NaCl also provides subsets of proteins with characteristic electrophoretic profiles. Figure 2 shows the densitometric tracings of the protein fractions eluting from the DNA column at progressively higher salt concentrations. Proteins of the TNP_1 class (molecular weight 44,000) appear to be DNA-binding proteins, and they require high ionic strengths for their elution. In contrast, most of the TNP_2 class has little or no affinity for DNA and emerges from the column at very low ionic strengths. (Control experiments using Sephadex G-25 columns that had been treated with the coupling reagent, but not reacted with DNA, did not bind nuclear proteins, and both TNP_1 and TNP_2 were recovered in the 0.05 M NaCl "run-off" peak.)

We conclude that the TNP_1 class of tumor nuclear proteins, although acidic in nature (as judged by amino acid composition [Boffa *et al.* 1975] and low isoelectric point range [between 4.85 and 5.25]) binds strongly to DNA at physiological pH values. (Further evidence to support this view is presented below.) Whether the binding involves strong electrostatic interactions between regions of the polypeptide chains that are enriched in basic amino acids and DNA phosphate groups remains to be determined, but the dissociation of the complex by salt would suggest that TNP_1 binding to DNA probably has an electrostatic component.

Evidence for an association of TNP_1 proteins with DNA in vivo has been obtained by studies of protein released during limited DNase I digestion of tumor nuclei.

Selective Release of TNP_1 by Limited DNase I Digestion

Limited digestion of avian erythrocyte chromatin by DNase I has been shown to result in a rapid and selective degradation of the globin genes, but these genes are not preferentially degraded in a nonerythroid cell, such as the fibroblast of the same organism (Weintraub and Groudine 1976). Similarly, the ovalbumin gene in oviduct chromatin is selectively degraded by DNase I, but such sensitivity is not detected in liver nuclei (Garel and Axel 1976). The differential sensitivity to DNase I of transcriptionally active DNA sequences, regardless of their rate of transcription (Garel *et al.* 1977), implies an altered conformation of the genes that are programmed for activity in a particular cell type. The reasons for the differential DNase I sensitivity of "active" DNA sequences will be discussed in more detail later; the present discussion focuses on the use of DNase I as a probe for the identification of proteins likely to be components of the transcription complex.

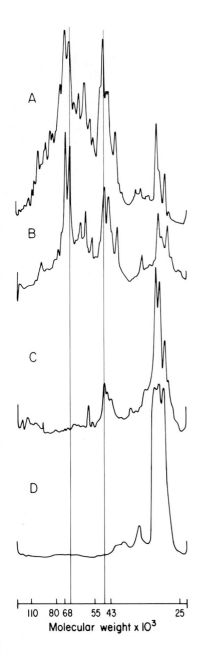

FIG. 3. Selective release of TNP_1 proteins during a limited digestion of adenocarcinoma nuclei by DNase I. Aliquots of the nuclear suspension were incubated in the presence (B and C) or absence (A and D) of pancreatic DNase I for five minutes. After centrifugation to separate the "resistant" chromatin fraction from more degraded chromatin fragments in the supernate, the proteins in both fractions were extracted and analyzed by electrophoresis in SDS polyacrylamide gels. Densitometric tracings of the protein banding patterns are shown, with vertical lines indicating the positions of TNP_1 and TNP_2. Note that DNase I digestion releases proteins of molecular weight similar to that of the TNP_1 class, but no loss of TNP_2 is observed. The "resistant" chromatin fraction after DNase I digestion is depleted in TNP_1, as is evident in comparisons of the profile of the DNase I-digested sample in (B) with the enzyme-free control in (A). Nuclei incubated in the absence of DNase I lose very little protein; the pattern shown in (D) was obtained after a 10-fold concentration of the supernate.

Nuclei isolated from DMH-induced adenocarcinomas were incubated with DNase I under conditions that released only $10 \pm 2\%$ of the total DNA. After this limited digestion, the nuclei were sonicated briefly, and the suspension was centrifuged to separate the residual "resistant" chromatin fraction from more highly degraded chromatin fragments in the supernatant fraction. The proteins of both fractions were analyzed by SDS-polyacrylamide gel electrophoresis, with the results shown in Figure 3. The limited digestion of tumor chromatin by DNase I releases some histones together with a class of nuclear proteins of molecular weight corresponding to that of TNP_1 (43,000–45,000 daltons). A smaller peak at 56,000 daltons is also observed (Figure 3C). It is significant that tumor nuclei incubated in the absence of DNase I do not release proteins of the TNP_1 class (Figure 3D), nor is there any indication of a selective release of TNP_2 from tumor nuclei incubated in the presence or absence of DNase I (Figure 3C and D). Examination of the electrophoretic profiles of the proteins remaining in the "resistant" chromatin fraction of control and DNase I-treated tumor nuclei (shown in panels A and B of Figure 3) indicates that limited DNase I digestion has not diminished the proportion of TNP_2 remaining in the nuclei but has released a considerable amount of TNP_1. This again indicates that the two major protein classes of the tumor are not alike in their nuclear localizations. The experiments confirm the chromatographic evidence summarized in Figure 2 that TNP_1 includes a set of DNA-binding proteins. The presence of such proteins on actively transcribing genes is also indicated (but not proved) in these experiments. (Because all incubations were performed in the presence of the protease inhibitor, PMSF, we conclude that the differential release of nuclear proteins by DNase I digestion is not likely to be an artefact of proteolysis.)

The basis for the selective release of proteins associated with transcriptionally active DNA sequences was next investigated—and evidence was obtained that the selective degradation of "active" genes correlates with the level of acetylation of the associated nucleosomal histones.

THE ROLE OF HISTONE ACETYLATION IN THE DIFFERENTIAL SENSITIVITY OF TRANSCRIPTIONALLY ACTIVE DNA SEQUENCES TO DNase I

It has been repeatedly observed that DNA sequences with the potential for transcription in a particular cell type are selectively degraded during brief digestions of the nuclei with DNase I. The corresponding sequences are not selectively degraded during DNase I digestions of nuclei from cells in which they are not expressed (Weintraub and Groudine 1976, Garel and Axel 1976, Garel et al. 1977, Levy-W. and Dixon 1977). What is the basis for the conformational difference between "active" and "inactive" chromatin?

On the premise that an altered conformation of the nucleosomes in transcription complexes might be due to postsynthetic modifications of the histones associated with the DNA template, we have studied the effects of histone acetylation on the DNase I sensitivity of tumor chromatin. There are many reasons why this premise warrants investigation. Since the discovery of histone acetylation (Allfrey 1964, Allfrey et al. 1964), numerous correlations have been noted between increased acetylation of the histones and gene activation, as induced by hormones, mitogens, and developmental stimuli, and decreased acetylation of the histones when transcription is suppressed during development of erythrocytes (Ruiz-Carrillo *et al.* 1974) and sperm cells (Wangh *et al.* 1972) (or inhibited by carcinogens such as aflatoxin B_1 [Edwards and Allfrey 1973]). Much of the evidence for temporal and spatial correlations between histone acetylation and gene activity has been reviewed recently (Allfrey 1977, Johnson and Allfrey 1978). Of particular relevance to the present study of changes in nuclear proteins during carcinogenesis are observations that histones associated with the DNA of transforming viruses, such as SV-40 and polyoma virus, are much more acetylated than the corresponding histones of the host cells (Schaffhausen and Benjamin 1976). The correlation between a high acetyl content of polyoma virus histones and malignant transformation is strengthened by the finding that nontransforming host-range mutants of the virus do not show a high level of histone acetylation. The transcriptionally active sequences of integrated adenovirus-5 genes in transformed hamster cells have recently been shown to be DNase I sensitive (Flint and Weintraub 1977), and although the level of acetylation of the histones associated with the integrated viral genome has not been determined, the results on SV-40 and polyoma viruses suggest that viral gene activity may be generally associated with a high level of acetylation of the associated histones.

It has been proposed that increased acetylation of the nucleosomal histones, by neutralizing the positive charges on the epsilon-amino groups of the modified lysine residues, may release the constraints upon the enveloping DNA strand (Allfrey 1977, Johnson and Allfrey 1978). A direct test of this hypothesis became possible when it was observed that in vivo levels of histone acetylation could be increased experimentally by exposing HeLa cells to 5 mM Na butyrate (Riggs *et al.* 1977). The postsynthetic acetylation of histones involves a transfer of acetyl groups from acetyl-coenzyme A (Allfrey 1964) to the epsilon-amino groups (Gershey *et al.* 1968, DeLange *et al.* 1969) of specific lysine residues in the amino-terminal regions of the polypeptide chain (DeLange *et al.* 1969, Candido and Dixon 1972a,b). Histones H3 and H4, which play a key role in the organization of the nucleosome (Camerini-Otero *et al.* 1976, Sollner-Webb *et al.* 1976, Moss *et al.* 1977), each have four sites of internal acetylation; and in most cell types, each of these histones comprises a mixture of polypeptide chains containing 0 to 4 epsilon-N-acetyllysine residues. The various acetylated forms are separated from each other and from the parent polypeptide chain by high resolution gel electrophoretic techniques (Panyim and Chalkley 1969, Wangh *et al.* 1972, Ruiz-Carrillo *et al.* 1974). Acetate uptake into histones in vivo is known to be reversible, and the overall level of acetylation involves an equilibrium between acetate uptake, as catalyzed by acetyl transferases, and acetate removal, as catalyzed by histone deacetylases. The ability to modify the level of acetylation by exposing cells to butyrate is due to the inhibition of histone deacetylases (Vidali *et al.* 1978, Boffa *et al.* 1978).

The inhibitory effects of butyrate on the deacetylation of histones has been established using the purified deacetylase of calf thymus lymphocyte nuclei (Vi-

dali *et al.* 1972) and purified histone H4 which had been labeled in situ with
³H-acetate. The effects of increasing concentrations of Na butyrate on the kinetics
of ³H-acetate release from the histone substrate are shown in Figure 4. It is
clear that 5 mM butyrate, the concentration used by Riggs *et al.* (1977) to
raise the level of acetylation of HeLa cell histones, effectively inhibits the deacetylation reaction.

We have confirmed the observation that butyrate treatment increases the
proportions of the acetylated forms of histones H3 and H4 in HeLa cells and
further established that the modification occurs at the nucleosomal level (Vidali
et al. 1978). Mono-nucleosomes were prepared from control and butyrate-treated
cells by digestion with staphylococcal nuclease and gradient centrifugation. The
monosome fractions were compared with regard to their contents of acetylated
and nonacetylated forms of histones H3 and H4. Figure 5 shows the densitometric tracings of the histone banding patterns in the chromatin monomer particles
of control and butyrate-treated HeLa cells, and it is clear that exposure to 7
mM Na butyrate leads to a massive accumulation of the acetylated forms of
these two key nucleosomal histones. As expected, this accumulation of acetylated
histones is due to the inhibition of histone deacetylation. We have shown that
7 mM butyrate has little or no effect on the rate of incorporation of radioactive
acetate into HeLa histones (Boffa *et al.* 1978); its major effect is to block the
removal of previously incorporated acetyl groups. This is shown by the double-
labeling experiments summarized in Figure 6. In these experiments, cells were
prepared containing histones labeled with either ¹⁴C-acetate or ³H-acetate. Cells
containing ¹⁴C-acetylated histones were washed, resuspended in nonradioactive
medium containing 7 mM Na butyrate and incubated at 37°C. Aliquots were
withdrawn at regular intervals for extraction of the histones, which were purified

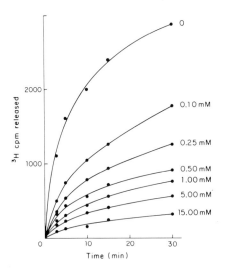

FIG. 4. Inhibition of a purified nuclear histone deacetylase by Na butyrate. The enzyme was purified from isolated calf thymus nuclei as described by Vidali *et al.* (1972) and tested on purified H4 histone that had been labeled in situ with ³H-acetate to a specific activity of 10,200 cpm/mg. The same preparation of histone deacetylase was used in all experiments comparing the kinetics of ³H-acetate release at different concentrations of Na butyrate in the reaction medium.

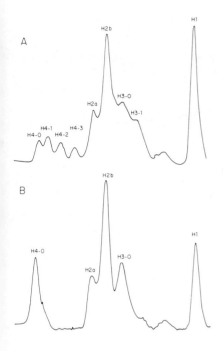

FIG. 5. Increased acetylation of nucleosomal histones H3 and H4 following a 21-hour exposure of HeLa S3 cells to 7 mM Na butyrate in the culture medium. The nucleosomes of control and butyrate-treated cells were prepared by digestion of the isolated nuclei with staphylococcal nuclease, and the mono-nucleosome peaks were purified by sucrose density gradient centrifugation. The histones were extracted and analyzed by electrophoresis in 25 cm, 12% polyacrylamide gels containing acetic acid and urea. Densitometric tracings of the stained histone bands are shown for the mono-nucleosomes of butyrate-treated cells in panel A, and for the control mono-nucleosomes in panel B. Note that increased substitution of the histone lysine residues by acetylation diminishes the electrophoretic mobility of the parent polypeptide chains. The mono- and multi-acetylated forms of histone H4 are present in high amounts after butyrate treatment, as compared with their relatively low proportions in the control nucleosomes. Butyrate treatment also increases the level of acetylation of histone H3 in the mono-nucleosomes.

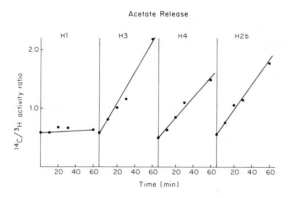

FIG. 6. Suppression of histone acetyl group "turnover" in HeLa cells exposed to 7 mM Na butyrate. Cells containing ^3H-acetyl-labeled histones were incubated at 37°C in nonradioactive, butyrate-free medium, while cells containing ^{14}C-acetyl-labeled histones were incubated in nonradioactive medium containing 7 mM Na butyrate. The retention of acetyl-^3H and acetyl-^{14}C groups in histones H1, H2b, H3, and H4 of control and butyrate-treated cells was compared at successive times during the "cold-chase." The progressive increase in the $^{14}C/^3H$ ratio of the nucleosomal histones H2b, H3, and H4 indicates a suppression of acetyl group "turnover" in butyrate-treated cells. The constancy of the $^{14}C/^3H$ ratio for histone H1 shows that the amino-terminal acetyl-serine is not affected by the presence of butyrate in the growth medium.

electrophoretically and measured for their residual ^{14}C-content. In parallel experiments, cells containing ^{3}H-acetylated histones were incubated in the absence of butyrate, and samples were withdrawn at the same times for isolation of the histones and measurement of the remaining ^{3}H-acetate content. (Because the cells in both experiments were mixed at each time point during the "cold-chase" experiment before isolation of the nuclei and extraction of the histones, all radioactively modified histones were exposed to the same conditions throughout their isolation, and differences in acetate retention must reflect differences in acetyl group "turnover" in the living cells due to the presence of butyrate in the medium.) After electrophoretic separation of histones H1, H2b, H3, and H4, the ratio ^{14}C/^{3}H was determined for each histone at each time point. The progressive increase in this ratio for the nucleosomal histones H2b, H3, and H4 (Figure 6) indicates that the ^{3}H-acetate content of the control histones declines rapidly during the "cold-chase," which the ^{14}C-acetate content of the corresponding histones in butyrate-treated cells remains high. The contrast between the rates of acetate release in control and butyrate-treated cells is illustrated by the decrease in the specific activities of the total histone fraction after a one-hour "cold-chase": from 5,710 cpm/mg to 2,420 cpm/mg (a decrease of 58%) in the control cells and from 6,190 cpm/mg to 5,200 cpm/mg (a decrease of only 16%) in the butyrate-treated cells. (No change in the ^{14}C/^{3}H ratio was seen for histone H1, in agreement with the view that acetate incorporation at the amino-terminal serine residue of H1 is essentially irreversible and takes place in the cytoplasm at the time of histone synthesis [Liew et al. 1970].) The invariant ^{14}C/^{3}H ratio in this case indicates that butyrate has no detectable influence on H1 synthesis during the time interval studied.)

What are the consequences of increased levels of histone acetylation for chromatin structure? We have compared the nucleosomes generated by digestion of control and butyrate-treated HeLa cell nuclei with staphylococcal nuclease. The monomer peaks were purified on sucrose density gradients and compared with regard to sedimentation coefficient, circular dichroic spectra, and DNA-melting curves. No significant differences were noted in any of these physical properties for nucleosomes differing as markedly in their contents of acetylated histones as those shown in Figure 5. Failure to detect such differences may simply be due to the fact that the nucleosome fractions analyzed represent populations of particles differing widely in their degree of acetylation, and only a small fraction of the total population may exhibit major structural alterations.

We next compared the chromatins of control and butyrate-treated HeLa cells for their sensitivity to DNase I. In these experiments, the cells were labeled with radioactive thymidine in the following protocol: The control cells were incubated with ^{3}H-thymidine for 5 hours, washed, and then grown for 20 hours in nonradioactive medium. An equivalent cell suspension was labeled with ^{14}C-thymidine for 5 hours, washed, and also grown for 20 hours in nonradioactive medium; these cells were then placed in a medium containing 7 mM Na butyrate and incubated for an additional 21 hours, thus increasing the level of acetylation of their histones. The control cells and butyrate-treated cells were harvested and mixed prior to isolation of the nuclei. The mixed nuclear suspension was then treated with DNase I, and the kinetics of release of ^{3}H-DNA fragments and ^{14}C-DNA fragments were compared. The results are summarized in Figure 7, which plots the time course of degradation of the control (^{3}H) and highly acetylated (^{14}C) chromatins. The figure also plots the ratio of ^{14}C/^{3}H for each time point during the DNase I digestion. The change in the ^{14}C/^{3}H ratio at early times is particularly revealing, because it indicates that chromatin containing the highly acetylated histones is more susceptible to DNase I attack (Vidali *et al.* 1978).

Similar experiments using staphylococcal nuclease in place of DNase I did not show this striking difference in the rates of degradation of chromatins from control and butyrate-treated HeLa cells. This result, taken with the knowledge that staphylococcal nuclease initially cleaves the DNA strands between the nu-

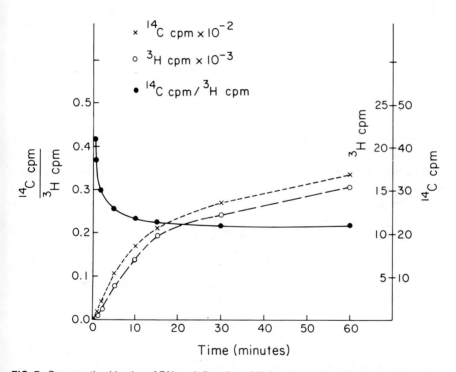

FIG. 7. Comparative kinetics of DNase I digestion of HeLa chromatins differing in their content of acetylated histones. Cells were labeled with ^{3}H-thymidine or with ^{14}C-thymidine. The ^{3}H-cells were harvested, while the ^{14}C-cells were incubated in 7 mM Na butyrate to increase the level of histone acetylation. Both cell populations were then mixed, and nuclei were isolated. The mixed nuclear suspension was incubated with DNase I, and the kinetics of release of ^{3}H-DNA fragments and ^{14}C-DNA fragments were compared. The ratio of ^{14}C/^{3}H was calculated for each time point. The early decrease in this ratio (solid line) indicates a preferential attack by DNase I on the highly acetylated chromatin from butyrate-treated cells.

cleosomes, whereas DNase I can attack the 140 nucleotide-pair strand that envelops the nucleosome core, strongly supports the view that acetylation of the nucleosomal histones H3 and H4 alters DNA interaction with the core histones and increases the susceptibility to DNase I attack.

The previous conclusion is based on the assumption that the DNA sequences that are preferentially degraded by DNase I are associated with highly acetylated forms of the histones. This has been confirmed by analysis of the histones remaining in the nuclei of butyrate-treated cells after a brief incubation in the presence of DNase I. The proportions of the multiacetylated forms of histone H4 were found to be significantly lowered after removal of only 10% of the DNA (Vidali *et al.* 1978). It follows that the most highly acetylated H4 molecules must have been released together with the most rapidly degraded DNA sequences. Similar conclusions have been drawn from studies of the release of ^{3}H-acetylated histones H3 and H4 during brief DNase I digestions of avian erythrocyte nuclei (Vidali *et al.* 1978).

Our observation that hyperacetylation of HeLa histones labilizes the associated DNA sequences to DNase I digestion suggests that a significant structural change has occurred at the nucleosomal level, at least for nucleosomes containing a high proportion of multiacetylated H3 and H4 molecules. A plausible structural model that explains these results is based on the known structures and sites of modification of the histones and the predictable consequences of charge neutralization by acetylation of their lysine residues. The distribution of epsilon-N-acetyllysine residues is not random; all of the modifiable lysines in histones H3 and H4 occur in the amino-terminal region of the polypeptide chain, which by virtue of its clustering of the basic amino acids—lysine, arginine, and histidine—carries a high net positive charge. Similar structural considerations apply to histones H2a and H2b. Thus, all of the histone classes in the octet comprising the nucleosome core (Kornberg 1977) are structured to favor DNA binding through their amino-terminal regions. These positively charged regions would be expected to interact electrostatically with the negatively charged phosphate groups of the DNA helix which envelops the nucleosome core (Baldwin *et al.* 1975). There are many indications that the amino-terminal arms of the histones are responsible for DNA binding (Boublik *et al.* 1971, Li and Bonner 1971, Lilley and Tatchell 1977, Weintraub and van Lente 1974, Whitlock and Simpson 1977, Wong and Marushige 1976, Ziccardi and Schumaker 1973). The selective digestion of the arms by trypsin (Weintraub and van Lente 1974) increases the rate of nuclease attack on the DNA of the nucleosome particle (Lilley and Tatchell 1977, Weintraub and van Lente 1974, Whitlock and Simpson 1977), changing the accessibility of certain sites without destroying the 10-nucleotide spacing of the cuts (Lilley and Tatchell 1977, Whitlock and Simpson 1977).

We believe that similar changes in DNase I-sensitivity, which reflect conformational changes in chromatin structure, are achieved by acetylation of the amino-terminal regions of the histones. The relatively high rate of acetylation of histones H3 and H4, in comparison with other histone fractions (Allfrey *et al.* 1964,

Edwards and Allfrey 1973, Ruiz-Carrillo *et al.* 1976) is consistent with the key role played by H3 and H4 in nucleosome organization (Camerini-Otero *et al.* 1976, Sollner-Webb *et al.* 1976, Moss *et al.* 1977). The release of constraints on the enveloping DNA helix may result in a relaxation of DNA twists within the nucleosome to favor a more extended configuration of the template. This structural change, which clearly influences DNA accessibility to DNase I, may favor DNA interactions with other enzymes and regulatory proteins involved in transcription. This would account for the many spatial and temporal correlations between histone acetylation and RNA synthesis (Allfrey 1977, Johnson and Allfrey 1978) and for observations that chemical acetylation of the histones increases the transcriptional activity of cell-free systems (Allfrey *et al.* 1964, Marushige 1976).

Histone Deacetylation as a Control Mechanism

Of particular interest in relation to acetylation as a structural control mechanism in chromatin are a number of observations that point to a regulatory role of histone deacetylases. A heirarchy of controls over histone deacetylation is indicated by changes in enzyme activity during embryonic muscle development (Boffa *et al.* 1971) and by the apparent loss of an inhibitor during purification of the histone deacetylase from thymus nuclei (Vidali *et al.* 1972). Two observations relevant to malignant transformation are the suppression of histone deacetylation in viral (SV-40) chromatin but not in host cell chromatin (Vidali and Vesco, manuscript in preparation) and evidence that the transcribing segments of intergrated viral genomes are selectively attacked by DNase I (Flint and Weintraub 1977).

The effects of a chemical carcinogen aflatoxin B_1 on histone acetylation are particularly suggestive. The administration of this hepatocarcinogen to rats leads to a sudden increase in the rate at which acetyl groups are released from histones H3 and H4 in the liver. The increase in histone deacetylation occurs within 15 minutes, without any effect on the kinetics of acetate uptake into liver histones in vivo or in vitro (Edwards and Allfrey 1973). It is known that aflatoxin B_1 has multiple inhibitory effects on RNA synthesis in the liver. In part, these reflect an inhibition of RNA polymerase II activity, but it has also been established that there is a direct impairment of DNA template function (Yu 1977). The latter observation is fully consistent with a tighter restructuring of chromatin as a consequence of the deacetylation of histones H3 and H4.

It remains to be seen whether similar effects on histone modification are produced by other chemical carcinogens and whether changes in the acetylation levels of nucleosomal histones provide an early signal of the disruption of transcriptional controls induced by carcinogens. A recent report that butyrate causes a reversible suppression of the neoplastic state in fibroblast lines transformed in vitro by chemical carcinogens (Leavitt *et al.* 1978) lends additional support to the relevance of this approach.

ACKNOWLEDGMENTS

This work was supported in part by grants from the U.S. Public Health Service, National Institutes of Health (CA-14908 and GM-17383), the American Cancer Society (NP-228H), the National Foundation-March of Dimes (1-440), and the Rockefeller Foundation Program in Reproductive Biology.

REFERENCES

Allfrey, V. G. 1964. Structural modifications of histones and their possible role in the regulation of ribonucleic acid synthesis. Can. Cancer Conf. 6:313–335.

Allfrey, V. G. 1977. Post-synthetic modification of histone structure: A mechanism for the modulation of histone-DNA interactions, *in* Chromatin and Chromosome Structure, H. J. Li and R. A. Eckhardt, eds., Academic Press, New York, pp. 167–191.

Allfrey, V. G., L. C. Boffa, and G. Vidali. 1978. Changes in composition and metabolism of nuclear non-histone proteins during chemical carcinogenesis. Association of tumor-specific DNA-binding proteins with DNase I-sensitive regions of chromatin and observations on the effects of histone acetylation on chromatin structure, *in* Differentiation and Development, J. Schultz and F. Ahmad, eds., 10th Miami Winter Symposia, Academic Press, New York (In press).

Allfrey, V. G., R. Faulkner, and A. E. Mirsky. 1964. Acetylation and methylation of histones and their possible role in the regulation of RNA synthesis. Proc. Natl. Acad. Sci. USA 51:786–794.

Allfrey, V. G., and A. Inoue. 1977. Affinity chromatography of DNA-binding proteins on DNA covalently attached to solid supports, *in* Methods in Cell Biology, D. Prescott, ed. Vol. 17. Academic Press, New York, pp. 253–270.

Allfrey, V. G., A. Inoue, J. Karn, E. M. Johnson, and G. Vidali. 1974. Phosphorylation of DNA-binding nuclear acidic proteins and gene activation in the HeLa cell cycle. Cold Spring Harbor Symp. Quant. Biol. 38:785–801.

Arnold, E. A., M. M. Buksas, and K. E. Young. 1973. A comparative study of some properties of chromatin from two "minimal deviation" hepatomas. Cancer Res. 33:1169–1176.

Austoker, J., D. Cox, and A. P. Mathias. 1972. Fractionation of nuclei from brain by zonal centrifugation and a study of the ribonucleic acid polymerase activity in the various classes of nuclei. Biochem. J. 129:1139–1155.

Baldwin, J. P., P. G. Boseley, E. M. Bradbury, and K. Ibel. 1975. The subunit structure of the eukaryotic chromosome. Nature 253:245–249.

Boffa, L. C., and V. G. Allfrey. 1976. Characteristic complements of nuclear nonhistone proteins in colonic epithelial tumors. Cancer Res. 36:2678–2685.

Boffa, L. C., and V. G. Allfrey. 1977. Changes in chromosomal proteins in colon cancer. The complexity and DNA-binding properties of tumor-associated proteins and evidence for their association with the malignant state in human colonic epithelium. Cancer 40:2584–2591.

Boffa, L. C., E. L. Gershey, and G. Vidali. 1971. Changes in the histone deacetylase activity during chick embryo muscle development. Biochim. Biophys. Acta 254:135–143.

Boffa, L. C., G. Vidali, and V. G. Allfrey. 1975. Selective synthesis and accumulation of nuclear non-histone proteins during carcinogenesis of the colon induced by 1,2-dimethylhydrazine. Cancer 36:2356–2363.

Boffa, L. C., G. Vidali, and V. G. Allfrey. 1976. Changes in nuclear non-histone protein composition during normal differentiation and carcinogenesis of intestinal epithelial cells. Exp. Cell Res. 98:396–410.

Boffa, L. C., G. Vidali, and V. G. Allfrey. 1978. Suppression of histone deacetylation in vivo and in vitro by Na butyrate. J. Biol. Chem. 253:3364–3366.

Boublik, M., E. M. Bradbury, C. Crane-Robinson, and H. W. E. Rattle. 1971. Proton magnetic resonance studies of the interactions of histones F1 and F2B with DNA, Nature New Biol. 229:149–150.

Camerini-Otero, R. D., B. Sollner-Webb, and G. Felsenfeld. 1976. The organization of histones and DNA in chromatin: Evidence for an arginine-rich histone kernel. Cell 8:333–347.

Candido, E. P. M., and G. H. Dixon. 1972a. Acetylation of trout testis histones in vivo. Site of the modification in histone IIb1. J. Biol. Chem. 247:3868–3873.

Candido, E. P. M., and G. H. Dixon. 1972b. Amino-terminal sequences and sites of in vivo acetylation of trout-testis histones III and IIb$_2$. Proc. Natl. Acad. Sci. USA 69:2015–2019.

Chae, C. B., M. C. Smith, and H. P. Morris. 1974. Chromosomal non-histone proteins of rat hepatomas and normal rat liver. Biochem. Biophys. Res. Commun. 60:1468–1474.

Chang, W. W. L., and C. P. Leblond. 1970. Renewal of the various types of epithelial cells in the descending colon of the mouse, *in* Carcinoma of the Colon and Antecedent Epithelium, W. J. Burdette, ed., Charles C Thomas, Springfield, Illinois, pp. 197–212.

DeLange, R. J., D. M. Fambrough, E. L. Smith, and J. Bonner. 1969. Calf and pea histone IV. II. The complete amino acid sequence of calf thymus histone IV. Presence of epsilon-N-acetyllysine. J. Biol. Chem. 244:319–334.

Deschner, E. E., C. M. Lewis, and M. Lipkin. 1963. In vitro study of human rectal epithelial cells. J. Clin. Invest. 42:1922–1928.

Deschner, E. E., M. Lipkin, and L. Solomon. 1966. Study of human rectal endothelial cells in vitro. II. ^{3}H-thymidine incorporation into polyps and adjacent mucosa. J. Natl. Cancer Inst. 36:844–855.

Druckrey, H. 1970. Production of colonic carcinoma by 1,2-dimethylhydrazine and azoxyalkanes, *in* Carcinoma of the Colon and Antecedent Epithelium, W. J. Burdette, ed., Charles C Thomas, Springfield, Illinois, pp. 267–279.

Druckrey, H., R. Preussmann, R. Matzkies, and S. Ivanovic. 1967. Selektive erzeugung von darm-krebs durch 1,2-dimethylhydrazin. Naturwissenschaften 54:285–286.

Edwards, G. S., and V. G. Allfrey. 1973. Aflatoxin B$_1$ and actinomycin D effects on histone acetyla-tion and deacetylation in the liver. Biochim. Biophys. Acta 299:354–366.

Flint, S. J., and H. Weintraub. 1977. An altered subunit configuration associated with the actively transcribing DNA of integrated adenovirus genes. Cell 12:783–794.

Garel, A., and R. Axel. 1976. Selective digestion of transcriptionally active ovalbumin genes from oviduct nuclei. Proc. Natl. Acad. Sci. USA 73:3966–3970.

Garel, A., M. Zolan, and R. Axel. 1977. Genes transcribed at diverse rates have a similar conforma-tion in chromatin. Proc. Natl. Acad. Sci. USA 74:4867–4871.

Garrard, W. T., and J. Bonner. 1974. Changes in chromatin proteins during liver regeneration. J. Biol. Chem. 249:5570–5579.

Gershey, E. L., G. Vidali, and V. G. Allfrey. 1968. Chemical studies of histone acetylation. The occurrence of epsilon-N-acetyllysine in the f2al histone. J. Biol. Chem. 243:5018–5022.

Gonzales-Mujica, F., and A. P. Mathias. 1973. Proteins from different classes of liver nuclei in normal and thioacetamide-treated rats. Biochem J. 133:441–455.

Gronow, M., and T. M. Thackrah. 1974a. Nuclear protein changes during the nitrosamine-induced carcinogenesis of rat liver. Chem. Biol. Interact. 9:225–236.

Gronow, M., and T. M. Thackrah. 1974b. Changes in the composition of rat liver chromatin during nitrosamine carcinogenesis. Eur. J. Cancer 10:21–25.

Hawks, A., R. M. Hicks, J. W. Holsman, and P. N. Magee. 1974. Morphological and biochemical effects of 1,2-dimethylhydrazine and 1-methylhydrazine in rats and mice. Br. J. Cancer 30:429–439.

Johnson, E. M., and V. G. Allfrey. 1978. Post-synthetic modifications of histone primary structure: Phosphorylation and acetylation as related to chromatin conformation and function, *in* Biochemical Actions of Hormones, G. Litwack, ed. Vol. 5. Academic Press, New York, pp. 1–56.

Johnson, E. M., J. Karn, and V. G. Allfrey. 1974. Early nuclear events in the induction of lymphocyte proliferation by mitogens. J. Biol. Chem. 249:4990–4999.

Kornberg, R. 1977. Structure of chromatin. Annu. Rev. Biochem. 46:931–954.

Laemmli, U. 1970. Cleavage of structural proteins during assembly of the head of bacteriophage T4. Nature 227:680–686.

Leavitt, J., J. C. Barrett, B. D. Crawford, and P. O. P. Ts'o. 1978. Butyric acid suppression of the in vitro neoplastic state of Syrian hamster cells. Nature 271:262–265.

Levy-W., B., and G. H. Dixon. 1977. Renaturation kinetics of cDNA complementary to cytoplasmic polyadenylated RNA from rainbow trout testis. Accessibility of the transcribed genes to pancreatic DNase. Nucleic Acids Res. 4:883–898.

Li, H. J., and J. Bonner. 1971. Interaction of histone half-molecules with deoxyribonucleic acid. Biochemistry 10:1461–1470.

Liew, C. C., G. W. Haslett, and V. G. Allfrey. 1970. N-acetyl-seryl-tRNA and polypeptide chain initiation during histone biosynthesis. Nature 226:414–417.

Lilley, D. M. J., and K. Tatchell. 1977. Chromatin core particle unfolding induced by tryptic cleavage of histones. Nucleic Acids Res. 4:2039–2055.

Lipkin, M. 1974. Phase 1 and phase 2 proliferative lesions of colonic epithelial cells in diseases leading to colonic cancer. Cancer 34:878–888.

Lipkin, M., and H. Quastler. 1962. Cell population kinetics in the colon of the mouse. J. Clin. Invest. 41:141–146.

Martin, M. S., F. Martin, R. Michiels, H. Bastien, E. Instreba, M. Bordes, and B. Viry. 1973. An experimental model for cancer of the colon and rectum: Intestinal carcinoma induced in the rat by 1,2-dimethylhydrazine. Digestion 8:22–34.

Marushige, K. 1976. Activation of chromatin by acetylation of histone side-chains. Proc. Natl. Acad. Sci. USA 73:3937–3941.

Moss, T., R. M. Stephens, C. Crane-Robinson, and E. M. Bradbury. 1977. A nucleosome-like structure containing DNA and the arginine-rich histones H3 and H4. Nucleic Acids Res. 4:2477–2485.

O'Farrell, P. H. 1975. High resolution two-dimensional gel electrophoresis of proteins. J. Biol. Chem. 250:4007–4021.

Orrick, L. R., M. O. J. Olson, and H. Busch. 1973. Comparison of nucleolar proteins of normal rat liver and Novikoff hepatoma ascites cells by two-dimensional polyacrylamide gel electrophoresis. Proc. Natl. Acad. Sci. USA 70:1316–1320.

Panyim, S., and R. Chalkley. 1969. High resolution acrylamide gel electrophoresis of histones. Arch. Biochem. Biophys. 130:337–346.

Riggs, M. G., R. G. Whittaker, J. R. Newmann, and V. R. Ingram. 1977. n-butyrate causes histone modification in HeLa and Friend erythroleukemia cells. Nature 268:462–464.

Ruiz-Carrillo, A., L. J. Wangh, and V. G. Allfrey. 1976. Selective synthesis and modification of nuclear proteins during maturation of avian erythroid cells. Arch. Biochem. Biophys. 174:273–290.

Ruiz-Carrillo, A., L. J. Wangh, V. C. Littau, and V. G. Allfrey. 1974. Changes in histone acetyl content and in nuclear non-histone protein composition of avian erythroid cells at different stages of maturation. J. Biol. Chem. 249:7358–7368.

Schaffhausen, B. S., and T. L. Benjamin. 1976. Deficiency in histone acetylation in non-transforming host-range mutants of polyoma virus. Proc. Natl. Acad. Sci. USA 73:1092–1096.

Sollner-Webb, B., R. D. Camerini-Otero, and G. Felsenfeld. 1976. Chromatin structure as probed by nucleases and proteases: Evidence for the central role of histones H3 and H4. Cell 9:179–193.

Stein, G. S., W. E. Criss, and H. P. Morris. 1974. Properties of the genome in experimental hepatomas. Variations in the composition of chromatin. Life Sci. 14:95–105.

Teng, C. S., C. T. Teng, and V. G. Allfrey. 1971. Studies of nuclear acidic proteins. Evidence for their phosphorylation, tissue-specificity, selective binding to deoxyribonucleic acid, and stimulatory effects on transcription. J. Biol. Chem. 246:3597–3609.

Thunherr, N., E. E. Deschner, E. H. Stonehill, and M. Lipkin. 1973. Induction of adenocarcinomas of the colon in mice by weekly injections of 1,2-dimethylhydrazine. Cancer Res. 33:940–945.

Vidali, G., L. C. Boffa, and V. G. Allfrey. 1972. Properties of an acidic histone-binding protein fraction from cell nuclei. Selective precipitation and deacetylation of histones F2A1 and F3. J. Biol. Chem. 247:7365–7373.

Vidali, G., L. C. Boffa, and V. G. Allfrey. 1978. Suppression of histone deacetylation by butyrate leads to accumulation of multi-acetylated forms of histones H3 and H4 and increased DNase I-sensitivity of the associated DNA sequences. Proc. Natl. Acad. Sci. USA (in press).

Wangh, L. J., A. Ruiz-Carrillo, and V. G. Allfrey. 1972. Separation and analysis of histone subfractions differing in their degree of acetylation: Some correlations with genetic activity in development. Arch. Biochem. Biophys. 150:44–56.

Weintraub, H., and M. Groudine. 1976. Chromosomal subunits in active genes have an altered conformation. Globin genes are digested by deoxyribonuclease I in red blood cell nuclei but not in fibroblast nuclei. Science 193:848–856.

Weintraub, H., and F. van Lente. 1974. Dissection of chromosome structure with trypsin and nucleases. Proc. Natl. Acad. Sci. USA 71:4249–4253.

Whitlock, J. P., Jr., and R. T. Simpson. 1977. Localization of sites along nucleosome DNA which interact with NH_2-terminal histone regions. J. Biol. Chem. 252:6516–6520.

Wilson, B., M. A. Lea, G. Vidali, and V. G. Allfrey. 1975. Fractionation of nuclei and analysis of nuclear proteins of rat liver and Morris hepatoma 7777. Cancer Res. 35:2954–2958.

Wong, T. K., and K. Marushige. 1976. Modification of histone binding in calf thymus chromatin and in the chromatin-protamine complex by acetic anhydride. Biochemistry 15:2041–2053.

Yeoman, L. C., C. W. Taylor, and H. Busch. 1974. Two-dimensional gel electrophoresis of acid-extractable nuclear proteins of regenerating and thioacetamide-treated rat liver, Morris 9618A hepatoma and Walker 256 carcinoma. Cancer Res. 34:424–428.

Yu, F. L. 1977. Mechanism of Aflatoxin B_1 inhibition of rat hepatic nuclear RNA synthesis. J. Biol. Chem. 252:3245–3251.

Ziccardi, R., and V. Schumaker. 1973. Interaction of histone f2al with T7 deoxyribonucleic acid. Cooperativity of histone binding. Biochemistry 12:3231–3235.

Carcinogens: Identification and Mechanisms of Action, edited by A. Clark Griffin and Charles R. Shaw. Raven Press, New York © 1979.

Retinoids and Cancer Prevention: The Importance of the Terminal Group of the Retinoid Molecule in Modifying Activity and Toxicity

Michael B. Sporn, Dianne L. Newton, Joseph M. Smith, Nancy Acton,* Arthur E. Jacobson,* and Arnold Brossi*

*National Cancer Institute, and *National Institute of Arthritis, Metabolism, and Digestive Diseases, National Institutes of Health, Bethesda, Maryland 20014*

The efficacy of retinoids in prevention of cancer of the lung, skin, bladder, and breast in experimental animals has been shown by several groups of investigators in recent years (Saffiotti *et al.* 1967, Bollag 1972, 1974, Sporn *et al.* 1976b, 1977, Grubbs *et al.* 1977a,b, Moon *et al.* 1977). In all of these studies, the retinoids have been given to animals after initiation of carcinogenesis has been completed, and it would appear that the retinoids are working as antipromoting agents (Verma and Boutwell 1977) to prevent the further progression of preneoplastic lesions to malignant, invasive carcinomas. In some studies, a definite increase in the latency period for development of tumors has been shown with the use of retinoids (Grubbs *et al.* 1977a, Moon *et al.* 1977), and it has been suggested that pharmacological extension of the latency period for development of cancer represents a valid approach to prevention of human cancer. However, the usefulness of this approach in man has yet to be demonstrated. It will involve new considerations in chronic administration of drugs, because people at risk for development of cancer would require intake of retinoids for very prolonged periods of time, as a preventive measure. In such situations, the therapeutic safety of a drug, as well as its therapeutic efficacy, must be assured. Since retinoids have been known for many years to have the potential for causing undesirable toxic reactions in both man (Smith and Goodman 1976) and experimental animals (Moore 1967), this concern for safety is a paramount consideration in the practical development of these agents for cancer prevention.

It is already well established that *all-trans*-retinol and its esters, as well as *all-trans*-retinoic acid, have serious limitations as potential agents for chemoprevention of cancer in man. Retinol and retinyl esters accumulate in the liver, principally as retinyl esters, where they may eventually cause severe hepatic dysfunction (Smith and Goodman 1976). Furthermore, this ability of the liver to sequester retinol or retinyl esters may prevent these retinoids from reaching a threshold plasma concentration to achieve the desired effects at a target site, such as bladder epithelium or intestinal epithelium. The chronic administration of high doses of retinol, retinyl esters, or retinoic acid may also result in severe general systemic toxicity, characterized by destabilization of membranes, rupture of lysosomes (with release of proteolytic and other degradative enzymes), and consequences as severe as increased intracranial pressure or bone fractures (Dingle and Fell 1963, Moore 1967). Were it not for these undesirable toxic effects, retinol, retinyl esters, or *all-trans*-retinoic acid would certainly be candidates for prevention of certain types of human cancers. The classical pharamcological solution for this type of problem is to develop synthetic analogs, and the great success of synthetic steroids as antiinflammatory and antifertility agents is an excellent example of the usefulness of synthetic modification of natural molecules to achieve pharmacological agents with greater activity and lesser toxicity.

Since the retinoids are hormone-like agents that control epithelial cell differentiation (in many ways resembling steroidal estrogens and androgens in their mechanism of action on target cells), a similar approach to synthetic modification of the basic retinoid molecule has a definite rationale. There are three regions of the retinoid molecule (Figure 1) which can be considered for synthetic modification, namely, the ring, side chain, and polar terminal group, and thus, an extremely large number of analogs can be considered for synthesis. A practical problem is where to begin and to determine if any rationale exists for consideration of synthetic efforts in a particular area. This article will briefly review the data which indicate that the polar terminal group of the retinoid molecule is a particularly important determinant in modifying activity, toxicity, metabolism, and tissue distribution and will describe some recent advances in the synthesis and properties of a class of retinoids whose biological properties have not previously been evaluated, namely the condensation products of *all-trans*-retinal and 1,3-diketones.

The importance of the terminal group of the retinoid molecule in determining the metabolic fate and disposition of the molecule has been known for over 30 years, since the original studies of Arens and van Dorp (1946), who showed that retinoic acid, although it had biological activity (growth promotion of the rat) equivalent to retinol or retinyl esters, was not stored in the liver, as occurs with retinol or retinyl esters. Other classical studies by Dowling and Wald (1960) confirmed that retinoic acid could not be reduced in vivo to retinal and retinol; they found that rats maintained on retinoic acid as their sole retinoid

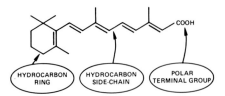

FIG. 1. Components of the retinoid molecule. The structure shown is *all-trans*-retinoic acid. The following retinoids result if the terminal –COOH group is changed to –CH_2OH, retinol; –CH_2OCOCH_3, retinyl acetate; –CH_2OCH_3, retinyl methyl ether.

grew normally and were in general good health, except for becoming night-blind and, then, eventually totally blind. The failure to form visual pigments confirmed that the body was incapable of reducing the terminal carboxyl group to an aldehyde group; clear indication of the metabolic importance of the terminal group has thus been known for almost 20 years. These data are shown diagrammatically in Figure 2. Similarly, there have been data in the literature for a long time which indicate that modifying the polar terminal group of the retinoid molecule can diminish toxicity without lessening biological activity (growth promotion of the rat). Retinyl methyl ether was synthesized by two groups of researchers in the late 1940's and was found to have growth-promoting activity essentially identical to that of retinol or retinyl esters (Hanze *et al.* 1948, Isler *et al.* 1949). In 1951, Wolbach and Maddock reported the important finding that retinyl methyl ether was significantly less active than retinol or retinyl esters in causing bone fractures in rats. However, they did not fully appreciate the significance of their discovery, since they were working under the assumption, now known to be incorrect, that activity and toxicity of retinoids always paralleled each other. The basis for the lesser toxicity of retinyl methyl ether was not investigated further by Wolbach and Maddock, and little more was done with their significant finding.

The recent development of new in vitro systems for studying structure-function relationships has made possible a more quantitative assessment of the role of the polar terminal group of the retinoid molecule in determining activity and toxicity. In these in vitro systems, activity has been assayed by measuring the ability of retinoids to control cell differentiation and reverse keratinization in tracheal organ cultures (Sporn *et al.* 1976a), while toxicity has been evaluated by measuring the lysis of either ear or tracheal cartilage in organ culture (Goodman *et al.* 1974, Sporn *et al.* 1976a, Bard and Lasnitzki 1977). These assays have confirmed the importance of the terminal group for determining both activity and toxicity. Retinoic acid has been found to be significantly more active than retinol, retinyl acetate, and retinyl methyl ether, all three of which are approximately equal in activity. In this series of retinoids, toxicity appears to be related to the nature of the terminal group, with retinoic acid found to be the most toxic. Retinol and retinyl acetate were found to be of an intermediate degree of toxicity, and retinyl methyl ether was markedly less toxic than the other three retinoids. Since retinoids have a detergent-like action in disrupting membrane structure (Dingle and Fell 1963), the lesser toxicity of retinyl methyl ether would appear to be a result of the diminished terminal polarity resulting

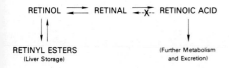

FIG. 2. Metabolism of the natural retinoids.

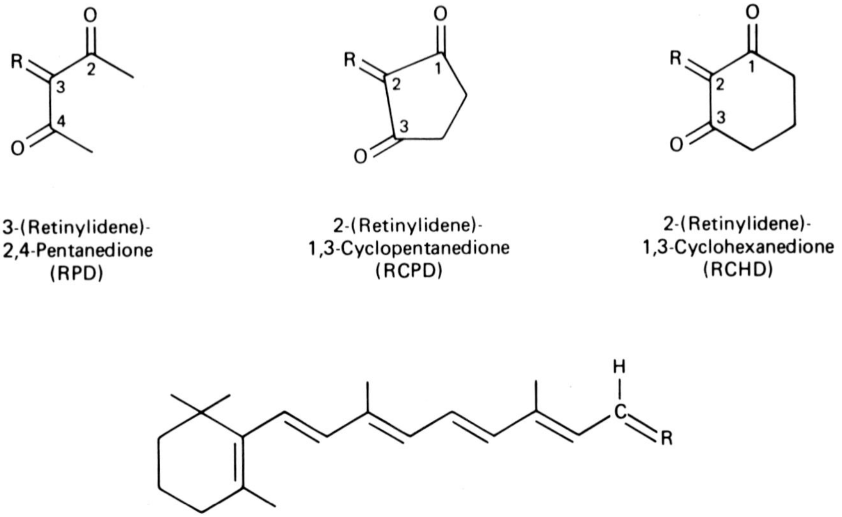

3-(Retinylidene)-
2,4-Pentanedione
(RPD)

2-(Retinylidene)-
1,3-Cyclopentanedione
(RCPD)

2-(Retinylidene)-
1,3-Cyclohexanedione
(RCHD)

Fig. 3. Structures of retinylidene 1,3-diketones.

in reduced detergency. In addition to the above in vitro studies, retinyl methyl ether has recently been found to have enhanced uptake into the mammary gland of the rat when compared to retinyl acetate (Sporn *et al.* 1976a) and greater effectiveness than retinyl acetate in preventing mammary cancer in experimental animals (Grubbs *et al.* 1977a). The change in tissue distribution is presumably the result of enhanced lipophilicity resulting from diminished polarity of introducing a methyl ether function as a terminal group.

All of these studies have suggested that further synthesis of new classes of retinoids, with modified terminal groups, might generate useful new structures. One such class of compounds is the set of retinylidine 1,3-diketones, formed by aldol condensation of retinal with 1,3-diketones. Although the synthesis of one such compound, 3-(*all-trans*-retinylidene)-2,4-pentanedione (retinylidene acetylacetone) had been reported more than 10 years ago (Haeck *et al.* 1966), no data were available regarding biological activity. We have modified the original synthesis to obtain better yields, and a large number of new 1,3-diketone adducts has been synthesized (Acton, Jacobson, and Brossi, unpublished results, details will be published elsewhere). Here we report a comparison of the biological properties of three retinylidine diketones (Figure 3), namely, 3-(*all-trans*-retinylidene)-2,4-pentanedione (RPD), 2-(*all-trans*-retinylidene)-1,3-cyclopentanedione (RCPD), and 2-(*all-trans*-retinylidene)-1,3-cyclohexanedione (RCHD).

All three compounds were assayed in vitro for control of cell differentiation and reversal of keratinization in tracheal organ culture, using a total of 371 hamster tracheas (Table 1 and Figure 4). The 2,4-pentanedione adduct, RPD,

TABLE 1. *Reversal of keratinized squamous metaplastic lesions of retinoid deficiency in tracheal organ cultures treated with retinoids*

Treatment of cultures (number of cultures)		% of cultures with respective amounts of squamous metaplasia					% of cultures with keratin and keratohyaline granules
		None	Minimal	Mild	Marked	Severe	
No Retinoid, collected day 3	(55)	7	7	44	20	22	74
No Retinoid, collected day 10	(49)	0	4	14	43	39	96
Retinoic Acid							
10^{-8} M	(11)	27	45	27	0	0	0
10^{-9} M	(49)	14	45	29	12	0	2
10^{-10} M	(23)	13	9	26	17	35	30
RPD							
10^{-7} M	(16)	31	31	25	12	0	0
10^{-8} M	(25)	24	4	40	28	4	0
10^{-9} M	(18)	0	0	11	44	44	67
10^{-10} M	(14)	0	0	14	57	29	100
RCPD							
10^{-8} M	(12)	0	0	17	75	8	92
10^{-9} M	(12)	8	0	58	17	17	92
RCHD							
10^{-8} M	(24)	38	42	21	0	0	0
10^{-9} M	(26)	19	12	35	31	4	0
10^{-10} M	(37)	11	0	30	41	19	51

All tracheas were cultured for the first three days in medium without retinoid. At this time, some tracheas were collected, while the rest were cultured for a further week in medium containing either no retinoid or retinoid added at the concentrations shown. These tracheas were collected on the 10th day of culture. Cultures were graded as to the percentage of their total epithelium showing squamous metaplasia on eight cross-sections from the middle of each trachea. If more than 40% of the total epithelial length was squamous, it was graded as having severe squamous metaplasia; between 10–40% was graded as marked; between 2–10% was graded as mild; and less than 2% was graded as minimal.

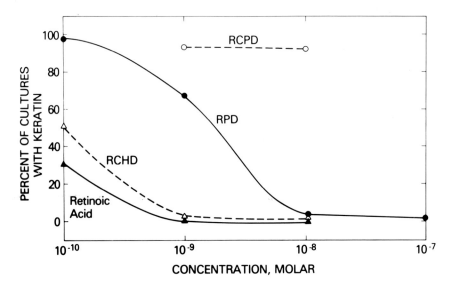

FIG. 4. Dose-response curves for reversal of keratinization in organ cultures of retinoid-deficient tracheal epithelium by application of retinoids. Tracheas (one per culture dish) were treated with retinoids for seven days before scoring for the presence of both keratin and keratohyaline granules. Numbers of tracheas used in these experiments are shown in Table 1.

was found to be less active than retinoic acid (its activity is approximately equal to that of retinyl acetate), while the 1,3-cyclopentanedione adduct, RCPD, was essentially inactive. In contrast, the 1,3-cyclohexanedione adduct, RCHD, was the most active, with a potency in tracheal organ culture approaching that of retinoic acid. Both RPD and RCHD were found to be markedly less toxic than retinyl acetate when administered in high doses for two weeks to weanling rats (Tables 2 and 3, Figures 5 and 6). Oral doses of retinyl acetate were given in an amount that killed one-half or more of the rats and caused total failure to gain weight in the survivors; equivalent molar doses of RPD and RCHD caused no fatalities, and weight gain in animals fed RPD and RCHD was essentially the same as found in control rats receiving the vehicle alone. The low toxicity of RPD and RCHD when given orally is not due to a total failure of absorption, since a major increase in metabolites of these two compounds was found in mammary tissue after oral administration, as seen in Figures 7 and 8, and Table 4. The trifluoroacetic acid (TFA) reaction (Dugan *et al.* 1964) has been used to detect RPD, RCHD, or their metabolites in mammary tissue or liver. Figure 7 shows reference TFA spectra for retinoic acid, retinyl acetate, retinal, RCHD, and RPD, and Figure 8 shows the TFA spectra of mammary tissue extracts after rats have been treated with retinyl acetate, RCHD, or RPD. Although the TFA spectrum of the tissue extracts from rats treated with retinyl acetate shows peak absorbance at the peak wavelength of the parent

TABLE 2. *Comparison of toxic effects of large doses of RPD and retinyl acetate given to rats**

Treatment	Survivors at 7 days	Mean weight, grams, at 7 days, ± S.E.	Survivors at 14 days	Mean weight, grams, at 14 days, ± S.E.
Vehicle alone 0.2 ml, 5x/week	6/6	102 ± 2	6/6	127 ± 3
RPD 30.4 μmoles, 5x/week	6/6	107 ± 2†	6/6	135 ± 4†
Retinyl acetate 30.4 μmoles, 5x/week	6/6	88 ± 5	6/6	109 ± 5
Vehicle alone 0.3 ml, 5x/week‡	5/5	101 ± 1	5/5	132 ± 2
RPD 45.6 μmoles, 5x/week	6/6	105 ± 2†	6/6	139 ± 3†
Retinyl acetate 45.6 μmoles, 5x/week	6/6	68 ± 4	3/6	65 ± 8

* Sprague-Dawley 4-week-old female rats, fed Wayne lab chow, were randomized into six groups, each containing six rats, with each group having a mean weight of 65–67 grams. They were treated five times per week (Monday–Friday), orally, as shown. Vehicle was ethanol:trioctanoin (1:3). The experiment was terminated at the end of 14 days.

† Significantly different from respective group treated with retinyl acetate, $p < 0.005$.

‡ This group consisted of only five animals.

TABLE 3. Comparison of toxic effects of large doses of RCHD and retinyl acetate given to rats*

Treatment	Survivors at 7 days	Mean weight, grams, at 7 days, ± S.E.	Survivors at 14 days	Mean weight, grams, at 14 days, ± S.E.
Vehicle alone				
0.2 ml, 5x/week	6/6	89 ± 2	6/6	133 ± 4
RCHD				
30.4 μmoles, 5x/week	6/6	87 ± 2†	6/6	130 ± 5†
Retinyl acetate				
30.4 μmoles, 5x/week	6/6	66 ± 3	6/6	79 ± 9
Vehicle alone				
0.3 ml, 5x/week	6/6	87 ± 3	6/6	135 ± 4
RCHD				
45.6 μmoles, 5x/week	6/6	85 ± 3†	6/6	126 ± 3†
Retinyl acetate				
45.6 μmoles, 5x/week	6/6	55 ± 1	2/6	48 ± 3

* Sprague-Dawley 4-week-old female rats, fed Wayne lab chow, were randomized into six groups, each containing six rats, with each group having a mean weight of 55–57 grams. They were treated five times per week (Monday–Friday), orally, as shown. Vehicle was ethanol:trioctanoin (1:3). The experiment was terminated at the end of 14 days.
† Significantly different from respective group treated with retinyl acetate, $p < 0.005$.

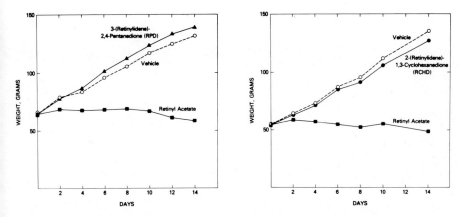

FIG. 5, left. Weights of rats treated with large oral doses of RPD and retinyl acetate. Groups of six rats received 10 doses, each 45.6 μmoles, of either RPD or retinyl acetate over a two-week period.

FIG. 6, right. Weights of rats treated with large oral doses of RCHD and retinyl acetate. Groups of six rats received 10 doses, each 45.6 μmoles, of either RCHD or retinyl acetate over a two-week period.

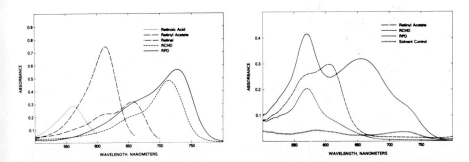

FIG. 7, left. Spectra of retinoids in the presence of trifluoracetic acid (TFA). Three milliliters of TFA reagent (1 part TFA plus 2 parts chloroform) was added to 0.3 ml aliquots of retinoids in chloroform; the solutions were scanned rapidly (total time to complete scans from addition of TFA was 50–72 seconds) in a Cary spectrophotometer. Concentrations (micromolar) of retinoids in 3.3 ml final volume were retinoic acid, 7.1; retinyl acetate, 7.4; retinal, 8.1; RCHD, 7.1; RPD, 8.3.

FIG. 8, right. Trifluoroacetic acid (TFA) spectra of ether extracts of mammary tissue of rats treated nine times with retinyl acetate, RCHD, or RPD. Rats were treated with retinoids as shown in Table 4. Samples of mammary tissue were taken and ground with five parts anhydrous sodium sulfate. The dried tissue powders were extracted with 10 ml of anhydrous ether, and 4 ml aliquots of the ethereal extracts were evaporated to dryness with nitrogen. These aliquots were redissolved in 0.3 ml of chloroform; 3.0 ml of TFA reagent was added, and the solutions scanned rapidly as described in Figure 7. The weights of the original tissue samples were as follows: solvent control, 0.22 grams; retinyl acetate, 0.30 grams; RPD, 0.28 grams; RCHD, 0.26 grams.

TABLE 4. *Comparison of tissue levels of retinoids 24 hours after the last of nine oral doses*

Retinoid	Number of Rats*	Liver	Breast
Solvent control	6	60†	1.2†
Retinyl acetate	6	1870†	11.8†
RPD	6	90†	18.7‡
RCHD	6	170†	14.4‡

* Sprague-Dawley female rats were dosed orally with retinoids (30 μmoles each dose), dissolved in 0.4 ml of ethanol:trioctanoin (1:3). The rats were treated three times weekly and killed 24 hours after the final dose. Tissue levels were determined with the trifluoroacetic acid method after extraction of tissue with ethyl ether. Figures are expressed as total optical density units of retinoid found per gram wet weight tissue.
† Read at 616 nanometers.
‡ Read at 570 nanometers.

compound (616 nanometers), the TFA spectra of the tissue extracts from rats treated with either RCHD or RPD are very different from those of the parent compounds. This indicates that both RCHD and RPD have been metabolized to new compounds, whose structures are at present unknown. High pressure liquid chromatographic (HPLC) analysis (Frolik *et al.* 1978) of extracts of mammary tissue from rats treated with either RCHD or RPD confirms this metabolism; substantial peaks representing materials that do not correspond to the parent substances were found for both RCHD and RPD (Figure 9). Whether these metabolites are formed in situ in mammary tissue or whether they are formed in the liver or some other organ is unknown at present. If these metabolites are formed in the liver, they are cleared rapidly, since liver levels of retinoids were not appreciably increased by repeated administration of either RCHD or RPD (Table 4), in contrast to the large accumulation of retinoid in the liver caused by administration of retinyl acetate.

In summary, the total set of data thus far obtained with the retinylidene 1,3-diketones indicates that these compounds have interesting biological properties. We have no explanation as yet for the large differences in activity between RCHD, RPD, and RCPD in the tracheal organ cultures. It is already clear that both RCHD and RPD can be actively metabolized by the rat and that both compounds are markedly less toxic in vivo than retinyl acetate. Whether RPD, RCHD, or other retinylidene 1,3-diketones which we are presently evaluating will have any use in cancer prevention in the experimental animal, or eventually in man, remains to be determined. However, the work which we have described here lends further support to the thesis that modification of the terminal polar group of the retinoid molecule can have important results in modifying activity, toxicity, metabolism, and tissue distribution of this class of molecules. Hopefully, such a rational approach to structure-function relationships will eventually yield pharmacological agents of practical benefit for cancer prevention.

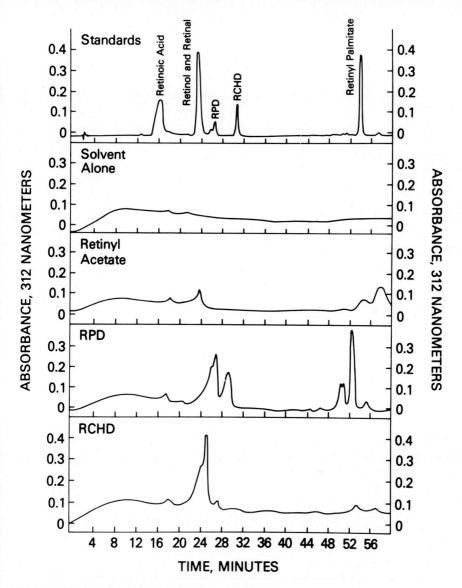

FIG. 9. HPLC analysis of retinoids and their metabolites found in ether extracts of mammary tissue after dosing with retinyl acetate, RPD, or RCHD. Rats were treated with retinoids as shown in Table 4. Samples of mammary tissue were taken and ground with five parts anhydrous sodium sulfate. The dried tissue powders were extracted with 10 ml of anhydrous ether, and 4 ml aliquots of the ethereal extracts were evaporated to dryness with nitrogen. These aliquots were redissolved in 400 μl of chloroform, to which 500 μl of acetonitrile was subseqently added. Aliquots of 100 μl of these redissolved extracts were then applied to 10 micron Spherisorb ODS colums, 3 × 250 mm. A linear gradient beginning with 67.8% methanol and ending with 97% methanol was run over a period of 48 minutes, with a flow rate of 1.2 ml per minute. The weights of the original tissue samples were as follows: solvent control, 0.26 grams; retinyl acetate, 0.20 grams; RPD, 0.17 grams; RCHD, 0.28 grams. Gradient artifact during the first 10 minutes has not been plotted. Absorbance values for the tissue samples have been multiplied by 25 (0.04 AUFS).

ACKNOWLEDGEMENTS

We thank BASF AG, Ludwigshafen, Germany; Hoffmann-La Roche Inc., Nutley, New Jersey; and Johnson and Johnson, New Brunswick, New Jersey; for generous gifts of retinyl acetate and retinoic acid. William Henderson and Larry Mullen have provided expert help with the animal experiments, and Doris Little has given valuable secretarial assistance.

REFERENCES

Arens, J. F., and D. A. van Dorp. 1946. Activity of vitamin A-acid in the rat. Nature 158:622–623.

Bard, D. R., and I. Lasnitzki. 1977. Toxicity of anti-carcinogenic retinoids in organ culture. Br. J. Cancer 35:115–119.

Bollag, W. 1972. Prophylaxis of chemically induced benign and malignant epithelial tumors by vitamin A acid (retinoic acid). Eur. J. Cancer 8:689–693.

Bollag, W. 1974. Therapeutic effects of an aromatic retinoic acid analog on chemically induced skin papillomas and carcinomas of mice. Eur. J. Cancer 10:731–737.

Dingle, J. T., and H. B. Fell. 1963. Studies on the mode of action of excess Vitamin A. 6. Lysosomal protease and the degradation of cartilage matrix. Biochem. J. 87:403–408.

Dowling, J. E., and G. Wald. 1960. The biological function of vitamin A acid. Proc. Natl. Acad. Sci. USA 46:587–608.

Dugan, R. E., N. A. Frigerio, and J. M. Siebert. 1964. Colorimetric determination of Vitamin A and its derivatives with trifluoroacetic acid. Anal. Chem. 36:114–117.

Frolik, C. A., T. E. Tavela, and M. B. Sporn. 1978. Separation of the natural retinoids by high-pressure liquid chromatography. J. Lipid Res. 19:32–37.

Goodman, D. S., J. E. Smith, R. M. Hembry, and J. T. Dingle. 1974. Comparison of the effects of vitamin A and its analogs upon rabbit ear cartilage in organ culture and upon growth of the vitamin A-deficient rat. J. Lipid Res. 15:406–414.

Grubbs, C. J., R. C. Moon, M. B. Sporn, and D. L. Newton. 1977a. Inhibition of mammary cancer by retinyl methyl ether. Cancer Res. 37:599–602.

Grubbs, C. J., R. C. Moon, R. A. Squire, G. M. Farrow, S. F. Stinson, D. G. Goodman, C. C. Brown, and M. B. Sporn. 1977b. 13-cis-retinoic acid: Inhibition of bladder carcinogenesis induced in rats by N-butyl-N-(4-hydroxybutyl)nitrosamine. Science 198:743–744.

Haeck, H. H., T. Kralt, and P. H. van Leeuwen. 1966. Synthesis of carotenoidal compounds. Rec. Trav. Chim. 85:334–338.

Hanze, A. R., T. W. Conger, E. C. Wise, and D. I. Weisblat. 1948. Crystalline vitamin A methyl ether. J. Am. Chem. Soc. 70:1253–1256.

Isler, O., R. Ronco, W. Guex, N. C. Hindley, W. Huber, K. Kialer, and M. Kofler. 1949. Über die Ester und Äther des synthetischen Vitamins A. Helv. Chim. Acta 32:489–505.

Moon, R. C., C. J. Grubbs, M. B. Sporn, and D. W. Goodman. 1977. Retinyl acetate inhibits mammary carcinogenesis induced by N-methyl-N-nitrosourea. Nature 267:620–621.

Moore, T. 1967. Pharmacology and toxicology of vitamin A, in The Vitamins. Vol. 1, 2nd ed. W. H. Sebrell and R. S. Harris, eds., Academic Press, New York pp. 280–294.

Saffiotti, U., R. Montesano, A. R. Sellakumar, and S. A. Borg. 1967. Experimental cancer of the lung. Inhibition by vitamin A of the induction of tracheobronchial squamous metaplasia and squamous cell tumors. Cancer 20:857–864.

Smith, F. R., and D. S. Goodman. 1976. Vitamin A transport in human vitamin A toxicity. N. Engl. J. Med. 294:805–808.

Sporn, M. B., N. M. Dunlop, D. L. Newton, and W. R. Henderson. 1976a. Relationships between structure and activity of retinoids. Nature 263:110–113.

Sporn, M. B., N. M. Dunlop, D. L. Newton, and J. M. Smith. 1976b. Prevention of chemical carcinogenesis by vitamin A and its synthetic analogs (retinoids). Fed. Proc. 35:1332–1338.

Sporn, M. B., R. A. Squire, C. C. Brown, J. M. Smith, M. L. Wenk, and S. Springer. 1977. 13-*cis*-retinoic acid: Inhibition of bladder carcinogenesis in the rat. Science 195:487–489.

Verma, A. K., and R. K. Boutwell. 1977. Vitamin A acid (retinoic acid), a potent inhibitor of 12-0-tetradecanoyl-phorbol-13-acetate induced ornithine decarboxylase activity in mouse epidermis. Cancer Res. 37:2196–2201.

Wolbach, S. B., and C. L. Maddock. 1951. Hypervitaminosis A: An adjunct to present methods of vitamin A identification. Proc. Soc. Exp. Biol. Med. 77:825–829.

Carcinogens: Identification and Mechanisms of Action, edited by A. Clark Griffin and Charles R. Shaw. Raven Press, New York © 1979.

Concluding Remarks on Chemicals and Chemical Carcinogenesis

James A. Miller

McArdle Laboratory for Cancer Research, University of Wisconsin Center for Health Sciences, Madison, Wisconsin 53706

As all of us expected and desired, each of the previous speakers provided valuable discussion of facts and concepts on important aspects of carcinogenesis. For me, these discussions have eased the burden of keeping abreast of this broad and very puzzling field. Dr. Becker's keynote speech (1979, see pages 5 to 17, this volume) presented an erudite and penetrating overview of the complexities of the analysis of carcinogenic processes. He characterized the present state of chemical carcinogenesis as being data- and theory-rich, but answer-poor. I agree. We need far more data and theories with much better predictive value before we can be answer-rich. However, the present situation, although far from ideal, is a great improvement over the time not many years ago when we were very limited with respect to data, theories, *and* answers. As workers in other sciences have found, we must learn to ask the proper questions in order to get meaningful answers. This will require new concepts and new techniques.

Since an attempt to summarize the preceding talks would have no point, my remarks are directed to some issues that I find of particular interest and that supplement the remarks of other speakers.

ON THE NATURES OF CARCINOGENIC AGENTS

Although we have heard discussions of chemical carcinogens and of the other main classes of carcinogenic agents (i.e., the oncogenic viruses and the physical carcinogens) (Huebner 1979, see pages 277 to 298, Paterson 1979, see pages 251 to 276, this volume), it is clear that chemical carcinogens are in center-stage at present. Currently they are the carcinogens of major interest to epidemiologists, laboratory investigators, and the lay public.

I have assembled some information on the number, kinds, and origins of carcinogens in our environment. Table 1 broadly categorizes those carcinogens that arise from human activities. The majority of these carcinogens are synthetic organic chemicals (Category I), and they are primarily nonpolar lipid-soluble compounds. At least a dozen different chemical classes are represented. The

TABLE 1. *Carcinogens arising from human activities*

I. Synthetic chemical carcinogens
   (Some research compounds, some economic poisons, some drugs, some compounds of technological value, and many analogs of parent chemical carcinogens)
II. Chemical carcinogens formed as unintentional by-products
   (Some pyrolysis and combustion products and certain combinations of chemicals; some free radicals?)
III. Various carcinogenic electromagnetic and particulate radiations
   (UV light, X-rays, α- and β-particles, neutrons, and γ-rays from synthetic elements)

carcinogenic activities of a few of these chemicals were discovered from epidemiological leads, and some were found to be carcinogens through tests designed for other purposes. However, most of these chemicals were tested as structural analogs of known carcinogens, and the large number of compounds synthesized primarily for analyses of structure-activity relationships has highly inflated the list of known chemical carcinogens. Relatively few chemicals are known to fall into Category II, the unintentional carcinogenic by-products of human activities. The known examples are primarily pyrolysis products and, possibly, free radicals. While additional members of this group will surely be found, the rate of increase will probably be far less than for those in Category I. Most, if not all, of the members of Category III, the particulate and electromagnetic radiations, are presumably known, and it is to be hoped that the exposures of human populations to these radiations will not increase greatly.

A wider variety of carcinogens occurs in our natural environment (Table 2); the term "naturally occurring" is used here in its broadest sense. The great majority of these agents have undoubtedly been present throughout evolution; some may even have facilitated the speciation of living systems. The organic cellular components (Group I) include both carcinogenic viral components of cells and low molecular weight, relatively nonpolar organic carcinogens. At present about 30 of the latter group of naturally occurring carcinogens are known. They are primarily metabolites of certain green plants and fungi, and it seems likely that many more members of this class will be found among the many thousands, if not more, of low molecular weight organic compounds in green plants and microorganisms. Many such compounds certainly remain

TABLE 2. *Carcinogenic agents in the natural environment*

I. Certain cellular components
   A. Nonviral
   B. Viral
II. Certain nonradioactive inorganic compounds
III. Some products arising from interactions of organic and inorganic compounds (e.g., nitrosamines and nitrosamides)
IV. Some products derived from physical decomposition of organic cellular components (e.g., pyrolysis and irradiation products)
V. Certain physical agents (UV light, ionizing particulate and continuous radiations)

to be isolated, characterized chemically, and tested for biological activity; relatively few have been analyzed for their mutagenic and carcinogenic properties. It is worth noting that our natural foods and the microorganisms in the gastrointestinal tract form major quantitative and qualititative contacts with our environment.

The naturally occurring chemical carcinogens also include the small number of known inorganic carcinogens (Table 2, Group II). The ions and compounds of about eight elements are currently included in this class, but many elements and their compounds have not yet been adequately tested for their carcinogenic potentials. Although some inorganic fibers, especially asbestos, are frequently included as chemical carcinogens, the physical properties of asbestos and fiber glass (e.g., the diameter and length of the fibers), rather than their chemical compositions, appear to determine their carcinogenic activities (Stanton and Wrench 1972). Accordingly, these fibers should probably be considered as physical carcinogens.

In addition, certain mixtures of inorganic and organic compounds can react to yield chemical carcinogens (e.g., nitrosamines and nitrosamides) (Group III) (Magee *et al.* 1976). Similarly, the pyrolysis (Kipling 1976) and irradiation of organic compounds (Black and Douglas 1972) can give rise to carcinogens (Group IV). The polycyclic aromatic hydrocarbons have long been recognized as examples of carcinogenic pyrolysis products. As shown recently by Sugimura and his associates (Sugimura *et al.* 1977, Takayama *et al.* 1977), the pyrolysis of certain free or protein-bound amino acids at the high temperatures that occasionally occur in cooking (charring) yields heterocyclic amine derivatives with considerable mutagenic and, probably, carcinogenic activity. Finally, a variety of physical carcinogens, UV light and particulate and ionizing radiations, occur naturally.

ON THE NUMBER OF KNOWN CHEMICALS

The magnitude of the task of identifying carcinogens among the chemicals in human environments can be appreciated by considering the efforts of chemists, primarily the organic chemists, during the past century. Recent computer-based studies from the Institute of Scientific Information (Garfield *et al.* 1973) and the Chemical Abstracts Service of the American Chemical Society (Maugh 1978) have shown the rate of development of new chemical compounds (Figure 1). From the time that the foundations of modern chemistry were established in the early 1800's to the end of World War II in 1945 about one million new organic compounds were recorded. In the first fourteen years after 1945 the second million new compounds were reported, and in two subsequent nine-year periods, the third and fourth million new compounds were recorded. As one who appreciates the beautiful intellectual and practical basis of organic chemistry, I would emphasize that this increase in numbers was not just an accumulation of chemicals. Instead, many of the new chemicals resulted from

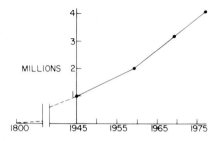

FIG. 1. The rate of development of new chemical compounds from the beginnings of modern chemistry to the present. (From Garfield *et al.* 1973 and Maugh 1978)

explosions of basic research in organic chemistry, especially the development of a wide range of new synthetic methods and of a series of sophisticated, rapid, and sensitive spectroscopic methods for characterization. It is most unlikely that the great advances in the last four years on the metabolic activation of the polycyclic aromatic hydrocarbons to electrophilic and mutagenic ultimate carcinogens (Weinstein 1979, see pages 399 to 418, this volume) could have been accomplished without this new background in organic chemistry. Dr. Sporn's report (1979, see pages 441 to 453, this volume) similarly reflected the important role of modern organic chemistry in making possible his elegant structure-function studies on the retinoids.

A great majority of the presently known four million chemicals are organic compounds of relatively low molecular weight (<1,000) (Table 3). I have not been able to find a good estimate of the number of known naturally occurring organic compounds in this group. However, it seems unlikely that it is more than 100,000, although the actual number of these compounds in all living species probably exceeds this number. Thus, it is evident that the majority of the 3.9 million known organic compounds are synthetic laboratory products.

TABLE 3. *Data on the total number of chemical compounds and the number in "common use"* *

I. Total chemicals (Data from the Chemical Abstracts Service, American Chemical Society)
   A. 4,039,907 total distinct entries as of November 7, 1977; the entries are accruing at the rate of 6,000/week
   B. Of this total
      1. 96% contain carbon; by difference, 4% or about 160,000 are apparently inorganic.
      2. 84% (3.4 million) are fully defined organic or inorganic compounds.
      3. 74% (3 million) contain at least one ring system.
      4. No estimate of the number of known naturally occurring compounds.
II. Number of compounds in "common use"; total estimate is about 63,000
   A. EPA estimate of number of compounds in common use
      1. 50,000 not including pesticides, pharmaceuticals, and food additives.
      2. About 1,500 different ingredients in pesticides.
   B. FDA estimate of number of compounds in drugs and foods
      1. About 4,000 active ingredients and 2,000 excipients in drugs.
      2. About 25,000 food additives that are used for nutritional value and flavorings.
      3. About 3,000 food additives that promote product life.

---

* See Maugh 1978

Most of them were prepared in only small amounts for research and remain in laboratories; thus, the great majority never reach the human environment. However, as outlined in Table 3, many of them have been sufficiently useful to lead to their "common use" (Maugh 1978). A total of 63,000 chemicals in common use seems too large, and I think there is good reason to doubt that all, or even a majority, of these compounds are really in "common use," even though they are certainly commonly available. It is of some interest that an EPA official has referred to this list of chemicals as the "strawman list" (Greenstreet 1978). In any case, it is evident that several thousand of these chemicals are in use in the human environment and that some individuals may make daily contact with many of them. The number of chemicals and the amounts of each that an individual may encounter will differ between members of the population as a consequence of their different job-related activities, social habits, intake of medicinal drugs, etc.

ON THE IDENTIFICATION OF CHEMICAL CARCINOGENS

The above discussion highlights the problems of identifying carcinogens among the large number of chemicals in the environment. A second problem follows from the finding that chemical carcinogens belong to over a dozen structural classes that share no common features (Miller 1970, Weisburger and Williams 1975). Some representative synthetic organic chemical carcinogens are shown in Figure 2, and the rather exotic structures of some of the naturally occurring chemical carcinogens are depicted in Figure 3. The carcinogens shown in these last two figures, like the majority of the known chemical carcinogens, are not directly reactive with cellular constituents. The meaning of this great variability in the structures of compounds with similar biological activity will be discussed below.

The great variety and number of essentially untested compounds in our environment emphasize the importance of the use of epidemiological leads in the detection of human carcinogens among the environmental chemicals. Fortunately, as we have heard at this meeting, the tools in modern cancer epidemiology have become much more sophisticated and more effective for the development of leads that can be further examined in the laboratory. Dr. Higginson, in his Rosenhaus lecture (Higginson 1976), put it very clearly and forcefully: "The present period is transitional as we dwell in a world with a wondrous variety of environments. If we as scientists do not study the experiments that have been begun by nature or by man through partial ignorance, and if we do not establish the facts we shall lose a unique opportunity to provide more rational guidelines to the future." One impressive example is the decrease in the incidence of primary stomach cancer that has occurred in the United States and other developed countries in the past four decades. The same effect is now apparent is Japan, which has traditionally been an area with a high incidence of primary stomach cancer. Hirayama, a leading Japanese epidemiologist, has shown a

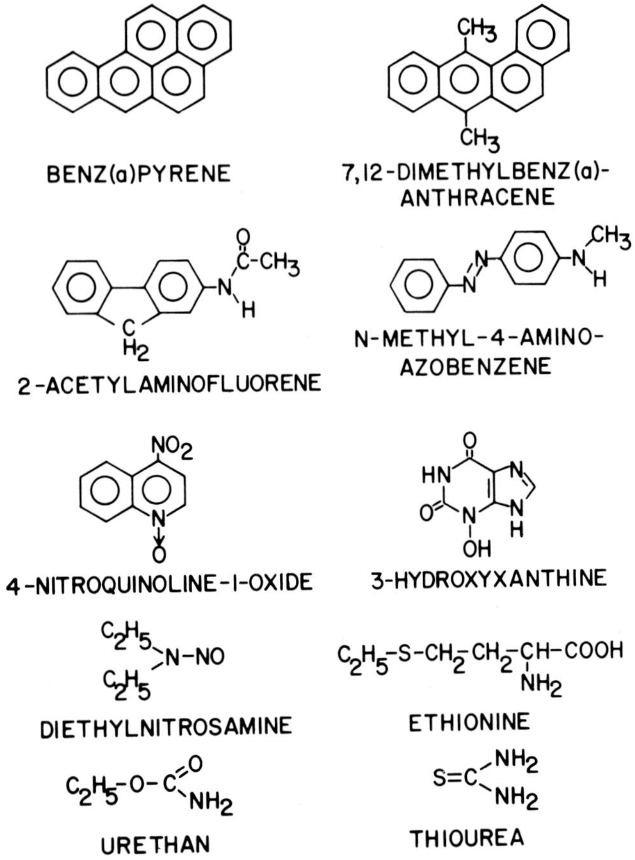

FIG. 2. The structures of some synthetic chemical carcinogens.

25% decrease in the level of this important tumor in Japan in the past 20 years (Hirayama 1977). This decrease is presumably associated with the increasing Westernization of Japan, but we have little information on the critical changes that have taken place in Japan or the U.S.

Higginson (1976, 1978) has further emphasized that for the immediate future the greatest reductions in cancer incidence can be obtained by individuals who establish personal action plans based on the facts already established in cancer epidemiology. These plans would include an individual's smoking, drinking, and eating habits and the individual's occupation. The relevant public education for the development of such personal plans is clearly an essential part of any national cancer plan, since it is evident from epidemiological data that as much as one fourth to one third of the burden of human cancer could be prevented or greatly delayed (Wynder and Mabuchi 1972). The effectiveness of these plans was noted by Dr. Higginson (1979, pages 187 to 208, this volume), who pointed

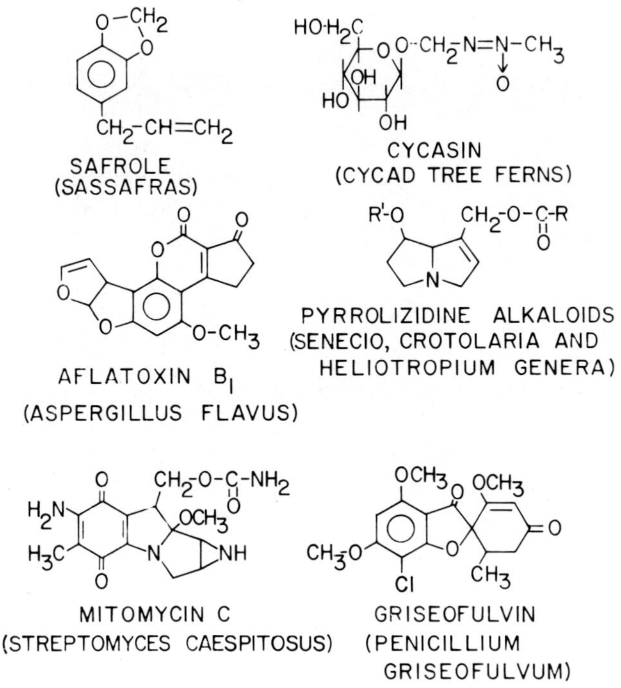

FIG. 3. The structures of some naturally occurring chemical carcinogens.

to the lower risks of professional people as compared to the general public for certain important human cancers. These individuals perhaps took the data more seriously or were better informed than the general public.

It is also evident that full use of the principles of cancer prevention requires that we be able to identify chemical carcinogens in our environment. Since both ethical and logistic considerations prevent deliberate tests in the human, animal models have provided most of our knowledge of chemical carcinogenesis. Both of this year's distinguished Bertner Awardees, Dr. Isaac Berenblum and Dr. Philippe Shubik, have dealt comprehensively with animal models for the detection of chemicals that possess carcinogenic and tumor-promoting activities. Tumors comparable to those important in the human can be produced in animals, and, as emphasized at these meetings, tumor formation and growth in animals are not fundamentally different from these processes in the human. Animal models will probably be needed for the indefinite future as final evidence for the potential carcinogenicity of chemicals, especially when the conditions (e.g., route) simulate human exposures. The suggestion by Drs. Saffiotti and Harris (1979, pages 67 to 84, this volume) at this meeting that data obtained with organ cultures of human tissues can improve the extrapolations from animal models to humans is particularly important.

In spite of the fact that limitations of the sizes of experimental groups make animal models relatively insensitive indicators of carcinogenicity, moderate increases in the amounts of compound administered permit examination of carcinogens of widely different activities. For example, the induction of liver tumors in the rat with aflatoxin B_1 or safrole shows that at least a 6-log range of activity can be accommodated by this model. Continued research is needed to improve these animal models, but the ones we have will continue to provide useful data on the carcinogenic potentials of environmental chemicals.

SHORT-TERM TESTS FOR POTENTIAL CARCINOGENIC ACTIVITY

The forbidding logistics of testing all environmental chemicals in conventional animal tests has led to extensive research during the past decade on more rapid assays for biological activities that might be indicators of carcinogenic activity. These prescreens are still being refined, and the results are still being evaluated. However, none of the tests currently appears to have a sufficiently low incidence of false-positive and, especially, of false-negative results to permit their use as definitive measures of carcinogenic potential. The tests do provide very valuable information for the selection of the chemicals to be tested and for the determination of their priorities for testing in the limited facilities available for animal assays.

At the present time, a battery of mutagenicity tests, which utilize either bacterial or mammalian cells, seems most suitable as a prescreen for the selection of chemicals for further testing. However, other test systems, especially those that assess the ability of chemicals to cause malignant transformation of cells in culture, are developing rapidly, as discussed by Dr. Heidelberger (1979, pages 85 to 94, this volume) and Dr. Pienta (1979, pages 123 to 144, this volume) at this meeting. Perhaps it is not too foolish to dream that the malignant transformations of a variety of human cells may eventually be valuable prescreens for carcinogenic activity. These tests might utilize a wide range of genetic backgrounds, for, as we noted at this meeting, one cannot ignore the modulating effects of this variable on carcinogenesis by chemicals and by other agents (Paterson 1979, pages 251 to 276, Nebert 1979, pages 159 to 187, this volume).

Of fundamental importance to the success of these rapid test systems is provision for the conversion in situ of chemical carcinogens to their active forms. As mentioned repeatedly during these meetings and as discussed in more detail for aromatic amines by Dr. Irving (1979, pages 211 to 227, this volume), the majority of the chemical carcinogens require metabolism in vivo for conversion to their active or ultimate carcinogenic forms (Figure 4). Thus, most chemical carcinogens, as administered to the animal, appear to be pre- or procarcinogens; frequently one or more proximate chemical carcinogens are intermediates in their conversion to ultimate carcinogens. Furthermore, some, perhaps many, chemical carcinogens may yield more than one ultimate carcinogenic metabolite.

The unifying feature for chemical carcinogens, despite the wide structural differences between the classes of precarcinogens, is that the ultimate carcinogens are electronically similar; they all appear to be strong electrophiles, i.e., electron-deficient reagents. The small groups of alkylating and acylating chemical carcinogens are strong electrophiles *per se* and are therefore ultimate carcinogens in the forms administered. These highly reactive electron-deficient species form covalent adducts nonenzymatically and relatively indiscriminately with a wide variety of nucleophilic or electron-rich sites in cellular molecules. The important informational macromolecules, the nucleic acids and proteins, have received the most attention in this regard, and covalent binding in vivo of chemical carcinogens to macromolecules is now regarded as a common finding. In view of this reactivity with nucleic acids it is not surprising to find that the ultimate carcinogenic forms of chemical carcinogens are mutagenic (Miller and Miller 1971, McCann *et al.* 1975).

Many chemical carcinogens are both activated and inactivated by oxidases in the endoplasmic reticulum and, at least in some cases, also in the nuclear membranes of mammalian cells. Since bacteria generally lack these mixed-function oxidases, bacterial mutagenicity test systems for potential carcinogens must be supplemented with these enzymes (generally from liver) in the form of fortified microsomes, with or without cytosol, or with whole cells.

The balance between the activation and inactivation of chemical carcinogens determines the amount of the ultimate reactive carcinogenic electrophiles formed in a tissue. This point has been emphasized at this meeting, especially by Dr. Wattenberg (1979, pages 299 to 316, this volume); he has shown that chemical carcinogenesis in animals can be inhibited by administration of a variety of synthetic and naturally occurring chemicals as anticarcinogens. It is important to realize that inactivation often also occurs in the microsome-mediated mutagenicity test systems. However, the balance between activation and inactivation in these systems may be different, both qualitatively and quantitatively, as compared to whole animal systems. In the mutagenicity test systems the amount of substrate available to the activation enzymes may be much higher than those that occur in vivo. While this situation may demonstrate the mutagenic potential of a carcinogen, it also may not accurately reflect the carcinogenic potential in vivo. The in vivo situation may present far more nucleophilic targets for reaction with the electrophiles that are formed; in addition, the pharmaco-dynamic systems of conjugation and excretion may further limit the levels of the ultimate chemical carcinogens that can be achieved in vivo. Inducers of the microsomal enzymes generally inhibit chemical carcinogenesis in vivo (Wattenberg 1979, pages 299 to 316, this volume), while they may markedly accentuate mutagenesis in tissue-mediated mutagenicity systems.

MECHANISMS OF ACTION OF CHEMICAL CARCINOGENS

In spite of the rapid development of knowledge of chemical carcinogenesis in the past two decades, we still lack detailed knowledge of the mechanisms

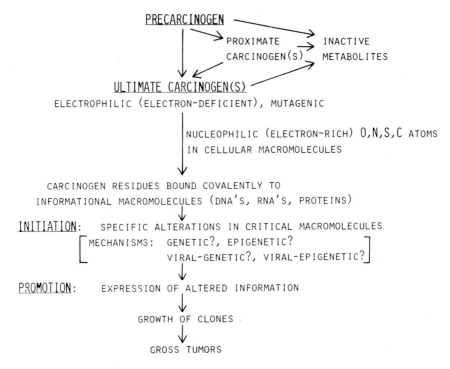

FIG. 4. The processes involved in carcinogenesis by chemical carcinogens.

of tumor induction. Thus, both genetic and epigenetic events, with or without the participation of viral oncogenic information, may be involved in tumor induction by chemicals. However, as denoted by the question marks in Figure 4, definitive data are not available in any case. The presumed mutational aspects of initiation have been emphasized repeatedly at this meeting. It has also been noted several times that covalent binding of the ultimate carcinogens occurs with cellular RNA's and proteins, as well as with DNA's. The mutational nature of initiation has not been demonstrated unequivocally, and, accordingly, it is too early to adopt, consciously or unconsciously, any unitary theory of chemical carcinogenesis.

Tables 4 and 5 outline some of the basic data that support both genetic and epigenetic mechanisms of the initiation of carcinogenesis. We have reviewed these data previously (Miller and Miller 1976, Miller 1978), so I will not discuss them in detail here. However, I would note the extremely interesting observations by Hart *et al.* (1977) on the induction of tumors in fish cells by ultraviolet light and on its prevention by postirradiation with visible light. These experiments provide strong data in support of a mutational mechanism of carcinogenesis by ultraviolet light. I would also mention the very important experimental contributions made by Dr. Pierce (Pierce and Cox 1978) with regard to possible

TABLE 4. *Support for genetic mechanisms of carcinogenesis*

—DNA is the primary source of heritable information in cells.
—The ultimate reactive forms of chemical carcinogens are mutagenic.
—Human xeroderma pigmentosum patients are very prone to the development of skin cancer and have defective DNA repair systems.
—Induction of tumors by UV in fish cells is inhibited by postirradiation with visible light.
—Susceptibilities for some cancers are heritable.

TABLE 5. *Support for epigenetic mechanisms of carcinogenesis**

—Differentiations to yield normal tissues appear to be epigenetic phenomena.
—Development of swimming tadpoles after implantation of tumor nuclei into enucleated frog eggs.
—Differentiation of malignant cells from mouse teratocarcinomas and squamous cell carcinomas to nonmalignant tissues.
—Differentiation of plant teratoma cells to yield apparently normal plants.
—Development of chimeric mice after implantation of single cells from teratocarcinomas into mouse blastulas.

* See Saunders 1978.

epigenetic mechanisms. In introducing this session, he mentioned that he might be the only epigeneticist at the meeting. I join him to a considerable degree in the emphasis of epigenetic events as possible key events in carcinogenesis (Saunders 1978); this emphasis is made in part to offset the tendency for uncritical acceptance of the mutational theory of initiation. We must think much harder about the possible importance of both genetic and epigenetic mechanisms as a stimulation to the generation of more decisive data.

APPROACHES TO THE REDUCTION OF EXPOSURE TO CHEMICAL CARCINOGENS

Table 6 outlines some approaches to the reduction of exposures to chemical carcinogens. Many of these approaches have already been discussed in my remarks and previously in this Symposium; other approaches should be added. We have heard at this Symposium about the probable importance of DNA repair (Paterson 1979, pages 251 to 276, Strauss 1979, pages 229 to 250, this volume), of the possible use of anticarcinogenic compounds, and about the possibility of chemoprevention of chemical carcinogenesis through the administration of retinoids (Wattenberg 1979, pages 299 to 316, Sporn 1979, pages 441 to 453, this volume).

Because of my own interests, I would emphasize the possible utility of Point IIA in Table 6 for the prevention or delay of chemical carcinogenesis. I feel that more use could be made of the formation of macromolecular-bound forms of chemicals in the whole animal, in cell culture, and in organ cultures as measures of the effective levels of reactive electrophiles under conditions of

TABLE 6. *Approaches to the detection of carcinogens in the environment*

I. Epidemiological leads.
II. Examination of man-made and natural chemicals in foods, drugs, cosmetics, water, air, industrial products, etc. for
  A. Structures metabolically convertible to electrophiles.
  B. Host-tissue mediated mutagenicity. These tests are based on the common electrophilicity of active forms of most chemical mutagens and carcinogens. The tests are sensitive, rapid, and inexpensive.
  C. Host-tissue mediated malignant transformation of mammalian cells in culture. These tests are still being developed.
  D. Carcinogenicity in rodents. These conventional assays have low sensitivity and are time consuming and expensive. However, they measure the key endpoint, i.e., carcinogenesis in whole animals.

exposure. Likewise, the information on structures that can or cannot be metabolically converted to electrophiles should be used in the synthesis of technologically useful substances. We now know a good deal about the possible routes of metabolic activation of chemical carcinogens. Accordingly, we should be able to avoid, in the synthesis and use of new compounds for technological and medical use, those compounds with molecular structures that are likely to be converted to electrophiles in vivo.

CONCLUSIONS

In conclusion, it is useful to recount some of the advances in the study of carcinogenesis in recent years. One major advance has been the recognition that carcinogenesis in many mammalian tissues is a multistage process; this point has been discussed by Drs. Berenblum, Shubik, Becker, and Farber, who have been pioneers in these important studies. A second important accomplishment has been the development of rapid procedures for the prediction of carcinogenic activity of chemicals. Third, the ability to cause malignant transformation in mammalian cell cultures by chemicals has been and will continue to be of considerable value in quantitative studies of the mechanisms of chemical carcinogenesis. A fourth area of advancement has been in the study of the interactions of carcinogens with cell constituents at the molecular level, as highlighted by Drs. Hewitt, Irving, Strauss, and Weinstein at this meeting. Fifth, the developments in our knowledge of the removal of promutagenic and possible procarcinogenic lesions in DNA, as reported by Dr. Strauss, is having and will continue to have a major impact on our understanding of the effects of carcinogens on DNA. Sixth, we have heard much at this meeting about the prevention and inhibition of specific stages of chemical carcinogenesis. Lastly, we have heard from Drs. Fraumeni and Higginson about new approaches to the study of the epidemiology of cancer.

We all look forward to further advances in the above-mentioned areas. We also hope that the future will bring decisive data on the molecular natures of initiation and of promotion, especially by chemicals. This information could obviously have great practical value. We look forward to significant advances in pharmacology and oncology in relation to the rational extrapolation of animal data on chemical carcinogens to the estimation of human risk. We would hope for much clearer identification of those humans at especially high risk to environmental carcinogens. We look forward to much better assessments of the roles of environmental factors, either as initiators or promoters, in the causation of specific human cancers. And, we *must* have a far better understanding and interplay, between scientists, government, industry, and the lay public in responsibly weighing risks, benefits, and costs of the reduction of possible carcinogenic hazards in our environment.

I will close with a brief personal comment. One of the very nice things about this Symposium has been the many bright and eager young oncologists in attendance. On behalf of us older oncologists, I hope that in their research they initiate successfully, promote wisely, and progress to glorious answers.

ACKNOWLEDGMENT

The author's research has been supported by Grants CA-07175 and CA-09135 from the National Cancer Institute.

REFERENCES

Becker, F. F. 1979. Keynote address: Evolution, chemical carcinogenesis, and mortality: The cycle of life, *in* Carcinogens: Identification and Mechanisms of Action (The University of Texas System Cancer Center 31st Annual Symposium on Fundamental Cancer Research, 1978), A. C. Griffin and C. R. Shaw, eds., Raven Press, New York, pp. 5–17.

Black, H. S., and D. R. Douglas. 1972. A model system for the evaluation of the role of cholesterol-α-oxide in ultraviolet carcinogenesis. Cancer Res. 32:2630–2632.

Garfield, E., G. S. Revesz, and J. H. Batzig. 1973. The synthetic chemical literature from 1960 to 1969. Nature 242:307–309.

Greenstreet, W. 1978. Chemicals: The "strawman list." Science 199:599.

Hart, P. W., R. B. Setlow, and A. D. Woodhead. 1977. Evidence that pyrimidine dimers in DNA can give rise to tumors. Proc. Natl. Acad. Sci. USA 74:5574–5578.

Heidelberger, C. 1979. In vitro chemical carcinogenesis, *in* Carcinogens: Identification and Mechanisms of Action (The University of Texas System Cancer Center 31st Annual Symposium on Fundamental Cancer Research, 1978), A. C. Griffin and C. R. Shaw, eds., Raven Press, New York, pp. 85–94.

Higginson, J. 1976. A hazardous society? Individual *versus* community responsibility in cancer prevention. Am. J. Public Health 66:359–366.

Higginson J. 1979. Perspectives and future developments in research on environmental carcinogenesis, *in* Carcinogens: Identification and Mechanisms of Action (The University of Texas System Cancer Center 31st Annual Symposium on Fundamental Cancer Research, 1978), A. C. Griffin and C. R. Shaw, eds., Raven Press, New York, pp. 187–208.

Hirayama, T. 1977. Changing patterns of cancer in Japan with special reference to the decrease in stomach cancer mortality, *in* Origins of Human Cancer, H. H. Hiatt, J. D. Watson, and J. A. Winsten, eds., Cold Spring Harbor Laboratory, Cold Spring Harbor, New York, pp. 55–75.

Huebner, R. J., and D. Fish. 1979. Sarc and leuk oncogene-transforming proteins as antigenic determinants of cause and prevention of cancer in mice and rats, *in* Carcinogens: Identification and Mechanisms of Action (The University of Texas System Cancer Center 31st Annual Symposium on Fundamental Cancer Research, 1978), A. C. Griffin and C. R. Shaw, eds., Raven Press, New York, pp. 277–298.

Irving, C. C. 1979. Species and tissue variations in the metabolic activation of aromatic amines, *in* Carcinogens: Identification and Mechanisms of Action (The University of Texas System Cancer Center 31st Annual Symposium on Fundamental Cancer Research, 1978), A. C. Griffin and C. R. Shaw, eds., Raven Press, New York, pp. 211–227.

Kipling, M. D. 1976. Soots, tars, and oils as causes of occupational cancer, *in* Chemical Carcinogens, ACS Monograph 173, C. E. Searle, ed., American Chemical Society, Washington, D.C., pp. 315–323.

Magee, P. N., R. Montesano, and R. Preussmann. 1976. N-nitroso compounds and related carcinogens, *in* Chemical Carcinogens, ACS Monograph 173, C. E. Searle, ed., American Chemical Society, Washington, D.C., pp. 491–625.

Maugh, T. H., II. 1978. Chemicals: How many are there? Science 199:162.

McCann, J., E. Choi, E. Yamasaki, and B. N. Ames. 1975. The detection of carcinogens as mutagens in the *Salmonella*/microsome test: Assay of 300 chemicals. Proc. Natl. Acad. Sci. USA 72:5135–5139.

Miller, E. C. 1978. Some current perspectives on chemical carcinogenesis in humans and experimental animals: Presidential address. Cancer Res. 38:1479–1496.

Miller, E. C., and J. A. Miller. 1971. The mutagenicity of chemical carcinogens: Correlations, problems, and interpretations, *in* Chemical Mutagens—Principles and Methods for Their Detection, A. Hollaender, ed. Vol. 1. Plenum Press, New York, pp. 83–119.

Miller, E. C., and J. A. Miller. 1976. The metabolism of chemical carcinogens to reactive electrophiles and their possible mechanisms of action in carcinogenesis, *in* Chemical Carcinogens, ACS Monograph 173, C. E. Searle, ed., American Chemical Society, Washington, D.C., pp. 737–762.

Miller, J. A. 1970. Carcinogenesis by chemicals: An overview—G. H. A. Clowes Memorial Lecture. Cancer Res. 30:559–576.

Nebert, D. W., R. C. Levitt, and O. Pelkonen. 1979. Genetic variation in metabolism of chemical carcinogens associated with susceptibility to tumorigenesis, *in* Carcinogens: Identification and Mechanisms of Action (The University of Texas System Cancer Center 31st Annual Symposium on Fundamental Cancer Research, 1978), A. C. Griffin and C. R. Shaw, eds., Raven Press, New York, pp. 159–187.

Paterson, M. C. 1979. Environmental carcinogenesis and imperfect repair of damaged DNA in *Homo sapiens:* Causal relation revealed by rare hereditary disorders, *in* Carcinogens: Identification and Mechanisms of Action (The University of Texas System Cancer Center 31st Annual Symposium on Fundamental Cancer Research, 1978), A. C. Griffin and C. R. Shaw, eds., Raven Press, New York, pp. 251–276.

Pienta, R. J. 1979. A hamster embryo cell model system for identifying carcinogens, *in* Carcinogens: Identification and Mechanisms of Action (The University of Texas System Cancer Center 31st Annual Symposium on Fundamental Cancer Research, 1978), A. C. Griffin and C. R. Shaw, eds., Raven Press, New York, pp. 123–144.

Pierce, G. B., and W. F. Cox, Jr. 1978. Neoplasms as caricatures of tissue renewal, *in* Cell Differentiation and Neoplasia (The University of Texas System Cancer Center 30th Annual Symposium on Fundamental Cancer Research, 1977), G. F. Saunders, ed. Raven Press, New York, pp. 57–66.

Saffiotti, U., and C. C. Harris. 1979. Carcinogenesis studies on organ cultures of animal and human respiratory tissues, *in* Carcinogens: Identification and Mechanisms of Action (The University of Texas System Cancer Center 31st Annual Symposium on Fundamental Cancer Research, 1978), A. C. Griffin and C. R. Shaw, eds., Raven Press, New York, pp. 67–84.

Saunders, G. F., ed. 1978. Cell Differentiation and Neoplasia (The University of Texas System Cancer Center 30th Annual Symposium on Fundamental Cancer Research, 1977), Raven Press, New York.

Sporn, M. B., D. L. Newton, J. M. Smith, N. Acton, A. E. Jacobson, and A. Brossi. 1979. Retinoids and cancer prevention: The importance of the terminal group of the retinoid molecule in modifying activity and toxicity, *in* Carcinogens: Identification and Mechanisms of Action (The University of Texas System Cancer Center 31st Annual Symposium on Fundamental Cancer Research, 1978), A. C. Griffin and C. R. Shaw, eds., Raven Press, New York, pp. 441–453.

Strauss, B. S., M. Altamirano, K. Bose, R. Sklar, and K. Tatsumi. 1979. Carcinogen-induced damage to DNA, *in* Carcinogens: Identification and Mechanisms of Action (The University of

Texas System Cancer Center 31st Annual Symposium on Fundamental Cancer Research, 1978), A. C. Griffin and C. R. Shaw, eds., Raven Press, New York, pp. 229–250.

Sugimura, T., T. Kawachi, M. Nagao, T. Yahagi, Y. Seino, T. Okamoto, K. Shudo, T. Kosuge, T. Tsuji, K. Wakabayashi, Y. Iitaka, and A. Itai. 1977. Mutagenic principle(s) in tryptophan and phenylalanine pyrolysis products. Proc. Japan. Acad. 53:58–61.

Stanton, M. F., and C. Wrench. 1972. Mechanisms of mesothelioma induction with asbestos and fibrous glass. J. Natl. Cancer Inst. 48:797–821.

Takayama, S., Y. Katoh, M. Tanaka, M. Nagao, K. Wakabayashi, and T. Sugimura. 1977. *In vitro* transformation of hamster embryo cells with tryptophan pyrolysis products. Proc. Japan. Acad. 53:126–129.

Wattenberg, L. W. 1979. Inhibitors of chemical carcinogenesis, *in* Carcinogens: Identification and Mechanisms of Action (The University of Texas System Cancer Center 31st Annual Symposium on Fundamental Cancer Research, 1978), A. C. Griffin and C. R. Shaw, eds., Raven Press, New York, pp. 299–316.

Weinstein, I. B., H. Yamasaki, M. Wigler, L-S. Lee, P. B. Fisher, A. Jeffrey, and D. Grunberger. 1979. Molecular and cellular events associated with the action of initiating carcinogens and tumor promoters, *in* Carcinogens: Identification and Mechanisms of Action (The University of Texas System Cancer Center 31st Annual Symposium on Fundamental Cancer Research, 1978), A. C. Griffin and C. R. Shaw, eds., Raven Press, New York, pp. 399–418.

Weisburger, J. H., and G. M. Williams. 1975. Metabolism of chemical carcinogens, *in* Cancer: A Comprehensive Treatise, Vol. 1. Etiology: Chemical and Physical Carcinogens. F. F. Becker, ed., Plenum Press, New York, pp. 185–234.

Wynder, E. L., and K. Mabuchi. 1972. Etiological and preventive aspects of human cancer. Prev. Med. 1:300–334.

Author Index*

A
Acton, Nancy, 441
Allfrey, Vincent G., 419
Allison, James P., 381
Altamirano, Manuel, 229
Arnott, Marilyn S., 145

B
Baldwin, Robert W., 365
Becker, Frederick F., 5
Berenblum, Isaac, 25
Boffa, Lidia C., 419
Bose, Kallol, 229
Brossi, Arnold, 441
Brusick, David, 93

C
Cameron, Ross G., 319
Clark, R. Lee, 1, 21

D
Davis, Edward M., 381

E
Embleton, Michael J., 365
Emmelot, P., 337

F
Farber, Emmanuel, 319
Fish, Donald C., 277
Fisher, Paul B., 399
Fraumeni, Joseph F., Jr., 51

G
Grunberger, Dezider, 399

H
Harless, Julie, 107

Harris, Curtis C., 65
Heidelberger, Charles, 83
Hewitt, Roger R., 107
Higginson, John, 187
Hixson, Douglas C., 381
Huebner, Robert J., 277

I
Irving, Charles C., 211

J
Jacobson, Arthur E., 441
Jeffrey, Alan, 399
Johnston, Dennis A., 145

L
Laishes, Brian, 319
Lee, Lih-Syng, 399
Levitt, Roy C., 157
Lin, Jung-Chung, 319
Lloyd, R. Stephen, 107
Love, Jack, 107

M
Medline, Alan, 319
Miller, James A., 455
Mondal, Sukdeb, 83

N
Nebert, Daniel W., 157
Newton, Dianne L., 441

O
Ogawa, Katsuhiro, 319

P
Paterson, M. C., 251
Pelkonen, Olavi, 157

See also List of Contributors, pp. vii–ix.

Subject Index